T0324157

A HISTORICAL PERSPECTIVE ON EVIDENCE-BASED IMMUNOLOGY

Dedication

This book is dedicated to

- Students, past, present, and future; and
- My wife, Jane Adrian, who provided encouragement, enthusiastic support, and confidence in this project. Without her the book would never have been completed.

A HISTORICAL PERSPECTIVE ON EVIDENCE-BASED IMMUNOLOGY

EDWARD J. MOTICKA, PhD
Professor and Chair, Basic Medical Sciences
School of Osteopathic Medicine in Arizona
A.T. Still University
Mesa, AZ, USA

ELSEVIER

AMSTERDAM • BOSTON • CAMBRIDGE • HEIDELBERG • LONDON
NEWYORK • OXFORD • PARIS • SAN DIEGO • SAN FRANCISCO
SINGAPORE • SYDNEY • TOKYO

Elsevier
Radarweg 29, PO Box 211, 1000 AE Amsterdam, Netherlands
The Boulevard, Langford Lane, Kidlington, Oxford OX5 1GB, UK
225 Wyman Street, Waltham, MA 02451, USA

ISBN: 978-0-12-398381-7

British Library Cataloguing-in-Publication Data
A catalogue record for this book is available from the British Library

Library of Congress Cataloging-in-Publication Data
A catalog record for this book is available from the Library of Congress

For Information on all Elsevier publications
visit our website at http://store.elsevier.com/

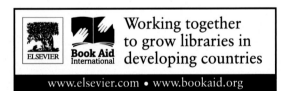

Working together
to grow libraries in
developing countries

www.elsevier.com • www.bookaid.org

Publisher: Janice Audet
Acquisition Editor: Linda Versteeg-Buschman
Editorial Project Manager: Mary Preap
Production Project Manager: Julia Haynes
Designer: Mark Rogers

Typeset by TNQ Books and Journals
www.tnq.co.in

Contents

40. The Future of Immunology

Foreword

Students and others initiating the study of immunology are confronted with numerous details about the immune system and immune responses that need to be assimilated into their knowledge base. These details are currently accepted by the community of immunologists; however, upon initial publication, the experiments and supporting data often engendered controversy. Examples include the notion that the lymphocyte is the primary immunocompetent cell, the validity of the clonal selection theory and its displacement of instruction theories, the role of central lymphoid organs (thymus, bursa of Fabricius, bone marrow) in maturation of immunocompetent B and T lymphocytes, and the requirement for cell interactions in the initiation of effective adaptive immune responses. Without some knowledge of the background to these facts, the student misses out on the rich history and compelling stories that bring immunology to life. It is to provide a sample of these stories that *A Historical Perspective on Evidence Based Immunology* was written.

Several realities about immunology and immunological research emerged during the preparation of this book:

- Immunology is an international endeavor. Scientists and clinicians from six of the seven continents performed experiments and observations that are included in this volume.
- Students and postdoctoral fellows produce a significant number of findings including the following:
  - George Nuttall's description of a serum substance (antibody) induced in rabbits injected with *Bacillus anthracis* that killed the bacteria. At the time Nuttall was a medical student in Germany.
  - Jacques Miller's discovery, shortly after receiving his PhD, that the thymus plays a critical role in the maturation of lymphocytes responsible for fighting infections.
  - Bruce Glick's observation during his graduate training that the bursa of Fabricius in chickens is required for the maturation of antibody-forming lymphocytes.
  - Don Mosier's experiments while a medical student demonstrating that optimal antibody production requires both plastic adherent cells (macrophages) and plastic nonadherent cells (lymphocytes).

  - The discovery by two hematology fellows, William Harrington and James Hollingsworth, that idiopathic thrombocytopenia purpura is an autoimmune disorder produced by antibodies specific for the patient's platelets.
  - Georges Köhler was a postdoctoral fellow in César Milstein's laboratory when these two scientists developed the technique leading to the production of monoclonal antibodies.
- Immunology is a young discipline. While anecdotal evidence existed for millennia that recovery from an infectious disease protects an individual from subsequent development of the same disease, the study of immunology as a scientific and clinical discipline dates from the late eighteenth century.
- The reach of immunology into medicine has evolved from attempts to prevent infectious disease to a discipline that is intimately involved in virtually every aspect of contemporary medicine.

The idea for this book had a long gestation. As a graduate student, I enrolled in an immunochemistry course taught by Alfred Nisonoff at the University of Illinois, Chicago. His approach to teaching included reading the primary literature, discussing the experiments performed and the conclusions reached, and determining what might be the next experiment to pursue. This course took place in the late 1960s shortly after the establishment of the basic structure of the immunoglobulin molecule. The journal articles read in this course led eventually to division of the heavy and light chains of immunoglobulin into constant and variable regions. This, in turn, was critical for determining the genetic makeup of the molecule and the mechanisms responsible for generation of diversity of both immunoglobulins and T cell receptors.

In 2011, my wife and I visited the Walter and Eliza Hall Institute for Medical Research in Melbourne, Australia, where we spent a fabulous afternoon discussing immunology with Jacques Miller. Following this experience, the desire to proceed with this volume was reenforced.

In addition to Drs Nisonoff and Miller, I am indebted to several other individuals who provided encouragement for the project and/or read various chapters prior to publication. These include J. John Cohen, MD; David Scott, PhD;

Max Cooper, MD, PhD; Katherine Knight, PhD; Jay Crutchfield, MD; Sharon Obadia, DO; Robin Pettit, PhD; Milton Pong, PhD; and Katherine Brown, PhD. I also thank the deans at A.T. Still University including Drs Doug Wood, Thomas McWilliams, Kay Kalousek, and Jeffrey Morgan who provided me the time to pursue this activity.

Other individuals critical to the successful completion of this project include the following:

- the librarians at Arizona State University and A.T. Still University particularly Catherine Ryczek who tirelessly filled my numerous requests for copies of journal articles from both the United States and the rest of the world,
- David Gardner, PhD, geneticist/molecular biologist, a colleague and a good friend who patiently read and commented on virtually every chapter. Our discussions improved the accuracy of the information contained although any errors of fact or omission are the authors alone,
- the editors, Mary Preap, Julia Haynes, and Linda Versteeg-Buschman for their patience and encouragement, and
- my wife, Jane Adrian, EdM, MPH. Jane read the entire manuscript several times and we discussed it extensively. During these discussions, she advocated for students and encouraged clarity in the description of the experiments and the interpretation of their results. Without her scientific expertise as a clinical laboratory scientist, her skill as an educator, and her experience as a published author, this book would not have been possible.

Glossary of Historical Terms

Investigators often assigned unique names for identical structures or molecules. This dichotomy of terms is confusing for students as they read some of the older literature. To assist in understanding these older terms, this glossary provides a list of several of these terms with contemporary equivalents.

19S gamma globulin—IgM

7S gamma globulin—IgG

Alexin—an original term for complement

Amboceptor—an original term for an antibody that bound to a pathogen and to complement (alexin) thereby destroying the pathogen

Arthus reaction—a skin reaction originally induced by repeated injections of horse serum into rabbit skin. The skin reaction is due to formation of antigen–antibody complexes that activate the complement system and induce inflammation.

B cell-activating factor (BAF)—name given to a culture supernatant that activated B lymphocytes in vitro: IL-1

B cell-differentiating factor (BCDF)—a factor in culture supernatants that induces antibody synthesis but not mitosis in B lymphocytes: IL-6

B cell growth factor—a factor in culture supernatants that induces mitosis in B lymphocytes: IL-4

B cell-stimulating factor 1—IL-4

B cell-stimulating factor 2—IL-6

Cluster of differentiation (CD)—a system of nomenclature for molecules expressed primarily on peripheral blood white blood cells originally devised by an international workshop on Human Leukocyte Differentiation Antigens. Initially it was used to classify monoclonal antibodies produced by different laboratories. Over 300 different CD markers are currently recognized.

Copula—something that connects; used to refer to the molecule that connects a pathogen with complement—antibody

Costimulator—an early term for antibody

CTLA4—cytotoxic T lymphocyte antigen 4; CD152

Desmon—an early term for antibody

Dick test—a skin test used to determine if an individual is immune to scarlet fever. Toxin from a culture of *Streptococcus pyogenes* is injected intradermally. A positive test, characterized by an erythematous reaction within 24h, indicates the individual is not immune to the pathogen.

Fixateur—a substance (antibody) that connects a pathogen with complement

Helper peak 1 (HP-1)—IL-1

Hepatocyte-stimulating factor—IL-1

Horror autotoxicus—a hypothesis proposed by Paul Ehrlich that the immune system was incapable of producing pathological reactions to self (autoimmune disease)

Hybridoma growth factor—IL-6

Immunokörper—immune body—German term used for antibody

Interferon β-2—one of the original designations of IL-6

I_R—immune response gene(s); genes to which immune response are linked; counterpart of class II genes

I_S—immune suppressor genes; genes thought to code for suppressive factors synthesized and secreted by T suppressor lymphocytes

Killer cell helper factor—IL-2

Ly antigens—antigens expressed on mouse lymphocytes used to develop polyclonal antibodies allowing characterization of subpopulations of T lymphocytes

Lymphocyte-activating factor (LAF)—IL-1

Pfeiffer phenomenon—the killing of *Vibrio cholerae* in the guinea pig peritoneal cavity when the microbe is injected along with antibody specific for *V. cholerae*. An early demonstration of complement activity.

Phylocytase—antibody

Prausnitz-Küstner (P-K) reaction—demonstration of type I (IgE-mediated) hypersensitivity induced by passive transfer of serum from an allergic to a nonallergic individual.

Reagin—term used to describe the antibody responsible for type I hypersensitivity; IgE

Schick test—a skin test devised to determine if a patient has sufficient antibody to protect against infection with *Corynebacterium diphtheriae*

Schultz–Dale reaction—in vitro assay to study type I hypersensitivity. Uterine smooth muscle removed from a sensitized guinea pig is exposed in vitro to the sensitizing antigen. The amount of muscle contraction is proportional to the degree of sensitization.

Secondary T cell-inducing factor—IL-2

Substance sensibilisatrice—antibody

T4—antigen expressed by helper lymphocytes; now CD4

T8—antigen expressed by cytotoxic lymphocytes; now CD8.

T cell growth factor (TCGF)—IL-2

T cell-replacing factor—IL-1

T cell-replacing factor 3 (TRF-III)—IL-1

T cell-replacing factor-μ—IL-1

T lymphocyte mitogenic factor—IL-2

Thymocyte-stimulating factor (TSF)—IL-2

Zwischenkörper—"between body"; antibody

β2A—original definition of IgA antibody based on electrophoretic mobility

γ-globulin—IgG

γ-M—IgM

1

Innate Host Defense Mechanisms and Adaptive Immune Responses

INTRODUCTION

All multicellular life forms, including plants, invertebrates, and vertebrates, have devised defense strategies that permit individuals to lead a healthy, relatively disease-free life. Knowledge about the mechanisms that have evolved to protect humans derives initially from anecdotal evidence that recovery from diseases such as smallpox or the plague protects the individual from developing the same disease a second time. The acceptance of Louis Pasteur's germ theory of disease in the mid-nineteenth century resulted in the concept of an immune response whose function is to provide this protection. Over the ensuing 150 years, many studies have addressed how our bodies deal with both pathogenic and nonpathogenic microbes in our environment. Analysis of these mechanisms, and the ability to manipulate them to our advantage, constitutes the discipline of immunology.

Two separate but interrelated host defense systems have evolved to defend the individual from attack by potential pathogens. In this text, pathogen is used in its broadest sense to refer to any external agent that can cause disease (pathology). Evolutionarily the first defense system to arise comprises innate or naturally occurring mechanisms. The components of this system are found in plants, invertebrates, and vertebrates. The second system, the adaptive immune response, evolved in vertebrates after divergence from the invertebrate lineage, about 500 million years ago. Interactions between the innate host defenses and the adaptive immune responses are generally successful in eliminating potential pathogens.

This chapter compares innate host defenses with adaptive immune responses as they function independently and interdependently to eliminate potential pathogens. The chapter reviews the historical evidence that provides the foundation for understanding the immune system and how the defense mechanisms at times defend us and at other times harm us.

INNATE DEFENSE MECHANISMS

Most potential pathogens are defeated by innate host defense mechanisms. Innate host defenses include physical barriers such as the skin and the mucous membranes along the gastrointestinal, respiratory, and genitourinary tracts, nonspecific cells such as macrophages and granulocytes, molecules including mediators of inflammation and proteins of the complement system, and effector mechanisms such as phagocytosis and inflammation. Recognition of a pathogen by the cells of this innate defense system results in the release of an array of antimicrobial molecules, such as lysozyme and defensins into the local environment. These molecules kill a variety of pathogenic microorganisms and are involved in enhancing ongoing inflammatory responses, a major effector mechanism of the innate system.

Innate host defense mechanisms and adaptive immune responses differ in three important characteristics in their response to pathogens:

- Cells of the innate host defenses are poised to respond immediately while the cells of the adaptive immune response require activation.
- Innate host defense mechanisms are not specific while adaptive immune responses produce cells and molecules that are highly specific for and target the pathogen.
- Innate host defense mechanisms lack memory of past responses should the host be invaded a second time by the same pathogen while adaptive immune responses display memory by mounting a more rapid response, resulting in an increased number of specific lymphocytes and a higher titer of antibodies to a second exposure.

Inflammation and phagocytosis are the two primary effector mechanisms by which the innate host defense system eliminates pathogens. Macrophages, a major phagocytic cell, migrate throughout the body, recognizing and engulfing foreign material. Phagocytosis, the ingestion of solid particles such as microorganisms, induces gene transcription in the phagocytes, resulting in the synthesis and secretion of mediators of the inflammatory response such as cytokines and chemokines. Inflammation recruits other cells into the local environment to play a role in eliminating the pathogen.

Innate host defense mechanisms depend on the presence of certain anatomical structures and cells, effector mechanisms, and recognition structures. In the following sections the history of each of these components is reviewed. It is noted when the historical background of a particular subject is covered in subsequent chapters of this book.

Anatomy

The main anatomical components of the innate host defense mechanisms include the skin and the mucous membranes lining the respiratory, gastrointestinal, and genitourinary tracts. These structures provide a barrier to invasion of the body by pathogens. The protective role performed by these structures remained unappreciated until general acceptance of the germ theory of disease in the second half of the nineteenth century. The development of the germ theory is generally credited to John Snow (1813–1858) who in 1849 studied an outbreak of cholera in London and traced it to a water well on Broad Street. Experimental proof of the germ theory was provided by Louis Pasteur (1822–1895). He demonstrated that microbes were responsible for fermentation of beer and wine as well as spoilage of beverages such as milk. He extended these observations to reveal that human and animal diseases could also be caused by microbes (Pasteur, 1880). Once the ubiquity of microorganisms was recognized, the interaction between the skin and mucous membranes with the environment became an area of biological research.

The presence of cilia on mucous membranes provides an additional barrier to the breaching of these surfaces by pathogens. Cilia and the presence of mucous enhance the protective function of these barriers by increasing the challenge for microbes attaching to and penetrating these membranes. Several antimicrobial substances, including lysozyme, phospholipase-A, and defensins, are found in secretions on these physical barriers. Lysozyme and phospholipase-A are present in tears, saliva, and nasal secretions while defensins and lysozyme are present along the mucous membranes lining the respiratory and gastrointestinal tracts.

Cells of the Innate Host Defenses

Three cell types provide protection against potential pathogens in the innate host defense system:

- granulocytes, including neutrophils, basophils, and eosinophils;
- phagocytic cells, including monocytes, macrophages, and dendritic cells; and
- a subset of lymphocytes with natural cytotoxicity potential.

These cells, classified as leukocytes, are found in the peripheral blood and distributed throughout the organs of the body. The initial morphological descriptions of leukocytes appeared in the 1840s when Gabriel Andral in France and William Addison in England reported the presence of white cells in peripheral blood (Hajdu, 2003). These observations were followed by reports of increased numbers of peripheral blood leukocytes that could be correlated with various diseases, including tuberculosis and sexually transmitted infections. In 1845 Rudolph Virchow (1821–1902) in Germany and John Hughes Bennett (1812–1875) in Scotland simultaneously described the peripheral blood cells of patients with leukemia (Chapter 35).

The functions of the cells of the innate host defense system became the focus of studies for the remainder of the nineteenth century. Two cell types, macrophages and granulocytes, are primarily involved in the removal of invading pathogens by the innate defense mechanisms. In 1879, Paul Ehrlich (1854–1915) initially described granulocytes based on staining characteristics using dyes he developed in his laboratory. Ilya Metchnikov (also Elie Metchnikoff) (1845–1916) provided descriptions of macrophages and developed his "phagocytic theory of immunity" in 1884 (Chapter 15).

In addition to macrophages and granulocytes, a third cell type, the NK (natural killer) lymphocyte, is considered a component of the innate host defenses. NK cells are a heterogenous population of lymphocytes characterized by their ability to lyse various cellular targets, particularly malignant cells and cells infected with a variety of intracellular pathogens. They were discovered in the early 1970s based on the destruction of tumor cells. Morphologically, many of these cells are large granular lymphocytes. NK lymphocytes exist in mice, humans, and other vertebrates. The experiments that characterized these cells are presented in Chapter 28.

Antimicrobial Molecules

In 1894, A.A. Kanthak and W.B. Hardy, working at Bartholomew Hospital in London and at Cambridge, injected rats and guinea pigs intraperitoneally with *Bacillus anthracis, Pseudomonas aeruginosa,* or *Vibrio cholerae.* At intervals they killed the animals, removed cells from their peritoneal cavities, and examined with a microscope. Kanthak and Hardy observed that granulocytes surrounded the bacteria and extruded their granules upon contact while macrophages phagocytized the microbes. Those bacteria that were contacted by the granulocytes were destroyed. One conclusion from this study was that the released granules must contain antimicrobial substances.

Numerous investigators attempted to characterize this antimicrobial material but were unsuccessful for more than 70 years. In 1966, H.I. Zeya and John Spitznagel at the University of North Carolina (1966a,b) isolated the contents of the granules using electrophoresis. They demonstrated that the antibacterial activity was found in at least three separate molecules. In 1984, Mark Selsted and colleagues at the University of California, Los Angeles purified the active material from rabbit granulocytes and demonstrated that it consisted of a group of molecules they termed defensins. Defensins are low molecular weight peptides that have antimicrobial activity. They are produced and stored in granulocytes of the peripheral blood and the Paneth cells of the intestine. Defensins are also found on the skin and along the mucous membranes of the respiratory, genitourinary, and gastrointestinal tracts.

In 1922, Alexander Fleming (1881–1955) described lysozyme (muramidase). While studying an individual with coryza (the common cold), he tried to isolate and culture a causative agent from the individual's nasal secretions. He was unsuccessful until day 4 when he noted growth of small colonies of large, gram-positive diplococcus that he termed *Micrococcus lysodeikticus.* This bacterium is now classified as *Micrococcus luteus* and is recognized as part of the normal flora. Application of a saline extract of nasal mucosa to cultures of *M. luteus* produced lysis of the bacteria. Lysozyme, as this extract is called, is present in many bodily fluids and tissues. Lysozyme is now known to provide protection against several gram-positive bacteria, especially on the conjunctiva of the eye and along mucous membranes.

Fleming received his early schooling in Scotland. In 1906 he was awarded the MBBS (MD) degree from St Mary's Hospital Medical School in London. He served as an assistant to Sir Almroth Wright (discoverer of complement—Chapter 12) at St Mary's and as an instructor in the medical school. Following service in World War I (1914–1918) Fleming returned to London to assume a professorship at the University of London.

Fleming is best known for his discovery of penicillin in 1929 when a fungus contaminated a culture of *Staphylococcus* while he was away from his laboratory. He returned from his summer holiday to find that the fungus had secreted a substance that inhibited the growth of *Staphylococcus* as well as other gram-positive bacteria. Fleming was unsuccessful in purifying this inhibitory substance; however, Howard Florey (1898–1968) and Ernst Boris Chain (1906–1979) succeeded and developed the fungal metabolite into the important antimicrobial drug, penicillin. Fleming, Florey, and Chain shared the Nobel Prize in Physiology or Medicine in 1945 "for the discovery of penicillin and its curative effect in various infectious diseases."

Effector Mechanisms

In immunological terms, effector mechanisms refer to the cells and/or molecules that are activated through interaction with a pathogen and subsequently inhibit the pathogen from causing disease. The innate host defenses employ four effector mechanisms:

- inflammation,
- phagocytosis,
- complement activation, and
- cell-mediated cytotoxicity.

Inflammation

More than 2400 years ago, Hippocrates developed a theory of the four cardinal humors to explain disease. These four humors, blood, phlegm, choler (yellow bile), and melancholy (black bile), needed to be in balance for a person to be healthy. Many disease treatments developed by early Greek physicians were aimed at restoring this balance. Well into the nineteenth century some physicians still attributed disease to an imbalance of the humors.

Celsus described the four cardinal signs of the inflammatory process, *calor*-warmth, *dolor*-pain, *tumor*-swelling, and *rubor*-redness, in his book *De Medicina* nearly 2000 years ago. Galen (130–200) described the beneficial effects of inflammation to injury and emphasized the role of the four humors in the process.

The development of the microscope in the 1700s revealed the existence of cells in the bodies of living organisms. These observations resulted in the development of the cell theory in the early 1800s. This theory included the tenets that organisms are composed of cells and that the cell is the fundamental building block of an individual. This theory influenced new generations of physicians during their training, including Rudolf Virchow.

Virchow (1821–1902), an experimental pathologist, received his medical training at the Friedrich Wilhelm Institute at the University of Berlin, Germany. Following military service, Virchow was appointed chair of pathology at the University of Wurzburg. Seven years later he assumed the chair of pathology at the University of Berlin where he remained until his death 45 years later.

Virchow made several contributions to pathology, including

- adding a third tenet to the cell theory that new cells arise from preexisting cells by division,
- proposing that the development of disease, particularly tumors, was due to a defect or malfunction of cells, and
- describing a fifth sign of inflammation, *function laesa*—loss of function.

Virchow investigated the cellular aspects of the inflammatory process and concluded that inflammation was a pathological proliferation of cells secondary to the leaking of nutrients from the blood vessels.

Phagocytosis

Interaction of the innate host defenses with a pathogen results in phagocytosis of foreign material and the induction of inflammation. In the 1880s Metchnikov originally described the process of phagocytosis (Chapter 15) when he observed wandering cells of a starfish engulfing material from a rose thorn introduced into the animal's body. This process is important in the innate host defenses against pathogens as well as in the initiation of the adaptive immune response (Chapter 14).

Complement

Several of the effector mechanisms of the innate host defense mechanisms are enhanced by activation of the complement system. The complement system consists of a group of serum proteins that are involved in eliminating potential pathogens. Activation of this system results in the release of biologically active mediators that augment

- phagocytosis,
- inflammation,
- chemotaxis (attraction of granulocytes and macrophages), and
- cell lysis.

There are three ways by which complement can be activated: the classical, alternate, and lectin pathways. The classical pathway requires antibody to bind an antigen (i.e., pathogen). In 1895 Jules Bordet (1870–1961) described complement when he reported that serum enhanced (complemented) the activity of specific antibodies to kill *V. cholerae*. Bordet was awarded the Nobel Prize in Physiology or Medicine in 1919 "for his discoveries relating to immunity."

The alternate pathway of complement activation results from the spontaneous cleavage of one of the components of complement termed C3. Cleavage of C3 results in a molecule that binds to the surface of pathogens and releases biologically active mediators to augment the innate host defense mechanisms. Louis Pillemer (1908–1957) described the alternate pathway of complement activation in 1954 when he isolated a new protein called properdin.

Experiments conducted during the 1970s and 1980s revealed the presence of a third pathway of complement activation, the lectin pathway. This pathway is initiated by lectins forming a bridge between carbohydrates on the pathogen surface and a component of complement termed C1. Both the lectin pathway and the alternate pathway are considered part of the innate host defenses. Additional information about the complement system is presented in Chapter 12.

NK Lymphocyte-mediated Cytotoxicity

Immunologists recognize three discrete populations of lymphocytes: NK, B, and T. NK lymphocytes are a component of the vertebrate innate host defense system that kill pathogens using cytotoxic mechanisms. These lymphocytes eliminate or control pathogens, such as intracellular bacteria and viruses that spend their life cycle within host cells. As described in Chapter 28, NK lymphocytes recognize their targets by cell surface receptors and contain cytotoxic chemicals in their cytoplasm that are released to the environment upon stimulation. These lymphocytes also participate in antibody-dependent cell-mediated cytotoxicity, a mechanism considered part of the adaptive immune response (Chapter 26).

Recognition of Pathogens

The mechanisms by which the host defense systems recognize foreign substances remained unknown until the last half of the twentieth century. Lymphocytes of the adaptive immune system recognize foreign material by unique, antigen-specific cell surface receptors (Chapter 17). B lymphocyte antigen receptors were described in the 1960s while antigen receptors of T lymphocytes were identified in the 1980s. Macrophages and other cells of the innate defense system recognize foreign molecules through a series of pattern recognition receptors (PRR) that were described in the 1990s.

Bruce Beutler and his colleagues at the University of Texas, Southwestern Medical School, Dallas (Poltorak et al., 1998) and Jules Hoffmann and his coworkers at the Institute of Molecular and Cellular Biology in Strasbourg, France (Lemaitre et al., 1996) described the role of a gene (Toll) in protecting fruit flies and mammals against potential pathogens. This gene codes for a cell surface molecule that recognizes molecular patterns present on the surfaces of microorganisms. Several additional PRRs have been identified subsequently. Binding of these receptors to pathogens initiates a series of intracellular signals that result in gene transcription and the production of inflammatory mediators. The discovery of PRRs was acknowledged by the presentation of the Nobel Prize in Physiology or Medicine in 2011 to Hoffman and Beutler "for their discoveries concerning the activation of innate immunity." Additional information about the investigations performed to identify these receptors is presented in Chapter 15.

ADAPTIVE IMMUNE RESPONSES

When a pathogen invades and eludes the innate host defense mechanisms, the adaptive immune system responds. The adaptive immune response relies on lymphocytes that provide the system with immunological specificity. Specificity is the ability of the adaptive immune response to discriminate between different foreign antigens. An immune response induced by one pathogen will, generally, not react with a different, closely related pathogen. This discrimination was obvious when ancient physicians realized that an individual who recovered from one disease such as the plague was protected from developing the plague a second time but was still susceptible to a second disease such as smallpox.

Lymphocytes provide a pool of potentially reactive cells each recognizing just one pathogen. Any pathogen stimulates only a few lymphocytes resulting in proliferation and differentiation of that lymphocyte into a clone, all the members of which have the same specificity. These clones of lymphocytes produce molecules (antibodies or cytokines) that kill or inactivate the pathogen.

Destruction of a pathogen by the adaptive immune response uses many of the same effector mechanisms employed by the innate host defenses. These include phagocytosis, inflammation, chemotaxis, and activation of the complement system. While the innate defense mechanisms are available within minutes of the introduction of a potential pathogen into the system, the adaptive immune response requires several days to be fully functional.

Adaptive immune responses, like innate host defenses, depend on the presence of certain anatomical structures and cells, effector mechanisms, and methods for recognizing potential pathogens.

Anatomy

Lymphocytes reactive to pathogens are housed in the lymphoid system consisting of the spleen, lymph nodes, and aggregates of lymphoid cells in virtually all organs. Two other organs of the lymphoid system, the thymus and the bone marrow (bursa in birds), are sites where these lymphocytes mature and differentiate (Chapters 9 and 10). Lymphocytes in these organs circulate by both the blood and lymphatic vascular systems. Lymphatic vessels drain extracellular fluid from the tissues of the body and connect the lymphoid organs with each other and with the blood vascular system.

Ancient Greeks first recognized lymph nodes. Hippocrates described palpable "glands" beneath the skin in several anatomical locations. During the next 2000 years various investigators detailed the thymus and spleen, lymphatic vessels including the lacteals draining the intestines, and the thoracic duct (Ambrose, 2006). By the mid-1600s, European anatomists defined the entire lymphatic system.

Three individuals, working independently, Jean Pecquet, Thomas Bartholin, and Olof Rudbeck, described the organization of the lymphatic system. Between 1650 and 1653, they reported three major findings (Ambrose, 2006):

1. the lacteals (lymphatic vessels) coming from the intestine drain into the thoracic duct;
2. the contents of the lacteals end up in the circulatory system rather than in the liver; and
3. lymphatic vessels exist throughout the body and not just in the mesentery of the abdominal cavity.

Jean Pecquet (1622–1674) studied medicine in Montpellier, France in the 1650s. During his medical studies he dissected dog hearts and noticed the presence of a milky white fluid emanating from the superior vena cava. He traced the origin of this fluid back through the thoracic duct and discovered a structure (the cysterna chyli) to which the intestinal lacteals drained. Further studies indicated that the lacteals do not empty into the liver (as had been claimed by numerous anatomists starting with Galen) but rather drain into the circulatory system that Harvey had recently described. Pecquet published his findings in 1651.

Thomas Bartholin (1616–1680), born in Denmark, studied at the University of Padua in Italy. He published an initial description of the human lymphatic system, including the lymphatic vessels that drained nonintestinal organs of the peritoneal cavity. He followed these vessels and determined that they drain into the thoracic duct and thus into the blood vascular system. In 1653 Bartholin published *Vasa lymphatica, nuper Hafaniae im animantibus inventa et hepatis exsequiae*. Bartholin argued that the lymphatic vessels did not drain into the liver but rather that lymphatic vessels drained from the liver to the circulatory system. Bartholin noted similar lymphatic vessels in other parts of the body, and he called them *vasa lymphatica*.

In the early 1650s, a Swedish medical student, Olof Rudbeck (1630–1702), also described the lymphatic circulation. He observed the presence of lymphatic vessels draining various organs of the body and concluded that the lacteals and other lymphatic vessels do not drain into the liver but rather drain into the thoracic duct, which conveys the contents of these vessels to the left subclavian vein. Rudbeck presented his findings to the faculty at the University of Uppsala, Sweden in May of 1652 and published a book (*Nova excercitatio anatomica exhibens Ductus Hepaticus Aquosus et Vasa Glandularum Serosa*) in the summer of 1653.

Three anatomists made similar discoveries within a few years of each other. The view of the lymphatic system that prevailed for over 1500 years was thus overturned. These near simultaneous discoveries were important to future advances in pathology and medicine during the next 250 years. The concurrent discoveries also led to a dispute of priority, particularly between Bartholin and Rudbeck, with charges of plagiarism by both sides. Today, over 350 years later, we appreciate the importance of these observations and give credit to all three scientists. Bartholin reflected this conclusion since he is purported to have said about this dispute, "[It] is … enough that the discovery is made; by whom it was done is only a vain and pretentious question" (Skavlem, 1921).

Lymphocytes of the Adaptive Immune Response

While the lymphatic system was described in the 1650s, surprisingly lymphocytes as a unique cell type were not recognized until the 1850s. For almost 100 years virtually nothing was known about their function. As recently as 1959, the soon to be Nobel Laureate, Sir Macfarlane Burnet, erroneously concluded that "an objective survey of the facts could well lead to the conclusion that there was no evidence of immunological activity in small lymphocytes" (Burnet, 1959).

However, the history of immunology during the last half of the twentieth century is filled with experiments demonstrating that lymphocytes are the central cell type of the adaptive immune response. Seminal studies demonstrating an immunological role for lymphocytes are presented in Chapter 4.

Immunologists have divided lymphocytes into functional subpopulations, including

- B lymphocytes, which mature in the bone marrow (bursa in chickens) and are responsible for providing protection against extracellular microorganisms through the production of antibody; and
- T lymphocytes, which mature in the thymus and are responsible for providing protection against intracellular microorganisms through the development of cytotoxic capabilities.

The experiments performed to reach this division are reviewed in Chapters 9 and 10. T lymphocytes have been further partitioned into several functional types, including

- T helper lymphocytes responsible for assisting both B and T lymphocytes to differentiate into competent effector cells (Chapters 13 and 23);
- T regulatory lymphocytes responsible for maintaining homeostasis in the adaptive immune response (Chapter 24); and
- cytotoxic T lymphocytes responsible for eliminating autologous cells that are altered by infection or malignant transformation (Chapter 27).

This division based on functional capabilities has been confirmed by the demonstration of phenotypic differences between these various subpopulations; the evidence for this is reviewed in Chapter 23.

Effector Mechanisms

The adaptive immune response employs many of the same effector mechanisms used by the innate host defenses to eliminate potential pathogens—inflammation, phagocytosis, complement activation, and cell lysis. Two products of the adaptive immune response, antibodies produced by B lymphocytes and sensitized T lymphocytes, direct these effector mechanisms to the pathogen.

Antibodies function to eliminate pathogens through a variety of methods. Antibodies neutralize pathogenic microorganisms and their toxic products by binding and inhibiting them from interacting with somatic cells. Antibody activates complement by the classical pathway leading to the release of biologically active molecules that are chemotactic and enhance inflammation. Antibodies alone or with components of the complement system serve as opsonins that enhance phagocytosis of pathogens by macrophages. Finally, antibody participates in antibody-dependent cell-mediated cytotoxicity, a process during which antibody serves as a link between a target and an NK lymphocyte with cytotoxic potential (Chapter 26).

Antigen-specific T lymphocytes eliminate pathogens and other "foreign" material such as tumors through several mechanisms, including cytotoxicity, induction of an inflammatory response, and secretion of cytokines (Chapter 27).

Recognition of Pathogens

Lymphocytes of the adaptive immune response express recognition receptors that enable them to identify specific markers (antigen) on pathogens. B lymphocytes express B cell receptors that mimic the specificity of the antibody molecules those cells will synthesize and secrete. T lymphocytes express T cell receptors that possess a similar degree of specificity. The DNA coding for these receptors is fashioned through the recombination of several gene segments leading to the expression of a vast number of different specific receptors on the lymphocyte surfaces. Details of the discovery of antigen-specific receptors on lymphocytes of the adaptive immune system are presented in Chapter 17. Chapter 18 describes the genetic mechanisms involved in generating the wide diversity in these receptors required for the adaptive immune system to recognize the considerable number of different pathogens it might encounter.

CONCLUSION

Two independent, yet interdependent, host defense mechanisms have evolved to provide protection against invasion by pathogens. Invertebrates and vertebrates both possess innate host defenses, including physical barriers (skin) that inhibit infiltration of the body by pathogens, cells (macrophages, granulocytes, NK lymphocytes, dendritic cells) that nonspecifically destroy intruders, and molecules (defensins, complement components) that inactivate or kill dangerous material. The components of this system are present at birth, do not require cell proliferation, and lack a memory of past exposure.

Vertebrates possess an adaptive immune system that consists of lymphocytes housed in unique anatomical structures making up the lymphatic system. Activation of the adaptive immune system results in the production of antigen-specific molecules (antibodies) by B lymphocytes or specifically sensitized effector T lymphocytes that employ the effector mechanisms of the innate system to destroy pathogens. The adaptive immune system is characterized by its ability to remember previous encounters with pathogens resulting in an enhanced response on reexposure.

Ninety-five percent of pathogens are eliminated by innate host defense mechanisms. If these mechanisms are overwhelmed, the adaptive immune system is activated.

Stimulation of the adaptive system requires presentation of the pathogen to lymphocytes (Chapters 14, 19, and 20). Once triggered, the adaptive system produces effector lymphocytes that employ the components of the innate defense system to eliminate the threat (Chapters 26 and 27).

This introductory chapter offers an overview of the experiments that identified the components of the innate host defenses and the adaptive immune responses. Many of the observations about the functions of both innate and adaptive systems derive from historically anecdotal evidence. These initial observations predate the realization that microorganisms exist and cause a large number of diseases that affect all life forms. Subsequent chapters provide the experimental evidence leading to the contemporary description of the immune system.

References

Ambrose, C.T., 2006. Immunology's first priority dispute—an account of the 17th century Rudbeck-Bartholin feud. Cell. Immunol. 242, 1–8.

Bordet, J., 1895. Les leucocytes et les proprieties actives du serum chez les vaccines. Ann. de L'inst. Pasteur 9, 462–506.

Burnet, F.M., 1959. The Clonal Selection Theory of Acquired Immunity. Vanderbilt University Press, Nashville, TN, p. 209.

Ehrlich, P., 1879. Methodologische Beitrage zur Physiologie und Pathologie der verschiedenen Rurmen der Luekocyten. Z. Klin. Med. 1, 553–560.

Fleming, A., 1922. On a remarkable bacteriolytic element found in tissues and secretions. Proc. Roy. Soc. Lond. B 93, 306–317.

Fleming, A., 1929. On the antibacterial action of cultures of a penicillium, with special reference to their use in the isolation of B. influenzae. Br. J. Exp. Pathol. 10, 226–236.

Hajdu, S.I., 2003. A note from history: the discovery of blood cells. Ann. Clin. Lab. Sci. 33, 237–238.

Kanthak, A.A., Hardy, W.B., 1894. The morphology and distribution of the wandering cells of mammalia. J. Physiol. 17, 81–119.

Lemaitre, B., Nicolas, E., Michaut, L., Reichart, J.M., Hoffman, J.A., 1996. The dorsoventral gene cassette spätzle/Toll/cactus controls the potent antifungal response in Drosophila adults. Cell 86, 973–983.

Metchnikoff, E., 1884. Uber eine Sprosspilzkrankheit der Daphnien. Beitrag zur Lehre uber den Kampf der Phagocyten gegen Krankheitserregen. Virchows Arch. 96, 177–195.

Pasteur, L., 1880. On the extension of the germ theory to the etiology of certain common diseases. Compt. Rend. Acad. Sci. 15, 1033–1044. http://ebooks.adelaide.edu.au/p/pasteur/louis/exgerm/complete.html.

Pillemer, L., Blum, L., Lepow, I.H., Ross, O.A., Rodd, E.W., Wardlaw, A.C., 1954. The properdin system and immunity. I. Demonstration and isolation of a new serum protein, properdin, and its role in immune phenomenon. Science 120, 279–285.

Poltorak, A., He, X., Smirnova, I., Liu, M-Y., Van Huffel, C., Du, X., Birdwell, D., Alejos, E., Silva, M., Galanos, C., Freundenberg, M., Ricciardi-Castagnoli, P., Layton, B., Beutler, B., 1998. Defective LPS signaling in C3H/HeJ and C57BL/10ScCr mice: mutations in Tlr4 gene. Science 282, 2085–2088.

Selsted, M.E., Szklarek, D., Lehrer, R.I., 1984. Purification and antibacterial activity of antimicrobial peptides of rabbit granulocytes. Infect. Immun. 45, 150–154.

Sklavem, J.H., 1921. The scientific life of Thomas Bartholin. Ann. Med. Hist. 3, 67–81.

Snow, J.D., 1849. On the mode of communication of cholera. J. Churchill, London, p. 31. http://resource.nlm.nih.gov/0050707.

Zeya, H.I., Spitznagel, J.K., 1966a. Cationic properties of polymorphonuclear leukocyte lysosomes. I. Resolution of antibacterial and enzymatic activities. J. Bacteriol. 91, 750–754.

Zeya, H.I., Spitznagel, J.K., 1966b. Cationic properties of polymorphonuclear leukocyte lysosomes. II. Composition, properties, and mechanism of antibacterial action. J. Bacteriol. 91, 755–762.

TIME LINE

ca 50 — Celsus describes the four cardinal signs of inflammation

1651–1653 — Jean Pecquet, Thomas Bartholin, and Olof Rudbeck independently report the anatomical structure of the lymphatic system

1843 — Gabriel Andral and William Addison independently describe leukocytes in the peripheral blood

1845 — Rudolph Virchow and John Hughes Bennett independently describe the peripheral blood cells of a patient with leukemia

1849 — John Snow postulates a germ theory of disease based on his study of a cholera epidemic

1858 — Rudolph Virchow publishes *Cellularpathologie* containing his description of the cellular basis of inflammation

1864 — Louis Pasteur provides experimental evidence in support of the germ theory of disease

1879 — Paul Ehrlich describes granulocytes in peripheral blood

1883 — Ilya Metchnikov develops the phagocytic theory of immunity

1894 — A.A. Kanthak and W.B. Hardy report on the antimicrobial activity of granulocyte granules

1895 — Jules Bordet discovers the complement system

1919 — Jules Bordet receives the Nobel Prize in Physiology or Medicine for his discoveries relating to immunity

1922 — Alexander Fleming describes the antimicrobial activity of lysozyme

1954 — Louis Pillemer and colleagues discover properdin and the alternate pathway of complement activation

1966 — H.I. Zeya and John Spitznagel isolate the antibacterial activity of granules from granulocytes using electrophoresis

1984 — Mark Selsted and coworkers characterize defensins from granulocyte granules

2011 — Jules Hoffman and Bruce Beutler share the Nobel Prize for Physiology or Medicine for their discovery of pattern recognition receptors and their role in innate host defense mechanisms

2

Hallmarks of the Adaptive Immune Responses

INTRODUCTION

Adaptive immune responses eliminate pathogens that evade innate host defenses. These protective mechanisms work in concert in two important ways:

- In the innate system, pattern recognition receptors on macrophages and dendritic cells recognize pathogen-associated molecular patterns. Recognition results in the phagocytosis and degradation of pathogens. In the adaptive system, these same cells serve as antigen-presenting cells, presenting small peptides to T lymphocytes. Presentation results in the activation of the T lymphocytes and the initiation of the adaptive response.
- The effector mechanisms, including complement activation, inflammation, phagocytosis, and cytotoxicity, used by the innate host defenses and the adaptive immune responses to eliminate potential pathogens are identical.

A distinction between innate host defense mechanisms and adaptive immune responses is the amount of time required for their activation. Innate host defenses, including inflammation and the release of antimicrobial substances, occur within minutes or hours of contact with a pathogen. Adaptive immune responses, characterized by the secretion of antibodies by B lymphocytes or activation of sensitized T lymphocytes, are detected only after a delay of several days following the initial encounter with the pathogen. While some of this delay may reflect the (in)sensitivity of the methods available for detecting activities of the adaptive immune response, immunologists agree that the generation of the adaptive response entails several discrete steps, including

- recognition of the foreign invader;
- interaction of various lymphocyte subpopulations;
- activation and proliferation of the responding cells;
- transcription of genes;
- synthesis of proteins; and
- generation of the specific end products (antibodies, cytokines, etc.).

Adaptive immune responses first emerged in the early vertebrates (hagfish and lamprey) with the appearance of new cell types (lymphocytes) and new effector molecules (i.e., antibodies). During vertebrate evolution lymphocytes further differentiated into functional subpopulations, while enhanced effector mechanisms arose, resulting in the immune system found in mammals.

A Historical Perspective on Evidence-Based Immunology
http://dx.doi.org/10.1016/B978-0-12-398381-7.00002-2

Three hallmarks differentiate the adaptive immune response from innate host defense mechanisms:

- immunologic specificity, the ability of the cells of the adaptive response to recognize subtle differences in pathogens;
- self–non-self-discrimination, the capability to recognize and act against foreign molecules while remaining inactive against self; and,
- memory, the potential to remember a previous encounter with a pathogen and to react in an amplified manner upon reexposure to the same challenge.

This chapter reviews the historical evidence for each of these characteristics.

IMMUNOLOGIC SPECIFICITY

Specificity is the ability of the adaptive immune response to discriminate between different pathogens. The products of an immune response (antibody or sensitized T lymphocyte) induced by one microorganism will, generally, not react with a different, closely related microorganism. Physicians over 1500 years ago recognized this phenomenon when they realized that patients who recovered from one disease (i.e., the plague) were protected from developing plague a second time but were still susceptible to a second disease such as smallpox. Similar instances of specificity have been demonstrated in antibody responses to biological molecules, including red blood cell antigens and potentially pathogenic microorganisms.

Specificity of the Adaptive Immune Response to Biological Pathogens

An example of the specificity of the adaptive immune response is the ability of antibodies to differentiate closely related molecules such as the ABO blood group antigens. Human erythrocytes express a number of unique cell-surface molecules (antigens) that can induce an antibody response in individuals who lack these markers. As a result, red blood cells used in blood transfusions must be matched between donor and recipient.

The ABO system represents one example of red blood cell antigens that require matching. Four different phenotypes (A, B, AB, or O) are present in the human population based on the expression of two antigens (A and B). A and B antigens are similar in structure. Both antigens consist of a carbohydrate backbone termed the H substance. The A antigen is formed by the addition of α-N-acetylgalactosamine to the H substance while the B antigen is formed by the addition of D-galactose to the H substance. Despite the similarity of these two antigens,

the immune system discriminates between the added sugars and produce two distinct antibodies. This is particularly evident in an individual lacking both A and B antigens (blood type O) who produces antibodies to both A and B blood group antigens.

Karl Landsteiner (1868–1943) discovered the ABO blood groups in 1900 (Rous, 1947). Landsteiner, received his MD in 1891 from the University of Vienna, Austria. He pursued a research career initially at several institutions in Vienna and Holland and, beginning in 1922, at the Rockefeller Institute in New York. The discovery of the blood groups derived from his observation that mixing blood from two individuals may result in agglutination of the red cells. This agglutination is due to the presence of naturally occurring antibodies in the serum of the individuals. Through testing a large number of blood specimens in this manner, Landsteiner discerned four groups of individuals based on their blood type.

The discovery of the blood groups rapidly led to the development of blood transfusions as a therapeutic intervention. Landsteiner was awarded the Nobel Prize in Physiology or Medicine in 1930 "for his discovery of human blood groups."

A second example of the specificity of the adaptive immune response is the ability to discriminate among microbial pathogens. This was an active area of study at the turn of the twentieth century, shortly after the discovery of antibodies. George Henry Falkiner Nuttall (1862–1937) is often credited with the initial description of antibodies. Nuttall received his MD from the University of California in 1884. In 1886 Nuttall moved to Germany to continue his education at the University of Gottingen. He demonstrated, while pursuing his PhD at the University of Gottingen, that serum derived from animals injected with *Bacillus anthracis* produced a substance that could kill the bacteria (Nuttall, 1888). Other investigators—Jozsef Fodor in Hungary and Karl Flügge and Hans Buchner in Germany— described the bactericidal effect of serum almost simultaneously (Schmalsteig and Goldman, 2009).

Shortly after the initial description of antibody, Rudolf Kraus (1868–1932), working at the State Institute for the Production of Diphtheria Serum in Austria, injected goats with filtrates from cultures of *Vibrio cholerae, Yersina pestis*, or *Salmonella typhi*. Serum from these animals reacted with an extract of the culture of the homologous bacteria but not with extracts of unrelated bacterial cultures (Kraus, 1897). Many studies performed in the initial decades of the twentieth century took advantage of this specificity of antibodies to identify and differentiate different types of bacterial pathogens.

Paul Uhlenhuth (1870–1957), working at the University of Greifswald in Germany, developed precipitin assays that demonstrated species specificity of antigens, including those associated with blood. He used rabbit antibodies to egg albumins to differentiate the albumins from several species of birds. He also demonstrated that a rabbit antibody against chicken blood precipitated chicken blood but would not react with blood from other animals, including horse, donkey, sheep, cow, or pigeon.

This observation led to the development of tests to determine the source of blood found at crime scenes. Rabbits injected with human blood produced an antibody that differentiated human blood from that of other species. Shortly after publication of this technique in 1901, Uhlenhuth was asked to determine the source of blood on the clothing of an individual suspected of killing and dismembering two young boys. The suspect denied involvement in the case although witnesses placed him in the vicinity when the murders were committed. The accused argued that the spots on his clothing were from wood stain or animal blood. Uhlenhuth demonstrated that at least some of the stains were from human blood. This evidence resulted in a guilty verdict, leading to the imposition of the death penalty for the convicted suspect. This use of antibody specificity laid the foundation "for the forensic method of distinguishing between different specimens of blood" (Uhlenhuth, 1911).

Specificity of the Response to Synthetic Pathogens

The emphasis of many of the investigations in the first decades of the twentieth century was on understanding the adaptive immune response to naturally occurring pathogens. During the 1920s and 1930s, Karl Landsteiner and his colleagues at the Rockefeller Institute of Medical Research extended these observations on specificity to the response induced by synthetic antigens. These elegant studies are summarized in the posthumously published monograph *The Specificity of Serological Reactions* (Landsteiner, 1945).

Landsteiner studied the antibody response induced by haptens (small molecular weight substances). Haptens are too small to induce an antibody response unless they are conjugated to a carrier protein such as albumin. While the haptens used by Landsteiner were chemicals synthesized in the laboratory, haptens also exist in nature. One example is urushiol, an oil found in the leaves of several plant species, including those of the genus *Toxicodendron*. This group of plants includes poison ivy, poison oak, and poison sumac. Urushiol is not immunogenic; however, it is reactive with some of the proteins of the skin. Once the protein–hapten complex forms, T lymphocytes are activated and induce an allergic rash (Chapter 33).

Landsteiner combined different synthetic haptens of known structure with the same carrier and immunized experimental animals with these complexes. Serum from these animals was mixed with the various hapten–carrier combinations in a precipitation assay.

Interpretation of the results of these assays allowed Landsteiner to conclude that

- animals produce antibodies specific for hapten–carrier complexes, including complexes containing synthetic haptens that are normally absent in the environment;
- antibodies synthesized against a hapten–carrier complex precipitated other complexes containing the same hapten; and
- antibodies distinguished between haptens that differed structurally only in minor ways.

As an example, rabbits immunized with one of four dipeptide haptens (glycyl-glycine; glycyl-leucine; leucyl-glycine; leucyl-leucine), each bound individually to the protein carrier ρ-aminonitrobenzoyl, produced antibodies that discriminated between the four haptens. The structure of these complexes is depicted in Figure 2.1. Precipitation assays using sera from these animals mixed with each of the antigens gave the results presented in Table 2.1. Under various conditions, each antiserum reacted with and precipitated only the immunizing antigen despite the fact that the four antigens appeared to be very similar structurally.

Landsteiner's results demonstrated the extensive repertoire of antibodies the immune system could synthesize. At the time these results were published in the mid-1940s, most immunologists favored an instruction theory of antibody formation in which the antigen imparted information to the antibody-forming cell. Landsteiner's results supported this theory since it was

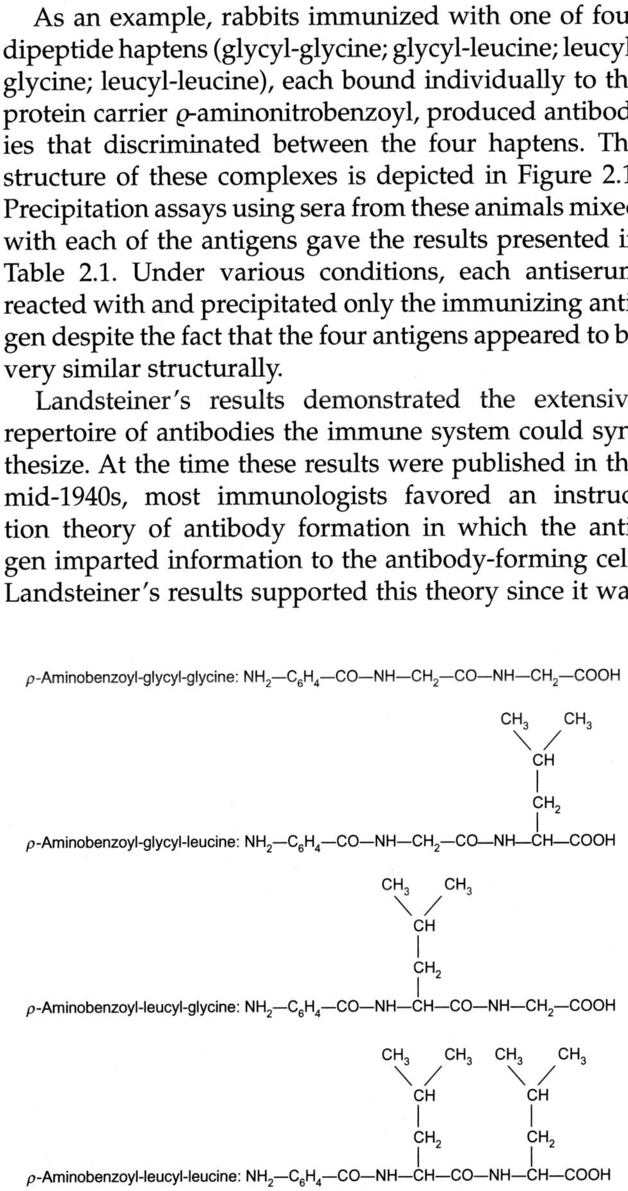

FIGURE 2.1 The chemical structure of the antigens used by Landsteiner and van der Scheer (1932) to study the specificity of antibodies. Four dipeptides served as haptens conjugated with the protein carrier ρ-aminonitrobenzyol served as immunogens injected into rabbits. Blood from these rabbits was tested in a precipitation assay for antibody activity; results are presented in Table 2.1.

TABLE 2.1　Ability of Antisera Induced by Various Antigens to Bind to the Immunizing Antigen and Other Closely Related Antigens. Individual Rabbits Were Injected With Glycyl-glycine (G.G.), Glycyl-leucine (G.L.), Leucyl-glycine (L.G.), or Leucyl-leucine (L.L.) Conjugated to ρ-aminonitrobenzoyl. The Resulting Antisera Were Tested in Precipitin Assays With Each of the Antigens and the Ability to Precipitate the Antigens Determined Semiquantitatively

Immune sera	Readings taken after	Antigens			
		G.G.	G.L.	L.G.	L.L.
G.G.	1 h at room temperature	++	0	0	0
	2 h at room temperature	++±	0	0	0
	Night in ice box	++++	0	Tr.	0
G.L.	1 h at room temperature	0	++	0	f.tr.
	2 h at room temperature	0	++±	0	Tr.
	Night in ice box	0	++++	0	+
L.G.	1 h at room temperature	f.tr.	0	++	0
	2 h at room temperature	+	0	+++	0
	Night in ice box	+	0	++++	0
L.L.	1 h at room temperature	0	±	0	+
	2 h at room temperature	0	+	0	++
	Night in ice box	0	++	0	+++

Five drops of immune serum were added to 0.2 cc of the 1:500 diluted antigens (prepared with chicken serum). Tr. = trace; f.tr. = faint trace.
From Landsteiner and van der Scheer (1932).

difficult to comprehend how the immune system could produce the large number of different antibodies, including to antigens not normally found in nature.

F. Macfarlane Burnet proposed an alternative explanation of antibody formation, the clonal selection theory, in 1959 (Chapter 6). This theory hypothesized that specific antibody-forming cells exist prior to exposure to antigen and that antigen "selects" and activates the appropriate cell. For the next 10 years the mechanism of antibody formation was debated. Landsteiner's findings provided an argument for those immunologists who rejected the clonal selection theory. This "Landsteiner problem" remained a conundrum for the acceptance of the clonal selection theory and was only explained after the mechanisms of genetic rearrangement occurring in developing lymphocytes were unraveled in the 1970s and 1980s (Chapter 18).

SELF–NON-SELF-DISCRIMINATION

A second hallmark of the adaptive immune response is self–non-self-discrimination. In 1901, Paul Ehrlich (1854–1915) and his associate Julius Morgenroth (1871–1924), working at the Center for Serum Research and Testing in Stieglitz, Germany, realized that an immunological response against self might result in disease, possibly leading to death. They developed the concept of "horror autotoxicus," literally that the body is prevented from acting against self, based on experiments in which they injected goats with their own erythrocytes or erythrocytes from other goats or other species. The antibodies that were produced lysed the red blood cells used for

stimulation. However, the injection of goats with their own red cells failed to induce antibody production.

Almost immediately after Ehrlich and Morgenroth developed the concept of "horror autotoxicus" other investigators provided conflicting observations. In 1903, Paul Uhlenhuth immunized rabbits with lens protein from cattle. The antibodies produced by these rabbits precipitated lens proteins from several animal species, including lens proteins from rabbits. This suggested that rabbits could respond immunologically to their own tissue. However, these autoantibodies failed to induce any pathology in the rabbits producing them.

The initial observation of antibodies to self causing pathology was reported in a patient with the rare disease paroxysmal cold hemoglobinuria (PCH). PCH is characterized by the spontaneous lysis in vivo of red cells, particularly in parts of the body where the ambient temperature is less than the core temperature. In 1904, William Donath and Karl Landsteiner, working in Germany, described antibody in patients with PCH that bound to the individual's own red cells and induced their destruction. The antibody is termed the Donath–Landsteiner antibody. Subsequently, other investigators have identified more than 80 diseases with a proven or suspected autoimmune etiology (Chapter 34).

While some individuals produce autoantibodies, most people do not develop autoimmune diseases. The mechanism responsible for inhibiting pathologic self-reactivity remained undiscovered for more than 50 years. Finally, in 1959, Macfarlane Burnet suggested a process by which the immune system distinguished between self and nonself when he proposed his clonal selection theory (Chapter 6). Experiments designed to test this theory demonstrated the existence of a critical time during the development of the immune system when immature lymphocytes "learned" or were trained to refrain from responding to self-antigens (Chapter 8).

The failure of self–non-self-discrimination leading to autoimmune diseases such as type I diabetes, rheumatoid arthritis, thyroiditis, systemic lupus erythematosus, and inflammatory bowel disease remains an important area of immunological investigation. Investigators aim to determine

- how an individual's genes interact with the environment in the initiation of autoimmunity,
- the mechanisms responsible for autoimmune pathology, and
- manipulations that might be used to restore the immune system's ability to differentiate self from nonself.

While many of the symptoms of autoimmune diseases are treatable (e.g., injection of insulin in type I diabetes), no cures have yet been identified.

IMMUNOLOGIC MEMORY

Immunologic memory or anamnesis refers to the phenomenon that an individual who has recovered from an infectious disease will not normally become ill upon subsequent exposure. This understanding represents the basis for the success of vaccines to stop the spread of communicable diseases during the past two centuries.

Early Anecdotal Evidence

Thucydides, a Greek scientist and historian, observed almost 2500 years ago that individuals who had survived the plague epidemic in Athens could care for others infected with the disease without recurring illness. In his *History of the Peloponnesian War*, Thucydides, 1904 describes an outbreak of plague, concluding that "it was with those who had recovered from the disease that the sick and the dying found most compassion. These knew what it was from experience, and had now no fear for themselves; for the same man was never attacked twice—never at least fatally."

Several cultures observed that once exposed to smallpox, an individual's body remembered and resisted further attack by smallpox. These observations led to attempts to artificially expose individuals to smallpox as a method of providing protection against the disease. More than 3000 years ago, the Chinese introduced dried powder from smallpox scabs to individuals, through a scratch in the skin or by inhalation, with the intent to induce a mild case of the disease and, consequently, immunity to further exposure. This process of rendering an individual resistant to a disease was utilized successfully prior to the development of the germ theory by Louis Pasteur (1822–1895) or the founding of the science of immunology, usually attributed to Edward Jenner (1749–1823).

Smallpox Vaccination Comes to Western Medicine

Lady Mary Worley Montagu (1689–1762), wife of the British ambassador to Istanbul, brought smallpox vaccination to Great Britain. In 1717 Lady Montagu wrote a letter to her friend Sarah Criswell describing the practice of the Turks in which they exposed their children by inoculating them with material derived from smallpox lesions. While the Turks termed this procedure engraftment, it was known as variolation when introduced to England. Variola is the Latin name for the smallpox virus and variolation is the process of exposing patients to smallpox virus subcutaneously. Variolation induced a (hopefully) mild case of smallpox, thereby stimulating immunological memory and rendering the patient immune to further exposure.

François-Marie Arout (Voltaire, 1694–1778) described variolation in his journal, published as *Letters Concerning the English Nation* (Voltaire, 1733). As recounted in Letter Number XI, Voltaire describes the practice of the residents of the island of Circassia. Young girls were routinely sold to the Sultans of Turkey and Persia and girls unscarred by smallpox commanded a higher price. Parents exposed their daughters to a mild case of smallpox when they were young, hoping to protect them from a more serious, potentially disfiguring case later in life. While admiring the British use of variolation, Voltaire ridiculed his French compatriots for failing to adopt the procedure in his country.

Variolation was risky due to the inclusion of live virus in the preparation that sometimes led to serious illness and death. Mortality from naturally occurring smallpox was approximately 20–30% of those who become infected while the death rate of individuals variolated was between 2% and 3%.

Ironically, during this same period, John Fewster (1738–1824), a surgeon in Gloucershire, England, observed that a person who had been naturally exposed to cowpox, a viral disease of cattle related to smallpox, did not exhibit the normal mild case of smallpox when variolated. Fewster presented this information to the London Medical Society in 1765 but never investigated further (Jesty and Williams, 2011), and the implications of this observation remained unappreciated for another 30 years.

Edward Jenner (1749–1823), a contemporary of Fewster, used this and other anecdotal evidence to develop the practice of vaccination (Jenner, 1798). Vaccination involved the inoculation of vaccinia virus, a variant of the cowpox virus, into an individual with the intent of inducing immunological memory, which could lead to a protective immune response should the vacinee be exposed to smallpox. Vaccination was significantly safer than variolation with an estimated mortality rate of approximately one to two deaths per million individuals vaccinated.

During the nineteenth and twentieth centuries, smallpox vaccination became a routine medical procedure, and the number of cases and deaths declined in the United States and Europe. Due to the concerted efforts of the World Health Organization (WHO), the last naturally occurring case of smallpox was reported in Somalia in 1977, and the smallpox virus was declared eradicated in 1980. At that time, two stockpiles of the variola virus were maintained, one by the United States and the other by the Soviet Union for future studies.

Development of Other Vaccines

Vaccines to more than 25 diseases, including rabies, yellow fever, diphtheria, and tetanus, were developed in the 200 years following Jenner's introduction of smallpox vaccination. Today the term vaccine describes any preparation used to induce a memory response to an infectious disease. Table 2.2 presents a list of vaccines currently available in the United States. The use of these vaccines to train an individual's immune system to remember and resist the infectious microbe has significantly decreased the morbidity and mortality associated with several infectious diseases.

The development of polio vaccines contributed significantly to the understanding of how the immune system remembers and responds to foreign antigens. Karl Landsteiner (1868–1943) and Erwin Popper (1879–1955) first identified the poliovirus in 1909. They isolated a "filterable agent" (something smaller than a bacteria, now known to be a virus) from the spinal cord of an individual who had died of polio and transferred that virus to a monkey who developed polio.

During the 1940s and 1950s, several competing groups worked to produce the first successful polio vaccine. In 1949, three American virologists, John Enders (1897–1985), Thomas Weller (1915–2008), and Frederick Robbins (1916–2003), developed a method for the large-scale cultivation of poliovirus in tissue culture (Enders et al., 1949). The development of two successful vaccines followed: one an inactivated virus developed by Jonas Salk (1914–1995) (the Salk vaccine licensed in 1955) and a second live, attenuated virus developed by Albert Sabin (1906–1993) (the Sabin vaccine licensed in 1960). The Salk vaccine is injected subcutaneously and provides systemic protection while the Sabin vaccine is administered orally and induces a local response. Both approaches induce

immunologic memory so that the individual is protected from future exposure to the poliovirus.

The different formulations and routes of exposure of these vaccines resulted in controversy and a feud between the two inventors. Salk's vaccine induces a systemic response and was instrumental in significantly decreasing the incidence of polio while it was the only vaccine available. However, the Sabin vaccine rapidly supplanted the Salk vaccine when it was introduced since it produced an antibody response in the gastrointestinal tract. Poliovirus is transmitted by the oral–fecal route, and hence the initial exposure to the virus is in the gastrointestinal tract. However, since the Sabin vaccine contains a live virus, cases of vaccine-induced polio were reported, particularly in immune-compromised patients and in unvaccinated contacts of newly vaccinated individuals. Consequently, as the number of naturally occurring cases of polio declined, the percentage of polio cases attributable to the vaccine increased. Eventually, the Salk vaccine became the preferred vaccine again because it has a lower risk of inadvertently causing polio. Since 2000, the recommended schedule of pediatric vaccination issued by the Centers for Disease Control and Prevention (CDC) includes a series of four injections of inactivated (Salk) polio vaccine. While the oral polio vaccine has been phased out in the United States, it is still used in other countries around the world.

Through the use of the Salk and Sabin vaccines, polio has been eliminated from the United States and most other countries and remains a target of the WHO for complete eradication. The Nobel Prize in Physiology or Medicine in 1954 was awarded to John Enders, Thomas Weller, and Frederick Robbins "for their discovery of the ability of the poliomyelitis virus to grow in cultures of various types of tissues."

The development of vaccines to infectious microorganisms has been one of the major contributions to health and a major accomplishment of immunologic research. Many of the childhood diseases, such as measles, mumps, chicken pox, and rubella, for which vaccines have been developed are only rarely seen in clinical practice today. Despite this impressive list of successes, vaccines against several diseases, including tuberculosis, malaria, and human immunodeficiency virus (HIV), remain in development.

Mechanisms to Explain Immunologic Memory

The success of all vaccines is due to the induction of immunologic recall that prepares the adaptive immune system to respond in a heightened manner upon reexposure to the microorganism. It is impossible to cite a single experiment that first demonstrated the phenomenon of memory in the adaptive immune response at the molecular level. Experimentally, immunologic

TABLE 2.2   Vaccines Currently Available in the United States; For Information on Recommendations for the Use of These Vaccines, Consult the CDC Website at http://www.cdc.gov/vaccines/

Vaccine preventable infections			
Microorganism	Disease	Notes	Year
Bacillus anthracis	Anthrax	Available to exposed individuals	1970
Bacillus calmette-guerin (BCG)	Tuberculosis	Not used in the US; available for infants in other countries	1921
Bordetella pertussis	Pertussis—whooping cough	Recommended pediatric vaccine	1926
Borrelia burgdorferi	Lyme disease	Discontinued—2002	
Clostridium tetani	Tetanus—lockjaw	Recommended pediatric vaccine	1927
Corynebacterium diphtheria	Diphtheria	Recommended pediatric vaccine	1923
Haemophilus influenza type B	Meningitis, pneumonia, epiglottitis	Recommended pediatric vaccine	1985
Hepatitis A virus (HAV)	Acute hepatitis	Recommended pediatric vaccine	1996
Hepatitis B virus (HBV)	Chronic hepatitis, cirrhosis, liver cancer	Recommended pediatric vaccine	1981
Human papillomavirus (HPV)	Genital warts, cervical, and other cancers	Recommended adolescent vaccine	2006
Influenza virus types A and B	Seasonal flu	Recommended yearly for all ages; reformulated yearly	1945
Japanese encephalitis virus	Encephalitis	Recommended for travelers to endemic areas	2009
Measles virus	Measles	Recommended pediatric vaccine	1954
Mumps virus	Mumps	Recommended pediatric vaccine	1967
Neisseria meningitides	Meningitis, septicemia	Recommended adolescent vaccine	2005
Polio virus	Poliomyelitis	Recommended pediatric vaccine	1995 1962
Rabies virus	Rabies	Available to exposed individuals	1885
Rotavirus	Gastroenteritis	Recommended pediatric vaccine	2006
Rubella virus	Fever, rash, birth defects	Recommended pediatric vaccine	1970
Salmonella typhi	Typhoid fever	Recommended for travelers to endemic areas	1896
Streptococcus pneumonia	Pneumonia, bacteremia, meningitis, otitis media	Recommended pediatric vaccine	2000
Vaccinia virus	Smallpox, monkeypox	Available to special populations	1792
Varicella zoster	Chicken pox	Recommended pediatric vaccine	1995
Herpes zoster	Shingles	Recommended senior vaccine	2006
Yellow fever virus	Yellow fever	Recommended for travelers to endemic area	1935

memory is demonstrated when an animal is injected two or more times with a pathogen. Multiple injections of an antigen result in the production of increased amounts of antibody specific to that antigen. During the 1920s and 1930s, most immunologic studies were performed with animals that had received multiple injections of antigen. As a result, most of these experiments

demonstrated what we today understand as memory responses.

F. Macfarlane Burnet (1899–1985), an Australian virologist and immunologist, and his colleague Frank Fenner (1914–2010), a virologist, were among the first to consider the differences between primary responses induced by an initial injection of antigen and memory or secondary immune responses (Burnet and Fenner, 1949). Rabbits injected intravenously or subcutaneously with antigen from *Staphylococcus* supplied blood to be tested for antibody activity. Results are presented in Figure 2.2 as antibody titers from individual animals injected either intravenously (top graph) or subcutaneously (bottom). The graphs presented in this figure demonstrate that antibody could be detected more rapidly after a secondary challenge (2 days) than after the primary injection (8–13 days). In addition, the quantity of antibody produced following a second injection of antigen was also increased.

Burnet and Fenner asked the following: What is the mechanism leading to the rapid increase in antibody titers following a second injection? They speculated that the increase in antibody resulted from "a phase in which the antibody forming units were multiplying at a relatively constant speed somewhere within the body." Although they did not know the identity of these "antibody-forming units," they considered that cells might be involved. Burnet and Fenner hypothesized that a primary antigenic challenge induces an increase in the number of cells and that the subsequent contact of antigen with these cells results in further cell proliferation followed by an increased and more rapid production of antibodies.

By the time Burnet and Fenner published *The Production of Antibodies*, immunologists agreed that a second exposure to an antigen resulted in the more rapid production of a greater amount of antibody. Still, several questions remained unanswered, including

- identification of the cell responsible for antibody synthesis (lymphocyte versus macrophage);
- the role of the antigen in determining antibody specificity; and
- the length of protection provided by vaccination.

Subsequent chapters provide information on the first two questions; studies on the length of protection against infectious diseases remain ongoing.

Duration of Immunologic Memory

Following recovery from an infectious disease or vaccination against an infectious microorganism, how long does that protection last? Many childhood vaccines are administered only during infancy, and a vaccinated individual is presumed "immune" for life, although this is not necessarily correct. Clinical observations have shown a requirement for revaccination against some pathogens. Some vaccines (i.e., tetanus toxoid) carry a recommendation for revaccination at prescribed intervals such as every 10 years, although these recommendations are not always based on scientific evidence. Our understanding of the duration of protection changes constantly, and periodic updates in vaccine recommendations are published by the CDC and the WHO. The most recent recommendations are available at http://www.cdc.gov/vaccines/ (CDC) and http://www.who.int/immunization/policy/immunization_tables/en/ (WHO).

The duration of immunological memory to smallpox vaccination is a case in point. Events in 2001 focused renewed, public attention on the possibility that smallpox might be used as a bioweapon. This is particularly worrisome in a population that is immunologically naïve to the virus. A study performed at the Oregon Health and Science University by Erika Hammarlund et al. (2003) assessed the level of the memory immune response to vaccinia virus. The last smallpox vaccinations were performed in 1971 so most people in the population studied were at least 30 years postvaccination. Hammarlund and colleagues collected blood samples from a representative group of individuals of different ages and separated the blood into serum and cells. Antibodies to the smallpox virus were measured in serum using an enzyme-linked immunosorbent assay. They measured antismallpox T lymphocytes (the cell type responsible for eliminating virally infected cells) by exposing peripheral blood lymphocytes to vaccinia antigen in vitro and measuring the synthesis and secretion of cytokines.

Results showed that "more than 90% of volunteers vaccinated 25–75 years ago still maintain substantial humoral (antibody) or cellular immunity...against vaccinia." Table 2.3 presents data on the number of virus-specific lymphocytes (CD4+ and CD8+ T cells) present in the peripheral blood as a function of time after vaccination. One amazing

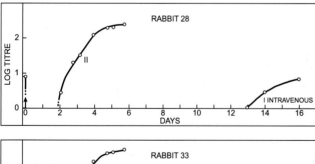
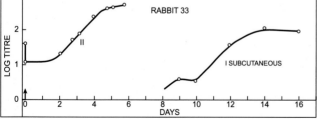

FIGURE 2.2 Primary and secondary antibody responses of two rabbits to injections of Staphylococcal toxin. Both primary and secondary injections were given on day 0; rabbit 28 received both injections intravenously while rabbit 33 received both injections subcutaneously. For both animals, curve I depicts the time course of the primary response while curve II depicts the time course of the secondary response. *From Burnet and Fenner (1949).*

TABLE 2.3 Percentage of Individuals Possessing CD4[+] and CD8[+] T Cells Specific for Smallpox 20–75 Years after Vaccination. Peripheral Blood Lymphocytes Isolated From Volunteers Were Cultured With Vaccinia and Their Ability to Synthesize and Secrete IFN-γ and TNF-α Was Assayed

	Volunteers with CD4[+] T-cell memory[a]			
Vaccinations	20–30 years[b]	31–50 years	51–75 years	$t_{1/2}$ of CD4[+] T cells[c]
1	100% (16/16)	89% (70/79)	52% (23/44)	10.6 (0–17)
2	83% (10/12)	78% (29/37)	57% (4/7)	8.3 (0–14.1)
3–14	82% (23/28)	91% (29/32)	ND[d]	12.4 (0–20.5)
	Volunteers with CD8[+] T-cell memory			
Vaccinations	20–30 years	31–50 years	51–75 years	$t_{1/2}$ of CD8[+] T cells
1	50% (8/16)	49% (39/79)	50% (22/44)	15.5 (0–27.1)
2	42% (5/12)	38% (14/37)	57% (4/7)	8.1 (0–16.9)
3–14	46% (13/28)	50% (16/32)	ND	9.0 (0–18.1)

[a] percentage of individuals possessing peripheral blood lymphocytes that proliferate in response to vaccinia antigen.
[b] number of years since the last smallpox vaccination.
[c] calculated half-life of vaccinia specific CD4[+] T lymphocytes.
[d] not determined.
From Hammarlund et al. (2003).

finding is that over 50% of individuals vaccinated more than 50 years previously possess both CD4[+] and CD8[+] T lymphocytes responsive to vaccinia antigens in vitro.

The effectiveness of these antibodies and lymphocytes specific for smallpox in protecting against infection remains unknown. Additional studies will clarify this question.

Cell Proliferation in Immunologic Memory

The mechanisms responsible for the changes observed in a memory response remain the subject of ongoing investigations. As early as 1949, Burnet and Fenner suggested that the induction of a memory response represents a proliferation of cells that had somehow been altered by primary immunization. An alternative explanation was that a large number of cells formed during the primary response remained in the animal, thus rendering proliferation unnecessary.

The availability of radioisotopes allowed investigators to study these two possibilities and to demonstrate the origin of cells appearing during a memory response. In 1962, Gus Nossal and Olaf Makela at Stanford University, California, injected groups of rats a single time with an antigen from Salmonella flagella. Either 2 or 40 weeks later they injected these rats with radioactive thymidine 2 h prior to receiving a second injection of the flagellar antigen. Radioactive thymidine can act as a precursor of DNA so that cells that proliferated in response to the second antigenic challenge would incorporate the radioisotope and could be detected by autoradiography. If antibody-forming cells remained from the primary reaction, these cells would not be radiolabeled.

Nossal and Makela removed spleens from the rats injected a second time with Salmonella flagella and determined the number of cells incorporating radioisotope. Virtually all the plasma cells formed during the first 5–6 days of the secondary response were labeled, indicating that they derived from the proliferation of a small number of cells rather than from differentiation of pre-existing cells without proliferation. Nossal and Makela concluded that antibody-forming cells remembered the initial antigenic exposure and divided following restimulation by antigen. This is most consistent with the hypothesis that "immunological memory depended on the persistence, following primary stimulation, of a continuously dividing stem line of primitive lymphocytes, reactive at all times to further antigenic stimulation." This hypothesis remains to be proven.

Studies on immunologic memory continue. In 2010 Susan Swain stated that "we know much less about the formation, maintenance and regulation of…memory cells than we do about the primary response of naïve lymphocytes." The studies reviewed in this section reflect the emphasis placed on B lymphocytes and antibody formation; however, similar studies have been performed using T lymphocytes and cell-mediated immune responses. Existing data provide evidence that antigenic activation alters the cell surface molecules expressed by lymphocytes. Current investigations are directed at understanding

- how long immunologic memory persists, particularly to vaccines;
- the identity of the genetic and molecular components required for the maintenance of immunologic memory;

- the differences of memory responses of various populations of lymphocytes involved in the adaptive immune response; and
- methods for enhancing or suppressing the memory response in a variety of clinical situations.

CONCLUSION

All life forms have evolved defense mechanisms to protect against an array of potential pathogens. Many of these defense mechanisms are innate; that is, they are naturally occurring, present at birth, nonspecific, and lack memory. A second defense mechanism, the adaptive immune response, evolved in mammals and other vertebrates to provide additional protection against potentially pathogenic microorganisms. Innate host defenses, characterized by phagocytosis and inflammation, eliminate most potential pathogens. Adaptive immune responses build on these innate mechanisms and are characterized by three hallmarks: immunologic specificity, self–non-self-discrimination, and immunologic memory.

Immunologic specificity refers to the ability of the cells of the adaptive immune response (B and T lymphocytes) to discriminate between different foreign antigens such as microorganisms or cells and proteins from other individuals or other species. Specificity is based on the presence of unique cell-surface receptors expressed by the lymphocytes of the adaptive immune response; the studies to identify these antigen-specific receptors are described in Chapter 17. The genetic mechanisms involved in generating sufficient diversity in these receptors so that the system can respond to virtually any antigen are presented in Chapter 18.

The adaptive immune system exercises a unique ability to protect the organism from life-threatening immune responses against self. Mechanisms that have evolved to provide this discriminatory function of the adaptive immune response are covered in Chapters 8, 20, and 21. The occurrence of autoimmune diseases (Chapter 34) demonstrates that these mechanisms are neither consistent nor foolproof.

Immunologic memory provides the rationale for the development of vaccines against microbes such as smallpox, polio, diphtheria, and measles that have historically caused epidemics responsible for altering social and economic history. Vaccine development efforts have been successful for many of these diseases, but additional investigations will add other debilitating diseases to the short list of those that have been eradicated. In particular, vaccines against several infectious diseases, including tuberculosis, malaria, dysentery, acquired immunodeficiency syndrome, and others are targets for ongoing studies. The concepts discovered during the development of successful vaccines against infectious microorganisms are currently under investigation in studies of noninfectious diseases such as cancer and autoimmunity (Chapter 38).

References

Burnet, F.M., 1959. The Clonal Selection Theory of Acquired Immunity. Vanderbilt University Press, Nashville, TN.

Burnet, F.M., Fenner, F., 1949. The Production of Antibodies, second ed. The Macmillan Company, Melbourne and London.

Donath, J., Landsteiner, K., 1904. Uber paroxysmile Hamoglobinurie. Munchen Med. Wochenschr. 51, 1590–1593.

Ehrlich, P., Morgenroth, J., 1901. Ueber Hämolysine. Berl. Klin.Wochenschr. 38, 251–257.

Enders, J.F., Weller, T.H., Robbins, F.C., 1949. Cultivation of the Lansing strain of poliomyelitis virus in cultures of various human embryonic tissues. Science 109, 85–87.

Hammarlund, E., Lewis, M.W., Hansen, S.G., Strelow, L.I., Nelson, J.A., Sexton, G.J., Hanifin, J.M., Slifka, M.K., 2003. Duration of antiviral immunity after smallpox vaccination. Nat. Med. 9, 1131–1137.

Jenner, E., 1798. An Inquiry into the Causes and Effects of the Variolae Vaccinae: A Disease Discovered in Some of the Western Counties of England, Particularly Gloucestershire, and Known by the Name of the Cow Pox. Sampson Low, London. Referenced in Jesty and Williams (2011).

Jesty, R., Williams, G., 2011. Who invented vaccination. Malta Med. J. 23, 29–32.

Kraus, R., 1897. Ueber specifische Reactionen in keim freien Filtraten aus Cholera, Typhus and Pestbouillon culturen, erzeugt durch homologes Serum. Wien. Klin. Wochenschr. 10, 736–738.

Landsteiner, K., 1945. The Specificity of Serological Reactions. Harvard University Press, Cambridge, MA.

Landsteiner, K., Popper, E., 1909. Übertragung der Poliomyelitis acuta auf Affen. Z. Immunitätsforsch. 2, 377–390.

Landsteiner, K., van der Scheer, 1932. On the serological specificity of peptides. J. Exp. Med. 55, 781–796.

Montagu, L.M.W., 1717. Letter to Sarah Criswell. http://pyramid.spd.louisville.edu/~eri/fos/lady_mary_montagu.html.

Nossal, G.J.V., Mäkelä, O., 1962. Autoradiographic studies on the immune response. I. The kinetics of plasma cell proliferation. J. Exp. Med. 115, 209–230.

Nuttall, G.H.F., 1888. Experimente über die bacterien feindlichen Einflüsse des thierischen Körpers. Zeitschr. für Hyg. 4, 853–894.

Rous, P., 1947. Karl landsteiner 1868–1943. Obit. Notices Fellows R. Soc. 5, 294–326.

Sabin, A.B., 1960. Oral, live poliovirus vaccine for elimination of poliomyelitis. Arc. Intern. Med. 106, 5–9.

Salk, J.E., 1955. Vaccination against paralytic poliomyelitis performance and prospects. Am. J. Pub. Health Nations Health 45, 575–596.

Schmalstieg, F.C., Goldman, A.S., 2009. Jules Bordet (1870–1961): a bridge between early and modern immunology. J. Med. Biog. 17, 217–224.

Swain, S., 2010. Grand challenges in immunological memory. Front. Immunol. 1, 103. http://www.frontiersin.org/Immunological_Memory/10.3389/fimmu.2010.00103/full (accessed 16.07.12.).

Thucydides, 1904. History of the Peloponnesian War, Translated by Richard Crawley. (chapter 9). https://ebooks.adelaide.edu.au/t/thucydides/crawley/

Uhlenhuth, P., 1901. Eine Methode zur Unterscheidung der verschiedenen Blutarten, im besonderen zum differentialdiagnostischen Nachweis des Menschenblutes. Dtsch. Med. Wochenschr. 27, 82–83.

Uhlenhuth, P., 1903. Zu Lehre von der Unterscheidung verschiedener Eiweissarten mit Hilfe spezifischer Sera, Festschrift zum 60. Geburtstage v. Robert Kock, Jena. Gustave Fischer Verlag. 48–74.

Uhlenhuth, P., 1911. On the biological differentiation of proteins by the precipitin reaction with special reference to the forensic examination of blood and meat. J. Roy. Inst. Pub. Health 19, 641–662.

Voltaire, F.-M.A., 1733. Letters on England. Letter XI – on Inoculation. http://www.online-literature.com/voltaire/letters_england/11/.

TIME LINE

430 BCE	Thucydides, Greek historian, reports that individuals who survived the plaque were immune from developing it a second time
1000	Chinese use dried scabs from smallpox lesions to protect against the disease
1718	Lady Montague introduces smallpox variolation to Great Britain
1765	John Fewster presents the initial description of cross-immunity to smallpox induced by cowpox
1796	Edward Jenner performs the first successful vaccination against smallpox
1887–1888	George Nuttall, Jozsef Fodor, Karl Flügge, and Hans von Buchner independently describe antibody activity in serum from animals injected with pathogenic microorganisms
1900	Karl Landsteiner discovers the ABO blood groups
1901	Paul Ehrlich and Julius Morgenroth introduce the concept of "horror autotoxicus"
1908	Karl Landsteiner and Erwin Popper isolate poliovirus
1930	Karl Landsteiner receives the Nobel Prize in Physiology or Medicine for the discovery of human blood groups
1945	Karl Landsteiner publishes *The Specificity of Serological Reactions*
1949	John Enders, Thomas Weller, and Frederick Robbins successfully culture poliovirus
1949	F. Macfarlane Burnet and Frank Fenner publish *The Production of Antibodies*
1954	Enders, Weller, and Robbins awarded the Nobel Prize in Physiology or Medicine
1955	Salk poliovirus approved
1960	Sabin poliovirus approved
1980	Smallpox declared eradicated

CHAPTER

3

Two Effector Mechanisms of the Adaptive Immune Response

INTRODUCTION

Most potential pathogens are deterred or destroyed by innate host defenses, including physical barriers (skin and mucous membranes), cells (macrophages and granulocytes), and molecules (inflammatory mediators and complement components). When pathogens circumvent these first-line host defenses, they trigger the adaptive immune response. Chapter 1 describes the basic components of both the innate host defenses and adaptive immune responses, while Chapter 2 details classic experiments that demonstrated the unique characteristics (specificity, memory, and self–non-self discrimination) of the adaptive response.

Immunological investigations in the first half of the twentieth century relied on measuring antibody in immunized animals and humans to demonstrate activity of the adaptive immune response. However, studies performed by Ilya Metchnikov and his colleagues in the 1890s as well as observations of graft rejection and skin sensitivity to antigens made 60 years later led investigators to suspect that some immune responses may involve cellular mechanisms. These suspicions were proven correct, and the role of cell-mediated immune responses in providing protection against pathogens is an important area of contemporary immunologic research.

The investigations presented in this chapter provide evidence that two independent yet interdependent mechanisms have evolved to respond to potential pathogens. Currently, immunologists divide adaptive immune responses into those involving antibody produced by B lymphocytes and those that are initiated by T lymphocytes, resulting in cell-mediated responses. This information helped develop immunology as a discipline and serves as the backdrop for studies unraveling a contemporary appreciation of the immune system.

ANTIBODY

In the late 1880s, several investigators reported that injection of experimental animals with bacteria (*Bacillus anthracis* or *Vibrio cholerae*) induced the production of a substance found in the serum that kill the bacteria (von Fodor, 1887; Nuttall, 1888; von Buchner, 1889; Schmalsteig and Goldman, 2009). The antibacterial substance is now termed antibody.

The demonstration that the body mounted an antibody response against potentially pathogenic microorganisms led to speculation that antibodies might be used to protect against bacterial infections. In 1890, Emil von Behring and Shibasaburo Kitasato provided the first

A Historical Perspective on Evidence-Based Immunology
http://dx.doi.org/10.1016/B978-0-12-398381-7.00003-4

21

evidence that passive transfer of antibodies (serotherapy) protected against infection. The successful development of serotherapy against two major infectious diseases, diphtheria and tetanus, established the field of immunology and demonstrated the usefulness of this discipline to medicine.

Development of Serotherapy

Corynebacterium diphtheriae causes a potentially fatal upper respiratory tract infection. Diphtheria is a contagious disease characterized by a sore throat, with a low-grade fever and the appearance of an adherent pseudomembrane on the tonsils and pharynx that may extend to the nasal cavity. This membrane, consisting of fibrin, bacteria, and leukocytes, may lead to difficulty in breathing, resulting in the disease being called the "strangling angel of children." Other complications of diphtheria include heart failure and paralysis. Prior to the development of an effective vaccine in 1921, the Centers for Disease Control and Prevention (CDC) recorded 206,000 cases of the disease with 15,520 deaths per year.

C. diphtheriae was first grown in the laboratory in 1884. A bacteria-free filtrate (exotoxin) of a culture of *C. diphtheriae* was identified as the cause of the pathology associated with infection (reviewed by Grundbacher, 1992). This exotoxin is produced by a bacteriophage infecting *C. diphtheria* and not by the bacterium itself. The exotoxin causes damage by inhibiting protein synthesis in the cells infected by the bacterium, resulting in the formation of the suffocating membrane.

Clostridium tetani, a bacterium present in the soil, can contaminate wounds and causes the disease tetanus. Tetanus is characterized by prolonged contraction of skeletal muscle that leads to tetani and death. *C. tetani* produces one of the most potent neurotoxins known (tetanospasmin), which binds irreversibly to neurons and interferes with the release of inhibitory neurotransmitters. As a result, motor neurons fire continually, leading to sustained and irreversible muscle contraction.

A few *C. tetani* organisms produce sufficient toxin to kill the individual. It is estimated that the minimal lethal dose in humans is 2.5 ng per kg. As a result, neither the toxin nor the number of *C. tetani* reach high enough levels to induce an immune response before the infected host dies. Thus, prior to the development of serotherapy (in the early 1900s) and a vaccine (in 1924), the mortality rate for patients infected with *C. tetani* approached 90%.

Both von Behring and Kitasato trained with Robert Koch at the University of Berlin. Robert Heinrich Herman Koch (1843–1910) developed a set of conditions (Koch's postulates) that are required prior to identifying a particular microorganism as the etiological agent of a disease.

Koch's postulates (http://www.medicinenet.com/script/main/art.asp?articlekey=7291) are as follows:

- the bacteria must be present in every case of the disease,
- the bacteria must be isolated from the host with the disease and grown in pure culture,
- the specific disease must be reproduced when a pure culture of the bacteria is inoculated into a healthy susceptible host, and
- the bacteria must be recoverable from the experimentally infected host.

Koch, born and educated in Germany, was awarded the MD degree from the University of Gottingen in 1866. During his research career, he isolated the causative agents of anthrax (*B. anthracis*), cholera (*V. cholerae*), and tuberculosis (*Mycobacterium tuberculosis*). Koch was awarded the Nobel Prize in Physiology or Medicine in 1905 "for his investigations and discoveries in relation to tuberculosis."

In the early 1890s, studies at the Hygiene Institute in Berlin led to the successful development of antibodies capable of neutralizing the exotoxins from both *C. diphtheriae* and *C. tetani*. Such antibodies are known as antitoxins. Emil von Behring (1854–1917) from Germany and Shibasaburo Kitasato (1852–1931) from Japan collaborated on this project (Behring and Kitasato, 1890; Behring, 1891). Von Behring and Kitasato immunized guinea pigs with diphtheria toxin that had been inactivated by heating. These injected animals produced a substance (an antitoxin) capable of neutralizing the toxic effects of *C. diphtheriae*. This antitoxin protected the animals against the disease when challenged with the bacteria. More importantly, animals exposed to diphtheria could be protected by treating them with serum from immunized donors. Such protection occurred even when the serum was given after the guinea pigs were infected.

This observation translated into the development of therapeutic intervention for patients infected with diphtheria. Horses injected with exotoxin from *C. diphtheriae* synthesized antibodies capable of neutralizing the toxin. This antitoxin was used to treat infected patients. In 1891, the first human patient to be treated with this antitoxin survived. Success led to further clinical use of the antitoxin and to what some consider the first controlled clinical trial (Hróbjartsson et al., 1998).

Johannes Fibiger (1867–1928), a Danish physician, earned his Ph.D. from the University of Copenhagen in 1895. He performed a trial on diphtheria-infected patients comparing standard treatment (observation and airway management) with standard treatment plus subcutaneous injections of antitoxin. The injections of antitoxin were given twice daily "until symptoms improved." Fibiger treated 239 patients in the experimental group with antitoxin plus standard therapy and 245 controls with standard therapy alone. Eight of the patients in the experimental group died (3.4%) while 30 of the patients in the control group died (12.3%).

Between 1890 and the early 1920s, serotherapy for diphtheria and tetanus became a standard treatment in many hospitals in Europe, Asia, and North and South America. The development of vaccines for diphtheria in 1921 and tetanus in 1924 decreased the need for serotherapy. Diphtheria antitoxin and tetanus antitoxin are still available from the CDC in the United States for emergency use in patients who have not previously been immunized.

The use of preformed antibodies as therapy, particularly following infection with C. diphtheriae, in the early part of the twentieth century decreased the morbidity and mortality of this disease. This success provided a patina of respectability to the emerging field of immunology and resulted in the awarding of the first Nobel Prize in Physiology or Medicine in 1900 to Emil von Behring "for his work on serum therapy, especially its application against diphtheria by which he has opened a new road in the domain of medical science and thereby placed in the hands of the physician a victorious weapon against illness and death."

Serum sickness emerged as an unintended consequence of serotherapy. As is presented in Chapter 33, the use of antibodies derived from horse serum for these treatments resulted in some patients producing antibodies to horse serum proteins. These newly formed antibodies, when bound to their antigen (horse serum proteins), produced antigen–antibody complexes that settled out in several different organs, most notably in the kidney. Immune complexes activated the complement system and resulted in a pathological reaction, glomerulonephritis, in the kidney glomeruli. This unexpected side effect was one of the first examples of pathology caused by aberrant immune responses.

Ehrlich's Side-Chain Theory of Antibody Formation

Paul Ehrlich (1854–1915), born in Germany, received his medical degree in 1878 from the University of Leipzig. He made major advances in the areas of bacteriology, hematology, and immunology (Kaufmann, 2008). As a medical student, he initiated the development of procedures for staining animal tissues. During the early part of his career, he refined and applied these techniques to blood and tissue cells. Using various dyes he discovered tissue mast cells, the cell type involved in allergic reactions, and the three types of granulocytes in the blood (neutrophils, basophils, and eosinophils).

The mechanism by which antibodies are produced was unknown at the turn of the twentieth century. Ehrlich contributed to the discussion of this issue by

hypothesizing the side chain theory of antibody formation (Ehrlich, 1900). This hypothesis is based on speculation concerning the way in which cells obtain nourishment. Ehrlich previously speculated that cells bind nutrients to cell surface side chains; this binding results in uptake. Extending this theory to the production of antibodies, he proposed that antibody-forming cells possess a variety of side chains that allow them to specifically bind noxious substances (i.e., toxins). This binding results in the release of the side chains, which are detected in serum as antibodies, and stimulation of the cell to synthesize additional copies of the neutralizing molecule. Figure 3.1 illustrates this process.

Most immunologists failed to embrace the side chain theory of antibody formation at the time. The introduction of the clonal selection theory of antibody formation by F. Macfarlane Burnet (1957) prompted a reevaluation of Ehrlich's ideas (Chapter 6).

Paul Ehrlich and his colleagues, working initially at Koch's Institute of Infectious Diseases in Berlin and later at his own Institute for Experimental Therapy in Frankfort-am-Main in Germany, pursued additional investigations of the immune system, including the

- specificity of the immune response,
- passive transfer of protective immunity from mother to offspring via breast milk,
- quantitation of antibody activity in serum, and
- the ability of an individual to produce autoantibodies.

Ehrlich shared the Nobel Prize in Physiology or Medicine in 1908 with Ilya Metchnikov "in recognition of their work on immunity" (Ehrlich, 1908).

CELL-MEDIATED IMMUNITY

Not all microorganisms can be eliminated by antibody-mediated effector mechanisms. Immunologists recognize a second type of adaptive immune response against foreign antigens, leading to specifically sensitized lymphocytes that participate in a process called cell-mediated immunity. The impetus for the study of the role of cells in an immune response can be traced to the work of Ilya Metchnikov (1845–1916) and his colleagues.

Metchnikov's most famous experiment involved inserting a rose thorn into the larvae of starfish (Tauber, 2003; Chapter 15). The foreign body stimulated local cells, phagocytes, to surround and break down the thorn. Initially, he considered the role of the phagocytes to be one of nutrition and intracellular digestion, though he soon realized that phagocytosis was a mechanism by which an animal defended itself against foreign intruders, including microorganisms.

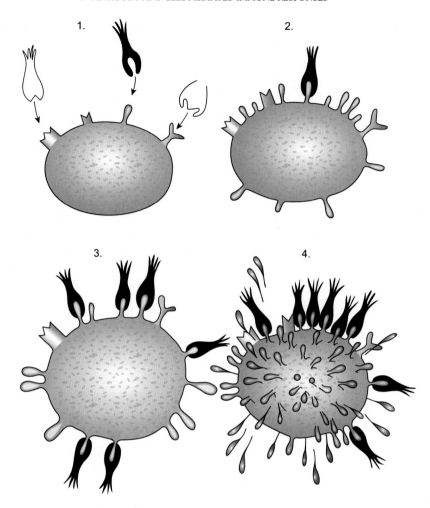

FIGURE 3.1 Ehrlich's side chain theory of antibody formation. In this hypothesis, foreign substances (black) would interact with complementary side chains on antibody-forming cells. This interaction would cause the production of additional side chains (antibody) and release of antibody into the cell's environment. *From Ehrlich (1900).*

Metchnikov, born and trained in Russia, worked in several institutes in Europe before accepting a position at the Pasteur Institute in Paris in 1888. By that time he had already made his initial observations on the uptake of foreign material by specialized cells in invertebrates, a process he termed phagocytosis. His phagocytic theory could explain all aspects of immunity known at the time, and he and his students, known as cellularists, vehemently disagreed with humoralists, who were investigating the role of soluble substances including antibody. The most prominent humoralist during this era was Paul Ehrlich.

Historians of immunology have commented on this dispute between the cellularists and the humoralists. Cellularists, led by Metchnikov, believed that all host defenses against pathogens could be explained by the action of phagocytes. Humoralists championed Ehrlich's theory that antibody was the primary mechanism for eliminating pathogens. This debate was a continuation of the debate between Robert Koch and Louis Pasteur

that started in 1881 (Gachelin, 2007). Koch and Pasteur both worked with *B. anthracis*, the causative agent of anthrax. Koch developed his set of postulates for determining the etiological agent responsible for an infectious disease based in part on this work. Koch felt that the chemical and biological characteristics of a microbe were specific and permanent. Pasteur used a low virulence strain of *B. anthracis* to develop a successful vaccine against anthrax in sheep. He considered that the virulence of microbes was variable and explained the historical appearance and disappearance of diseases such as smallpox, syphilis, and plague. Pasteur felt that this variation could be useful in developing vaccines against infectious microbes.

The disagreement between Ehrlich and Metchnikov was further influenced not only by the personalities of the two protagonists but also by the political differences of Germany and France resulting from the Franco-Prussian War of 1870. Even the awarding of the Nobel Prize for Physiology or Medicine jointly to Ehrlich and

Metchnikov in 1908 "in recognition of their work on immunity" failed to settle the dispute.

The presence of antibodies in mammals is easier to detect than specifically sensitized lymphocytes. Serum thought to contain antibodies can be mixed with antigen and the reaction visualized by precipitation, agglutination, cell lysis, or other phenomena. The detection of activated lymphocytes required the development of technology such as radioactive labeling of DNA (to detect proliferation) or quantitation of proteins synthesized as a result of stimulation. Accordingly, many studies during the first half of the twentieth century focused on antibodies as the major provider of protection against pathogens. The work of von Behring and others in transferring immunity against the exotoxins of diphtheria and tetanus to unimmunized individuals amply demonstrated the power of antibody in protecting against infectious microorganisms. However, several immunological phenomena described in the first half of the twentieth century could not be explained through the action of antibody alone.

For example, antibody activity failed to explain responses to transplanted foreign tumors, to grafts of normal tissue, and to intracellular microorganisms such as viruses and *Mycobacterium tuberculosis*. The effector mechanisms responsible for these reactions, termed cell-mediated immunity, involve the activity of a population of specialized lymphocytes (T cells). Studies on the hypersensitivity skin reactions induced to synthetic chemicals in immunized guinea pigs provided initial evidence for the activity of these lymphocytes.

Transfer of Skin Hypersensitivity Reactions

Merrill Chase (1905–2004) grew up in Providence, Rhode Island and received his undergraduate and graduate training at Brown University. In 1932 he was hired to work with Karl Landsteiner at The Rockefeller Institute for Medical Research in New York where he remained for the entirety of his career. Landsteiner and Chase injected guinea pigs and rabbits systemically with synthetic chemicals such as picryl chloride, 2-3 dinitrochlorobenzene, and *o*-chlorobenzoyl chloride. They evaluated the level of sensitization by injecting these same chemicals into the animal's skin. Inflammation (heat, redness, swelling, and pain) at the inoculation site signaled a positive reaction. Immunologists in the 1930s and 1940s considered that these skin reactions were due to the action of specific antibodies. Chase and Landsteiner designed experiments to transfer this skin reactivity and characterize the antibodies based on the idea that the antibodies would be present in serum. Despite numerous attempts using a variety of protocols, sensitization could not be transferred by injecting serum from a sensitized animal to a nonsensitized animal. This argued against the possibility that the serum contained antibodies.

Alternatively, Chase postulated that the responsible antibodies were cell bound rather than in the serum. He attempted several methods to isolate putative cell-bound antibodies from the skin of animals sensitized to picryl chloride, 2-3 dinitrochlorobenzene, and *o*-chlorobenzoyl chloride. The methods he used in attempts to mechanically dislodge antibodies from skin cells were described in a 1985 summary of his career:

> Extracts of 'sensitive skin' were prepared from skin scrapings taken from guinea pigs at various times during the sensitizing course. The scrapings were ground with quartz sand or glycerol-saline and passed through a Carver press at 200,000 lbs./sq. in., or first defatted with diethyl ether before freezing the tissue with dry ice. Then I partially pulverized the skin in a Graeser shock press by striking the cold steel plunger repeatedly with a sledgehammer.

Despite this heroic effort, the transfer of skin sensitivity to nonsensitized guinea pigs failed.

Using a different approach, Chase injected another group of guinea pigs with these same chemicals. He harvested cells from the peritoneal cavity of animals to determine if the antibodies might be bound to these cells. He disrupted the cells and harvested an extract that he injected into nonsensitized guinea pigs. This also failed to transfer the skin sensitivity.

In one experiment, Chase accidentally used a preparation that was contaminated with some cells from the peritoneal exudate. Injection of this cell-containing preparation into normal animals resulted in positive skin reactions (Landsteiner and Chase, 1942). This serendipitous finding, indicating that cells rather than antibody were involved in the transfer, is the historical basis for our contemporary appreciation of cell-mediated immune responses. Chase eventually demonstrated the ability of cells to transfer hypersensitivity to all the chemicals used in the original sensitization protocol (Chase, 1945).

Other investigators failed to confirm these results and, in fact, Chase in his 1985 reminiscence reported that he also had difficulty repeating his own observations. Acceptance of the role of cell-mediated immune responses in the adaptive immune system came from future investigations of graft rejection.

Transfer of Graft Rejection

Peter Medawar (1915–1987), born in Brazil, immigrated to England with his parents shortly after the end of the First World War. He studied at Oxford and earned a Ph.D. in zoology in 1937. During the next 10 years he served as a fellow and teacher at several of the colleges in Oxford University. In 1947 he moved to Birmingham University, and in 1951 he became the Jodrell Professor of Zoology at University College in London. In 1962 he assumed the position of director of the National Institute for Medical

Research. In addition to his studies on graft rejection, he discovered acquired immunological tolerance (Chapter 8) for which he and F. Macfarland Burnet were awarded the Nobel Prize for Physiology or Medicine in 1960.

During the Second World War, many patients, including members of the army and air force, were treated for severe burns. The transplantation of skin to cover the burn areas and protect against infections became an important part of the treatment plan. Most of the skin transplants failed. The Medical Research Council asked Medawar to investigate why skin taken from an individual failed to survive when transplanted to an unrelated recipient. Medawar observed that when donor and recipient were related, skin grafts exchanged between them were more likely to survive than when donor and recipient were unrelated. Analysis of the reaction leading to graft failure revealed characteristics similar to other adaptive immune responses, including specificity and memory (Medawar, 1944).

Gibson and Medawar (1943) reported the presence of antibodies in the serum of both humans and rabbits that had rejected foreign grafts. Medawar concluded that the immunological reaction responsible for graft rejection was due to the action of antibodies. Other investigators made similar observations and conclusions (reviewed in Hildeman and Medawar, 1959). Histological evaluation of graft rejection, however, revealed infiltration of the graft with lymphocytes, a picture resembling that seen in skin hypersensitivity reactions such as the ones reported by Chase and Landsteiner.

The role of lymphocytes in graft rejection received support in 1955 when Avrion Mitchison (1928–present) demonstrated the activity of these cells in rejection of tumor allografts. Mitchison, earned his Ph.D. at Oxford in Peter Medawar's laboratory and accepted an academic position at Edinburgh University.

Studies performed in the first half of the twentieth century demonstrated that tumors induce an immune response when transplanted to nonidentical (allogeneic) recipients (Chapter 37). In 1955, Mitchison showed that lymphocytes derived from the lymph nodes draining a tumor allograft transferred the immune response to the tumor to naive, syngeneic animals. Cells from other lymph nodes, the spleen, or whole blood did not transfer this response. In addition, serum from tumor-bearing animals failed to cause rejection. Mitchison's conclusion was that tumors are immunogenic and that the immune response induced by tumors involves the activation of cells.

If tumors are rejected through the activity of lymphocytes, is a similar mechanism responsible for the rejection of nonmalignant grafts? Medawar's group (Brent et al., 1958) continued searching for the mechanism of graft rejection using guinea pigs that had rejected a skin graft from an unrelated donor. Lymphocytes from these recipients were injected into the skin of the original graft donor. The rationale for this experimental design was that if the inoculum contained lymphocytes specific for antigens on the donor graft, injecting these lymphocytes would induce an inflammatory reaction. In fact, a reaction did occur at the site of injection within 5–8 h. Injection of serum from the animal that had rejected the graft into the skin donor failed to induce a similar reaction.

These results strongly suggested that graft rejection depended on the direct activity of cells rather than antibodies. To prove this conclusion, several research groups transferred lymphoid cells from animals rejecting a graft to naive animals. Injected animals received skin grafts from the original donor, and the grafts were observed. The prediction was that the grafts on the treated animals would be rejected in an accelerated fashion. The results of these investigations were equivocal.

Finally, Rupert Billingham (1921–2002) and his colleagues showed that lymphocytes, but not serum from mice that had rejected a skin graft, could transfer this reactivity to other mice (Billingham et al., 1963). Figure 3.2 outlines the experimental protocol used in these studies.

Neonatal mice of one inbred strain (A) injected with lymphocytes of a second inbred strain (the alien strain in Figure 3.2) became tolerant to antigens expressed by cells of the second strain (Chapter 8). Tolerant mice accept a skin graft from the alien strain indefinitely. Other A strain mice grafted with skin from the alien strain rejected the skin in 10–14 days. Billingham and colleagues harvested serum and lymphocytes from mice that had rejected a graft and transferred these cells or serum to tolerant A strain mice that had been transplanted with skin from the alien strain. If graft rejection involves antibody, then transfer of serum would cause graft destruction in the tolerant host. Alternatively, if graft rejection is due to lymphocytes, the transfer of serum alone would not result in rejection while lymphocytes would.

Table 3.1 presents the results of this experiment. Transfer of immune lymphocytes but not serum from mice that had rejected a skin graft to tolerant mice caused graft rejection in most recipients. Nonimmune lymphocytes injected into tolerant mice with successful grafts cause graft rejection only when large numbers of cells (240 million) were transferred.

Billingham and his group demonstrated two additional features using this transfer protocol:

- grafts on normal mice could be rejected by the transfer of immune lymphocytes, but this required higher doses than were required to cause rejection in tolerant mice; and
- grafts on normal and tolerant mice were not rejected following serum transfer.

The cell responsible for rejection is a lymphocyte, as demonstrated by studies in inbred strains of rats using thoracic duct cells rather than lymph node cells. Thoracic

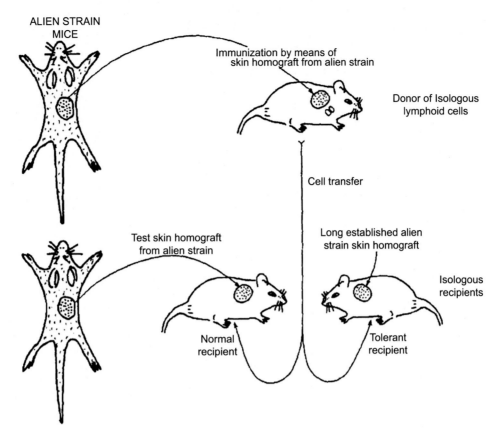

FIGURE 3.2 Experimental design used by Billingham et al. (1963) to demonstrate the ability of lymphocytes to transfer sensitivity to foreign skin grafts. Neonatal mice of one inbred strain (A) were injected with lymphocytes of a second strain (the alien strain) to induce immunologic tolerance. Normal strain A mice received skin grafts from alien strain mice. At various times during the rejection of this graft, lymphocytes from the grafted mice were harvested and injected into normal or tolerant strain A mice bearing skin grafts from the alien strain. The fate of the grafts on the injected mice was followed. *From Billingham et al. (1963).*

duct cells contain primarily lymphocytes that are the antigen-reactive cell in the adaptive immune response (Chapter 4). Thoracic duct lymphocytes were as effective at transferring sensitivity to skin grafts in unresponsive (tolerant) animals as were lymph node cells (Billingham et al., 1963). This observation argues that lymphocytes rather than other cell types present in lymph nodes are involved in graft rejection.

These results confirmed the investigations of Chase and Landsteiner that a second effector mechanism exists in the adaptive immune response. Studies performed during the second half of the twentieth century validated the role of cell-mediated immunity in the rejection of tumors and grafts as well as in providing protection against pathogens, including viruses and intracellular bacteria such as *Mycobacterium tuberculosis*.

CONCLUSION

The experiments presented in this chapter demonstrate that the adaptive immune response consists of antibody-mediated and cell-mediated mechanisms. Antibodies, produced by B lymphocytes, are responsible for providing protection against extracellular pathogens such as most bacteria and many protozoal parasites. Antibody helps eliminate these pathogens by activating several effector mechanisms, including the complement system, phagocytosis, neutralization, and antibody-dependent cell-mediated cytotoxicity (Chapter 26). Cell-mediated responses involve T lymphocytes that perform several functions in providing protection against intracellular pathogens such as viruses, fungi, and intracellular bacteria. T lymphocytes eliminate these pathogens through cell lysis and the induction of an inflammatory response (Chapter 27).

Patients with various immunodeficiencies (Chapter 32) have reinforced this dichotomy. Patients diagnosed with X-linked agammaglobulinemia have a history of recurrent bacterial infections. These patients lack antibodies in their serum and B lymphocytes in their peripheral lymphoid tissue. Other patients presenting with a history of recurrent viral infections have been

TABLE 3.1   Ability of Lymphocytes to Transfer Skin Graft Rejection to Normal or Tolerant Mice. Tolerant A Strain Mice Bearing a Successful Allogeneic Skin Graft Were Injected with Various Numbers of Lymph Node Cells from Syngeneic Mice That Were Either Unmanipulated (Normal) or Rejecting a Skin Graft (Sensitized)

Abolition of tolerance of CBA skin in A strain mice by the intraperitoneal transfer of isologous node cells					
Isologous donors			Tolerant A strain mice		
Status	Immunizing stimulus	No. of cells transferred (×10⁶)	No. tested	Survival times of grafts after cell transfer (days)	MSTᵃ (days)
Normal	–	240	3	12 (2)ᵇ, 14	12
		120	3	20, >100 (2)	
		30	6	>100 (6)	
		15	5	18, 19, 56, >100 (2)	
		5	6	>100 (6)	
Sensitizedᶜ	CBA skin	240	5	9 (4), 10	9
		120	5	8 (3), 10 (2)	8
		60	8	9 (4), 10 (4)	9
		30	6	11 (3), 14, 17, 25	12
		20	5	9 (5)	9
		15	8	10 (2), 11 (2), 17, 18, 22 (2)	12
		10	8	10, 11 (3), 24, 25, 55, >100	12
		5	12	15 (2), 16, 17, 19 (2), 20, 24, 25, 39 (2), 45	21

ᵃMedian survival time.
ᵇNumbers in parentheses indicate number of animals.
ᶜSuspensions of regional node cells were prepared from sensitized donors 11 days after they had been grafted with CBA skin.
From Billingham et al. (1963).

found to have a congenital defect in the development of T lymphocytes.

Despite the division of the adaptive immune response into antibody-mediated and cell-mediated components, all foreign pathogens stimulate both B and T lymphocytes. The relative level of response by antibody or T lymphocytes dictates the eventual outcome of any interaction with a pathogen. The two arms of the system function concurrently and cooperatively in recognizing non-self and in providing defense against foreign invaders.

The identification of two types of adaptive immune responses led to studies to identify the cells responsible for antibody-mediated and cell-mediated reactions. Chapter 4 recounts the beginning of these studies, leading to the identification of lymphocytes as the antigen-reactive cell. Subsequent chapters recount the experiments that identified B lymphocytes (Chapter 10) and T lymphocytes (Chapter 9).

References

Behring, E.A., 1891. Untersuchungen über das Zustandekommen der Diphtherie-immunität bei Thieren. Dtsch. Med. Wochenschr. 50, 1145–1148.

Behring, E.A., Kitasato, S., 1890. Über das Zustandekommen der Diphtheria-immunität and der Tetanus-immunität bei Thieren. Dtsch. Med. Wochenschr. 49, 1113–1114.

Billingham, R.E., Silvers, W.K., Wilson, D.B., 1963. Further studies on adoptive transfer of sensitivity to skin homografts. J. Exp. Med. 118, 397–419.

Brent, L., Brown, J., Medawar, P.B., 1958. Skin transplantation immunity in relation to hypersensitivity. Lancet 272, 561–564.

Burnet, F.M., 1957. A modification of Jerne's theory of antibody production using the concept of clonal selection. Aust. J. Sci. 20, 67–68.

Chase, M.W., 1945. The cellular transfer of cutaneous hypersensitivity to tuberculin. Proc. Soc. Exp. Biol. Med. 59, 134–135.

Chase, M.W., 1985. Immunology and experimental dermatology. Annu. Rev. Immunol. 3, 1–29.

Ehrlich, P., 1900. Croonian lecture: on immunity with special reference to cell life. Proc. Roy. Soc. Lond. 66, 424–448.

Ehrlich, P., 1908. Partial cell functions. In: Nobel Lectures, Physiology or Medicine, 1901–1921. Elsevier Publishing Co., Amsterdam. 1967; accessed at http://nobelprize.org/nobel_prizes/medicine/laureates/1908/ehrlich-lecture.html.

Gachelin, G., 2007. The designing of anti-diphtheria serotherapy at the Institut Pasteur (1881–1900): the role of a supranational network of microbiologists. Dynamis 27, 45–62.

Gibson, T., Medawar, P.B., 1943. The fate of skin homografts in man. J. Anat. 77, 299–310.

Grundbacher, F.J., 1992. Behring's discovery of diphtheria and tetanus antitoxins. Immunol. Today 13, 188–190.

Hildemann, W.H., Medawar, P.B., 1959. Relationship between skin transplantation immunity and the formation of humoral isoantibodies in mice. Immunology 2, 44–52.

Hjóbjartsson, A., Gøtzsche, P.C., Gluud, C., 1998. The controlled clinical trial turns 100 years: Fibiger's trial of serum treatment of diphtheria. Brit. J. Med. 317, 1243–1245.

Kaufmann, S.H., 2008. Immunology's foundation: the 100-year anniversary of the nobel prize to Paul Ehrlich and Elie Metchnikoff. Nat. Immunol. 9, 705–712.

Landsteiner, K., Chase, M.W., 1942. Experiments on transfer of cutaneous sensitivity to simple compounds. Proc. Soc. Exp. Biol. Med. 49, 688–690.

Metchnikov, I., 1908. On the present state of the question of immunity in infectious diseases. In: Nobel Lectures, Physiology or Medicine 1901–1921. Elsevier Publishing Co., Amsterdam. 1967; accessed at http://nobelprize.org/nobel_prizes/medicine/laureates/1908/mechnikov-lecture.html.

Medawar, P.B., 1944. The behavior and fate of skin autografts and skin homografts in rabbits. A report to the war wounds committee of the medical research council. J. Anat. 78, 176–199.

Mitchison, N.A., 1955. Studies on the immunological response to foreign tumor transplants in the mouse. J. Exp. Med. 102, 157–177.

Nuttall, G.H.F., 1888. Experimente über die bacterien feindlichen Einflüsse des thierischen Körpers. Zeitschr. für Hyg. 4, 853–894.

Schmalstieg, F.C., Goldman, A.S., 2009. Jules Bordet (1870–1961): a bridge between early and modern immunology. J. Med. Biog. 17, 217–224.

Tauber, A.I., 2003. Metchnikoff and the phagocytosis theory. Nat. Rev. Mol. Cell. Biol. 4, 897–901.

Von Buchner, H., 1889. Über die bacterioentődtende wirkung des zellfreien blutserums. Zbl. Bakt. (Naturwiss) 5, 817–823.

Von Fodor, J., 1887. Die Fähigkeit des Bluts Bakterien zu vernichten. Dtsch. Med. Wochenschr. 13, 745–746.

TIME LINE

1880	Ilya Metchnikov develops the phagocytic theory of immunity
1887–88	Jozsef von Fodor, George Nuttall, Karl Flügge, and Hans von Buchner independently describe antibacterial activity (antibody) in serum from rabbits injected with pathogenic microorganisms
1890–91	Emil von Behring and Shibasaburo Kitasato develop serotherapy for diphtheria and tetanus
1900	Nobel Prize in Physiology or Medicine awarded to Emil von Behring
1900	Paul Ehrlich proposes the side chain theory of antibody formation
1908	Nobel Prize in Physiology or Medicine awarded to Paul Ehrlich and Elia Metchnikoff
1921	Development of vaccine against diphtheria
1924	Development of vaccine against tetanus
1942	Karl Landsteiner and Merrill Chase report the transfer of tuberculin sensitivity and skin sensitization to chemicals to naïve animals by lymphoid cells
1955	Avrion Mitchison transfers tumor immunity to a naïve host using lymphocytes
1958	Peter Medawar reports the transfer of sensitization induced by skin graft rejection by lymph node cells
1960	Nobel Prize in Physiology or Medicine awarded to Peter Medawar and F. Macfarlane Burnet
1963	Rupert Billingham and coworkers demonstrate the abrogation of tolerance to skin grafts by transfer of sensitized lymphocytes

CHAPTER

4

The Small Lymphocyte Is the Antigen Reactive Cell

INTRODUCTION

By 1950, immunologists accepted the classic characteristics of the adaptive immune response: memory, specificity, and self–nonself-discrimination. However, the identity of the cell or cells responsible for the adaptive immune response remained a mystery. Many immunologists suspected that cells of the reticuloendothelial (RE) system produced antibody. The RE system includes cells with the ability to take up and sequester foreign material, such as macrophages, monocytes, endothelial cells of the liver, spleen, and bone marrow, and reticular cells of the lymphatic system. The early studies of Metchnikoff and the prevalence of instructional theories of antibody formation failed to challenge this conclusion.

Evidence that the lymphocyte is the principal cell involved in adaptive immune responses derived from studies on the "disappearing lymphocyte" phenomenon, the observation that chronic drainage of the thoracic duct depletes the animal of most of its small lymphocytes. In the 1950s, James Gowans (1924 to present) and his colleagues working at Oxford initiated a series of experiments designed to understand this phenomenon. Gowans' studies demonstrated a circulatory path for lymphocytes between the vascular and lymphatic systems and showed that lymphocytes following antigenic challenge are active in many immune reactions.

Lymphocytes exist morphologically as both small and large cells. While the thoracic duct contains a preponderance of small lymphocytes, large lymphocytes are found in the peripheral blood and in the organized lymphoid tissues (spleen and lymph nodes). The relationship of small and large lymphocytes to each other and to antibody-forming plasma cells was unknown in 1950. This chapter reviews studies that support the role of the small lymphocyte as the antigen-reactive cell and as the precursor cell of large lymphocytes and plasma cells. In this text, an antigen-reactive cell is defined as a cell that interacts with and responds in an immunologically specific manner to pathogens.

THE SMALL LYMPHOCYTE

Twenty-first century immunology revolves around the functional division of small lymphocytes into subpopulations: T lymphocytes (responsible for cell-mediated immunity) and B lymphocytes (responsible for antibody production). A long and convoluted path has led to our current understanding that the small lymphocyte

A Historical Perspective on Evidence-Based Immunology
http://dx.doi.org/10.1016/B978-0-12-398381-7.00004-6

represents the keystone to protection against infectious microorganisms and to homeostasis in the immune system.

For the first half of the twentieth century, the identity of the cell responsible for initiating the adaptive immune response eluded detection. Winston Churchill, recovering from an infection during World War II, is said to have looked at his hospital chart and asked his physician, "What are these lymphocytes?" His physician responded, "We do not know, Mr Prime Minister," to which Churchill replied, "Then why do you count them?" This comment reflects the dismissive attitude many physicians and scientists had about the small lymphocyte.

While lymphocytes are observed in the peripheral blood (Figure 4.1) and in histological sections of the spleen, lymph nodes, and other lymphatic organs, the function of these cells remained unknown. Arnold Rich (1893–1968), a pathologist at Johns Hopkins and an expert on the immune response elicited by *Mycobacterium tuberculosis,* underscored this deficit when he remarked that "our complete ignorance of the function of the lymphocytes is a serious gap in medical knowledge" (Rich, 1936). Alexander Maximow and William Bloom erroneously speculated in the fifth edition of *A Textbook of Histology* (1949) that the function of the small lymphocyte was hematopoietic, phagocytic, and/ or fibrocytic in nature. Other views of small lymphocytes mistakenly concluded that they were end-stage cells in the process of dying subsequent to having performed their (unknown) function. In fact as recently as 1959, the soon to be Nobel Laureate, Sir Macfarlane Burnet, opined that "an objective survey of the facts could well lead to the conclusion that there was no evidence of immunological activity in small lymphocytes" (Burnet, 1959). This opinion was soon to be overturned.

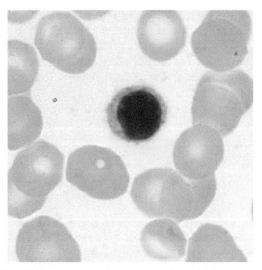

FIGURE 4.1 Small lymphocyte in a blood smear stained with Giemsa. *From the CDC Image Library* http://www.dpd.cdc.gov/dpdx/html/imagelibrary/A-F/Artifacts/body_Artifacts_il8.htm.

James Murphy (1884–1950), a cancer specialist, studied the role of the small lymphocyte in the response to tuberculosis and in transplanted tumors. Murphy trained as a physician at Johns Hopkins University and spent most of his career pursuing research at the Rockefeller Institute. In 1926, Murphy summarized his observations on the response to *M. tuberculosis* and transplanted tumors:

- Cells from lymph nodes or spleen placed on the membranes of an embryonated egg near an explant of a successfully growing tumor would destroy that tumor.
- Lymphoid tissue placed on the chorioallantoic membrane of an embryonated egg produced splenomegaly in the embryo and accumulations of cells (pocks) on the membrane, an early example of graft-versus-host (GvH) reaction.
- Immunization, low levels of irradiation, or dry heat increased the number of lymphocytes in an animal and enhanced the resistance of the animal to the growth of a transplanted tumor. Conversely, large doses of irradiation caused a lymphopenia and a decreased ability of the animal to resist a transplanted tumor.
- Immunization, low levels of irradiation, or dry heat enhanced the resistance of mice to infection with tubercle bacilli while higher doses of irradiation decreased the animal's resistance to infection.

Murphy published the importance of the lymphocyte in tumor graft rejection and in providing resistance to tuberculosis during the 1920s. However, these observations remained unacknowledged for almost a quarter century. Jacques Miller concludes, "Murphy's experiments show only that changes in lymphoid tissue, in the local cellular infiltrate and in the level of blood lymphocytes are associated with 'resistance'" and that he "never stated that this 'resistance' was immunological" (Miller, 2003). Art Silverstein attributes the lack of support for this work to the inability/unwillingness of the leaders of the field of immunology to appreciate the contributions of a clinical pathologist (Silverstein, 2003).

Despite this disregard, Murphy's results were rediscovered by a series of experiments performed during the 1950s and 1960s. Four complementary lines of research provided conclusive evidence that the small lymphocyte is the central player in the adaptive immune response:

- passive transfer experiments,
- migratory pathways of small lymphocytes,
- depletion experiments, and
- immunocompetence of small lymphocytes.

Subsequent chapters consider the evidence that there are, in addition, different functional subpopulations of lymphocytes that act individually and in concert to perform the immune responses with which we now work.

PASSIVE TRANSFER EXPERIMENTS

In the early 1940s, Karl Landsteiner (1868–1943) and Merrill Chase (1905–2004), working at the Rockefeller Institute for Medical Research in New York, injected guinea pigs with synthetic chemicals (Chapter 3). These guinea pigs generate an immune response that can be evaluated by inoculating the chemicals into the animal's skin. A positive response is characterized by the appearance of an inflammatory response at the injection site; such animals are considered sensitized. Attempts to transfer this skin reaction were based on the assumption that the guinea pigs produced antibody to the chemical. This antibody was postulated to exist either in the serum or bound to cells.

Chase removed serum from one sensitized guinea pig and injected it into a second, naïve guinea pig. This maneuver failed to transfer the sensitization. He then removed cells from the peritoneal cavity of a sensitized guinea pig and prepared a cell-free supernatant. The peritoneal cavity contains a mixed population of macrophages and lymphocytes. Chase reasoned that the cells might release antibody into a supernatant that could then transfer the skin activity. Injection of this preparation likewise failed to transfer the reactivity.

However, in one experiment, Chase inadvertently used a supernatant that had not been as rigorously prepared as other preparations. The guinea pigs who received this supernatant demonstrated skin reactivity to the chemicals injected into their skin, showing that the less pure supernatant had transferred the chemical sensitivity to naive guinea pigs. Microscopic evaluation revealed that this supernatant was not cell free but contained lymphocytes (Landsteiner and Chase, 1942).

Landsteiner and Chase concluded "that the sensitivity is produced by an activity in the recipient of the surviving cells, if not by antibodies carried by these". Immunologists now agree that the skin sensitization to the chemicals transferred in this experiment is due to the activity of lymphocytes, particularly T lymphocytes, and that antibodies play no role in sensitization.

Chase further investigated the mechanism of the transferred sensitivity reaction as well as the skin reaction induced by products of *M. tuberculosis* and concluded that both reactions are due to lymphocyte activity. For these observations Chase is credited with discovering cell-mediated immunity (Chapter 3).

Other investigators developed protocols based on the Landsteiner and Chase experiments. Frank Dixon

and coworkers at the University of Pittsburgh (Roberts and Dixon, 1955; Roberts et al., 1957) described the morphology of the cells responsible for the production of antibodies to a foreign protein. Roberts and co-workers injected rabbits with bovine gamma globulin (BGG) or bovine serum albumin (BSA). They harvested cells from lymph nodes or peritoneal cavities and transferred them to two groups of naive rabbits. Both groups were exposed to a dose of radiation known to inhibit immune reactivity. One group of irradiated rabbits received cells from antigen-injected donors, while the other group received cells from uninoculated donors. Both groups of rabbits were subsequently injected with the original antigens, and their antibody response was measured.

Rabbits receiving cells from immunized animals produced a memory or secondary response characterized by a rapid production of large amounts of antibody while recipients of cells from naïve donors produced a primary response. The responses of rabbits receiving lymph node cells (90% lymphocytes) and those receiving peritoneal exudate cells (70% macrophages and 11% lymphocytes) were similar, leading the authors to conclude that "lymphocytes in the case of lymph node cells and macrophages in the case of peritoneal exudate cells—were most likely responsible for the antibody responses" (Roberts et al., 1957). The fact that these investigators mentioned the role of macrophages in antibody production demonstrates the reluctance of immunologists to abandon RE cells as antibody producers.

Future studies focused increasingly on the lymphocyte as the antigen-reactive cell. James Gowans performed seminal studies in the 1950s and 1960s that confirmed our current perception of the role of lymphocytes in the adaptive immune response.

MIGRATORY PATHWAYS OF SMALL LYMPHOCYTES

Gowans received his MB (Bachelor of Medicine) and PhD from Oxford and spent a year in the Pasteur Institute in Paris prior to joining the Florey laboratory at the Sir William Dunn School of Pathology at Oxford in 1953. Howard Florey (1898–1968) shared the Nobel Prize in Physiology or Medicine in 1945 (with Ernst Boris Chain and Sir Alexander Fleming) for his role in the development of penicillin into an effective treatment for bacterial infections. Florey suggested to Gowans that he tackle the "disappearing lymphocyte" phenomenon, the observation that chronic drainage of the thoracic duct depletes an animal of most of its small lymphocytes. Florey, who was not an immunologist, thought this might answer the question of whether lymphocytes were end-stage cells or if they had some function.

In 1948, Jesse Bollman and colleagues at the Mayo Clinic, Rochester, Minnesota, first described a technique for cannulating the thoracic duct of the rat. The thoracic duct contains greater than 90% small lymphocytes, and consequently the development of the cannulation technique provided investigators with a source of almost pure lymphocytes. If the cannula draining the thoracic duct remained open for several days, the number of recovered lymphocytes in the lymph approached zero. These observations led to two questions:

- What happened to these lymphocytes in a normal animal?
- What was the source of the lymphocytes in the thoracic duct?

Small lymphocytes are found almost everywhere in the body: the peripheral blood, the thoracic duct, lymph nodes, spleen, and thymus as well as in isolated nodules in virtually every organ system. The thoracic duct empties into the left subclavian vein, continually delivering a significant number of small lymphocytes to the vascular system. While the existence of a separate lymphatic circulatory system was described in the 1700s (Chapter 1), the role of this system in the circulation of lymphocytes was unknown.

In his initial studies, Gowans (1957) collected lymphocytes from the thoracic duct of rats and then reinjected them intravenously. This manipulation allowed him to continue collecting lymphocytes from the thoracic duct and suggested to Gowans that small lymphocytes traveled not only from the thoracic duct to the peripheral blood but also from the peripheral blood back to the thoracic duct.

To test this hypothesis, Gowans labeled the DNA of thoracic duct lymphocytes in vitro with the radioisotope ^{32}P and reinfused the labeled cells intravenously. The labeled cells appeared in the small lymphocyte pool recovered from the thoracic duct a short time later (Gowans, 1959). When Gowans presented at a hematology meeting, his results were met with skepticism. The attendees asked Gowans about the life span of the small lymphocyte. Discussants at the meeting argued that lymphocytes were short-lived cells and that the labeled DNA was possibly reutilized by newly formed lymphocytes that appeared in the thoracic duct. One of the referees of the original manuscript submitted by Gowans made similar arguments and recommended against publishing the paper (Gowans, 1996).

To answer these criticisms, Gowans and Knight (1964) labeled thoracic duct lymphocytes in vitro with a radioactive precursor of RNA prior to reinfusing them. In vivo, RNA is formed de novo in every cell thus eliminating possible reuse of the radioisotope. Labeled cells,

detected by autoradiography, were found in the thoracic duct as well as in all of the lymphoid organs with the exception of the thymus. Thus the investigators concluded that lymphocytes recirculate from the circulatory system through lymph nodes and other lymphoid tissues to the thoracic duct.

The discovery of the circulatory path for small lymphocytes proved that small lymphocytes did not really disappear with thoracic duct drainage, thereby solving the "disappearing lymphocyte" phenomenon. These data did not, however, answer the question concerning what small lymphocytes do. As Gowans points out in a 1996 review, "the demonstration that lymphocytes re-circulated from blood to lymph gave no clues to their function." Unraveling the function of the small lymphocyte required additional studies to evaluate the immunological capabilities of rats depleted of their lymphocytes and to determine the immunocompetence of thoracic duct lymphocytes.

DEPLETION EXPERIMENTS

By the early 1960s investigators agreed that the small lymphocyte played a role in the adaptive immune response. In 1961 Jacque Miller, working at the Chester Beatty Research Institute in London, demonstrated that neonatal removal of the thymus, an organ consisting of almost pure small lymphocytes, depressed the ability of the thymectomized animal to respond to subsequent antigenic challenge (Chapter 9). Gowans, aware of these studies, hypothesized that a similar immunodeficient state might occur in rats subjected to thoracic duct drainage. Adult rats depleted of small lymphocytes by chronic drainage from a cannula implanted in their thoracic duct showed decreased numbers of peripheral blood lymphocytes, a reduction in lymph node weight, and a lymphopenia in their spleen and lymph nodes (McGregor and Gowans, 1963).

McGregor and Gowans injected normal and lymphocyte-depleted rats with sheep erythrocytes (SRBC) and measured serum antibody levels at intervals using an in vitro assay. Results, depicted in Figure 4.2, demonstrate an inverse correlation between the number of days the rats were subjected to thoracic duct drainage and the amount of antibody they could subsequently produce; that is, as the duration of thoracic duct drainage increased, the amount of antibody produced decreased. Since thoracic duct drainage depleted the rats of lymphocytes, one could postulate that the decreased lymphocyte numbers led to decreased antibody production.

This experiment was repeated with a protein antigen, tetanus toxoid. Antibody titers to tetanus toxoid were determined by a tanned cell hemagglutination assay. In this assay, erythrocytes are treated with tannic acid and

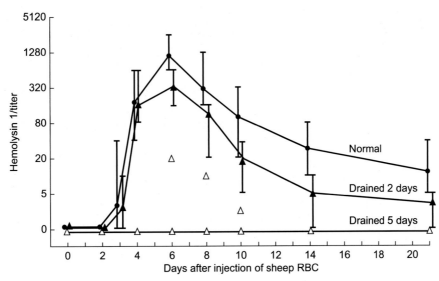

FIGURE 4.2   Antibody (hemolysin) response of rats injected a single time with SRBC following 0 (filled circles), 2 (filled triangles), or 5 days (open triangles) of thoracic duct drainage. In the group subjected to 5 days of thoracic duct drainage, 9 of 10 animals had no measurable antibody in their serum; the tenth animal is depicted by the open triangles on days 6, 8, and 10. *McGregor and Gowans (1963). Originally published in J. Exp. Med. 117, 303–320.*

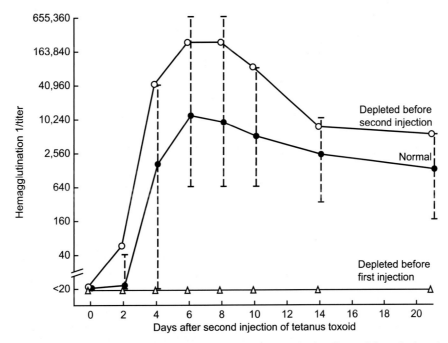

FIGURE 4.3   Serum antibody titers in rats receiving two injections of tetanus toxoid. The effects of thoracic duct drainage for 5 days on the primary response (open triangles) and secondary or memory response (open circles) are compared to the response of normal, nondepleted rats (filled circles). *McGregor and Gowans (1963). Originally published in J. Exp. Med. 117, 303–320.*

mixed with tetanus toxoid. Serum containing antibodies specific for tetanus toxoid agglutinate these cells. Results, depicted in Figure 4.3, show that rats depleted of lymphocytes lost their ability to produce antibodies to tetanus toxoid.

McGregor and Gowans used this protocol to further characterize the circulation of lymphocytes. Two groups of rats depleted of lymphocytes by 5 days of thoracic

duct drainage were used. One group was injected with tetanus toxoid immediately following removal of the thoracic duct cannula and again 3 weeks later. These animals produced no antibodies, suggesting that the removal of the small lymphocytes depleted the cells that could respond to the antigen. A second group of rats, injected with toxoid 2 weeks before the initiation of thoracic duct drainage and again immediately following cannula removal, produced antibody to tetanus toxoid in an amount equivalent to control animals. Two conclusions can be made from these results:

- In the intact animal, the first injection of tetanus toxoid activated the lymphocytes. Thoracic duct drainage does not remove these activated lymphocytes.
- Lymphocytes capable of responding to antigen circulate freely prior to antigenic challenge while these same cells leave the circulatory path once they have been activated.

These studies provide indirect evidence that the small lymphocyte is a precursor to cells producing antibodies to foreign antigens. The next series of studies determined directly the immunocompetence of small lymphocytes removed from the thoracic duct.

IMMUNOCOMPETENCE OF THORACIC DUCT LYMPHOCYTES

The Gowans' laboratory continued to study the immune capability of thoracic duct lymphocytes (Gowans, 1962; Gowans et al., 1962). Three measures of immunocompetence were employed: antibody formation, rejection of a foreign (allo)graft, and GvH reactions.

Chronic thoracic duct drainage led to a decreased antibody response to SRBC and tetanus toxoid (Figures 4.2 and 4.3). Antibody production was reconstituted by injecting depleted rats with thoracic duct lymphocytes derived from other rats of the same inbred strain (Figure 4.4). Since thoracic duct lymphocytes are mainly small lymphocytes, these results indicate that the small lymphocyte is the precursor of antibody-forming cells (Gowans et al., 1962; McGregor and Gowans, 1963). Thoracic duct lymphocytes also restored responses in rats that had been irradiated (McGregor and Gowans, 1963).

Thoracic duct lymphocytes also participate in skin allograft rejection (Gowans et al., 1962). Gowans and his group induced immunological tolerance to antigens expressed by a second inbred strain of rats. Immunological tolerance (the inability of the rats to respond immunologically to a normally immunogenic stimulus) was evaluated by the ability of a skin allograft to survive upon transplantation.

Gowans and colleagues injected rats bearing tolerated skin allografts with normal thoracic duct cells (>99% small lymphocytes) from rats of the same strain. The grafts were destroyed in the injected animals in a manner similar to that seen with allografts placed on nontolerant rats.

The rejection of allografts is a function of a population of T lymphocytes (Chapter 36). A similar reaction is observed when immunocompetent cells are injected into a host who, based on genetics or immune incompetence, is unable to reject the cells (Simonsen et al., 1958; Billingham, 1958). The injected cells initiate an immune response against the cells of the host and, in essence, reject the host. This is termed a graft-versus-host (GvH) reaction and is seen occasionally in the clinic when immunocompromised patients receive a bone marrow transplant.

Gowans used the GvH reaction to evaluate the immunocompetence of thoracic duct lymphocytes. F_1 hybrid rats, produced by mating individuals from two inbred strains, possess genes from both parents and hence express antigens (proteins) unique to each parent. As a result, these F_1 animals fail to react immunologically to cells from either parent. Gowans and coworkers injected thoracic duct lymphocytes from one of the parent strains into F_1 hybrid rats. These parental lymphocytes reacted against the antigens present in the F_1 animal from the second parent. This initiated a graft (parental cells) versus host (F_1) reaction. If sufficient parental cells are injected, the F_1 hosts are killed.

Results, presented in Table 4.1, show that injection of 200 million parental cells into F_1 animals killed all the hosts. These studies proved that the small lymphocytes found in the thoracic duct are capable of inducing a GvH reaction and thus are immunocompetent.

Gesner and Gowans performed similar studies using mice that had received a potentially lethal dose of radiation and were reconstituted using either autologous or heterologous thoracic duct lymphocytes. Animals receiving heterologous lymphocytes developed symptoms of GvH disease and died while those receiving autologous lymphocytes survived (Gesner and Gowans, 1962).

MORPHOLOGICAL CHANGES OF ACTIVATED SMALL LYMPHOCYTES

Lymphocytes involved in the GvH reaction and the rejection of allografts were radiolabeled and traced by autoradiography. The lymphocytes traveled initially to the lymph nodes where they underwent transformation into blast cells that subsequently gave rise to small lymphocytes. Similarly, thoracic duct lymphocytes involved in the initiation of an antibody response became large, pyroninophilic cells reminiscent of plasma cells. These unexpected observations mirror similar findings presented by Arnold Rich almost 30 years earlier. In his report to the annual meeting of the American Association of Pathologists, Rich described experiments demonstrating that the initial morphological reaction to foreign protein is "proliferation and marked cytological alteration of the lymphocytes." He speculated that these cellular activities might be related to antibody formation (Rich, 1936).

Taken together, the studies by Gowans' group during the 1950s and 1960s demonstrate that the small lymphocyte found in the thoracic duct is the antigen-reactive cell for various immunological reactions, including

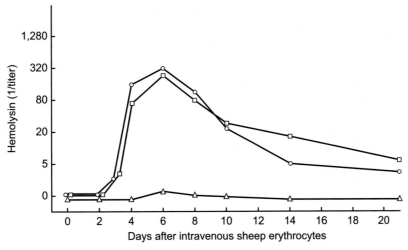

FIGURE 4.4 Hemolysin response to sheep erythrocytes in rats depleted of small lymphocytes by thoracic duct drainage and reconstituted with normal lymphocytes. Squares depict the response of rats injected with SRBCs after 2 days of thoracic duct drainage; triangles depict the response of rats injected with SRBCs after 5 days of thoracic duct drainage; circles depict the response of rats injected with SRBCs after 5 days of thoracic duct drainage and reinfusion with normal lymphocytes. *From Gowans et al. (1962). Originally published in Nature 196, 651–655.*

TABLE 4.1 Induction of Graft-Versus-Host Disease in F_1 Rats as the Result of Injecting Parental Strain Lymphocytes. Injections of More than 200 Million Cells Invariably Led to the Death of the F_1 Animal Regardless of the Initial Body Weight. Injections of Fewer than 200 Million Cells Induced Fatal GvH Disease in Small Recipients

	Lethal effect of parental thoracic duct lymphocytes on F_1 hybrid rats of varying body weight			
	F_1 recipients			
Intravenous dose of parental lymphocytes $\times 10^4$	**No. deaths/no. injected**	**Initial body wt (g)**	**Sex**	**Time of death[a]**
205	10/10	176–204	M	16–20
204	6/6	127–134	F	20–21
104	0/5	244–256	M	
106	0/7	138–160	F	
104	0/3	76–79	M	
109	6/6	57–69	F	15–23
109	12/12	45–52	M	15–19

[a]*Number of days after injection.*
From Gowans, 1962.

antibody formation, graft rejection, and GvH reactions. As described by McGregor and Gowans (1963)

> The simplest hypothesis would be as follows. Primary immune responses are initiated by the interaction of small lymphocytes with antigen....After contact with antigen the small lymphocytes become fixed in lymphoid tissue and no longer circulate between blood and lymph...In the lymphoid tissue the fixed lymphocytes enlarge and give rise to a dividing cell line which perpetuates itself and produces a small number of plasma cells...These speculations rest on the assumption that small lymphocytes participate in primary responses by generating the cells which eventually synthesize antibody.

The small lymphocyte is now established as the progenitor cell for every antigen-reactive cell. Immunologists agree that the small lymphocyte is not a single cell population but rather encompasses a large number of cell types, including T lymphocytes and B lymphocytes that are involved in a myriad of immune reactions. The small lymphocyte derives from lymphoid stem cells in hematopoietic tissues such as the bone marrow. Differentiation and maturation occur in the bone marrow (for antibody-producing B lymphocytes) or in the thymus (for T lymphocytes). Small lymphocytes emerging from these two sites join the circulating pool described by Gowans and others. Once activated by interaction with antigen, the small lymphocyte proliferates and becomes a large lymphocyte localized to the organized lymphoid tissues such as the spleen and lymph nodes. Further differentiation stimulates additional changes, resulting in the formation of plasma cells that produce antibody or small lymphocytes that perform the many functions of T lymphocytes. The experiments that resulted in this contemporary vision of the immune system are presented in subsequent chapters.

CONCLUSION

James Gowans and his colleagues working at Oxford over a period of more than 15 years provided a preponderance of evidence that the small lymphocyte is the cell central to the adaptive immune response. Starting with the question of the "disappearing lymphocyte" phenomenon, Gowans and his colleagues pursued a number of experimental protocols that led them to conclude that the small lymphocyte travels between the blood circulatory system and the lymphatic system and is responsible for all immune reactivity in mammals. These studies derived from a remark by Howard Florey made to Gowans as he began his research career.

During the decades following the discovery of the role of the small lymphocyte in the adaptive immune response advances based on this insight include

- identification of the plasma cell as the antibody producing cell (Chapter 5);
- differentiation of immunocompetent cells into functionally distinct populations of B and T lymphocytes;
- division of T lymphocytes into several functional subpopulations including helper (CD4[+]) and cytotoxic (CD8[+]) T cells (Chapter 23) and identifying them by their cell surface antigens;
- separation of CD4[+] T lymphocytes into subpopulations based on the cytokines they secrete (Chapter 23);
- understanding the role of the thymus (Chapter 9) and the bursa of Fabricius (Chapter 10) in the development of antigen-reactive cells;
- deciphering the role of cell collaboration in the initiation of adaptive immune responses (Chapters 13 and 14); and
- identification of the cell surface receptors responsible for pathogen recognition (Chapter 17).

References

Billingham, R.E., 1958. Reactions of grafts against their hosts. Science 130, 947–953.
Bollman, J.L., Cain, J.C., Grindlay, J.H., 1948. Techniques for the collection of lymph from the liver, small intestine or thoracic duct of the rat. J. Lab. Clin. Med. 33, 1349–1352.
Burnet, F.M., 1959. The Clonal Selection Theory of Acquired Immunity. Vanderbilt University Press, Nashville, TN, p. 209.
Gesner, B.M., Gowans, J.L., 1962. The fate of lethally irradiated mice given isologous and heterologous thoracic duct lymphocytes. Br. J. Exp. Pathol. 43, 431–440.
Gowans, J.L., 1957. The effect of the continuous re-infusion of lymph and lymphocytes on the output of lymphocytes from the thoracic duct of unanaesthetized rats. Brit. J. Exp. Path. 38, 67–78.
Gowans, J.L., 1959. The recirculation of lymphocytes from blood to lymph in the rat. J. Physiol. 146, 54–69.
Gowans, J.L., 1962. The fate of parental strain lymphocytes in F1 hybrid rats. Ann. N.Y. Acad. Sci. 99, 432–455.
Gowans, J.L., 1996. The lymphocyte—a disgraceful gap in medical knowledge. Immunol. Today 17, 288–291.
Gowans, J.L., Knight, E.J., 1964. The route of re-circulation of lymphocytes in the rat. Proc. R. Soc. London Ser. B 159, 257–282.
Gowans, J.L., McGregor, D.D., Cowan, D.M., Ford, C.D., 1962. Initiation of immune responses by small lymphocytes. Nature 196, 651–655.
Landsteiner, K., Chase, M.W., 1942. Experiments on transfer of cutaneous sensitivity to simple compounds. Proc. Soc. Exp. Biol. Med. 49, 688–690.
Maximow, A.A., Bloom, W., 1949. A Textbook of Histology. W.B. Saunders, Philadelphia, PA.
McGregor, D.D., Gowans, J.L., 1963. The antibody response of rats depleted of lymphocytes by chronic drainage from the thoracic duct. J. Exp. Med. 117, 303–320.
Miller, J.F.A.P., 1961. Immunological function of the thymus. Lancet 278, 748–749.
Miller, J.F.A.P., 2003. How important was Murphy? Nat. Immunol. 2, 981.
Murphy, J.B., 1926. The Lymphocyte in Resistance to Tissue Grafting, Malignant Disease, and Tuberculosis Infection. Rockefeller Institute for Medical Research, New York, NY.
Rich, A.R., 1936. Inflammation in resistance to infection. Am. J. Pathol. 12, 723–733.
Roberts, J.C., Dixon, F.J., 1955. The transfer of lymph node cells in the study of the immune response to foreign proteins. J. Exp. Med. 102, 379–392.
Roberts, J.C., Dixon, F.J., Weigle, W.O., 1957. Antibody-producing lymph node cells and peritoneal exudate cells. AMA Arch. Pathol. 64, 324–332.
Silverstein, A.M., 2003. The lymphocyte in immunology: from James B. Murphy to James L. Gowans. Nat. Immunol. 2, 569–571.
Simonsen, M., Engleberth-Holm, J., Jensen, E., Poulsen, H., 1958. A study of the graft-versus-host reaction in transplantation to embryos, F1 hybrids, and irradiated animals. Ann. N.Y. Acad. Sci. 73, 834–841.

TIME LINE

1926	James Murphy publishes studies demonstrating that lymphocytes play a role in tumor rejection and response to tubercle bacilli
1936	Arnold Rich describes the initial cytological reaction to foreign protein, including proliferation and alteration of lymphocytes
1942	Karl Landsteiner and Merrill Chase report that lymphocytes from the peritoneal cavity can transfer skin sensitization to simple chemicals
1948	Jesse Bollmer and colleagues describe the "disappearing lymphocyte phenomenon" induced by thoracic duct drainage
1957–1964	James Gowans demonstrates migration of lymphocytes between blood and lymphatic circulations
1961	Jacques Miller provides the initial evidence that neonatal thymectomy decreases response to antigenic challenge
1962	James Gowans reports that thoracic duct lymphocytes are active in antibody formation, graft rejection, and initiation of GvH reactions
1963	D.D. McGregor and James Gowans publish studies showing that thoracic duct drainage decreases antibody responses to several antigens

5

Lymphocytes Transform into Plasma Cells and Produce Antibodies

INTRODUCTION

As recounted in Chapter 4, small lymphocytes are antigen-reactive cells. The resulting immune reactivity as measured by antibody production or skin sensitization to foreign antigens can be transferred from immunized to naïve animals by small lymphocytes. Animals depleted of small lymphocytes by thoracic duct drainage fail to generate an effective adaptive immune response. Animals rendered immune incompetent by draining lymphocytes from the thoracic duct or by irradiation can be reconstituted by the transfer of small lymphocytes. These small lymphocytes produce antibodies, reject foreign tissue grafts, and participate in graft-versus-host reactions. While immunologists agreed with these conclusions, the identity of the specific cell ultimately responsible for antibody formation remained unknown.

During the first half of the twentieth century, most immunologists favored the instruction theory of antibody formation. The instruction theory assumed that antigen was phagocytized by a cell with antibody-synthesizing capacity. Once engulfed, the antigen altered the proteins that the cell produced, resulting in synthesis and secretion of antibody that bound specifically to the antigen. The cells that met these criteria included cells of the reticuloendothelial system: macrophages, monocytes, endothelial cells of the liver, spleen, and bone marrow, and reticular cells of the lymphatic system. Consequently, at the time, the small lymphocyte seemed an unlikely participant in antibody production since it lacked phagocytic capability and appeared to be metabolically inactive.

At the same time, other researchers occasionally noted morphological changes in small lymphocytes during the activation of the immune response that they attributed to antibody formation. For example, Arnold Rich (1936), in his studies on the cutaneous response to tuberculin, described proliferation of and cytologic changes in lymphocytes that he speculated might be an early sign of immune activation. Likewise, James Gowans and his group noted similar morphological changes in the small lymphocytes when animals were injected with antigen.

The resolution of these differing views of the cell type or types responsible for antibody synthesis required the development of new research techniques such as immunofluorescence and tissue culture.

CELLS AND ANTIBODIES

In the late 1880s, several investigators injected experimental animals with bacteria (*Bacillus anthracis* or *Vibrio cholerae*), resulting in the appearance of a serum substance

A Historical Perspective on Evidence-Based Immunology
http://dx.doi.org/10.1016/B978-0-12-398381-7.00005-8

that could kill the immunizing microbe (von Fodor, 1887; Nuttall, 1888; von Buchner, 1889). This serum substance became the focus of numerous studies and was called several different names including Immunkörper, Zwischenkörper, amboceptor, substance sensibilatrice, fixator, Desmon, philocytase, Immunisin, and copula (Lindenmann, 1984). Eventually the term antibody, first used by Emil von Behring and Shibasaburo Kitasato in 1890 and by Ehrlich in 1891, was accepted by all investigators. Antibodies assumed a central role in studies of the immune response during the first half of the twentieth century. Several reasons for this focus include

- antibody activity as measured by precipitation and agglutination could be readily detected in the serum of an immunized animal;
- serological techniques provided clinical evaluation of immune competence and identification of microorganisms;
- serotherapy, particularly against diphtheria, had proven the practical application of immunology; and
- many functional studies of the immune response centered on the activity of antibodies.

Composition of Antibodies

Introduced in the 1890s, sera-containing antibodies against bacterial toxins as well as bacterial pathogens evolved into a standard treatment protocol in the early twentieth century. Passive transfer of antibodies was used to treat infections caused by *Corynebacterium diphtheria, Clostridium tetanii, Streptococcus pneumonia, Neisseria meningitidis, Hemophilus influenza,* and group A *Streptococcus* (Casadevall, 1996). The antibodies used in these serum therapies were developed primarily in horses. Today we understand that the injection of foreign (horse) serum into a human may result in unintended side effects, primarily the production of antibodies directed against the horse serum itself. These antibodies may induce pathology characterized by fever, skin rash, joint pain, cardiac abnormalities, and kidney malfunction. This constellation of symptoms, termed serum sickness, was eventually shown to be due to the formation of antigen–antibody complexes (Chapter 33). Attempts to purify and concentrate the antibodies used in these protocols resulted in important information about the composition of antibody molecules.

Oswald Avery (1877–1955) pursued studies designed to enhance the potency of antibodies produced in horses against *S. pneumonia* while simultaneously decreasing the incidence or severity of serum sickness and other adverse reactions. These investigations led to the demonstration that the antibody activity to *S. pneumonia* is in the globulin fraction of the horse serum.

Avery treated horse serum with various concentrations of ammonium sulfate, a commonly used method for precipitating proteins from serum. He solubilized the precipitates and injected these solutions into mice infected with a lethal dose of *S. pneumonia*. The fractions providing the greatest protection precipitated with 38–42% ammonium sulfate, a fraction known to contain globulins and to exclude albumin and euglobulins. Moreover, the globulin fraction was also the most active in related agglutination and precipitation assays (Avery, 1915).

In 1939 Arne Tiselius and Elvin Kabat further analyzed serum with antibody activity to *S. pneumonia* using the recently developed technique of serum electrophoresis—a method for separating a solution into components based on the electrical charge of the particles (Tiselius, 1937). This method separates serum into albumin and three globulin fractions; alpha, beta, and gamma; antibodies migrate with the gamma globulin fraction.

At the time, the cellular source of these gamma globulins was unknown. Instruction theories of antibody formation postulated that invading pathogens induced conformational changes in naturally occurring serum globulins that conferred antigen-binding capability. Immunologists considered that these conformational changes could occur in a variety of cells as opposed to a single cell type.

The identity of the plasma cell as the antibody-synthesizing unit required another 30 years and several lines of investigation, including

- localization of antigens and antibodies in lymph nodes, draining a site of pathogen injection,
- passive transfer studies, and
- direct visualization of antibody inside lymphocytes and plasma cells.

ANTIGENS AND ANTIBODIES IN LYMPHOID ORGANS

In 1933, two investigators at the Rockefeller Institute, Stephen Hudack and Phillip McMaster, injected themselves with isotonic dyes intradermally and noted that these dyes were taken up by a network of lymphatic vessels that led to local lymph nodes. When they injected dyes intradermally into mouse ears, they obtained similar results (McMaster and Hudack, 1934). These observations led Hudack and McMaster to hypothesize that bacteria entering the body through a breach in the skin would also end up in the local lymph node, that, therefore, might be a site of antibody formation.

They tested this hypothesis by injecting killed bacteria (*Salmonella* spp.) intradermally into the ears of mice. At various intervals, they removed the draining (cervical) lymph nodes and aseptically ground them with sand. This procedure extracted any antibodies that may have been present in the organs. McMaster and Hudack (1935) tested this extract for agglutination of *Salmonella* and detected specific bacterial agglutinins approximately 7 days after immunization. They concluded that antibody formed in response to antigenic challenge is located in the same organ that drained the site of pathogen entry.

The presence of antibodies in the draining lymph node, however, did not prove that antibodies were formed there. This experiment also failed to identify the specific cell or cells responsible for antibody formation and, in fact, McMaster and Hudack erroneously speculated that "cells of this (reticuloendothelial) system which are present in the lymph nodes or elsewhere may be responsible for agglutinin (antibody) formation."

Seven years later, in 1942, William Ehrich and T.N. Harris at the University of Pennsylvania studied the events occurring in the draining lymph node during the initiation of an antibody response. They injected either typhoid vaccine or sheep erythrocytes (SRBC) into rabbit footpads. Antibody production to typhoid vaccine and to SRBC was assayed by agglutination and hemolysin assays, respectively. The investigators further determined the number of lymphocytes in the lymph and recorded histological changes in the lymph node itself.

Increased numbers of lymphocytes appeared in the lymph during the first days following immunization. Antibodies appeared in the efferent lymph 2–4 days later with maximal antibody levels present at day 6. The lymph node was infiltrated by granulocytes and monocytes, following which a hyperplasia of lymphocytes occurred. The authors concluded that "the fact that the tissue response accompanying the formation of antibodies was chiefly a lymphocytic one points to the lymphocyte as a factor in the formation of antibodies."

The role of the lymphocyte in antibody production was strengthened by correlating the concentration of antibody present in extracts of lymphocytes from the popliteal lymph node with the concentration found in the draining lymph (Harris et al., 1945). The titer of antibody in extracts of lymphocytes was 8–16 times higher than the titer measured in the lymph. Several control experiments ruled out the possibility that the antibody present in the lymphocyte extracts had merely been adsorbed from the lymph. Histological changes in the lymph node that preceded or accompanied the presence of antibody included the proliferation of lymphocytes, appearance of lymphoblasts, and an increase in the number of lymphocytes exiting the node. A companion study using the same experimental protocol demonstrated that macrophages do not contain significant amounts of

antibodies at the time most agglutinating activity could be measured (Ehrich et al., 1946).

LYMPHOCYTE–PLASMA CELL DEBATE

The studies reviewed in the previous section provided significant evidence that the lymphocyte played an important role in the production of antibodies. However, a number of investigators, particularly from the Scandinavian countries (i.e., Bing and Plum, 1937; Bing, 1940; Bjoerneboe and Gormsen, 1943), argued that the important cell for antibody formation is the plasma cell. Many investigators in the United States remained unaware of these results due to difficulties in scientific communication during World War II. In 1948, Astrid Fagraeus (1913–1997) published the definitive study in this area, demonstrating that antibodies are synthesized by plasma cells.

Fagraeus received her MD from the Karolinska Institute in Stockholm in 1943 and earned her PhD from the same institution in 1948. She presented the studies that demonstrated the function of the plasma cells to the Karolinska Institute as her PhD dissertation. Fagraeus injected rabbits with *Salmonella typhi* twice, 14–25 days apart. Using an agglutination assay, she determined serum antibody levels. She also prepared spleens for microscopic evaluation.

Histological examination of spleen sections revealed an increase in the number of plasma cells that directly correlated with the amount of antibody present in the serum. To confirm this correlation, Fagraeus excised portions of the spleens containing predominately plasma cells and placed them in tissue culture. Control cultures contained lymphoid follicles consisting primarily of lymphocytes. She stimulated both sets of cultures with *S. typhi*. The amount of antibody secreted in the plasma cell cultures was greater than the amount produced by cultures of lymphoid follicles (Figure 5.1). She concluded that antibodies are produced by cells that morphologically resemble plasma cells at various stages of maturation. Unfortunately, Fagraeus erroneously hypothesized that plasma cells develop from cells of the reticuloendothelial system and concluded that "nothing has emerged which speaks directly in favor of the participation of the lymphocytes in the formation of antibodies."

Fagraeus' results convinced a significant number of investigators that the plasma cell produced antibodies. Within a year, William Ehrich, a major supporter of the view that lymphocytes secreted antibodies, published a paper (Ehrich et al., 1949) demonstrating that plasma cells produce antibodies.

Ehrich and colleagues injected typhoid vaccine into rabbit footpads. They removed draining popliteal lymph

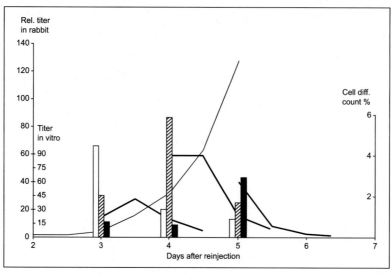

_____ relative increase in serum titer (of table 3).
_____ rate of antibody production in vitro in 12-hour intervals. Cultures initiated
on 3rd, 4th and 5th day respectively.
Differential cell counts in imprints on the days indicated.
White column—transitional cells.
Shaded column—immature plasma cells.
Black column—mature plasma cells.

FIGURE 5.1   Comparison of antibody present in serum (relative titer in rabbit—thin solid line), with the types of cells present in the spleen (cell difference count %, bars) and the amount of antibody produced by spleen cells in culture (titer in vitro—thicker solid line starting on days 3, 4, and 5). As the amount of serum antibody increased, the proportion of cells identified as immature and mature plasma cells also increased. *From Fagraeus (1948).*

nodes, weighed the nodes, and prepared single cell suspensions. The amount of DNA and RNA was measured using a colorimetric method (Schneider, 1946). Injection of the typhoid vaccine induced an increase in lymph node weight and an increase in antibody production. The increase in lymph node weight was directly proportional to an increase in DNA content while the increase in antibody corresponded to an increase in RNA. Histologically, the initial increase in cell number in the lymph node revealed plasmablasts and mature plasma cells, while the number of lymphocytes increased later in the response after the peak of antibody production. Interestingly, most of the RNA present in the lymph nodes was contained in the plasma cells. In summary, Ehrich and his collaborators concluded "these results are interpreted as indicating that the plasma cell and not the lymphocyte is responsible for antibody formation."

PASSIVE TRANSFER STUDIES

While Fagraeus and Ehrich concluded that the plasma cell synthesized antibody, other investigators continued to promote the role of lymphocytes. Several experimental protocols using passive transfer of adaptive immune responses were employed to demonstrate this point:

- Ragweed sensitivity as well as allergic reactivity to rabbit epithelium were transferred from a sensitized donor to a naïve recipient using leukocytes from peripheral blood (Walzer and Glazer, 1950).
- Karl Landsteiner and Merrill Chase transferred antibody-synthesizing capability from sensitized to naïve animals, primarily guinea pigs, using several different cell types, including lymphocytes (Landsteiner and Chase, 1942). Chase (1953) reported that both the ability to make antibodies capable of producing anaphylaxis as well as delayed hypersensitivity could be transferred to naive guinea pigs using lymphocytes from sensitized guinea pigs. Antibody activity in this system was demonstrated by using serum from the recipients of the lymphocytes to induce the contraction of intestinal smooth muscle in vitro. This is the basis for the Schultz–Dale reaction that was used for many years as a clinical test to detect the presence of antibodies responsible for anaphylaxis (Chapter 33).
- Finally, in 1954 Harris and colleagues transferred antibody production from immunized rabbits to naïve animals using lymph node cells. These investigators injected rabbits subcutaneously with several pathogens (dysentery bacilli, typhoid, and influenza virus) and harvested their popliteal lymph nodes. They injected

lymphocytes from these lymph nodes intravenously into normal rabbits. Serum collected from the recipients at various intervals after injection was tested for the presence of specific antibodies. Antibody appeared as early as day 1 after injection and was detectable for up to 3 weeks. Lymphocytes that were killed by freezing and thawing, lysing with distilled water, or heating to 52°C lost the ability to produce antibody. The authors present several possible explanations and conclude that "the transferred cells might contain a mechanism of antibody formation."

VISUALIZATION OF ANTIBODY-FORMING CELLS

Although correlations between cell types, the presence of antibody, and the synthesis of DNA and RNA are suggestive, final proof of the cell type responsible for antibody production depended on the development of new technology that would allow visualization of antibodies in the cells producing them: bacterial immobilization and immunofluorescence.

Erik Reiss, working in William Ehrich's laboratory at the University of Pennsylvania School of Medicine, developed the bacterial immobilization technique in 1950. Reiss and colleagues injected the O antigen of *S. typhi* into the hind footpads of rabbits. They harvested popliteal lymph nodes and incubated individual cells with the microorganism. Cells that produced antibody to the O antigen and immobilized the bacteria were selected and characterized morphologically. Using this technique, Reiss and colleagues concluded that most antibody-forming cells are plasma cells.

Observations Using Immunofluorescent Stains

The bacterial immobilization technique to detect cells producing antibody was limited to motile bacteria. In the early 1950s, Albert Coons and colleagues at Harvard Medical School developed a technique that directly visualized the location of proteins within tissue. Using a modification of this technique, Coons provided final validation that plasma cells synthesize antibody.

Albert Coons (1912–1978) received his MD in 1937 from Harvard where he spent virtually his entire career. His research interest was labeling antibody molecules so that they could be used to localize antigens in tissues. His first attempts entailed chemically binding various dyes to antibodies. When these initial attempts met with marginal success, he turned to fluorescent molecules to label antibodies. A complex of a specific antibody chemically coupled with fluorescein, a green emitting molecule, provided Coons a reagent with which he could readily detect antigens in tissue (Coons, 1961). He fixed

tissues on microscope slides and treated them with the fluorescein–antibody complex. Using a fluorescent microscope he visualized the structural details of the cells and the localization of the fluorescent probe.

Coons adapted the fluorescent antibody technique to visualize antibody-forming cells using a two-step procedure known as the sandwich technique (Coons et al., 1955). He treated sections or tissues from immunized animals first with antigen and then with a fluorescent-labeled antibody specific for that antigen. Coons reasoned that cells synthesizing specific antibody would bind the antigen and that the antigen would bind the tagged antibody. This technique allowed enumeration of the cells producing antibody to a particular antigen as well as morphologically identifying those antibody-forming cells.

Rabbits, injected intravenously with either human gamma globulin (HGG) or ovalbumin (OVA), served as the source of lymphoid tissues that were frozen, sectioned, and fixed on glass microscope slides. Coons and coworkers incubated these preparations with either HGG or OVA, after which they were washed to eliminate unbound antigen. This step provided a target for the antibodies specific for either HGG or OVA that had been tagged with fluorescein isocyanate. The investigators added fluorescent antibodies to the preparations, incubated them, and localized the tagged antibody using a fluorescent microscope. Negative controls included sections treated with no antigen or with an antigen different from the one used for immunization; these controls showed virtually no staining. In the original studies antibody was detected initially within relatively large cells with a basophilic cytoplasm and a large nucleus. Morphologically these cells were plasma cells (Leduc et al., 1955).

TRANSFORMATION OF SMALL LYMPHOCYTES INTO PLASMA CELLS

Identification of the plasma cell as the antibody-forming cell stimulated a search for the origin of this cell. This search revealed the relationship of plasma cells to lymphocytes. James Gowans and his group demonstrated that plasma cells derived from small lymphocytes (Chapter 4) using a transfer protocol. Gowans (1962) concluded that small lymphocytes can become large pyroninophilic cells that appear to be identical to plasma cells.

McGregor and Gowans (1963) depleted rats of lymphocytes through thoracic duct drainage. They injected these rats with small lymphocytes derived from the thoracic duct and determined the ability of the reconstituted rats to produce antibodies. Injection of small lymphocytes from the thoracic duct reconstituted the ability of these rats to respond to sheep erythrocytes and tetanus with the appearance of large, plasmacytoid cells in lymphoid tissue.

From these observations, McGregor and Gowans hypothesized that "primary immune responses are initiated by the interaction of small lymphocytes with antigen…After contact with antigen the small lymphocytes become fixed in lymphoid tissue…enlarge and give rise to a dividing cell line which perpetuates itself and produces a small number of plasma cells." Today immunologists concur with this hypothesis, and the small lymphocyte is acknowledged as the central cell type involved in the adaptive immune response.

CONCLUSION

The studies described in this chapter demonstrate that lymphocytes, which are the antigen-reactive cells, are transformed into plasma cells. This morphological transformation correlates with the synthesis and secretion of antibodies. The development of the immunofluorescent staining technique to demonstrate antibody synthesis by individual cells confirmed that plasma cells are the primary source of antibody production.

Issues that remained for subsequent investigations included

- the identity of the anatomical site where lymphocytes mature to antibody-producing cells (Chapter 10);
- the mechanism by which potential antibody-forming cells recognize foreign antigen (Chapter 17);
- the stimuli required to activate antibody-forming cells to synthesize and secrete antibodies (Chapter 19);
- the mechanisms involved in inhibiting these cells from producing antibodies to self-antigens (Chapter 21) or from producing too much or too little antibody (Chapter 24); and
- the mechanism responsible for determining the antigen specificity of the antibody-forming cells and their products (Chapter 18).

The studies described in this and the previous chapters were performed in the midst of the debate between instruction and selection theories of antibody formation. Burnet formulated the clonal selection theory of antibody formation (Chapter 6) in 1957, almost a decade after many of the investigations described here had been published. The coming decades would provide answers to many of the questions about antibody-producing cells, including the genetic determination of antibody structure and specificity and the role of ancillary cells in the activation of antibody production, which were not yet obvious. These important questions and others were addressed by investigators who were pioneers in the developing field of cellular immunology.

References

Avery, O., 1915. The distribution of the immune bodies occurring in antipneumococcus serum. J. Exp. Med. 21, 133–145.

Behring, E.A., Kitasato, S., 1890. Über das Zustandekommen der Diphtheria-immunität and der Tetanus-immunität bei Thieren. Dtsch. Med. Wochenschr. 49, 1113–1114.

Bing, J., 1940. Further investigation on hyperglobulinemia. Acta Med. Scand. 103, 547–583.

Bing, J., Plum, P., 1937. Serum proteins in leucopenia. Acta Med. Scand. 92, 415–428.

Bjoerneboe, M., Gormsen, H., 1943. Experimental studies on the role of plasma cells as antibody producers. Acta Path. Microb. Scand. 20, 649–692.

von Buchner, H., 1889. Über die bakterioentődtende wirkung des zellfreien blutserums. Zbl. Bakt. (Naturwiss) 5, 817–823.

Casadevall, A., 1996. Antibody-based therapies for emerging infectious diseases. Emerg. Inf. Dis. 2, 200–208.

Chase, M.W., 1953. Immunological reactions mediated through cells. In: Pappenheimer, A.M. (Ed.), The Nature and Significance of the Antibody Response. Columbia University Press, New York, NY.

Coons, A.H., 1961. The beginnings of immunofluorescence. J. Immunol. 87, 499–503.

Coons, A.H., Leduc, E.H., Connolly, J.M., 1955. Studies on antibody production. I. A method for the histochemical demonstration of specific antibody and its application to a study of the hyperimmune rabbit. J. Exp. Med. 102, 49–60.

Ehrich, W.E., Drabkin, D.L., Forman, C., 1949. Nucleic acids and the production of antibody by plasma cells. J. Exp. Med. 90, 157–168.

Ehrich, W.E., Harris, T.N., 1942. The formation of antibodies in the popliteal lymph node in rabbits. J. Exp. Med. 76, 335–347.

Ehrich, W.E., Harris, T.N., Mertens, E., 1946. The absence of antibody in the macrophages during maximum antibody formation. J. Exp. Med. 83, 373–381.

Fagraeus, A., 1948. The plasma cellular reaction and its relation to the formation of antibodies in vitro. J. Immunol. 58, 1–13.

von Fodor, J., 1887. Die Fähigkeit des Bluts Bakterien zu vernichten. Dtsch. Med. Wochenschr. 13, 745–746.

Gowans, J.L., 1962. The fate of parental strain small lymphocytes in F1 hybrid rats. Ann. N.Y. Acad. Sci. 99, 432–455.

Harris, T.N., Grimm, E., Mertens, E., Ehrich, W.E., 1945. The role of the lymphocyte in antibody formation. J. Exp. Med. 81, 73–83.

Harris, S., Harris, T.N., Farber, M.B., 1954. Studies on the transfer of lymph node cells. I. Appearance of antibody in recipients of cells from donor rabbits injected with antigen. J. Immunol. 72, 148–160.

Hudack, S.S., McMaster, P.D., 1933. The lymphatic participation in human cutaneous phenomena: a study of the minute lymphatics of the living skin. J. Exp. Med. 57, 751–774.

Landsteiner, K., Chase, M.W., 1942. Experiments on transfer of cutaneous sensitivity to simple compounds. Proc. Soc. Exp. Biol. Med. 49, 688–690.

Leduc, E.H., Coons, A.H., Connolly, J.M., 1955. Studies on antibody formation. II. The primary and secondary responses in the popliteal lymph nose of the rabbit. J. Exp. Med. 102, 61–72.

Lindenmann, J., 1984. Origin of the terms "antibody" and "antigen". Scand. J. Immunol. 19, 281–285.

McGregor, D.D., Gowans, J.L., 1963. The antibody response of rats depleted of lymphocytes by chronic drainage from the thoracic duct. J. Exp. Med. 117, 303–320.

McMaster, P.D., Hudack, S.S., 1934. The participation of skin lymphatics in repair of the lesions due to incisions and burns. J. Exp. Med. 60, 479–501.

McMaster, P.D., Hudack, S.S., 1935. The formation of agglutinins within lymph nodes. J. Exp. Med. 61, 783–805.

Nuttall, G.H.F., 1888. Experiment uber die bacterien feindlichen einflusse des thierischen Korpers. Zeitschr. F. Hyg. 4, 853–894.

Reiss, E., Marten, E., Ehrich, W.E., 1950. Agglutination of bacteria by lymphoid cells in vitro. Proc. Soc. Exp. Biol. Med. 74, 732–735.

Rich, A.R., 1936. Inflammation in resistance to infection. Am. J. Pathol. 12, 723–733.

Schneider, W.C., 1946. Phosphorous compounds in animal tissues. III. A comparison of methods for the estimation of nucleic acids. J. Biol. Chem. 164, 747–751.

Tiselius, A., 1937. A new apparatus for electrophoretic analysis of colloidal mixtures. Trans. Faraday Soc. 33, 524–531.

Tiselius, A., Kabat, E.A., 1939. An electrophoretic study of immune serum and purified antibody preparations. J. Exp. Med. 69, 119–131.

Walzer, M., Glazer, I., 1950. Passive transfer of atopic hypersensitivities in man by means of leukocytes. Proc. Soc. Exp. Boil. Med. 74, 872–876.

TIME LINE

1880s	George Nuttall, Jozsef von Fodor, Karl Flügge, and Hans von Buchner report the presence of antibody-like activity in serum of animals injected with bacteria
1890	Emil von Behring and Shibasaburo Kitasato first use the term antibody
1915	Oswald Avery demonstrates that antibodies are serum globulins
1935	Phillip McMaster and Stephen Hudack prove that the lymph node was the site of antibody formation
1939	Arne Tiselius and Elvin Kabat use electrophoresis to show that antibodies were gamma globulins
1942	William Ehrich and T.N. Harris argue that antibodies are produced by lymphocytes
1948	Astrid Fagraeus demonstrates that cultures containing predominately plasma cells produced more antibody than cultures made up of lymphocytes
1950	Matthew Walzer and Israel Glazer transfer ragweed sensitization by peripheral blood leukocytes
1950	Erik Reiss and colleagues develop the bacterial immobilization technique and show that most antibody-forming cells are plasma cells
1953	Merrill Chase shows that lymph node cells (lymphocytes) from sensitized guinea pigs could transfer the ability to produce antibodies active in the Schultz–Dale phenomenon
1955	Albert Coons and colleagues demonstrate that antibody-forming cells were relatively large cells with a basophilic cytoplasm (plasma cells)
1962	James Gowans concludes that small lymphocytes can transform into plasma cells

6

The Clonal Selection Theory of Antibody Formation

INTRODUCTION

Immunology originally developed as a branch of microbiology to study the body's response to potentially pathogenic microorganisms. In the 1950s, immunology incorporated principles of molecular biology, biochemistry, and genetics and emerged as a unique discipline distinct from microbiology. Landsteiner and others demonstrated that both microbial and nonmicrobial antigens such as synthetic molecules induce immune responses. Based on these observations, investigators speculated about the mechanisms by which the immune system recognized foreign pathogens and yet refrained from reacting to self. As part of these studies, immunologists focused on the mechanism of antibody formation.

Until the late 1940s, most immunologists accepted instruction or antigen template models of antibody formation. These hypotheses required antigen to be engulfed by cells of the reticuloendothelial system. Once phagocytized, the pathogen instructed the cell to alter the structure of its synthesized proteins to make an antibody molecule that was complementary in shape to the pathogen. This information transfer depended on either

- the three-dimensional structure of the antigen serving as a template for the formation of the antibody, in which case all antibodies would have an identical amino acid sequence; or
- the antigen provided information to the genetic material of the antibody-synthesizing cell, altering the nucleotide sequence.

By contrast, biochemists and geneticists made observations that challenged instruction theories:

- The amino acid sequence of a protein dictates its tertiary and quaternary configuration. Thus it became difficult to reconcile how a molecule with a set amino acid sequence could bind to a multitude of differently shaped antigens.
- The amino acid order of a protein is determined by the sequence of nucleotides in the cell's DNA. Francis Crick detailed the "central dogma of molecular biology" in 1958, which postulated that the flow of genetic information in a cell is unidirectional (DNA makes RNA makes protein).

A Historical Perspective on Evidence-Based Immunology
http://dx.doi.org/10.1016/B978-0-12-398381-7.00006-X

This hypothesis, which stated that information could not flow from protein to nucleotides, is inconsistent with instruction theories of antibody formation (Crick, 1970).

Crick was criticized for using the term "dogma" in his formulation of this idea, as he relates in his autobiography:

> I called this idea the central dogma, for two reasons, I suspect. I had already used the obvious word hypothesis in the sequence hypothesis, and in addition I wanted to suggest that this new assumption was more central and more powerful. ... As it turned out, the use of the word dogma caused almost more trouble than it was worth. Many years later Jacques Monod pointed out to me that I did not appear to understand the correct use of the word dogma, which is a belief that cannot be doubted. I did apprehend this in a vague sort of way but since I thought that all religious beliefs were without foundation, I used the word the way I myself thought about it, not as most of the world does, and simply applied it to a grand hypothesis that, however plausible, had little direct experimental support.

During the decade between 1949 and 1958, three models of antibody formation were proposed to address challenges to instruction theories:

- Burnet and Fenner's modified enzyme hypothesis;
- Jerne's natural selection hypothesis; and
- Burnet's clonal selection hypothesis.

Burnet originally proposed the clonal selection hypothesis in 1957. This model postulates that antigen selects from a population of cells already genetically pre-committed to produce an antibody molecule to which the antigen bound. Since the original publication of this idea, a plethora of experiments have been designed to disprove the model; none has succeeded, and the preponderance of evidence generated in subsequent studies of the immune system is consistent with the tenets of this hypothesis. By the late 1960s the community of immunologists accepted Burnet's model, and the clonal selection hypothesis is now referred to as the clonal selection theory.

EARLY MODELS OF ANTIBODY FORMATION

The clonal selection theory may be the single most important advance in immunology in the past hundred years. The acceptance of the tenets of this theory marked a turning point in thinking about the interaction of the immune system with the environment. Most previous models of antibody formation attributed an instructional role to the antigen.

The selection hypotheses of antibody formation developed during the 1950s were not the first attempt at explaining antibody synthesis based on a process of selection. Paul Ehrlich (1854–1915) originally suggested a selection hypothesis in 1900. His side-chain model proposed that cells of the body possessed surface receptors (side chains) that resembled the antibodies they could produce. The binding of a pathogen to these side chains caused the cell to release the side chains. This in turn stimulated the production of additional molecules (antibodies) identical to these side chains. The newly synthesized molecules secreted into the serum resulted in an increase in serum antibody levels (Figure 6.1).

Ehrlich's side-chain hypothesis engendered a great deal of criticism because at the time the structure and source of antibodies were unknown. Immunological studies in the first decades of the twentieth century focused on categorization of the types of antigens against which antibodies could be induced. The first antibodies detected were against potentially pathogenic microorganisms; however, Karl Landsteiner (1868–1943) and other investigators showed that antibodies could be synthesized against an apparently enormous number of different antigens, including synthetic molecules (Landsteiner, 1945; see Chapter 2). The observations that the immune system synthesized such a vast array of antibodies to molecules that do not normally occur in nature led many investigators to question the validity of a selection mechanism such as Ehrlich's that required the presence of preformed cell surface receptors for every possible pathogen.

An antigen template or instruction mechanism, however, appeared to better explain the ability of animals to form the vast array of antibodies. Several instruction models of antibody formation hypothesized that precursors to antibodies existed either in the serum or on the surface of cells. The interaction of an antigen with these prototypical antibodies resulted in changes to the molecule that caused it to assume a configuration capable of binding the eliciting antigen. This new configuration would be communicated to the cells responsible for antibody production, and new antibodies with the same specificity would be produced. Influential proponents of instruction models included Felix Haurowitz and Linus Pauling.

Felix Haurowitz (1896–1987), born and educated as a physician in Prague, earned the Doctor of Science degree in 1923 for studies on hemoglobin. During his career, which spanned more than 50 years, Haurowitz spent time in academic institutions in Germany, Turkey, and the United States. His final position was as professor of chemistry at Indiana University.

Haurowitz switched to the study of immunology in 1930 and developed a model of antibody formation shortly thereafter. Fritz Breinl and Haurowitz (1930) initially proposed that the antigen altered the sequence

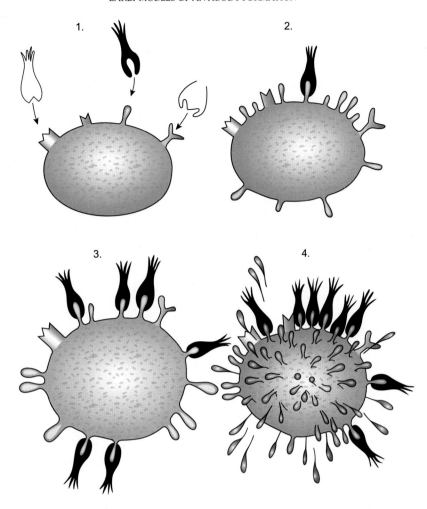

FIGURE 6.1　Ehrlich's side-chain theory of antibody formation. This is the original formulation of a selection hypothesis. Cells capable of synthesizing antibodies possessed on their surface a variety of receptors. Antigen would bind to (select) one of these receptors and cause it to dissociate from the cell. This process in turn would result in the synthesis of additional antibody of the same specificity. *From Ehrlich (1900).*

of amino acids in the binding site and that antibody-forming cells incorporated this information when they synthesized more antibody molecules. Subsequently, Haurowitz developed the template hypothesis of antibody formation that proposed that "the antigen acts directly as a mold, the antibody being formed as a negative print of the determinant group of the antigen" (Haurowitz, 1953). This hypothesis is similar to Pauling's model (see below) and included the idea that the amino acid sequences of antibodies and normal serum globulins are the same or very similar. Although most immunologists abandoned instruction models of antibody formation during the 1960s, Haurowitz continued to publish papers supporting the idea throughout his career (Haurowitz, 1978).

Linus Pauling (1901–1994), born in Oregon, earned a PhD in chemistry in 1925 from the California Institute of Technology where he spent virtually his entire career. He is the only person to be awarded two Nobel Prizes

individually—in Chemistry in 1954 "for his research into the nature of the chemical bond and its application to the elucidation of the structure of complex substances" and the Nobel Peace Prize in 1963. As a scientist interested in the structure of complex molecules, including antibodies, he developed a model of "the structure and process of formation of antibodies" (Pauling, 1940).

Pauling's model of antibody formation was similar to the template hypothesis of Haurowitz. According to this model, antibody developed the capability to bind antigen by being molded around the antigenic molecule. This is illustrated in Figure 6.2, where the antigen serves as a template around which the tertiary structure of the antibody molecule is formed. In this model, all antibody molecules have the same primary amino acid sequence; specificity for different antigens is conferred by changes in conformation induced by the antigen.

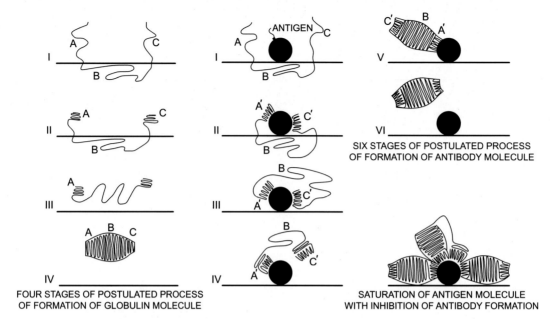

SIX STAGES OF POSTULATED PROCESS
OF FORMATION OF ANTIBODY MOLECULE

FOUR STAGES OF POSTULATED PROCESS
OF FORMATION OF GLOBULIN MOLECULE

SATURATION OF ANTIGEN MOLECULE
WITH INHIBITION OF ANTIBODY FORMATION

FIGURE 6.2   Diagrams representing four stages in the process of formation of a molecule of normal serum globulin (left side of figure) and six stages in the process of formation of an antibody molecule as the result of interaction of the globulin polypeptide chain with an antigen molecule. There is also shown (lower right) an antigen molecule surrounded by attached antibody molecules or parts of molecules, thus inhibiting further antibody formation. *From Pauling (1940).*

CHALLENGES TO INSTRUCTION MODELS

As biochemists unraveled protein structure and the role that amino acid sequence plays in determining the tertiary configuration of the antibody binding site, evidence mounted against instruction models of antibody formation. Similarly, the finding that the order of amino acids in a protein is determined by DNA sequence argued against antigen altering the primary structure of antibody. In addition to these issues, several other immunological phenomena could not easily be explained by instruction models (Burnet and Fenner, 1949; Jerne, 1955):

1. Immunological memory (the booster effect): When antigen is injected a second time, the ability of an individual to produce antibodies is greatly enhanced. If antigen were responsible for driving the production of antibody, as hypothesized by instruction models, a second stimulus with antigen would induce a response proportional to the dose injected. Thus, if the second dose were the same as the first, the prediction would be that the level of antibody produced would be approximately the same after each exposure.

2. Immunologic maturation: As an immune response matures, the average avidity of an antiserum (the strength of binding between antigen and several antibody molecules) increases. This reflects changes

in the binding affinity of individual antibody molecules, most likely due to changes in the amino acids present in the antigen-binding site. These changes occur due to mutations in the DNA coding for the individual chains of the antibody molecules. Antibodies produced as a result of being molded by antigen, as proposed by instruction hypotheses, would not be expected to change their amino acid sequence.

3. Rate of antibody formation: During the primary immune response, the amount of antibody produced increases exponentially until a plateau is reached. Predictions based on instruction hypotheses require that maximal antibody formation occurs early in the response when antigen concentration is highest.

4. The production of antibodies in the absence of antigen: Many studies describe the continued production of antibodies even after all injected antigen has been cleared. The stimulus for this prolonged antibody production cannot be accounted for by instruction hypotheses that require the continued presence of antigenic templates. In addition, the synthesis of natural antibodies (antibodies present in an animal without apparent antigenic stimulation) is difficult to explain with instruction models.

5. Amount of antibody produced: Rabbits injected a second time with *Salmonella* produce approximately 100,000 antibody molecules per second per bacterium injected. This rate is continued for several

weeks, and the antibody produced is directed primarily against cell surface determinants. As Jerne argues, "if we imagine that the bacteria serving as antigen templates were not broken down but resided in toto each in an antibody producing cell, this would entail impossible quantitative implications. If, however, the bacteria were broken down into many fragments, how would a cell in which one of these fragments served as antigen template be able to distinguish what part of the fragment had originally been at the surface of the intact bacterium?"

6. Occurrence of a lag phase during the primary response: Typically antibody cannot be detected in peripheral blood until several days after antigen injection. This delay is termed the lag phase. If instruction models were correct, antibody should be detected in the plasma almost immediately after antigen injection without a lag.

7. Production of antibodies directed against pathogens but not to self: If antibodies are produced following phagocytosis, autoantibodies would be a common occurrence since tissues of the body are continually being catabolized and recycled.

PARADIGM SHIFT: FROM INSTRUCTION TO SELECTION

These challenges to instruction hypotheses prompted the development of three new models to explain how antigen induces the synthesis of specific antibody.

The Modified Enzyme Concept

During the 1940s and 1950s, Jacques Monod, François Jacob, and Andre Lwoff described the presence of inducible (or adaptable) enzymes in bacteria and yeast. These enzymes are expressed only under conditions when they are useful for the survival of the microorganism. Genes coding for these enzymes are activated by environmental stimuli such as the presence (or absence) of certain nutrients. Studies of these enzymes stimulated a change in the way that biologists considered gene regulation and resulted in the awarding of the 1965 Nobel Prize in Physiology or Medicine to these three investigators "for discoveries concerning genetic control of enzyme and virus synthesis." These results led Macfarlane Burnet and Frank Fenner in 1949 to propose that a similar mechanism is involved in the production of antibody.

F. Macfarlane Burnet (1899–1985) spent most of his professional career at the Walter and Eliza Hall Institute (WEHI) of Medical Research in Melbourne, Australia. He was trained as a physician in Melbourne (1924) and earned his PhD from the University of London in 1928. Early in his career he studied the nature of bacterial

viruses (bacteriophages) and their replication. In 1928, he returned to the WEHI as assistant director and pursued various virology projects, primarily focused on the isolation and epidemiology of canary pox and influenza. He also investigated the epidemiology of herpes and Q fever. The causative agent for Q fever, *Coxiella* burnetii was named in his honor. In 1944, he became director of WEHI, and in the mid-1950s he declared that immunology be the research emphasis of the institute.

Burnet and Fenner's modified enzyme hypothesis proposed that cells that phagocytize antigen contain enzymes active in removing cellular debris and dead cells. Phagocytosis of antigen induces the formation of new enzymes specific for, and proficient at, destroying that antigen. Some of these induced enzymes are secreted by the cell. In the extracellular environment, these induced enzymes are modified, maintaining the ability to bind antigens but losing their enzymatic activity, thus acting as antibodies.

This hypothesis explained the continued production of antibody in the absence of antigen as well as the development of a memory response upon subsequent exposure to the same antigen. To explain the capacity of the adaptive immune response to differentiate self from non-self, the theory postulated a "self-marker" enzyme that could not be adapted into antibody molecules.

The mechanism responsible for changing the amino acid sequence of the enzymes to lose enzymatic activity and become specific antibodies remained unexplained. This model was also formulated prior to an understanding of the molecular biology of protein synthesis.

The Natural Selection Hypothesis of Antibody Formation

In 1955, Niels Kaj Jerne (1911–1994) introduced the natural selection model of antibody formation in an attempt to "provide simple explanations" to the challenges faced by instruction models. Jerne's hypothesis provided a conceptual leap in that the role of the antigen went from functioning as an instructor of antibody production to selecting the antibody needed. Jerne was born in England of Danish parents. He was raised and educated in the Netherlands, trained as a physician at the University of Copenhagen, and earned his PhD in 1951. Jerne worked at an array of institutions, including the Danish National Serum Institute, the World Health Organization, the University of Pittsburgh, and the Johann Wolfgang Goethe University. He was the director of the Paul Ehrlich Institute in Germany and the Basel Institute for Immunology in Switzerland.

In the 30 years following the development of his natural selection model of antibody formation, Jerne made significant contributions to the field of immunology by postulating that tolerance to self occurs in the thymus and that T and B lymphocytes communicate with each other through a network of antibodies and antiantibodies (idiotypes and anti-idiotypes) on their cell surface. Although this latter idea has been proven incorrect, he was awarded the Nobel Prize in Physiology or Medicine in 1984 for "theories concerning the specificity in development and control of the immune system." This prize was shared with Georges J.F. Kohler and Cesar Milstein, who were awarded the prize for "the discovery of the principle for production of monoclonal antibodies."

Jerne's natural selection model of antibody formation (Jerne, 1955) postulated that serum of an animal contained antibodies of every specificity that the animal could possibly produce. These antibodies were spontaneously synthesized during the production of natural globulins. When foreign pathogen entered the system, the antigen bound to natural antibodies that possessed affinity for the particular antigen. The antigen–antibody complexes were subsequently phagocytized and dissociated within the cell. The presence of the selected globulin molecule in the cell signaled that cell to produce additional identical antibodies. This theory required that the system produce large numbers of "natural" antibodies of various specificities in the absence of antigenic challenge. It also necessitated that information about the amino acid sequence of the selected antibody somehow be transmitted from the engulfed antigen–antibody complex to the genetic material coding for the amino acid sequence of the antibody.

The natural selection hypothesis succeeded in answering several of the criticisms of instruction models. Immunologic memory developed from an alteration in the antibody-forming cell produced by uptake of antigen–antibody complexes. The lag phase in the antibody response was attributed to the processing required following interaction of antigen with natural antibodies. Self–non-self discrimination was explained by postulating that self-reactive, natural antibodies produced early in life would bind to self-antigens and be eliminated, thus resulting in the absence of circulating antibodies specific for self.

At the time this hypothesis was under development, the "central dogma of molecular biology" was emerging. Based on the proposition that genetic information flowed in one direction from nucleic acids to protein, geneticists and molecular biologists found Jerne's natural selection model of antibody formation difficult to accept. Supposedly, James Watson is reported to have remarked about the hypothesis that "it stinks" (Söderqvist, 2003). Many immunologists also rejected Jerne's hypothesis because it required the existence of millions of antibody specificities, some of which were specific for synthetic molecules and many of which would never be used during an immune response. Immunologists also had difficulty accepting the natural selection model of antibody formation due to the lack of information of how the targeted antibody-forming cells are selected.

THE CLONAL SELECTION THEORY

Burnet continued the assault on instruction models of antibody formation as he developed his clonal selection theory. Burnet initially published this theory in an Australian medical journal (Burnet, 1957) and later expanded his thoughts in a book based on a series of lectures presented at Vanderbilt University in Nashville (Burnet, 1959). Like Jerne, Burnet postulated that antigen selects the antibody to be produced from a population of preexisting molecules. In Burnet's hypothesis the primary unit of selection for antigen was the lymphocyte-expressing antibody on its surface rather than antibody circulating in the peripheral blood. The idea that potential antibody-forming lymphocytes possessed cell surface receptors to which antigen bound was reminiscent of Ehrlich's side-chain theory.

Postulates that differentiate Burnet's clonal selection theory from Jerne's natural selection hypothesis and from other models of antibody formation include the following:

- Antigen-binding receptors exist on the surface of antibody-forming lymphocytes prior to introduction of antigen. Thus when antigen binds to these cell surface receptors the lymphocyte is activated and produces antibody of that same binding specificity.
- An individual lymphocyte expresses receptors, all of which are the same specificity. Accordingly, a lymphocyte, once selected, produces large quantities of antibody, all of which possess the same antigen specificity.
- Potential antibody-forming lymphocytes go through a developmental stage during which they are exquisitely sensitive to elimination if they interact with self-antigens. This interaction results in the destruction of these lymphocytes and the development of self-tolerance (the ability to differentiate self from non-self). While Burnet was unable to demonstrate the induction of immunological tolerance, the formulation of the clonal selection theory correctly predicted the mechanism responsible for tolerance induction and helped explain the findings published by Billingham et al. (1953) (Chapter 8).

Almost simultaneously with the publication of Burnet's original description of the clonal selection theory, David Talmage published a similar theory in the *Annual Reviews of Medicine* (1957). Talmage (1919–2014) trained as a physician at Washington University in St. Louis and spent his career as faculty at several medical schools. At the time of this publication he was a faculty member at the University of Chicago. He described the various models of antibody production in vogue at that time as (1) the antigen-template theory, where the antigen serves as the template by which the antibody develops a complementary configuration; (2) the adaptive enzyme theory, in which the antigen induces an enzymatic change in the cellular mechanism responsible for producing antibodies; and (3) the natural selection theory, where the antigen selects serum globulins (natural antibody) and the resulting antigen–antibody complex induces cells to produce more of the antibody. After considering the pros and cons of each of these theories, Talmage opted for a modification of Ehrlich's side-chain hypothesis in which antigen selects cells based on cell surface receptors. He stated

> The process of natural selection requires the selective multiplication of a few species out of a diverse population. As a working hypothesis it is tempting to consider that one of the multiplying units in the antibody response is the cell itself. According to this hypothesis only those cells are selected for multiplication whose synthesized product has affinity for the antigen injected.

This speculation is very similar to the clonal selection theory published by Burnet and introduced the important concept that antigen selection occurred at the level of the cell. While it has been argued that Talmage should have received more recognition for the development of the clonal selection theory than he did (Ada, 1989), it is of note that he did not include the notion that an individual cell produced antibody of a single specificity, a major contribution of Burnet's theory.

An Attempt to Disprove the Clonal Selection Theory

The development of the clonal selection theory generated studies designed to prove it incorrect. Gus Nossal joined the WEHI shortly after Burnet presented the clonal selection theory and set out to refute it. He speculated that if antibody-forming cells were competent to produce antibodies of more than a single specificity, the clonal selection theory would be disproved. In 1958, Nossal, along with Joshua Lederberg, devised a technique allowing them to determine antibody secretion by single cells. The design of the experiment and the results are presented in Chapter 7. Nossal as well as other investigators failed to demonstrate that an antibody-forming cell produced antibodies of two specificities. This failure to detect multispecific antibody-forming lymphocytes strengthened one of the basic tenets of the theory.

Extension of the Clonal Selection Theory to T Lymphocytes

At the time the clonal selection theory was presented, virtually all immunologic studies involved the measurement of antibody. The role of cell-mediated immunity in the adaptive immune response was virtually unknown. Likewise, the cells of the adaptive immune response had not yet been separated into subpopulations of T and B lymphocytes. Once the division of antigen-reactive cells into T and B lymphocytes was confirmed in the 1960s, studies were designed to determine if T lymphocytes were also selected by antigen and followed the rules of the clonal selection theory. Evolving technologies and understanding of the immune system resulted in this question being answered only after several additional facts had been uncovered. These included the following:

1. The identity of the cell surface receptor on T lymphocytes: While initial speculation focused on the antigen-specific T lymphocyte receptor being an immunoglobulin molecule, investigations using monoclonal antibodies and genetic clonal techniques demonstrated that the structures of the receptors on B and T lymphocytes were unique (Chapter 17).
2. The mechanism by which T lymphocytes recognize antigen: The receptors on B lymphocytes directly bind antigens of various chemical compositions. T lymphocytes can only bind protein antigens that have been processed (digested) by specialized cells and displayed on the surface of those cells bound to major histocompatibility complex-encoded molecules (Chapters 16 and 20).
3. The process of self-tolerance induction in T lymphocytes: The thymus is the site for T lymphocyte maturation and elimination of potentially self-reactive cells. T lymphocytes, like B lymphocytes, are specific for a single antigen and go through a developmental stage during which they are eliminated if they interact with self-antigens (Chapters 8 and 22).

The convergence of investigations performed by molecular immunologists on the molecular biology and genetics of the T-cell receptor and by cellular immunologists on the mechanisms by which T lymphocytes recognize antigen resulted in a final understanding of the universality of clonal selection in the immune system. Both T and B lymphocytes recognize foreign antigen through the binding of antigenic determinants to cell surface receptors. While the molecular structures of these receptors differ, the level of specificity and discrimination between the two systems is remarkably similar.

Sir Macfarlane Burnet was awarded the Nobel Prize in Physiology or Medicine in 1960 for the development of the clonal selection theory, particularly the speculation of the mechanism by which unresponsiveness to self (tolerance) arises. He shared the prize with Sir Peter Medawar for their "discovery of immunological tolerance."

CONCLUSION

The development of the clonal selection theory advanced the understanding of the adaptive immune response into the twenty-first century and generated research addressing a multitude of important questions. The clonal selection theory motivated studies leading to the

- identification of the lymphocyte as the antigen-reactive cell (Chapter 4);
- differentiation of separate populations of T and B lymphocytes responsible for cell-mediated and antibody-mediated responses (Chapters 9 and 10);
- recognition of the interaction of T and B lymphocytes in the initiation of an adaptive immune response (Chapter 13);
- identification of antigen-specific receptors on B and T lymphocytes (Chapter 17); and
- deciphering of the mechanism by which potentially self-reactive lymphocytes are eliminated (Chapters 8, 21, and 22).

Since the publication of Burnet's original paper in 1957, the clonal selection theory has driven the interpretation of most new findings in cellular and molecular immunology. The theory has successfully incorporated new observations, and all experimental data that have been presented are consistent with the basic tenets of the clonal selection theory.

References

Ada, G.L., 1989. The conception and birth of Burnet's clonal selection theory in immunology. In: Mazumdar, P.M. (Ed.), Theory in Immunology 1930-1980: Essays on the History of Immunology. Wall and Thompson, Toronto, pp. 33–40.

Billingham, R.E., Brent, L., Medawar, P.B., 1953. 'Actively acquired tolerance' of foreign cells. Nature 172, 603–606.

Breinl, F., Haurowitz, F., 1930. Chemische untersuchung des Präzipitates aus Hämoglobin und anti-hämoglobin serum und bemerk ungenüber die natur der antikorper. Hoppe-Seyler's Z. Physiol. Chem. 192, 45–57. Referenced in Podolsky, S.H., Tauber, A.I. (1997). The Generation of Diversity. Clonal Selection Theory and the Rise of Molecular Immunology. Harvard University Press, Cambridge, MA.

Burnet, F.M., 1957. A modification of Jerne's theory of antibody production using the concept of clonal selection. Aust. J. Sci. 20, 67–68.

Burnet, F.M., 1959. The Clonal Selection Theory of Acquired Immunity. Vanderbilt University Press, Nashville, TN.

Burnet, F.M., Fenner, F., 1949. The Production of Antibodies, second ed. Macmillan, London. p. 149.

Crick, F., 1970. Central dogma of molecular biology. Nature 227, 561–563.

Ehrlich, P., 1900. On immunity with special reference to cell life. Proc. Roy. Soc. 66, 424–428.

Haurowitz, F., 1953. The immunological response. Annu. Rev. Micro. 7, 389–414.

Haurowitz, F., 1978. Mechanism of antigen-induced antibody biosynthesis from antibody precursors, the heavy and light immunoglobulin chains. Proc. Natl. Acad. Sci. U.S.A. 75, 2434–2438.

Jerne, N.K., 1955. The natural selection theory of antibody formation. Proc. Natl. Acad. Sci. U.S.A. 41, 849–857.

Landsteiner, K., 1945. The Specificity of Serological Reactions. Harvard University Press, Cambridge, MA.

Nossal, G.J.V., Lederberg, J., 1958. Antibody production by single cells. Nature 181, 1419–1420.

Pauling, L., 1940. A theory of the structure and process of formation of antibodies. J. Am. Chem. Soc. 62, 2643–2657.

Söderqvist, T., 2003. Science as Autobiography: The Troubled Life of Niels Jerne. Yale University Press, New Haven, CT.

Talmage, D.W., 1957. Allergy and immunology. Annu. Rev. Med. 8, 239–256.

TIME LINE

1900	Paul Ehrlich proposes the "side-chain theory" of antibody formation
1930	Fritz Breinl and Felix Haurowitz propose an instruction model of antibody formation
1940	Linus Pauling publishes his instruction hypothesis of antibody formation
1949	Macfarlane Burnet and Frank Fenner publish the modified enzyme hypothesis of antibody formation
1953	James Watson and Francis Crick publish the double helix model of DNA
1953	Felix Haurowitz develops the template hypothesis of antibody formation
1953	Rupert Billingham, Leslie Brent, and Peter Medawar demonstrate the induction of immunological tolerance in neonatal mice
1955	Niels Jerne postulates a natural selection model of antibody formation
1957	Macfarlane Burnet proposes the clonal selection theory of antibody formation
1957	David Talmage describes a selection theory of antibody formation similar to Burnet's
1958	Francis Crick proposes the "central dogma of molecular biology," postulating that the flow of information in a cell is unidirectional
1958	Gus Nossal and Joshua Lederberg demonstrate that an antibody-forming cell synthesizes antibodies of a single specificity
1960	Nobel Prize in Physiology or Medicine awarded to F. Macfarlane Burnet and Peter Medawar

7

Plasma Cells Produce Antibody of a Single Specificity

INTRODUCTION

Plasma cells, derived from lymphocytes, synthesize and secrete antibodies (Chapter 5). At the time Astrid Fagraeus (1948) and Albert Coons et al. (1955) provided evidence to support this conclusion, the mechanism responsible for antibody production was under debate. Most immunologists favored instruction theories of antibody formation although the first selection theories were being developed. Instruction theories postulated that cells of the reticuloendothelial system phagocytized antigen that instructed those cells to synthesize an antibody with a binding site complementary to the configuration of the antigen (Pauling, 1940); these theories assumed that a single antibody-forming cell could produce antibodies of several different specificities.

During the 1950s, new information about protein structure and configuration emerged that led several researchers to question the instruction theories. F. Macfarlane Burnet and Frank Fenner published a modified enzyme theory of antibody formation in 1949, and selection theories were advanced by Niels Jerne in 1955 and Burnet in 1957 (Chapter 6). The modified enzyme theory of Burnet and Fenner as well as the natural selection theory of Jerne were consistent with plasma cells producing antibodies of multiple specificities. Burnet's clonal selection theory, however, required that an antibody-forming cell expresses a single specificity.

To differentiate between the two theories, instruction and selection, investigators designed experimental models to determine the number of different antibody specificities synthesized by a single antibody-forming cell. If instruction theories were correct, a single cell should be able to synthesize antibodies of multiple specificities since each antigen taken up by the cell would instruct the cell to alter the configuration of the binding site to match that antigen. In contrast, Burnet's clonal selection theory predicted that a single antibody-forming cell would synthesize antibody of a single specificity, all of which would bind the same antigen. This prediction was contingent on the premise that the antigen selected and activated specific lymphocytes based on the antibody that cell was genetically preprogrammed to synthesize.

To test the hypothesis that a single cell could produce antibodies of more than a single specificity (and in an attempt to disprove Burnet's clonal selection hypothesis), Gus Nossal and Joshua Lederberg designed an experiment to detect antibody formation by single cells. Results from their studies demonstrated that each activated lymphocyte produces a unique antibody of a single specificity.

SINGLE CELL EXPERIMENTS: DEVELOPMENT OF THE MICRODROP TECHNIQUE

Gus Nossal (1931 to present) entered the world of immunology when he joined the Walter and Eliza Hall Institute (WEHI) in 1957. He was born in Austria but immigrated to Australia in 1939 with his parents. He graduated from the University of Sydney as a physician in 1954. His arrival at WEHI coincided with the development of the clonal selection theory by Burnet who at that time was director of the Institute. Nossal eventually succeeded Burnet as the director of WEHI in 1965.

As described by Nossal in a review (2002), upon arrival at WEHI, he hypothesized that if he "could show that a single cell from a multiple immunized animal were to secrete two or three antibody specificities simultaneously," the clonal selection theory could be disproved. Nossal realized that the experiment he envisioned required a technique that could detect antibody produced by individual cells.

Fortuitously, Joshua Lederberg (1925–2008) arrived at the University of Melbourne as a Fulbright Visiting Professor of Bacteriology in 1957. Lederberg, a geneticist who had made major contributions to molecular genetics as a student and professor at the University of Wisconsin, would be awarded the Nobel Prize in Physiology or Medicine (shared with George Beadle and Edward Tatum) in 1958 "for his discoveries concerning genetic recombination and the organization of the genetic material of bacteria."

In 1954, Lederberg developed a technique involving micromanipulation whereby a single bacterium could be isolated and studied in a microdrop of culture medium. Nossal adapted this technique to determine the antibody specificities secreted by individual cells from animals immunized with two different antigens.

Nossal and Lederberg (1958) injected *Salmonella adelaide* and *Salmonella typhi* into the hind footpads of rats. Three injections were given over a 3-week period; 3 days after the last injection Nossal and Lederberg dissected the popliteal lymph nodes draining the injection sites and dissociated them, creating single cell suspensions. Aliquots of this suspension containing one cell were micromanipulated onto glass slides and incubated for 4 h. Antibody production was assayed by introducing approximately 10 bacteria of one or the other strain into each microdrop; the presence of antibody resulted in the loss of bacterial motility.

Salmonella adelaide and *Salmonella typhi* flagella are antigenically distinct as measured by serum antibody. Thus, Nossal and Lederberg could distinguish cells producing antibodies to one or both strains. Droplets positive for antibody to one of the *Salmonella* strains were subsequently tested for their ability to inhibit the activity of the second bacterium.

Nossal and Lederberg predicted that if the clonal selection hypothesis was incorrect, some of the cells in the microdrop cultures would produce antibodies directed against both antigens. The results are presented in Table 7.1. Droplets contained between 1 and 10 cells; only those containing a single cell were evaluated. Of a total of 274 droplets examined, 57 contained a single cell. Thirty-nine of the droplets containing a single cell received *S. adelaide* to test for the presence of antibodies. Six of these 39 droplets possessed antibody that inhibited the motility of *S. adelaide*; none inhibited the motility of *S. typhi*. Similarly, 3 of 18 droplets containing a single cell possessed antibody activity directed against the flagella of *S. typhi*; none of these droplets inhibited the movement of *S. adelaide*. Control droplets containing no cells or cells from unimmunized animals failed to inhibit the motility of either bacterium.

These data supported the interpretation that a single cell taken from an animal stimulated with two antigens produced antibody of a single specificity. Based on these data, the clonal selection theory could not be rejected.

Other investigators performing similar experiments, however, were obtaining conflicting results. A group at Washington University and the University of Illinois led by Mel Cohn and Edwin Lennox injected rabbits with two different bacteriophages, T2 and T5, both of which infect *E. coli*. A single cell suspension of lymph nodes draining the site of injection was mixed with the T2 and T5 bacteriophages and distributed into microdroplets on cover slips. Following 48 h of incubation, culture fluid was recovered by adsorption on filter paper and added to cultures of *E. coli* to determine if phage activity had been inhibited. Ninety-five of 925 lymphocytes tested (10.3%) showed activity against one of the bacteriophages, while 21 of the 95 positive droplets (22%) neutralized both phages. The authors (Attardi et al., 1959) claimed that their results support the hypothesis that a single cell can synthesize antibodies of two (or more) discrete specificities. They concluded that these data "do not support the theories which postulate only one antibody potentiality per cell."

The reason for these disparate results remains unexplained. As Nossal (2002) states in a review, "We will probably never know the reason why such excellent and respected scientists obtained such incorrect results." Two possibilities have been suggested:

1. The experimental protocol used by the Attardi group may have been biased toward detection of incomplete allelic exclusion—that is, antibodies were being coded for by both alleles of the immunoglobulin genes (Viret and Gurr, 2009).
2. Cells used to set up the microdrops may not have been sufficiently washed to remove cell fragments or antibodies passively attached to the cells prior to testing (Nossal, 2002).

TABLE 7.1 Antibody Production by Isolated Cells (*From Nossal and Lederberg, 1958*). Lymph Node Cells Isolated from Rats Injected with Both *Salmonella adelaide* and *Salmonella typhi* Were Tested for Their Ability to Immobilize the Immunizing Bacteria. Drops Containing Single Cells Were Also Tested for Immobilizing Activity Against the Alternative Bacteria and Were Negative

No. of cells in drop	No. of drops inhibitory	No. of drops tested
FIRST TESTED VERSUS S. ADELAIDE		
1	6[a]	39
2	5	25
3	7	24
4	6	21
5	6	10
6–10	17	33
FIRST TESTED VERSUS S. TYPHI		
1	3[a]	18
2	6	26
3	0	14
4	3	14
5	1	8
6–10	22	42

Lymph node cells from rats presensitized to *S. adelaide* plus *S. typhi* were dispensed in microdroplets and incubated for 4h. They were then tested by the introduction of motile bacteria.

[a]*These droplets were also tested for any activity against the alternative serotype and were negative.*

Nossal and his laboratory continued to assay single cells for their ability to produce antibodies of multiple specificities. At the time of a review published in 1962 (Nossal and Makela, 1962), more than 7000 cells from doubly immunized rats had been evaluated. Of the 38% of these cells that produced detectable antibody, 98.2% synthesized antibody of a single specificity. Characterization of those cells that appeared to produce antibodies of two different specificities showed that most reacted strongly against one of the antigens and only weakly against the second antigen. Only two of these cells secreted antibodies reactive with both antigens. Nossal concluded that these were most likely cross-reactions not detectable when assaying serum antibacterial antibodies.

IMMUNOFLUORESCENT STUDIES

In 1958, R.G. White, working at London Hospital, used immunofluorescence to confirm that an antibody-forming lymphocyte produces antibody of a single specificity. Rabbits injected with two antigens (*Streptococcus*

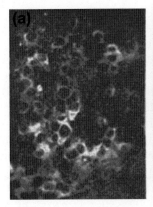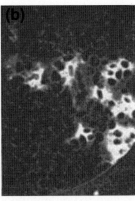

FIGURE 7.1 Immunofluorescence staining of a rabbit spleen producing antibodies to two different antigens. Panel (a) shows cells producing antibody to *Streptococcus pneumonia* while panel (b) shows the same section following quenching of the fluorescence and restaining to demonstrate antibody production to ovalbumin. *From White (1958).*

pneumonia and ovalbumin) provided lymph nodes and spleens for these studies. The lymphoid tissues were frozen, sectioned, and exposed to a mixture of the two antigens. The rationale for this approach was that cells that synthesized antibody to *S. pneumonia* would bind the microbe while cells synthesizing antibodies to ovalbumin would bind that antigen.

Unbound antigen was washed away and the sections incubated with antibodies to one or the other of the antigens coupled to fluorescein, a green fluorescent dye. Using a fluorescent microscope, the sections were photographed, the fluorescence was quenched (i.e., decreased in intensity), and the same section was exposed to fluorescein-conjugated antibodies to the second antigen. The sections were once again photographed and the two photos of the section were compared.

Figure 7.1 illustrates the results obtained by this procedure. The section on the left shows rabbit lymphocytes treated with *S. pneumonia* and stained with fluorescent-conjugated antibodies to the capsular polysaccharide of this *Streptococcus*. The photograph on the right is the same section of rabbit spleen treated with ovalbumin and stained with fluorescent-conjugated antibody to ovalbumin. This study showed that antibody-forming cells to both antigens existed; however, no cells synthesizing antibodies to both antigens were detected.

Baruj Benacerraf and his group at Harvard obtained similar results (Green et al., 1967) using cells from rabbits injected with a hapten–carrier conjugate. A hapten is a small molecule that is not immunogenic unless conjugated to a carrier protein. Rabbits or guinea pigs injected with the hapten 2,4 dinitrophenyl (DNP) conjugated to either bovine serum albumin (BSA) or bovine gamma globulin (BGG) served as the source of lymphoid tissues. Cells prepared on microscope slides were tested for antibody production using the same technique described above. A second immunofluorescent marker, rhodamine, was available, allowing the detection of two positive antibody-forming cells simultaneously.

Cell smears incubated with two different antigens (i.e., BSA and DNP-BGG) were subsequently exposed to antibodies specific for these two antigens (i.e., BSA and DNP) labeled with either fluorescein, which emitted green fluorescence, or rhodamine, which emitted red fluorescence. Since the fluorescent molecules emitted at different wavelengths, individual cells producing one or two different antibodies could be visualized.

Antibody-forming cells to both hapten and carrier were detected by immunofluorescence; however, no cells producing antibodies to both hapten and carrier antigens were revealed. While these results confirmed that a single cell produced antibody of a single specificity, additional studies appeared during the next 10 years that further supported the tenets of the clonal selection theory. These studies required identification of antigen-specific receptors on antibody-forming cells. All receptors on a B lymphocyte are of a single specificity and share antigen-binding ability with the antibody that the cell produces (Chapter 17).

ANTIGEN RECEPTORS ON B LYMPHOCYTES

Goran Möller in 1961, working in Sweden, provided the first evidence that antibody-forming B lymphocytes possess immunoglobulin on their surface when he treated mouse lymphocytes with fluorescein-conjugated antibodies specific for rabbit antimouse immunoglobulin. This was a negative control for other experiments he was performing; however, a small number of the lymphocytes bound to the fluorescent antibodies, demonstrating the presence of immunoglobulin on their surface.

During the ensuing decade other investigators confirmed these results. By 1971, Joseph Davie and William Paul, working at the National Institutes of Health in Bethesda, Maryland, concluded that some lymphocytes express immunoglobulin on their surface by which they bind antigen.

Discovery that lymphocytes express cell surface immunoglobulin spurred studies aimed at determining the role of these receptors. One method that became popular during the late 1960s and early 1970s involved treating lymphocytes with labeled antibodies to immunoglobulin under various conditions. A simple experiment in which lymphocytes were treated with fluorescein-conjugated antibodies to immunoglobulin at different temperatures produced an unexpected observation: the immunoglobulin molecules on the surface of B lymphocytes behave dissimilarly based on temperature. Treatment of B lymphocytes in vitro with antibodies to immunoglobulin at 4°C results in uniform labeling

of the lymphocyte surface. Treatment at 37°C causes the surface immunoglobulin to migrate to one pole of the cell (they are capped).

The presence of immunoglobulin molecules on the surface of antibody-forming lymphocytes led to the prediction that lymphocytes "recognized" foreign antigen by the binding of the antigen to these antibody molecules. Based on this prediction, Martin Raff et al. (1973), working at University College in London, demonstrated that all of the receptor molecules on a particular B lymphocyte are of a single specificity. Mouse spleen cells treated with antigen (polymerized flagellin of *S. adelaide*) under capping conditions (37°C), resulting in the redistribution of cell surface immunoglobulins to one pole of the lymphocyte, were subsequently treated with fluoresceinated antibodies to immunoglobulin under noncapping conditions (4°C). This two-step procedure was designed to detect any immunoglobulin receptors that remained after the initial exposure at physiological conditions. Specific antigen capped greater than 95% of the surface immunoglobulin on lymphocytes from both naïve and immunized animals, leaving few, if any, immunoglobulin molecules to be stained with antibodies to immunoglobulin. These results strongly supported the prediction that all of the receptors on a given lymphocyte are specific for one antigen.

Cell Surface Immunoglobulin and Secreted Antibody Possess the Same Specificity

The observation that all of the immunoglobulin receptors on antibody-forming lymphocytes shared the same specificity led to the speculation that this specificity was identical to the antibody that lymphocytes synthesized. Gus Nossal and Beverley Pike confirmed this hypothesis in 1976 using the microdrop technique to characterize the products of single cells. Spleen cells from mice injected with a hapten–carrier conjugate (4-hydroxy-3-iodo-5-nitrophenyl conjugated to polymerized flagellin (NIP-POL)) were harvested to provide a source of antibody-forming lymphocytes. Nossal and Pike incubated these lymphocytes on NIP conjugated to gelatin. Increasing the temperature of the gelatin resulted in the release of lymphocytes specific for NIP. They micromanipulated these isolated cells into microdrops to which NIP-POL was added to induce antibody synthesis. Antibody production to NIP and to POL was tested. Lymphocytes isolated based on their ability to bind NIP synthesized antibodies specific for NIP but not antibodies to POL.

These studies confirmed that each plasma cell produces antibody of a single specificity. This observation led to two important advances, one clinical and one industrial:

- establishment of the molecular basis of multiple myeloma, and
- development of the techniques resulting in the production of monoclonal antibodies.

MULTIPLE MYELOMA AND THE ONE CELL: ONE ANTIBODY CONCEPT

Multiple myeloma, a malignant disorder of plasma cells, was first described in 1844 by S. Solly (Chapter 35). Patients present with bone pain and a history of fractures as well as infection, renal failure, and/or anemia. In 1848, Henry Bence Jones (1814–1873) described a unique protein in the urine of a patient diagnosed with multiple myeloma (mollities ossium or softening of the bone). Bence Jones proteins precipitate when urine is heated to approximately 60 °C and become soluble when the urine boils. Abnormalities in serum and urine proteins serve as diagnostic clues to the disease.

The presence of a unique protein in the serum of myeloma patients was detected in 1939 by Lewis Longworth and colleagues working at the Rockefeller Institute for Medical Research. Analysis of serum proteins in patients and of proteins produced by myeloma cells by serum electrophoresis demonstrated that the abnormal serum proteins most likely were produced by the malignant cells (Miller et al., 1952). Henry Kunkel's group evaluated the serum proteins of myeloma patients and concluded that these proteins were related to normal gamma globulin. Each myeloma protein was immunologically unique, suggesting individual antigenic specificity (Slater et al., 1955). A large number of similar studies allowed Kunkel to conclude in 1968 that myeloma proteins "may actually represent antibodies for which in most instances the antigen is unknown."

Leonhard Korngold and Rose Lipari (1956), working at the Sloan Kettering Institute for Cancer Research, used a gel diffusion assay and determined that an antiserum against Bence Jones proteins also reacted against the myeloma protein from the same patient and against normal gamma globulin. These studies were performed prior to structural analysis of the immunoglobulin described in Chapter 11, and the relationship of these urinary proteins to the chains of antibody molecules was unclear. Eventually Gerald Edelman and Joseph Gally in 1962 showed that Bence Jones proteins and the light chains from the myeloma protein of the same patient had identical amino acid sequences. To honor the contributions of Korngold and Lipari to this field, the two types of light chains found in all immunoglobulin molecules are designated κ or λ based on the initial letter of their last names.

Myeloma proteins and antibodies are structurally identical, implying that the bone marrow cell that became malignantly transformed was, in fact, an antibody-forming cell. The electrophoretic mobility of the gamma globulins found in the serum of myeloma patients demonstrated that the product of the tumor cells was homogeneous. Nossal's laboratory (Marchalonis and Nossal, 1968) studied the electrophoretic mobility of antibody produced by single lymphocytes in microdrops. They concluded that "the product of nearly all single antibody-forming cells is just as restricted as that of a myeloma cell." Thus the observations made in the clinic and those from the experimental laboratory reinforced each other.

DEVELOPMENT OF MONOCLONAL ANTIBODIES

In 1975, Georges Köhler and Cesar Milstein made a major advance in immunology when they developed the technology for the production of monoclonal antibodies (Chapter 37). Monoclonal antibodies are produced by clones of antibody-forming cells (hybridomas) that have a defined specificity. Hybridomas are formed by the fusion of an antibody-forming B lymphocyte from an immunized animal with a nonimmunoglobulin secreting plasmacytoma. Selection in vitro results in the isolation of a cell line, producing a homogeneous antibody. The development of hybridomas requires that antibody-forming cells produce antibodies of a single specificity.

The availability of monoclonal antibodies specific for cell surface molecules, cytokines, and other components of the adaptive immune response stimulated the study of the molecular biology of the immune system. Clinically, the production of monoclonal antibodies provides a number of targeted therapies for a variety of diseases, including cancer and autoimmunity (Chapter 38). The development of the technology leading to cell lines synthesizing and secreting monoclonal antibodies resulted in the awarding of the Nobel Prize in Physiology or Medicine in 1984 to Georges J.F. Köhler and Cesar Milstein for "the discovery of the principle for production of monoclonal antibodies."

CONCLUSION

The studies reviewed in this chapter provide the evidence that resulted in the acceptance of the clonal selection theory. Antibody-forming lymphocytes synthesize antibodies of a single specificity, explaining several immunologic phenomena, including specificity and memory. At the time these studies were performed, the separation of lymphocytes into functionally discrete populations of T and B lymphocytes had not yet occurred. Accordingly, these experiments focused on the lymphocytes responsible for antibody production. Similar observations about the specificity of T lymphocytes have been made (Chapter 17).

These results allowed the design of experiments that answered the following questions:

- the mechanisms involved in activation of T and B lymphocytes (Chapters 19 and 20);
- the molecular biology of the generation of antibody and T lymphocyte diversity (Chapter 18);
- the mechanisms responsible for imposing self-nonself-discrimination on B and T lymphocytes (Chapters 21 and 22); and
- the regulation of the adaptive immune response maintaining homeostasis (Chapter 24).

References

Attardi, G., Cohn, M., Horibata, K., Lennox, E.S., 1959. Symposium on the biology of cells modified by viruses or antigens. II On the analysis of antibody synthesis at the cellular level. Bacteriol. Rev. 23, 213–223.

Bence Jones, H., 1848. On the new substance occurring in the urine of a patient with mollities ossium. Philos. Trans. R. Soc. Lond. 138, 55–62.

Burnet, F.M., 1957. A modification of Jerne's theory of antibody production using the concept of clonal selection. Aust. J. Sci. 20, 67–69.

Burnet, F.M., Fenner, F., 1949. The Production of Antibodies, second ed. Macmillan, London. p. 149.

Coons, A.H., Leduc, E.H., Connolly, J.M., 1955. Studies on antibody production. I. A method for the histochemical demonstration of specific antibody and its application to a study of the hyperimmune rabbit. J. Exp. Med. 102, 49–60.

Davie, J.M., Paul, W.E., 1971. Receptors on immunocompetent cells. II. Specificity and nature of receptors of dinitrophenylated guinea pig albumin 125I-binding lymphocytes of normal guinea pigs. J. Exp. Med. 134, 495–516.

Edelman, G.M., Gally, J.A., 1962. The nature of Bence-Jones proteins: chemical similarities to polypeptide chains of myeloma globulins and normal gamma-globulins. J. Exp. Med. 116, 207–227.

Fagraeus, A., 1948. The plasma cellular reaction and its relation to the formation of antibodies in vitro. J. Immunol. 58, 1–13.

Green, J., Vassalli, P., Nussenzweig, V., Benacerraf, B., 1967. Specificity of the antibodies produced by single cells following immunization with antigens bearing two types of antigenic determinants. J. Exp. Med. 125, 511–526.

Jerne, N.K., 1955. The natural selection theory of antibody formation. Proc. Natl. Acad. Sci. U.S.A. 41, 849–857.

Kohler, G., Milstein, C., 1975. Continuous cultures of fused cells secreting antibody of predefined specificity. Nature 256, 495–497.

Korngold, L., Lipari, R., 1956. Multiple myeloma proteins. III. The antigenic relationship of Bence Jones proteins to normal gamma-globulin and multiple-myeloma serum proteins. Cancer 9, 262–272.

Kunkel, H.G., 1968. The "abnormality" of myeloma proteins. Cancer Res. 28, 1351–1353.

Lederberg, J., 1954. A simple method for isolating individual microbes. J. Bacteriol. 68, 258–259.

Longworth, L.G., Shedlovsky, T., Mac Innes, D.A., 1939. Electrophoretic patterns of normal and pathological human blood, serum and plasma. J. Exp. Med. 70, 399–413.

Marchalonis, J.J., Nossal, G.J.V., 1968. Electrophoretic analysis of antibody produced by single cells. Proc. Natl. Acad. Sci. U.S.A. 61, 860–867.

Miller, G.L., Brown, C.E., Miller, E.E., Eitelman, E.S., 1952. An electrophoretic study on the origin of the abnormal plasma proteins in multiple myeloma. Cancer Res. 12, 716–719.

Möller, G., 1961. Demonstration of mouse isoantigens at the cellular level by the fluorescent antibody technique. J. Exp. Med. 114, 415–434.

Nossal, G.J.V., 2002. One cell, one antibody: prelude and aftermath. Immunol. Rev. 185, 15–23.

Nossal, G.J.V., Lederberg, J., 1958. Antibody production by single cells. Nature 181, 1419–1420.

Nossal, G.J.V., Makela, O., 1962. Elaboration of antibodies by single cells. Annu. Rev. Microbiol. 16, 53–74.

Nossal, G.J.V., Pike, B.L., 1976. Single cell studies on the antibody-forming potential of fractionated, hapten-specific B lymphocytes. Immunology 30, 189–202.

Pauling, L., 1940. A theory of the structure and process of formation of antibodies. J. Am. Chem. Soc. 62, 2643–2657.

Raff, M.C., Feldman, M., de Petris, S., 1973. Monospecificity of bone marrow-derived lymphocytes. J. Exp. Med. 137, 1024–1030.

Slater, R.J., Ward, S.M., Kunkel, H.G., 1955. Immunological relationships among the myeloma proteins. J. Exp. Med. 101, 85–108.

Solly, S., 1844. Remarks on the pathology of mollities ossium with cases. Med. Chir. Trans. Lond. 27, 435–461.

Viret, C., Gurr, W., 2009. The origin of the "one cell-one antibody" rule. J. Immunol. 182, 1229–1230.

White, R.G., 1958. Antibody production by single cells. Nature 182, 1383–1384.

TIME LINE

1956	Leonhard Korngold and Rose Lipari demonstrate that Bence Jones proteins are immunoglobulin light chains
1957	F. Macfarlane Burnet proposes the clonal selection theory of antibody formation
1958	Gus Nossal and Joshua Lederberg demonstrate that an antibody-forming cell synthesizes antibodies of a single specificity
1958	R.G. White uses immunofluorescence to demonstrate that antibody-forming cells are unispecific
1960	Henry Kunkel demonstrates that myeloma proteins are antibodies and are the product of a single-transformed B cell
1961	Göran Möller demonstrates that some lymphocytes express immunoglobulin as cell surface receptors
1973	Martin Raff reports that antigen-specific receptors on B cells are of a single specificity
1975	Georges Köhler and Cesar Milstein develop hybridoma technology
1976	Gus Nossal and Beverley Pike demonstrate that antibody produced by a B cell has the same specificity as the antigen-specific cell surface receptor
1984	Nobel Prize in Physiology or Medicine awarded to Köhler and Milstein

8

Self–Non-self Discrimination: How the Immune System Avoids Self-Destruction

INTRODUCTION

The three hallmarks of the adaptive immune response are immunologic specificity, memory of previous exposure, and self–non-self discrimination (Chapter 2). Of these, the ability of the immune system to differentiate between self and non-self (foreign) is critical to maintain homeostasis and to protect against the development of autoimmune disease.

Early in the history of immunology, the idea that an animal could produce antibodies against its own cells seemed counterintuitive and was considered impossible. During the late nineteenth and early twentieth centuries, most immunological studies focused on immune responses that could protect individuals from potentially pathogenic microorganisms. Paul Ehrlich (1854–1915) was one of the first scientists to investigate whether the immune system reacted to self. Based on studies involving goats injected with red blood cells, he formalized the idea that the immune system would not respond to self and introduced the concept of "horror autotoxicus"—literally the fear of self-toxicity.

Contemporaneously with Ehrlich's conclusions, however, other investigators were reporting that antibodies to foreign antigens could cause pathology. The concept that antibodies could both protect against disease (i.e., through the use of vaccines and passive serotherapy) and induce pathology was revolutionary. Examples of pathology caused by antibodies include the characterization of anaphylaxis in 1902 by Paul Portier and Charles Richet, working in Paris, the description of serum sickness in 1905 by Clemens von Pirquet and Bela Schick at the University of Vienna Children's Clinic, and the experimental induction of a localized immune complex reaction in 1903 by Nicholas Maurice Arthus at the Pasteur Institute, Paris. The observations leading to the discovery of these diseases/reactions are presented in Chapters 33 and 39.

Subsequent investigations in the first decade of the twentieth century revealed that an individual could produce an immune response against self that could lead to destructive autoimmune diseases. The history of autoimmunity and the pathologies induced by autoantibodies and autoreactive lymphocytes are covered in greater detail in Chapter 34. The current chapter will focus on the observations made during the first half of the twentieth century that led immunologists to understand the mechanisms by which the immune system differentiates self from non-self.

HORROR AUTOTOXICUS

The concept of horror autotoxicus derived from studies performed by Paul Ehrlich and Julius Morgenroth (1901) at the Institute for Sera Research and Serum Testing (now renamed the Paul Ehrlich Institute) in Frankfurt, Germany. Sera from goats injected with their own red blood cells with red blood cells from other goats or with red blood cells from other species were assayed for the presence of antibodies specific for red blood cells. Goats failed to produce antibodies against their own erythrocytes but did produce antibodies against red blood cells from other species and from other members of their own species. These results led Ehrlich and Morgenroth to postulate that normally an animal would not produce antibodies against self (autoantibodies) or, if formed, they would somehow be prevented from producing damage to self (Silverstein, 1986).

Ehrlich and Morgenroth suggested no mechanism by which the production or activity of autoantibodies was regulated. Knowledge of how antigens are recognized and the mechanism of antibody formation were both rudimentary. A significant amount of experimental work performed over several decades was necessary for our contemporary understanding of how the cells of the immune system discriminate foreign pathogens from self.

PRODUCTION OF AUTOANTIBODIES

Shortly after Ehrlich and Morgenroth introduced the idea of horror autotoxicus, reports of antibodies produced by humans and other species to autologous tissues (i.e., spermatozoa, brain, lens of the eye) appeared in the literature. Antibodies induced by injection of self-antigens in most of these studies failed to result in pathology. However, in 1904, Julius Donath and Karl Landsteiner presented evidence that autoantibodies were responsible for the pathology observed in a human disease, paroxysmal cold hemoglobinuria (PCH).

PCH is a rare clinical syndrome characterized by hemolytic anemia and the presence of large amounts of hemoglobin in the urine of patients exposed to the cold. In the early 1900s, 90% of the patients presenting with PCH had a positive test for syphilis a sexually transmitted disease caused by Treponema pallidum. With the introduction of antibiotics to treat syphilis, the incidence of PCH has significantly declined. Now the disease is seen primarily in infants following a viral infection.

Donath and Landsteiner, working with patients diagnosed with PCH at the University of Vienna, identified a substance in their serum (autoantibody) that bound their red blood cells and, under appropriate conditions,

resulted in the lysis of these cells (through activation of complement). This autoantibody has specificity for the P antigen found on human erythrocytes; it is thought that the molecular structure of this red cell antigen is similar to the molecular structure of an antigenic determinant found on the infecting pathogen (either *Treponema pallidum* or a virus) and that the autoantibody is induced due to molecular mimicry; that is, an antibody synthesized in response to the pathogen will react with the self-antigen.

Other anecdotal reports of pathology due to autoantibodies were published sporadically between 1910 and 1945 and include

- sympathetic ophthalmia (inflammation of the eye in a patient who had previously suffered a penetrating injury of the contralateral eye);
- renal pathology in rabbits injected with homologous kidney; and
- neurological pathology as a sequelae of rabies vaccination.

The initial rabies vaccine, developed by Louis Pasteur and Emile Roux in the mid-1880s, derived from the dried spinal cord of rabbits infected with rabies virus. These early vaccines contained some rabbit nervous tissue. The vaccine was administered to patients exposed to a rabid animal. The vaccination protocol involved a series of injections over several days; this protected most individuals who had been infected by the rabies virus. However, patients in whom the vaccine "failed" often received a second round of injections of the vaccine. Some of these individuals developed ascending paralysis (loss of muscle activity starting in the lower limbs and ascending throughout the body) with a mortality rate of approximately 30%.

An explanation for these clinical findings was that the vaccine activated the immune response of the patient to produce antibodies to the rabbit nervous tissue. These antibodies cross-reacted with human nervous tissue, inducing inflammation in both the peripheral and central nervous systems and leading to demyelination and the resulting paralysis.

In 1934, Francis Schwentker and Thomas Rivers, working at the Rockefeller Institute of Medical Research, tested the hypothesis that the neurological sequelae following rabies vaccine result from the formation of anti-brain antibodies. They injected rabbits repeatedly with brain extracts or emulsions, then quantitated antibodies specific for the brain. Injection of fresh emulsions of brain did not induce antibody, while injections of brain that had been allowed to sit for five or more days or that had been mixed with an immunological stimulant such as vaccinia virus induced significant concentrations of antibodies specific for myelin. Several of the injected rabbits that produced antibodies to myelin were also partially paralyzed. Histological observations of the brains of these animals revealed foci of perivascular infiltration and necrosis surrounded by inflammation.

These results prompted a search for a better rabies vaccine that would not induce encephalopathy. A new and improved vaccine was developed from rabies virus adapted to grow in fertile chicken eggs. However, this caused reactions in individuals with allergy to eggs. Virus was then grown in animal cell lines, but this also caused reactions in some individuals due to the presence of foreign animal proteins. Currently, vaccines are derived from virus grown in human diploid cells and are therefore free from many of the antigens that can induce unintended pathological immune responses.

Experimental Induction of Autoimmune Thyroid Disease

Noel Rose (1927 to present), working in the laboratory of Ernest Witebsky (1901–1969) at the State University of New York, Buffalo, demonstrated the ability of specific antibodies to the thyroid to produce autoimmune disease (Witebsky et al., 1957; Rose, 1991). Rose injected rabbits with relatively pure thyroglobulin from cows and other species. Thyroglobulin is a protein synthesized and used by the thyroid gland to produce the hormones of the gland. The antibodies induced by these injections were specific for the thyroid gland and often cross-reacted with the thyroid of other species. Injection of rabbits with rabbit thyroglobulin, however, failed to induce any antibodies specific for the thyroid.

Rose speculated that this lack of an antibody response to rabbit thyroglobulin was due to the presence in the rabbits of circulating thyroglobulin that interfered with the synthesis of antibodies to thyroglobulin. To investigate this postulate, Rose and his colleagues injected thyroidectomized rabbits with thyroglobulin isolated from the rabbit's own thyroids. Since the thyroid gland from a single animal yielded only a small amount of thyroglobulin, Rose increased the immunogenicity of the thyroglobulin by emulsifying the antigen with the immunostimulant complete Freund's adjuvant (CFA), a water-in-oil emulsion containing killed *Mycobacterium*. All rabbits injected subcutaneously with this mixture produced antibodies against their own thyroglobulin.

As a control, rabbits in which one lobe of the thyroid was removed were also injected with their own thyroglobulin incorporated in CFA. Unexpectedly, these hemithyroidectomized animals also produced antibodies specific for thyroglobulin. Even sham-thyroidectomized rabbits (rabbits subjected to a mock surgery without

removal of the thyroid gland) injected with rabbit thyroglobulin in CFA produced specific antibodies to thyroglobulin. This outcome reflected the fact that the immune system could be made to respond to "self" if appropriately stimulated. It also provided an experimental protocol for animal models of induced autoimmune disease.

Histological sections of thyroids from these animals revealed tissue heavily infiltrated with mononuclear cells. John Paine, a surgeon who had assisted with the thyroidectomies, noted similarities between thyroid glands from injected rabbits and thyroid glands from patients with Hashimoto thyroiditis. Sera from patients with Hashimoto thyroiditis tested positive for the presence of antithyroglobulin antibodies. This initial description of an induced autoimmune disease has formed the basis for a large number of investigations. These observations concerning the induction of autoimmune diseases will be described in greater detail in the chapter on autoimmune disease (Chapter 34).

AN EXPERIMENT OF NATURE

Ray Owen, a young faculty member in the departments of genetics and veterinary science at the University of Wisconsin, made an observation that would have major repercussions on understanding how the immune system distinguishes self from non-self. Owen (1915–2014) earned his PhD from the University of Wisconsin in 1941. As a junior faculty member, he investigated freemartin dizygotic twin cattle who shared circulatory systems in utero.

Owen was interested in consequences that may have resulted from this naturally occurring chimerism. The term chimera originates from Greek mythology and refers to a monstrous hybrid creature composed of the parts of more than one animal. Owen studied the blood types of bovine fraternal twins and demonstrated that the majority of such twins have identical blood types (Owen, 1945). The incidence of identical twins in cattle is rare, and the number of different, genetically determined blood groups is large (40 at the time of the study). Owen argued that the most likely explanation for his finding was that the twins shared a single blood supply as embryos. Based on these findings, Owen concluded that "an interchange of cells between bovine twin embryos occurs as a result of vascular anastomoses." Since most of the cattle studied were adults, he further concluded that the interchange involved hematopoietic stem cells that became resident in the bone marrow and continued to produce new cells throughout the life of the animal.

Several other observations were reported that are consistent with this interpretation:

- One of the chimeric bulls Owen studied did not transmit some of the blood group antigens he expressed to any of his 20 offspring. Thus, his germline genotype, as inferred from his progeny, seemed to lack genes coding for the blood groups he possessed. These blood groups were ones that were expressed in his twin, and the progenitor cells most likely came from that animal.
- Twins of opposite sex that had been sired by different bulls had identical blood types, including two antigens that could not have been inherited from either the mother or from the bull that sired them. The only logical source of the genetic material coding for these antigens was the other twin.
- Normally, all red cells in an animal express the same antigens since they derive from a common hematopoietic stem cell. Some of the twins studied by Owen possessed a mixture of two antigenically distinct types of red blood cells.

Evidence that Twin Cattle Are Immunological Chimeras

Peter Medawar (1915–1987) expanded these observations by investigating whether one twin could accept a skin graft from the other twin. Most grafts exchanged between cattle twins were accepted; this result was expected if the twins were monozygotic, but it was also true when the twins were known to be dizygotic (Anderson et al., 1951; Billingham et al., 1952). One possible explanation cited by the authors is that the dizygotic twins are somehow "desensitized" to skin antigens of their sibling. They further suggest that since the embryo is immunologically inactive (i.e., unable to synthesize antibodies), perhaps the "antigen confronts the embryo's gradually awakening faculty of immunological response," thereby altering the immune reactivity of the developing cells.

F. Macfarlane Burnet and Frank Fenner (1949) observed that animals did not respond to an immunogenic challenge until late in fetal life or shortly after birth. They hypothesized that the developing immune system could not respond to immunogenic material introduced during embryogenesis. The extension of this idea was that any immunogenic material with which cells of the immune system came in contact during embryogenesis would be treated as self. Antigens that were first experienced after this period would be treated as non-self and induce an immune response.

This idea that the immune system needs to "learn" the difference between self and non-self during development was a total change from the then contemporary understanding of the immune system. In the late 1940s, most immunologists still accepted instruction models of antibody formation (Chapter 6). In these models, antibody was synthesized by cells that first phagocytized antigen. In addition, antigens were defined as anything foreign to the individual. Therefore, self-components were not thought of as antigens, and the lack of a response to self could be explained by an inability to phagocytize self. While this is a circular argument, it appears that little thought was given at the time about why the immune system did not normally respond to self.

It would be another eight years before Burnet proposed his clonal selection theory that included the idea that lymphocytes passed through a stage in their development during which they could be inactivated through antigen contact.

ACQUISITION OF SELF–NON-SELF DISCRIMINATION

Peter Medawar and his colleagues provided conclusive evidence that immunocompetent lymphocytes go through a stage in their development during which interaction with antigen leads to the destruction or inhibition of that cell's specific ability to respond to that antigen (Billingham et al., 1953). Medawar (1915–1987), working at Oxford, studied immunological mechanisms responsible for skin graft rejection. During World War II, he focused his interest to determining improved methods for skin grafting and controlling graft rejection, particularly in individuals suffering from severe burns. The large number of burn victims resulting from bombings influenced his studies. The War Wounds Committee of the British Medical Council assigned Medawar to investigate why grafts between unrelated individuals invariably failed. At the time, graft failure was considered to reflect the surgeon's skill; however, Medawar demonstrated that the failure was due to an immunological reaction (Chapter 36).

In 1948, Medawar moved to Birmingham University, and in 1951 he became the Jodrell Professor of Zoology at University College in London. One of his former students at Oxford, Rupert E. Billingham (1921–2002), joined him at University College and they, along with Leslie Brent (1925 to present), focused on experiments based on the observations made by Ray Owen and the predictions of Burnet.

Billingham, Brent, and Medawar designed an experiment based on the principle "that mammals and birds never develop, or develop to only a limited degree, the power to react immunologically against foreign homologous tissue cells to which they have been exposed sufficiently early in foetal life" (Billingham et al., 1953). The basic outline of the protocol is depicted in Figure 8.1.

Billingham and colleagues injected a mixture of adult cells (testis, kidney, and spleen) from one inbred strain of mice (A) into embryonic mice of a second inbred strain

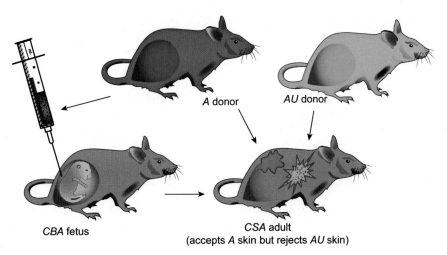

A donor

AU donor

CBA fetus

CSA adult
(accepts A skin but rejects AU skin)

FIGURE 8.1 Diagram of the experimental protocol used by Billingham and colleagues to demonstrate immunological tolerance. CBA embryos were injected with cells from a strain A mouse. Once these treated mice became adults, they accepted skin grafts from strain A animals but not from an unrelated strain (AU). *From Obhari and Lakkis (2004), Nature Medicine 10, 2265.*

(CBA) to mimic the naturally occurring vascular anastomosis observed in cattle twins. In their first experiment, five out of six treated embryos survived and appeared normal at birth. At 8 weeks of age, these treated CBA strain mice received skin grafts from A mice. Normally, such skin grafts survived 11.0 ± 0.3 days. At 11 days, two of the grafts were inflamed and necrotic (signs of rejection) while the other three grafts appeared normal. Since A strain mice are albinos, the grafted tissue could be distinguished from host CBA skin, which is agouti. Each of the successful grafts grew hair and appeared to be incorporated into the skin of the host.

The three successful grafts remained viable until two additional experiments were performed.

1. Fifty days after the original grafting, one of the mice with a successful graft received a second graft from an A strain mouse. This graft as well as the original graft continued to survive.
2. On days 77 and 101 following grafting, mice bearing successful skin grafts were injected with lymph node fragments from CBA mice that had rejected a skin graft from an A strain mouse. This experiment was performed to rule out the possibility that the skin grafts had modulated their antigens and were no longer foreign. The successful grafts on these two animals underwent rejection 2–3 days later.

Additional studies on other litters of mice and different strain combinations were reported in the original publication and provided further characterization of the phenomenon of immunological tolerance (unresponsiveness), including the following:

- the length of graft survival differs from animal to animal, with some mice accepting grafts indefinitely while others show only slight prolongation of graft survival;

- the acceptance of grafts is immunologically specific; that is, a skin graft from a third inbred strain to the treated mice is rejected in approximately 11 days;
- injection of several different tissues into embryos results in extended graft survival;
- induction of graft prolongation required the foreign cells to be injected prior to birth of the mice; and
- grafts removed from treated hosts after several weeks and transplanted to normal animals were rejected as normal transplants.

Billingham and colleagues also reported companion studies in which chicken embryos of one strain were injected, intravenously, with whole blood from a second strain. Fourteen days after hatching, the injected birds were grafted with skin from the blood donor. Five out of seven animals from this experiment showed prolonged graft survival.

Contemporaneously with this paper, a similar study was published by Milan Hašek (1953). Hašek (1925–1984) studied in Prague and received the MD degree from Charles University. He earned a PhD from the Czechoslovak Academy of Sciences where he soon became director of the Department of Experimental Biology and Genetics. At the time, Czechoslovakia was politically aligned with the Soviet Union, which had adopted a system of genetics based on concepts originally promulgated by Jean Baptiste Lamarck (1744–1829). Lamarck hypothesized that traits acquired during an individual's lifetime could be inherited by subsequent generations. In the 1930s, Trofim Lysenko developed a form of Lamarckism in the Soviet Union to satisfy the opposition of Joseph Stalin to Western (Mendelian) genetics. Lysenkoism was used to explain results of plant grafting developed by I.V. Michurin and became official doctrine of the state. The acceptance and teaching of Lamarckian genetics rather than Mendelian genetics in the Soviet bloc severely impeded the development of modern genetics in countries under Soviet influence in several fields, including agriculture and medicine (Ivanyi, 2003).

Hašek designed a protocol that he thought would demonstrate the inheritance of acquired characteristics in vertebrates (Figure 8.2). In several aspects, Hašek's experiments mimicked Owen's observations in cattle more closely than did Billingham's mouse experiment. Hašek had developed a method for parabiotically connecting the blood supply of developing birds while they were still in ovo. He achieved this parabiosis by exposing the egg membranes to each other using a bridge of blastoderm tissue removed from embryos incubated for 20–40h. This bridge allowed the development of blood vessels between the two embryos and the free mixing of the blood cells. In several experiments he produced chickens of one strain (White Leghorn) that had developed under the influence of the circulatory system of either a second strain of chicken (Rhode Island Red) or of Peking ducks.

Eggs incubated under these conditions and allowed to hatch resulted in birds that contained blood cells derived from both parabiotic partners. When the chickens that hatched from these eggs were injected with red blood cells from their partner, they failed to produce antibody to those erythrocytes although they did produce antibodies to the red cells of an unrelated chicken. Hašek concluded that "the presence of partner's agglutinogens (antigens) during parabiosis led to the lack of antibody response in adult age."

These two studies, using different experimental approaches, demonstrated that exposure of an embryo or fetus to foreign cells resulted in the inability to respond to these cells later in life. Billingham et al. (1953) concluded that this unresponsiveness was due to the induction of adaptively acquired tolerance, which they contrasted with the development of adaptively acquired immunity. Both tolerance and immunity are possible outcomes when antigen interacts with lymphocytes of the immune system. Hašek interpreted his findings as being due to some type of metabolic effects. Although the introduction to his paper summarizes Lysenko's doctrine, Hašek did not use this doctrine to interpret his results and never bred the chickens produced to determine if the acquired characteristic (immunologic unresponsiveness or tolerance) was heritable. Subsequent studies from Hašek's laboratory demonstrated that his parabionts accepted skin grafts from the foreign partner (Hašek et al., 1959). These results led Hašek to agree with the interpretation of Billingham and colleagues that lymphocytes developing in a particular environment accepted the antigens present in that environment as self.

The hypothetical work by Burnet and the experimental studies by Medawar's group advanced the understanding of how the immune system develops and matures. Burnet's prediction that antigen-reactive lymphocytes go through a stage in development during which they are sensitive to being inactivated by contact with foreign antigen was proven correct by the experimental studies performed in London by Billingham and his colleagues and in Prague by Hašek. These studies resulted in the awarding of the Nobel Prize in Physiology or Medicine in 1960 to Medawar and Burnet "for discovery of acquired immunological tolerance."

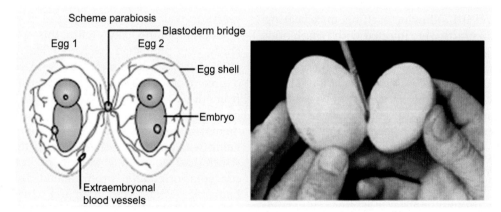

FIGURE 8.2   Diagram (on the left) of the process developed by Milan Hašek to produce parabiosis between two fertilized chicken eggs. Small holes are drilled into the shells of eggs after 8–12 days of incubation, exposing the chorioallantoic membranes. A bridge between the two embryos is constructed using blastoderm tissue from a 20–40h fertilized egg. Blood vessels grow across this bridge, providing a common vascular system for the two developing embryos. The photo on the right demonstrates the process of joining the eggs and sealing the vascular bridge with paraffin. *From Ivanyi (2003), Nature Rev. Immunol. 3, 591.*

CONCLUSION

Experiments described in this chapter advance our understanding of the way the immune system develops and functions. Immunologists now agree that antigen-reactive lymphocytes go through a developmental phase during which they are eliminated if they respond to self or to an artificially introduced foreign antigen. Lymphocytes that survive this process constitute the cells capable of protecting against infection by foreign pathogens.

Immunological tolerance is the lack of a response by an immunocompetent individual to antigens that normally elicit an adaptive immune response. The process of tolerance induction occurs in each individual during lymphocyte maturation. The concept of immunological tolerance describes the mechanism by which the immune system differentiates self from non-self. Abrogation of self-tolerance explains the development of autoimmune disease. The exact process responsible for eliminating self-reactive T and B lymphocytes is described in subsequent chapters (Chapter 21 for B lymphocytes and Chapter 22 for T lymphocytes). Autoimmune diseases are presented in Chapter 34.

These studies on the induction of immunologic tolerance were performed in an era when little was known about the genetics and structure of the histocompatibility antigens or about the roles of the thymus and bursa in the development of immunocompetent lymphocytes. They also were performed prior to Burnet's formulation of the clonal selection hypothesis (although he had proposed a mechanism for tolerance in his 1949 book, *The Production of Antibodies*). Clinically, an appreciation of immunologic tolerance was originally hailed as a breakthrough in providing methods to enhance survival of tissue and organ grafts. Unfortunately, the induction of immunologic tolerance in potential graft recipients has not succeeded as originally anticipated. However, this knowledge remains useful in developing therapeutic interventions for patients presenting with autoimmune diseases (Chapter 34) or other immune-mediated diseases such as allergy (Chapter 33).

References

Anderson, D., Billingham, R.E., Lampkin, G.H., Medawar, P.B., 1951. The use of skin grafting to distinguish between monozygotic and dizygotic twins in cattle. Heredity 5, 379–397.

Arthus, M., 1903. Injections répétées de serum du cheval chez le lapin. Compt. Rend. Soc. Biol. 55, 817–820.

Billingham, R.E., Brent, L., Medawar, P.B., 1953. 'Actively acquired tolerance' of foreign cells. Nature 172, 603–606.

Billingham, R.E., Lampkin, G.H., Medawar, P.B., Williams, L.L., 1952. Tolerance to homografts, twin diagnosis, and the freemartin condition in cattle. Heredity 6, 201–212.

Burnet, F.M., Fenner, F., 1949. Production of Antibodies, second ed. MacMillan, London.

Donath, J., Landsteiner, K., 1904. Uber paroxysmile Hamoglobinurie. Muchen. Med. Wochenschr. 51, 1590–1593.

Ehrlich, P., Morgenroth, J., 1901. Uber Haumlmolysine. Berl. Klin. Wochenschr. 38, 251–257.

Hašek, M., 1953. Vegetative hybridization of animals by joint blood circulation during embryonal development (Czech by Ivanyi, J., 2003, Trans.). Transplantation 76, 1412–1421.

Hašek, M., Hraba, T., Hort, J., 1959. Acquired immunological tolerance of heterografts. Nature 183, 1199–1200.

Ivanyi, J., 2003. Milan Hašek and the discovery of immunological tolerance. Nat. Rev. Immunol. 3, 591–597.

Obhari, J.S., Lakkis, F.G., 2004. Transplantation tolerance: babies take the first step. Nat. Med. 10, 1165–1166.

Owen, R.D., 1945. Immunogenetic consequences of vascular anastomoses between bovine twins. Science 102, 400–401.

Portier, P., Richet, C., 1902. De l'action anaphylactique de certains venins. Compt. Rend. Soc. Biol. 54, 170–172.

Rose, N.R., 1991. The discovery of thyroid autoimmunity. Immunol. Today 12, 167–168.

Schwentker, F.F., Rivers, T.M., 1934. The antibody response of rabbits to injections of emulsions and extracts of homologous brain. J. Exp. Med. 60, 559–574.

Silverstein, A.M., 1986. History of immunology. The Donath-Landsteiner autoantibody: the incommensurable languages of early immunologic debate. Cell. Immunol. 97, 173–188.

von Pirquet, C.E., Schick, B., 1905. Die Serumkrankheit. Franz Deuticke, Leipzig/Wien.

Witebsky, E., Rose, N.R., Terplan, K., Paine, J.R., Egan, R.W., 1957. Chronic thyroiditis and autoimmunization. J. Amer. Med. Assoc. 164, 1439–1447.

TIME LINE

1901	Paul Ehrlich and Julius Morgenroth develop concept of "horror autotoxicus"
1904	Julius Donath and Karl Landsteiner describe the role of antiself red blood cell antibodies in the pathogenesis of paroxysmal cold hemoglobinuria
1945	Ray Owen describes blood cell chimerism in freemartin cattle
1949	F. Macfarlane Burnet and Frank Fenner hypothesize that developing antigen-reactive cells are susceptible to tolerance induction
1951	Peter Medawar and colleagues prove that freemartin cattle permanently accept skin grafts from their twin
1953	Rupert Billingham, Leslie Brent, and Peter Medawar demonstrate the induction of immunological nonresponsiveness by injecting neonatal mice with foreign cells
1953	Milan Hašek reports on the induction of unresponsiveness between birds subjected to parabiosis as embryos
1957	Ernest Witebsky and Noel Rose publish the initial description of antiself antibodies, leading to an autoimmune disease (Hashimoto thyroiditis)
1960	Nobel Prize in Physiology or Medicine awarded to Peter Medawar and Macfarlane Burnet

CHAPTER

9

The Thymus in Lymphocyte Maturation

INTRODUCTION

For much of the first half of the twentieth century, biology textbooks and reviews of the thymus declared the function of the thymus unknown. As recently as 1954, Professor Geoffrey Keynes, presenting The Thomas Young Memorial Lecture to the Royal Society of London on "The Physiology of the Thymus Gland," decried his frustration at the lack of definitive information about the function of the thymus, concluding his lecture with the following paragraph:

> The pathological and clinical (may I even say surgical?) approach has thus furnished us with a working hypothesis on which the function of the thymus gland may eventually be elucidated. There are still many difficulties in the way of a final solution, and progress is likely to be slow. It may be thought safer to return for the present to Galen's belief that the thymus is just a cushion to protect the great vessels from contact with the sternum. This would certainly save us all a great deal of trouble (Keynes, 1954).

Today immunologists agree that the thymus is a central lymphoid organ, which, along with the bursa of Fabricius (in birds) and bone marrow (in mammals), is required for the development of immunocompetent lymphocytes. The thymus develops from the third and fourth pharyngeal pouches (which are also the origins of the parathyroid glands) and is located in the superior mediastinum. Lymphoid progenitor cells migrate initially from hematopoietic tissues in the fetus (the yolk sac and fetal liver) and then from the bone marrow during fetal and neonatal life

to populate the thymus. In the thymus, lymphoid precursors mature to immunocompetent T lymphocytes that express antigen-specific cell surface receptors. These lymphocytes respond to various pathogens, including bacteria, virally infected cells, and malignantly transformed cancer cells. The thymus represents an environment in which self–non-self-discrimination occurs, resulting in the elimination of potentially autoreactive T lymphocytes that could give rise to autoimmune disease.

EARLY HISTORY OF THE THYMUS

The thymus is largest, relative to total body size, at birth and involutes during adolescence. Histologically, the small lymphocyte is the predominant cell type in the thymus. John Beard (1900), an embryologist at the University of Edinburgh, Scotland, proposed that the thymus was the source of the small lymphocytes in circulation and in lymphoid organs such as the spleen and lymph nodes. Observations that the thymus is replaced with fibrous and adipose tissue in the adult led other investigators to disagree with this conclusion. In addition, the role of small lymphocytes in the immune system had yet to be deciphered (Chapter 4). As a result, textbooks written before 1961 treated the thymus as a part of the endocrine system or as a vestigial organ that had lost its primary function during the course of evolution.

Prior to 1960, investigators designed numerous experiments to determine the function of the thymus. One classical approach to study the function of any organ is

A Historical Perspective on Evidence-Based Immunology
http://dx.doi.org/10.1016/B978-0-12-398381-7.00009-5

to remove that organ surgically and describe the consequence on the physiology of the animal. Investigators surgically removed the thymus from various experimental animals but failed to uncover any consistent deficit. These negative results were most likely due to two aspects of experimental design:

- most investigators thymectomized animals as adults rather than early in life when the organ is performing its primary function, and
- the focus of many of these early studies was the endocrine system rather than the immune system.

We now know that the major role of the thymus is to provide T lymphocytes to the peripheral immune system and that this occurs prior to or shortly after birth.

A few early studies of animals thymectomized during the neonatal stage suggested the actual function of the organ. Noel Paton and Alexander Goodall (1904), working at the Royal College of Physicians in Edinburgh, Scotland, performed a large series of studies involving thymectomy of several different animal species. Among other findings, they report on two guinea pigs, one of which (A) was thymectomized on the day of birth while the littermate (B) served as control. Approximately 2 months later "they were then injected with streptococci, of which A died, but B lived." This particular observation received no further attention in their publication. Other investigators reported the occurrence of wasting disease in thymectomized animals or the inability of euthymic animals to clear infections, but the realization that the thymus played a role in the immune system evaded these scientists.

By the late 1950s, biologists noted that the thymus generated large numbers of small lymphocytes although the function of those lymphocytes was unknown. Small lymphocytes contain scant cytoplasm with no obvious functional organelles or granules as seen in other leukocytes of the peripheral blood. Small lymphocytes were thought to be end-stage cells waiting to die.

Additional findings that argued against the thymus having a role in providing immune protection included

- injection of antigen directly into the thymus did not produce the histological changes seen in other lymphoid organs,
- antibody-forming cells or plasma cells were not found in the thymus during either a systemic or local response to a foreign antigen,
- removal of the thymus at or after puberty did not affect the longevity of the animal or appear to alter its immunological capabilities, and
- transfer of thymic cells into an irradiated animal failed to reconstitute the antibody-forming capacity of that animal.

Our contemporary understanding that the thymus is a central lymphoid organ responsible for development of immunocompetent T lymphocytes is consistent with these results. Today immunologists agree that the thymus contains virtually no antibody-forming B lymphocytes and few mature immunocompetent cells.

SERENDIPITY AND NEONATAL THYMECTOMY

In 1958, Jacques Miller, a PhD student at the Chester Beatty Research Institute in London, serendipitously discovered that the thymus plays a significant role in the maturation of the adaptive immune response during his studies of the mechanism by which murine leukemia virus (MLV) induced leukemia in different strains of mice.

While working with mice with a low incidence of naturally occurring leukemia, Miller in 1959 demonstrated that the thymus is required for the development of leukemia. Mice injected with MLV as neonates and subsequently thymectomized at weaning failed to develop leukemia. Implantation of thymic tissue into these mice 6 months later resulted in the development of leukemia. Subsequent investigations showed that the virus remained latent and could be isolated from lymphoid tissues of the thymectomized animals, suggesting that the thymus was necessary to provide an anatomical repository for the oncogenic virus.

Miller next investigated the role the thymus played in allowing the virus to proliferate in nonthymic tissues. Since the virus had to be injected into the mice at birth to successfully induce leukemia, Miller thymectomized mice at birth prior to inoculation with the virus. At the time, Miller was housing his experimental animals in space he had been assigned in a decommissioned horse barn, which was likely contaminated with murine pathogens that probably played a role in his breakthrough. Although he was studying the growth of the virus, the key finding of this study was that more than 50% of mice thymectomized at 1 day of age died from infection within 2–4 months whether they had been injected with virus or not. These results led Miller to conclude that "the thymus at birth may be essential to life" (Miller, 1961a).

Subsequently, Miller altered the focus of his experiments to study the hypothesis that the thymus plays a critical role in the development of immune competence. In Miller's next study, mice 1–16 h of age were either thymectomized or sham-thymectomized (animals subjected to surgical manipulation without removal of the thymus) and allowed to recover. This protocol did not include injection with virus. Thymectomized mice had a significantly decreased number of lymphocytes in the peripheral blood and diminished histologic development of lymph nodes when compared with sham-operated controls. More exciting, as depicted in Table 9.1, nine of the 13 neonatally

TABLE 9.1   Survival of Allogeneic Skin Grafts in Thymectomized Mice *(From Miller, 1961b)*. Groups of Mice Were Thymectomized on the Day of Birth or at 5 Days of Age. Some of the Neonatally Thymectomized Mice Received a Syngeneic Thymus Graft at 3 Weeks of Age. Mice were Transplanted With Skin From Various Strains of Mice and the Survival of the Grafts Recorded. Controls Consisted of Mice That Were Sham-Thymectomized on the Day of Birth or Left Intact

Survival of allogenic skin grafts in mice thymectomized in the neonatal period						
Group	Age at operation	Strain of mice	Skin graft	Number grafted	Number tolerant	Median survival time of graft (days)
Thymectomized	1–16 h	C3H	Ak	7	5	45–101[a]
		Ak	C3H	6	4	41–90[a]
		(AkXT6)F$_1$	C3H	8	8	50–118[a]
Thymectomized	5 days	C3H	Ak	5	0	11 ± 0.7
Thymectomized and thymus-grafted 3 weeks later	5 h	C3H	Ak	5	0	11–15
Sham-thymectomized	1–16 h	C3H	Ak	6	0	11 ± 0.6
		Ak	C3H	3	0	10 ± 0.8
Intact		C3H	Ak	61	0	11 ± 0.6
		Ak	C3H	45	0	10 ± 0.9
		(AkXT6)F$_1$	C3H	10	0	11 ± 0.1

[a]These figures apply to the tolerant mice.

thymectomized mice accepted skin allografts indefinitely during the period of the study while the sham-operated animals rejected all such grafts (Miller, 1961b). Miller erroneously concluded that thymectomy had induced a state of immunologic tolerance to the allografts in these animals.

Miller used the term tolerance to refer to the lack of responsiveness induced by neonatal thymectomy. Immunologic tolerance was initially demonstrated in 1953 by Rupert Billingham and his colleagues (Chapter 8) and is defined as specific unresponsiveness to an antigen that would normally elicit an immune response. The immune deficiency following neonatal thymectomy is generalized, affecting the response to many, if not all, antigens.

Miller's initial publication provided the following additional insights about the effects of neonatal thymectomy on the adaptive immune response (Table 9.1):

* Most mice thymectomized during the first day of life accepted foreign skin grafts for 40 or more days while mice thymectomized at five days of life rejected foreign skin grafts (allografts) with a mean survival time (MST) of 11 days. This MST is similar to that seen when intact or sham-thymectomized animals were grafted with foreign skin. The interpretation of these results is that the thymus provides immunocompetent lymphocytes to peripheral lymphoid tissue prior to 5 days of life.
* Neonatally thymectomized mice could be rescued if they received a graft of fetal thymus tissue. These reconstituted mice rejected skin allografts within 11–15 days, indicating that the immunocompetence of these animals could be restored.

Confirmation of Thymus Function

Other immunologists soon confirmed and expanded Miller's findings. Karl Erik Fichtelius and his collaborators at the Histological Institute of the University of Uppsala, Sweden (1961), found that guinea pigs thymectomized shortly after birth had a slight but significant decrease in antibody production to foreign antigens. Similarly, Robert Good's group at the University of Minnesota published a series of papers (Dalmasso et al., 1962; Good et al., 1962; Martinez et al., 1962; Papermaster et al., 1962) that evaluated the immune system in thymectomized animals and cataloged the defects produced by neonatal thymectomy.

Robert A. Good (1922–2003) received both the MD and PhD degrees from the University of Minnesota and was trained as a pediatrician. He spent much of his professional career at the University of Minnesota with additional stops at the Sloan-Kettering Institute for Cancer Research in New York, the Oklahoma Medical Research Foundation, and the University of South Florida Medical School. Good pursued basic and clinical immunologic research focused on the ontogeny of the immune system and the identification and treatment of congenital immunodeficiency diseases.

Good's group studied mice, rabbits, and chickens thymectomized as neonates and showed that these animals had decreased numbers of lymphocytes in their peripheral blood and lymphoid organs. They accepted skin allografts for a prolonged period of time. When sensitized systemically with diphtheria toxoid and subsequently tested by an intradermal injection of the toxoid, the thymectomized animals failed to produce a delayed hypersensitivity reaction. Lymphocytes isolated from thymectomized animals failed to induce a graft-versus-host reaction when injected into immunoincompetent animals. These results as well as additional studies performed on bursectomized chickens (Chapter 10) led Good's group to postulate the existence of two functional populations of lymphocytes. Those that require an intact thymus for maturation are called T lymphocytes and are responsible for the various manifestations of cell-mediated immunity, including allograft rejection, delayed hypersensitivity reactions, and the ability to mount a graft-versus-host response, while those that mature in the absence of the thymus produce antibodies and are called B lymphocytes.

Extirpation experiments in several species provided evidence that the thymus is essential for the maturation of some immunocompetent lymphocytes. Confirmation came from parallel studies aimed at reversing the effect of surgical removal of the thymus by grafting the missing organ. Miller demonstrated in his initial experiments that thymectomized mice could be rescued with a thymus graft. Other investigators also designed studies aimed at restoring immune competence to thymectomized animals. Good's group demonstrated that grafting syngeneic thymus cells into neonatally thymectomized mice rescued most of the manipulated animals from early mortality and restored foreign graft rejection. The lymphoid organs of these reconstituted mice appeared histologically intact, and the peripheral blood lymphocytes from these thymus-grafted mice initiated a graft-versus-host reaction (Dalmasso et al., 1963).

A confounding observation made in the course of these reconstitution experiments was that allogeneic thymus grafts failed to restore immune reactivity to thymectomized animals. In an interview with Jacques Miller in January of 2011, Miller stated that not understanding the implications of this observation was the greatest disappointment of his career. The explanation for this outcome required more than a decade of additional studies and was not completely understood until the 1970s when the requirement for histocompatibility between cells collaborating in the adaptive immune response was demonstrated (Chapter 16).

NATURALLY OCCURRING EXAMPLES OF EUTHYMIC STATES

Shortly after the results of experimental thymectomy were published, clinical cases of individuals born lacking a thymus were reported. Undoubtedly, similar patients existed prior to the 1960s, but these individuals, born before the availability of antibiotics, failed to survive beyond infancy and succumbed to common bacterial infections. Antibiotics to treat infections in these patients and the appreciation of the role of the thymus in rodents resulted in renewed interest in these congenital anomalies (see Chapter 32). The clinical descriptions of two groups of euthymic patients confirmed the results derived from animal studies and serve as an example of the interaction between basic immunologic research and its application to clinical observations.

Christian Nezelof (1922–present), a pediatrician and pathologist at Necker Hospital, Paris, reported a case of a patient who presented with a congenital absence of the thymus (Nezelof et al., 1964). Nezelof syndrome, or thymic dysplasia, is a rare, congenital, autosomal recessive immunodeficiency, characterized by an absence of T lymphocyte activity in the presence of normal or near-normal levels of serum immunoglobulin. Patients born with this condition lack a thymic shadow on radiological examination and present with severe, recurrent infections within the first 6 months of life. The infections are primarily due to intracellular pathogens such as viruses, including those responsible for measles and mumps, and fungi such as *Histoplasma capsulatum* and *Cryptococcus neoformans*. Infections with these microbes are the type immunologists have come to expect in patients lacking T lymphocytes. Individuals with this disease invariably die before the age of two unless they receive a graft of fetal thymus.

Two similar patients were reported in 1964 by E.C. Allibone and colleagues in Leeds, England. These infants were siblings whose parents were first cousins. The first patient, a girl, developed pneumonia during the first year of life and died despite treatment with antibiotics. The causative agent was considered to be *Pneumocystis carinii* (*Pneumocystis jiroveci*), an opportunistic pathogen often seen in patients with defective cell-mediated immunity. Her brother succumbed to progressive vaccinia following immunization with smallpox vaccine. In both cases, the level of serum gamma globulin was within reference range although the number of lymphocytes in the peripheral blood and in lymphoid organs was depressed. In one of the cases, thymic tissue could not be found at autopsy.

Angelo DiGeorge (1921–2009), a pediatric endocrinologist at Temple University, was attending a lecture by Max Cooper at the 1965 meeting of the Society of Pediatric Research when he realized that Cooper's results obtained with thymectomized and bursectomized chickens helped make sense of some of the pediatric patients he had been treating. Subsequently, DiGeorge and his colleagues presented another example of infants born without a functional thymus (Lischner et al., 1967). The symptoms seen in these patients confirmed Cooper's data and supported the division of lymphocytes into distinct functional populations.

Patients with DiGeorge syndrome present at birth with life-threatening tetany due to a congenital absence of the parathyroid glands, resulting in a subsequent inability to regulate serum calcium levels. The parathyroid glands, like the thymus, develop embryologically from the third and fourth pharyngeal pouches. Despite therapeutic resolution of serum calcium levels, these infants fail to thrive, and all four original patients succumbed, most likely to microbial infections. On autopsy, no trace of the thymus gland could be found.

DiGeorge syndrome is now known to result from a deletion on chromosome 22. Depending on the extent of the chromosomal material lost, patients exhibit a range of symptoms. In its most severe form, patients with DiGeorge (22q11.2 deletion) syndrome lack T lymphocytes as revealed by a history of recurrent infections, an inability to mount a normal delayed hypersensitivity reaction, and a failure to produce antibodies following injection with several antigens. They also exhibit cardiac malformations and structural defects in the palate obvious at birth. Today pediatricians attribute these interrelated findings to the failure of embryological development of the third and fourth pharyngeal pouches (Fomin et al., 2010).

The discovery of a strain of mice with a congenital absence of the thymus provided additional confirmation that the thymus is essential for the proper development of the adaptive immune system. Nude (nu/nu) mice were first described in 1962 by N.R. Grist in Scotland (Flanagan, 1966). In 1968, E.M. Pantelouris of the University of Strathclyde in Glasgow reported that homozygous nude mice lacked thymuses and had low peripheral blood lymphocyte counts. Jørgen Rygaard, working at the State Serum Institute in Copenhagen, Denmark, reported in 1969 that these hairless mice failed to mount several adaptive immune responses, including delayed type hypersensitivity reactions and rejection of allogeneic tumor and skin grafts. Nude mice have become an important model for the study of the immune system and the role of T lymphocytes in immune responses, including graft rejection, killing of virally infected cells, cytolysis of malignant cells, delayed hypersensitivity, and regulation of antibody synthesis.

CONCLUSION

The research described in this chapter determined the role of the thymus in the adaptive immune response. The thymus had been an enigma for several centuries and was assigned several proposed functions by early investigators. Miller finally unraveled the physiological role of this organ in 1961; there are three reasons why he succeeded while previous investigators had failed:

- Timing—the age of the mice at thymectomy. Immunologists now agree that the thymus performs its most critical functions before and shortly after birth. T lymphocytes mature and migrate to the periphery throughout life, but the most critical time

for this activity is during the fetal and neonatal periods. Other investigators had removed the thymus of older mice (or rabbits or guinea pigs) and failed to detect any increase in the susceptibility of the animals to infections because mature T lymphocytes had already migrated to peripheral lymphoid organs.

- Experimental conditions—the conditions under which the animals were housed. Miller housed his thymectomized mice in a decommissioned horse barn. In this environment, the mice were likely exposed to infectious microorganisms that might have been responsible for their early demise. Other researchers housed their thymectomized animals in a dedicated animal facility that lacked the array of microorganisms found in the horse barn.
- The receptiveness of the investigator to interpreting his data. At the time when he made the observation, Miller had not had extensive training as an immunologist and was much more interested in pursuing research on the induction of leukemia by oncogenic viruses. As with several other important advances in immunology as well as in other areas of experimental science, the observations were made by an individual without preconceived ideas about the results and who was willing to consider unorthodox interpretations.

The discovery of the role of the thymus, along with the almost simultaneous description of the role of the bursa of Fabricius in chickens and the bone marrow in mammals (Chapter 10), in the maturation of immunocompetent lymphocytes provided a foundation for interpreting the mechanisms responsible for the typical adaptive immune response. These breakthroughs led to the development of novel therapies for autoimmune diseases, malignancies, and for overcoming immunological rejection of transplanted tissue and organs.

References

Allibone, E.C., Goldie, W., Marmion, B.P., 1964. *Pneumocystis carinii* pneumonia and progressive vaccinia in siblings. Arc. Dis. Child. 39, 26–34.

Beard, J., 1900. The source of the leukocytes and the true function of the thymus. Anat. Anz. 18, 550–560.

Billingham, R.E., Brent, L., Medawar, P.B., 1953. 'Actively acquired tolerance' of foreign cells. Nature 172, 603–606.

Cooper, M.D., Peterson, R.D.A., Good, R.A., 1965. A new concept of the cellular basis of immunity. J. Ped. 67, 907–908.

Dalmasso, A.P., Martinez, C., Good, R.A., 1962. Further studies of suppression of the homograft reaction by thymectomy in the mouse. Proc. Soc. Exp. Biol. Med. 111, 143–146.

Dalmasso, A.P., Martinez, C., Sjodin, K., Good, R.A., 1963. Studies on the role of the thymus in immunobiology. Reconstitution of immunologic capacity in mice thymectomized at birth. J. Exp. Med. 118, 1089–1109.

Fichtelius, K.E., Laurell, G., Philipsson, I., 1961. The influence of thymectomy on antibody formation. Acta Pathol. Micrbiol. Scand. 51, 81–86.

Flanagan, S.P., 1966. "Nude" a new hairless gene with pleiotropic effects in the mouse. Genet. Res. 8, 295–309.

Fomin, A.B.F., Pastorino, A.C., Kim, C.A., Pereira, A.C., Carneiro-Sampaio, M., Jacob, M.A., 2010. DiGeorge syndrome: a not so rare disease. Clinics 65, 865–869.

Good, R.A., Dalmasso, A.P., Martinez, C., Archer, O.K., Pierce, J.C., Papermaster, B.W., 1962. The role of the thymus in development of immunologic capacity in rabbits and mice. J. Exp. Med. 116, 773–796.

Keynes, G., 1954. The physiology of the thymus gland. Brit. Med. J. 2 (4889), 659–663.

Lischner, H.W., Punnett, H.H., DiGeorge, A.M., 1967. Lymphocytes in the absence of the thymus. Nature 214, 580–582.

Martinez, C., Kersey, J., Papermaster, B.W., Good, R.A., 1962. Skin homograft survival in thymectomized mice. Proc. Soc. Exp. Biol. Med. 109, 193–196.

Miller, J.F.A.P., 1959. Role of the thymus in murine leukemia. Nature 183, 1069.

Miller, J.F.A.P., 1961a. Analysis of the thymus influence in leukaemogenesis. Nature 191, 248–249.

Miller, J.F.A.P., 1961b. Immunological function of the thymus. Lancet 278, 748–749.

Nezelof, C., Jammet, M.L., Lortholary, P., Labrune, B., Lamy, M., 1964. Hereditary thymic hypoplasia: its place and responsibility in a case of lymphocytic, normoplasmocytic and normoglobulinemia aplasia in an infant. Arch. Fr. Pediat. 21, 897–920.

Pantelouris, E.M., 1968. Absence of thymus in a mouse mutant. Nature 217, 370–371.

Papermaster, B.W., Dalmasso, A.P., Martinez, C., Good, R.A., 1962. Suppression of antibody forming capacity with thymectomy in the mouse. Proc. Soc. Exp. Biol. Med. 111, 41–43.

Paton, D.N., Goodall, A., 1904. A contribution to the physiology of the thymus. J. Physiol. 31, 49–64.

Rygaard, J., 1969. Immunobiology of the mouse mutant, "nude". Preliminary investigations. Acta Pathol. Microbiol. Scand. 77, 761–762.

TIME LINE

1904	Noel Paton and Alexander Goodall report that a guinea pig thymectomized on the day of birth succumbed to an injection of streptococci
1961	Jacque Miller demonstrates that removal of the thymus in mice on the first day of life led to death within 2–4 months
1962	Robert Good and colleagues report that neonatally thymectomized mice fail to demonstrate a normal delayed type hypersensitivity response or rejection of foreign skin grafts
1963	Robert Good shows that deficiencies in the immune response resulting from thymectomy could be replaced by thymus grafts
1964	Christian Nezelof describes the first clinical example of thymic hypoplasia
1965	Max Cooper and colleagues demonstrate a division of function of lymphocytes using thymectomized and bursectomized chickens
1967	Angelo DiGeorge reports four patients born without a functional thymus
1968	E.M. Pantelouris reports that nude mice lack thymuses
1969	Jørgen Rygaard characterizes the immunological defect in nude (athymic) mice

10

The Bursa of Fabricius in Lymphocyte Maturation

INTRODUCTION

The bursa of Fabricius is a lymphoepithelial organ present in gallinaceous birds such as chickens, turkeys, pheasants, grouse, partridges, and quails. Although originally described in the 1600s, the function of this organ remained unknown well into the twentieth century. In 1956 Bruce Glick and Timothy Chang, graduate students at Ohio State University, reported that removal of the bursa from newly hatched chickens subsequently severely impaired antibody production when the chickens became adults.

Published in the peer-reviewed journal *Poultry Science*, these findings remained obscure for several years. One reason for this was the unavailability of electronic retrieval of scientific publications, thus delaying the discovery of this seminal finding until the early 1960s.

The rediscovery of the function of the bursa in lymphocyte development, at about the same time Jacques Miller demonstrated the role of the thymus (Chapter 9), stimulated inquiries regarding the ontogeny of immunocompetence. The concept of central versus peripheral lymphoid organs emerged. Central lymphoid organs are those in which lymphocytes mature and include the thymus, the source of T lymphocytes, and the bone marrow in mammals or bursa of Fabricius in birds, the source of B lymphocytes. Peripheral lymphoid organs, such as the spleen and lymph nodes, are where mature T and B lymphocytes reside and initiate adaptive immune responses. Chickens, unlike mammals, possess both a bursa and a thymus that can be surgically removed. They therefore provide a unique experimental model in which developing T and B lymphocytes can be individually manipulated.

The focus on an avian species in immunological research represented a shift for many investigators, most of whom used mammals such as mice, rats, rabbits, or guinea pigs. Mammals were preferred because they were relatively inexpensive, easy to handle, and could be housed in conventional animal facilities. Inbred strains of several mammalian species such as mice, rats, and guinea pigs were available. Inbred animals, all of whom are identical, eliminated much of the problem of interpreting results due to genetic heterogeneity.

A potential problem with experimental models relying on birds is that the results obtained may not be readily translated to mammals, which do not possess a bursa of Fabricius. Investigators spent several years searching

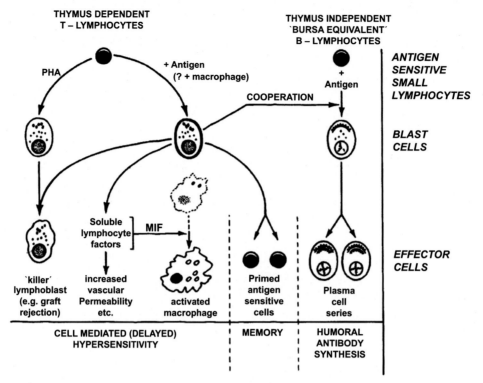

FIGURE 10.1   Functional division of T and B lymphocytes based on site of differentiation. This figure introduced the terms T lymphocyte and B lymphocyte and differentiated the roles of each in cell-mediated immunity (cytotoxicity, graft rejection, induction of inflammation, delayed-type hypersensitivity) and antibody-mediated immunity. PHA = phytohemagglutinin, a nonspecific mitogen capable of activating T lymphocytes; MIF = (macrophage) migration inhibition factor. *From Roitt et al. (1969).*

unsuccessfully for a bursa equivalent and concluded that mammals do not possess a discrete organ with functions analogous to those of the bursa. Instead those functions in mammals occur within the bone marrow.

Studies of the thymus and the bursa of Fabricius, along with clinical observations of patients presenting with congenital immunodeficiencies, demonstrated that the adaptive immune response employs two distinct populations of lymphocytes. These lymphocytes have different developmental histories and perform distinct functions in providing protection against foreign pathogens. Ivan Roitt compiled the data from these divergent clinical and basic science studies on the thymus and the bursa to provide an overview of lymphoid development that remains the basis for our understanding of cellular immunology today (Figure 10.1).

EARLY HISTORY OF THE BURSA OF FABRICIUS

Hieronymus Fabricius (1537–1619), a professor of anatomy and surgery at the University of Padua, Italy, from 1565 to 1604, made a number of contributions to the fields of embryology, anatomy, and surgery. Fabricius provided detailed descriptions of the development of the fetus, the structure of the gastrointestinal tract, and the presence of valves in veins. Among his students was Sir William Harvey, a British physician who is most widely known for his description of the blood circulatory system.

In 1621 Fabricius' lecture notes were published posthumously by one of his students (reviewed in Scott, 2004). These notes contained a description of a hindgut lymphoepithelial organ found in chickens and other gallinaceous birds. This organ has since been named the bursa of Fabricius in his honor. Initially, Fabricius postulated erroneously that the organ was a repository in the female for semen following copulation. William Harvey, among other anatomists, demonstrated that the bursa exists in both genders, thus arguing against this function.

During the next 300 years, several investigators proposed that the organ was part of the endocrine system. Even in the late 1950s and early 1960s researchers were injecting various hormones into bursectomized and intact chickens to compare effects (Perek and Eilat, 1960; Newcomer and Connally, 1960). This line of investigation failed to produce definitive data that the bursa had an endocrine function even though several groups reported a decrease in bursal weight following injection with adrenocorticotrophic hormone (ACTH) or in birds subjected to stress.

Ronald Meyer and colleagues at the University of Wisconsin made a surprising finding in 1959 from their studies on the possible endocrine role of the bursa. They exposed fertilized eggs to a solution containing testosterone and described how the chicks that hatched from the treated eggs lacked a bursa. This observation led to the development of the technique of hormonal bursectomy that proved significant for subsequent studies to determine the immunological role of the bursa.

SERENDIPITY AND BURSECTOMY

Bruce Glick (1927–2009), a graduate student in the Poultry Science Department at Ohio State University in the early 1950s, made the seminal discovery regarding the function of the bursa of Fabricius. His long-term interest in birds had been inspired by his fourth-grade teacher in Pittsburgh. Following military service during World War II, he pursued undergraduate and graduate degrees in poultry science and genetics, first at Rutgers University, then at the University of Massachusetts, and finally at Ohio State University. Early in his graduate career he watched his mentor, Dr R. George Japp, surgically remove an obscure organ from a goose. When asked, Dr Japp identified the organ as the bursa of Fabricius. Glick asked, "What is its function?" and Japp replied, "Good question, you find the answer" (Glick, 1979; Taylor and McCorkle, 2009).

Glick initially studied the growth rate of the cells of the chicken bursa and determined that the bursa grew most rapidly during the first 3 weeks after hatching. He reasoned that he could most easily approach functional studies by removing the bursa during this rapid growth phase. Accordingly, he performed surgical bursectomy on chickens shortly after hatching and evaluated a variety of functions, focusing on potential endocrine activities; he found no difference between bursectomized and control animals. Two years into his PhD studies, serendipity intervened when one of Glick's fellow graduate students, Timothy Chang, needed animals to produce antibodies against *Salmonella*. The only animals available were several 6-month-old chickens from Glick's experiments. These were injected with the *Salmonella* type O antigen but failed to produce any antibody. When the identification numbers assigned to the chickens were checked, all of them had been bursectomized during the first 3 weeks of life. Glick and his colleagues expanded these results by immunizing additional bursectomized and unmanipulated, control chickens with *Salmonella* and measuring antibodies produced to the O antigen. Table 10.1 summarizes the results obtained in these initial experiments and shows that 87% of control chickens produced antibodies while only 17% of bursectomized animals possessed measurable serum antibody levels.

Glick's mentor, George Jaap, realized the importance of this finding and urged Glick and Chang to write a paper and submit it for publication. *Science* rejected the

TABLE 10.1 Results of Immunizing Neonatally Bursectomized and Control Chickens with the O Antigen of *Salmonella typhimurium*

	Chickens possessing antibody to O antigen	Chickens lacking antibody to O antigen
Bursectomized	8	67
Control	63	10

Adapted from Taylor and McCorkle (2009).

manuscript and advised the authors to further elucidate the mechanism responsible for the defective antibody production. Glick and his colleagues subsequently submitted the work to the journal *Poultry Science* where it was published and has become a citation classic (Glick et al., 1956).

This paper was published 5 years before the landmark paper by Jacques Miller describing the role of the thymus in the development of immunocompetent lymphocytes (Chapter 9). Most immunologists were unaware of the role of the bursa until similar studies were reported by several groups, including August Mueller, Harold Wolfe, and Roland Meyer at the University of Wisconsin, Noel Warner and A. Szenberg at the Walter and Eliza Hall Institute in Melbourne, Australia, and Max Cooper working in the laboratory of Robert Good at the University of Minnesota.

REDISCOVERY OF THE ROLE OF THE BURSA OF FABRICIUS

Roland Meyer and his colleagues reported in early 1959 that exposure of fertilized chicken eggs to testosterone inhibited the lymphocytic development of the bursa. Within a year (Mueller et al., 1960), they published a comparison of the effects of hormonal and surgical bursectomy on the production of precipitating antibodies to bovine serum albumin (BSA). They treated embryonated eggs on the fifth day of incubation with 19-nortestosterone. Chickens that hatched 16 days later comprised the hormonal bursectomy group. Surgical bursectomies were carried out at 1, 2, 5, and 10 weeks posthatch. Meyer and his colleagues injected all chickens with BSA at 6, 12, or 22 weeks of age and bled 1–2 weeks later. Sera from these samples were tested for the presence of antibody to BSA.

Chickens exposed to testosterone as embryos failed to thrive, and all died by 11 weeks post-hatching. None of these birds produced antibody to the injected BSA. Surgical bursectomy at 1 or 2 weeks of age resulted in a decreased production of antibody 6, 12, and 22 weeks later while birds bursectomized at 10 weeks of age showed no decrease in antibody production.

Two years later, Warner and Szenberg, working with Sir Macfarlane Burnet in Melbourne, confirmed these observations and differentiated the roles of the thymus and bursa in lymphocyte maturation (Warner et al., 1962; Szenberg and Warner, 1962). These investigators injected 12-day-old chicken embryos with testosterone propionate to inhibit the development of the bursa. Chickens that hatched from these eggs were considered bursaless. About 30% of these chicks also showed some atrophy in the thymus. The investigators tested the immune capacity of two groups of animals (bursaless with intact thymus and bursaless with atrophic thymus). Both groups of animals failed to produce antibodies when injected with BSA. These birds lacked plasma cells in the peripheral lymphoid tissue, and their serum gamma globulin levels were decreased when compared with untreated birds. Skin allografts on hormonally bursectomized chickens with intact thymus were rejected in a normal time frame while skin grafts performed on chickens with atrophic thymus were accepted for the duration of the experiment.

Incorporating the studies on thymectomy published by Miller (1961) with these observations on the effects of hormonal bursectomy, Warner and Szenberg (1964) proposed the existence of two functionally different populations of immunologically competent lymphocytes: one dependent on the bursa for development and the other dependent on the thymus. They hypothesized that bursa-dependent lymphocytes produced antibodies while thymus-dependent lymphocytes participated in cell-mediated immune responses.

Max Cooper, a pediatrician trained in the 1950s at Tulane University in New Orleans, Louisiana, pursued several opportunities prior to becoming a researcher. He served as a house officer and research assistant in London, completed a fellowship in allergy and immunology at the University of California, San Francisco, and directed an allergy clinic at Tulane. In the early 1960s, he applied for a research fellowship in Robert Good's laboratory at the University of Minnesota based on their common interest in immunodeficiency diseases and other immunopathologies (Cooper, 2010).

Cooper joined a group of graduate students and postdoctoral fellows who were at the cutting edge of the new field of cellular immunology. When Cooper arrived at Good's laboratory in the early 1960s, several recent advances in the field made immunology intriguing. These included the following:

- the description of the role of the thymus in lymphocyte development by Jacques Miller in Melbourne (Chapter 8);
- the discovery of the circulation of lymphocytes between peripheral blood and the lymphatic system by James Gowans in London (Chapter 4);
- the identification of the lymphocyte as the precursor for antibody-producing plasma cells by Astrid Fragraeus in Stockholm (Chapter 5); and

- the elucidation of the four-chain structure of antibody molecules by Rodney Porter in London and Gerald Edelman in New York (Chapter 11).

Simultaneously, due to the use of newly discovered antibiotics, infants and children born with a variety of congenital immunodeficiencies such as agammaglobulinemia and thymic aplasia survived long enough for clinicians to study the underlying genetic defects. The initial description of an individual unable to produce antibody was published by Ogden Bruton in 1952. The original patient was an 8-year-old boy who presented with a long history of recurrent infections. Among other tests, Bruton sampled the boy's serum and sent it for analysis by the newly developed technique of serum electrophoresis. The laboratory reported a complete absence of gamma globulins. Bruton, thinking there was a lab error, sent a second sample, which provided the same result. Based on these data, Bruton inferred that the patient had no antibody-forming cells (the identity of which was unknown in 1952) and decided to treat the boy with periodic injections of normal human gamma globulin. This treatment resulted in an increased level of serum antibodies that helped protect the boy from additional microbial infections.

Subsequently, other patients have been diagnosed with this X-linked syndrome, which is one of the first of numerous congenital immunodeficiency diseases to be described (Chapter 32). The analysis of the immunological defects in these patients helped confirm the data published from concurrent animal studies.

As pediatricians, Cooper and Good focused their studies on immunodeficiency diseases that subsequently shed light on the functioning of the immune system. Researchers in Good's laboratory pursued a diverse group of investigations, including

- the ontogeny and phylogeny of the immune response,
- the biological basis of the antibody response,
- autoimmune diseases,
- malignancies of the lymphoid system,
- the complement system,
- transplantation, and
- the effects of thymectomy on immune responsiveness.

Cooper became aware of Glick's observations published 6 years previously. In addition, he read papers published by Harold Wolfe's group at the University of Wisconsin (Mueller et al., 1960) and by the Australian scientists (Warner et al., 1962) that confirmed Glick's observation that bursectomy of chickens early in life resulted in diminished antibody production. Cooper and his colleagues studied the chicken's immune system following surgical bursectomy, surgical thymectomy, or a combination of surgical bursectomy plus thymectomy in newly hatched birds to evaluate the existence of two populations of lymphocytes. The initial studies confirmed Glick's observations that surgical bursectomy decreased antibody production. However, they found no deficit in immune function as measured by graft rejection following thymectomy.

Despite these laboratory findings, but based on clinical observations of infants with congenital immunodeficiencies, Cooper postulated the existence of two functionally distinct populations of lymphocytes. In particular, he noted that boys with Wiskott–Aldrich syndrome, an X-linked disorder characterized by thrombocytopenia, eczema, and recurrent ear infections, sometimes succumbed to herpes simplex viral infections. He contrasted these clinical presentations with those of boys suffering from agammaglobulinemia, another X-linked disorder characterized by recurrent bacterial infections and an inability to synthesize antibody. Unlike boys with Wiskott–Aldrich syndrome, agammaglobulinemic patients cleared viral infections.

Cooper and his colleagues demonstrated the existence of two functionally distinct populations of lymphocytes by adding sublethal irradiation to the surgical manipulations of thymectomy or bursectomy in newly hatched chickens. The addition of sublethal irradiation to the experimental design clarified the dichotomy of the two cell lineages.

Cooper set up four different experimental groups of newly hatched chickens as follows:

1. bursectomized,
2. thymectomized,
3. thymectomized and bursectomized, or
4. unmanipulated controls.

Subgroups of each of these animals were subjected to sublethal irradiation.

A variety of different assays were performed to detect immunological competence in each of the groups:

- Antibody synthesis was measured in chickens injected with *Brucella abortus*.
- Delayed-type hypersensitivity was induced by sensitizing chickens with diphtheria toxoid and testing their responses to a subsequent injection of the antigen into their wattle.
- Transplantation immunity (host-versus-graft reactivity) was assessed by transplanting chickens with allogeneic and syngeneic skin grafts.
- Graft-versus-host reactivity was determined by injecting lymphocytes from manipulated animals intravenously into 14-day-old chick embryos of an allogeneic strain.

Table 10.2 summarizes some of the results of this series of experiments as reported in papers published

TABLE 10.2 Effect of Adding Irradiation to Thymectomy or Bursectomy on the Ability of Chickens to Respond to Various Immunologic Stimuli

Group	Allograft rejection[a]	DTH reactivity[b]	Antibody production[c]	GvH response[d]
Control irradiated [e,f]	15/15	10/10	15/16	74.0 mg
Thymectomized irradiated	7/12	2/14	7/12	43.0 mg
Bursectomized irradiated	15/15	ND	0/14	78.5 mg
Thymectomized bursectomized irradiated	ND	ND	0/8	ND

[a]*Rejection of allografts determined at day 27 after placement of grafts. Results presented as number of animals rejecting allograft/number grafted.*
[b]*Delayed-type hypersensitivity determined in chickens sensitized with diphtheria toxoid and complete Freund's adjuvant and tested 7 days later. Results presented as number of animals with a positive response/number injected.*
[c]*Antibody to* Brucella abortus *organisms 9 days after immunization. Results presented as number of chickens with a positive response/number tested.*
[d]*Graft-versus-host reactivity of cells derived from the various experimental groups tested by injection into allogeneic chick embryos. Results presented as spleen weight of the injected embryos. Spleens derived from uninjected chick embryos averaged 9.3 mg.*
[e]*Surgical procedures were performed on day of hatching.*
[f]*Surgically manipulated and control birds were irradiated one day after hatching.*
Cooper et al. (1965, 1966a).

during the mid-1960s (Cooper et al., 1965, 1967). Only the responses of the groups of chickens exposed to the sublethal irradiation are presented. The results confirmed that bursectomy performed shortly after hatching decreased the amount of antibody produced against a foreign antigen but did not alter rejection of foreign skin grafts. Thymectomy, particularly when accompanied with irradiation, inhibited graft rejection, delayed-type hypersensitivity, and graft-versus-host reactivity.

These findings as well as histological observations of lymphoid organs in the chickens led the authors to conclude that

The bursa of Fabricius and the thymus are 'central lymphoid organs' in the chicken, essential to the ontogenetic development of adaptive immunity in that species. Surgical removal of one or both of these organs in the newly hatched chicken, followed by sublethal X-irradiation the next day, has permitted recognition of two morphologically distinct cell systems in the 'peripheral lymphoid tissues' of the spleen, gut and other organs, and clear definition of the separate functions of each cell system. **Cooper et al., 1966a**

SEARCH FOR THE BURSA EQUIVALENT IN MAMMALS

Mammals, including humans, do not possess a bursa of Fabricius. Extrapolation of the conclusions from the work on chickens to mammals required the identification in mammals of a bursa equivalent. In the middle to late 1960s, researchers searched for an organ or organs in mammals that functioned analogous to the chicken bursa. Several groups investigated this question, focusing initially on other gut associated tissues such as the appendix, tonsils, and Peyer's patches (Sutherland et al., 1964; Cooper et al., 1966b; Fichtelius, 1967; Owen et al., 1974). Surgically removing these organs individually or as a group consistently failed to produce animals with a deficient antibody response. Eventually, studies revealing the sequential molecular events that occur during B lymphocyte development (Chapter 18) resulted in a recognition that B lymphocytes in mammals arise from hematopoietic stem cells in the fetal liver and bone marrow and undergo continued maturation in the bone marrow.

DIVISION OF LYMPHOCYTES INTO TWO FUNCTIONALLY DISTINCT POPULATIONS

By the late 1960s, two functionally distinct populations of lymphocytes with discrete developmental histories had been described. In 1969, Ivan Roitt and his colleagues at Middlesex Hospital Medical School in London reviewed the cellular basis of immunological responses and summarized the data available at that time:

- Two populations of lymphocytes exist: one thymus-dependent and the other thymus-independent (bursa-dependent).
- Both populations contain antigen sensitive cells that recognize foreign antigen.
- Interaction of thymus-independent cells with foreign antigen results in lymphocyte differentiation, proliferation, and maturation into plasma cells that produce antibodies.
- Interaction of thymus-dependent cells with foreign antigen results in transformation of the lymphocytes into blasts that are responsible for a variety of different functions, including
  - immunological memory (Chapter 2);
  - death of foreign cells, leading to graft rejection (cytotoxicity) (Chapter 36);
  - synthesis and secretion of soluble factors, inducing inflammation (Chapter 25); and
  - cooperation with thymus-independent cells in the production of antibody (Chapter 13).

Roitt and his colleagues (1969) introduced the terms T lymphocytes to refer to thymus-dependent cells and B lymphocytes to refer to thymus-independent (bursa-dependent) cells. A diagram describing the immune system as understood in the late 1960s is presented as Figure 10.1.

MARKERS TO DIFFERENTIATE T AND B LYMPHOCYTES

Prior to antigen stimulation, both B and T lymphocytes appear morphologically as small, nondescript cells with a large nucleus and scant cytoplasm (Figure 10.2) that cannot be differentiated histologically. Investigators developed several techniques to separate lymphocyte populations, including electrophoresis, centrifugation, separation on a gradient of a salt solution, sensitivity to drugs, and binding to erythrocytes from sheep and other animals to form rosettes. These studies failed to produce an easy and consistent method to differentiate functionally unique lymphocyte populations.

The development of antibodies specific to lymphocyte cell surface molecules provided a much more effective method for differentiating T lymphocytes from B lymphocytes. Investigators produced an array of antibodies specific for many different cell surface molecules. Initially these antibodies were produced by injecting mice from one inbred strain with leukemia cells from a different inbred strain. The resulting antibodies reacted not only with the leukemia cells of the donor strain but also with lymphocytes from nonleukemic mice (Boyse et al., 1968). The cell surface molecules detected by these antibodies were termed Ly since they were found on lymphocytes but not on other cells types. These antibodies were useful in differentiating different functional populations of T lymphocytes (Chapter 23).

Technology to produce cell lines, hybridomas, capable of secreting large quantities of monoclonal antibodies of a single specificity (Köhler and Milstein, 1975—Chapter 37) permitted differentiation of T lymphocytes from B lymphocytes as well as discrimination of functional

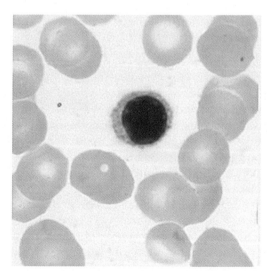

FIGURE 10.2 Small lymphocyte in a blood smear stained with Giemsa. *From the CDC image library* http://www.dpd.cdc.gov/dpdx/ html/imagelibrary/A-F/Artifacts/body_Artifacts_il8.htm.

subpopulations of T lymphocytes. For example, Kung et al. (1979) developed a series of monoclonal antibodies specific for human T lymphocytes. Human peripheral blood lymphocytes were isolated by incubation with sheep erythrocytes to form E-rosettes. Kung and coworkers injected these lymphocytes into mice, harvested spleen cells, and fused them with a mouse myeloma cell to produce hybridomas that could be maintained in long-term culture. Hybridomas that produced antibodies that reacted with human lymphocytes were cloned. Investigators depended on the resulting monoclonal antibody to characterize T lymphocyte subpopulations. By the early 1980s, a large number of different monoclonal antibodies reactive with cell surface molecules on an array of lymphocytes had been developed and subsequently employed to further differentiate and define subpopulations of lymphocytes. Georges Köhler and Ceasar Milstein were awarded the 1984 Nobel Prize in Physiology and Medicine (shared with Niels Jerne) for "the discovery of the principle for the production of monoclonal antibodies."

In the 1980s, each investigator independently named the antibody used in his or her laboratory: chaos reigned. To reduce the confusion in comparing studies from different laboratories, the International Union of Immunology Societies (IUIS) and the World Health Organization (WHO) sponsored the first international workshop on Human Leukocyte Differentiation Antigens in Paris in 1982. Participants at this meeting compared the specificity of 139 monoclonal antibodies submitted by 55 research groups from 14 countries. Using a panel of cultured cells, participants determined the specificity of the antibodies by immunofluorescence. The workshop defined 15 clusters of differentiation (CD) markers (IUIS-WHO nomenclature subcommittee, 1984). These CD antigens (CD1-11 and CDw12-w15) identified markers of various subsets of human leukocytes, including lymphocytes, granulocytes, and monocytes. The list has now been expanded to include more than 350 different CD antigens.

Investigators have identified antigens on the surface of lymphocytes in other animals that parallel the CD markers of humans. Monoclonal antibodies against many of these antigens now exist and enable investigators to target and design their research questions.

Clinically, several of the monoclonal antibodies that define CD markers are used to quantify the number of immunocompetent cells in normal and immunopathological states, including CD3 (pan T lymphocyte), CD4 (helper T lymphocytes), CD8 (cytotoxic T lymphocytes), CD16 (natural killer lymphocytes), and CD19 and CD20 (B lymphocytes). Quantification of the number of CD4+ T lymphocytes in patients presenting with human immunodeficiency virus (HIV) infection currently serves as a surrogate marker for the progression of the disease

Acquired Immunodeficiency Syndrome (AIDS). CD markers are also used to identify and classify tumors of lymphocytes (lymphomas and leukemias) and, in the case of B cell lymphomas, as a target for therapy (Chapter 38).

CONCLUSION

Glick in 1956 demonstrated that surgical removal of the bursa of Fabricius in chickens at or shortly after hatching leads to a profound decrease in antibody production in birds. This observation remained obscured from the wider immunological community for nearly 6 years. Rediscovery of this study, along with the results published by Miller on the role of the thymus in lymphocyte development, led to the identification of separate organs for the maturation of two functionally unique populations of lymphocytes involved in the adaptive immune response. These results provided the explanation for the division of the adaptive immune system into two separate but interrelated systems. This division into thymus-derived T lymphocytes and bursa (or bone marrow)-derived B lymphocytes spurred investigations in a number of important areas, including

- determination of the cell-associated structures used by T and B lymphocytes to recognize antigen (Chapter 17);
- identification of the molecular events involved in cell interactions in the immune response (Chapters 13 and 14);
- detection of the genes that control the acquisition of lymphocyte specificity and the mechanism involved in providing immunologic diversity (Chapter 18);
- description of functionally different subpopulations of lymphocytes (Chapter 23); and
- determination of the mechanisms that are active in the development and maintenance of self-tolerance (Chapters 21 and 22).

References

Boyse, E.A., Miyazawa, M., Aoki, T., Old, L.J., 1968. Ly-A and Ly-B: two systems of lymphocyte isoantigens in the mouse. Proc. Roy. Soc. B 170, 175–193.

Bruton, O.C., 1952. Agammaglobulinemia. Pediatrics 9, 722–728.

Cooper, M.D., 2010. A life of adventure in immunobiology. Annu. Rev. Immunol. 28, 1–19.

Cooper, M.D., Gabrielsen, A.E., Good, R.A., 1967. Role of the thymus and other central lymphoid tissues in immunological disease. Annu. Rev. Med. 18, 113–138.

Cooper, M.D., Peterson, R.D.A., Good, R.A., 1965. Delineation of the thymic and bursal lymphoid systems in the chicken. Nature 205, 143–146.

Cooper, M.D., Peterson, R.D.A., South, M.A., Good, R.A., 1966a. The functions of the thymus system and the bursa system in the chicken. J. Exp. Med. 123, 75–102.

Cooper, M.D., Perey, D.Y., McNeally, M.F., Gabrielsen, A.E., Sutherland, D.E.R., Good, R.A., 1966b. A mammalian equivalent of the avian bursa of Fabricius. Lancet 287, 1388–1391.

Fichtelius, K.E., 1967. The mammalian equivalent to bursa Fabricii of birds. Exp. Cell. Res. 46, 231–234.

Glick, B., 1979. This week's citation classic. Curr. Contents 22, 241.

Glick, B., Chang, T.S., Jaap, R.G., 1956. The bursa of Fabricius and antibody production in the domestic fowl. Poult. Sci. 35, 224–225.

IUIS-WHO monenclature subcommittee, 1984. Nomenclature for clusters of differentiation (CD) of antigens defined on human leukocyte populations. Bull. WHO 62, 809–811.

Köhler, G., Milstein, C., 1975. Continuous cultures of fused cells secreting antibody of predefined specificity. Nature 256, 495–497.

Kung, P.C., Goldstein, G., Reinherz, E.L., Schlossman, S.F., 1979. Monoclonal antibodies defining distinctive human T cell surface antigens. Science 206, 347–349.

Meyer, R.K., Rao, M.A., Aspinal, R.L., 1959. Inhibition of the development of the bursa of Fabricius in the embryos of the common fowl by 19-nortestosterone. Endocrinology 64, 890–897.

Miller, J.F.A.P., 1961. Immunological function of the thymus. Lancet 278, 748–749.

Mueller, A.P., Wolfe, H.R., Meyer, R.K., 1960. Precipitin production in chickens. XXI. Antibody production in bursectomized chickens and in chickens injected with 19-nortestosterone on the fifth day of incubation. J. Immunol. 85, 172–179.

Newcomer, W.S., Connally, J.D., 1960. The bursa of Fabricius as an indicator of chronic stress in immature chickens. Endocrinology 67, 264–266.

Owen, J.J.T., Cooper, M.D., Raff, M.C., 1974. In vitro generation of B lymphocytes in mouse fetal liver, a mammalian 'bursa equivalent'. Nature 249, 361–363.

Perek, M., Eilat, A., 1960. The bursa of Fabricius and adrenal ascorbic acid depletion following ACTH injections in chicks. J. Endocrinol. 20, 251–255.

Roitt, I.M., Greaves, M.F., Torrigiani, G., Brostoff, J., Playfair, J.H.L., 1969. The cellular basis of immunological responses. A synthesis of some current views. Lancet 294, 367–371.

Scott, T.R., 2004. Our current understanding of humoral immunity of poultry. Poult. Sci. 83, 574–579.

Sutherland, D.E.R., Archer, O.K., Good, R.A., 1964. Role of the appendix in development of immunological competence. Proc. Soc. Exp. Biol. Med. 115, 673–676.

Szenberg, A., Warner, N.L., 1962. Dissociation of immunological responsiveness in fowls with a hormonally arrested development of lymphoid tissues. Nature 194, 146–147.

Taylor, R.L., McCorkle, F.M., 2009. A landmark contribution to poultry science-immunological function of the bursa of Fabricius. Poult. Sci. 88, 816–823.

Warner, N.L., Szenberg, A., Burnet, F.M., 1962. The immunological role of different lymphoid organs in the chicken. I. Dissociation of immunological responsiveness. Aust. J. Exp. Biol. Med. Sci. 40, 373–387.

Warner, N.L., Szenberg, A., 1964. The immunological function of the bursa of Fabricius in chickens. Annu. Rev. Microbiol. 18, 253–266.

TIME LINE

1621	Publication of the first description of the bursa by Hieronymous Fabricius
1952	Ogden Bruton describes the first case of the B cell immunodeficiency, agammaglobulinemia
1956	Bruce Glick reports that removal of the bursa of Fabricius in newly hatched chickens severely depresses subsequent antibody formation
1960	August Mueller and colleagues demonstrate that hormonal bursectomy and surgical bursectomy decrease antibody production in chickens
1962	Noel Warner and A. Szenberg begin differentiation of the roles of the thymus and the bursa in the adaptive immune response
1966	Max Cooper and colleagues differentiate thymus-dependent and bursa-dependent lymphocytes
1969	Ivan Roitt introduces terms to refer to thymus-dependent T lymphocytes and bursa-dependent B lymphocytes
1975	Georges Köhler and Cesar Milstein develop hybridoma technology to produce monoclonal antibodies
1982	First international workshop on human leukocyte differentiation antigens; introduction of the cluster of differentiation (CD) nomenclature
1984	Köhler and Milstein awarded the Nobel Prize in Physiology or Medicine

11

Revealing the Structure of the Immunoglobulin Molecule

INTRODUCTION

In the late 1880s, several investigators reported that the injection of experimental animals with bacteria (*Bacillus anthracis* or *Vibrio cholerae*) induced the production of a serum substance that could kill the immunizing microbe (Von Fodor, 1887; Nuttall, 1888; Von Buchner, 1889; reviewed by Schmalsteig and Goldman, 2009). Today this substance is called antibody. Antibodies are glycoproteins synthesized in response to a foreign antigen that bind specifically to the inducing antigen and activate effector mechanisms to eliminate the foreign material.

Experiments performed between the late 1880s and the early 1960s revealed the relationships among antibody composition, molecular structure, and function. These investigations paralleled similar biochemical studies aimed at understanding the structure of other molecules of biological importance such as hormones (i.e., insulin), enzymes (i.e., trypsin, lipase), toxins from pathogenic microorganisms (i.e., diphtheria and tetanus), and drugs from plants or microbes (i.e., antibiotics).

Initial clues to antibody composition came from studies of the serum substances produced in response to bacterial pathogens, particularly to *Corynebacterium diphtheriae, Clostridium tetani,* and *Streptococcus pneumoniae.* These microorganisms caused significant morbidity and mortality in the first decades of the twentieth century. Studies beginning in the 1890s and continuing until the introduction of antibiotics were aimed at providing protective immunity against these microbes either by passive transfer of preformed antibodies or by the development of vaccines. As a result, the composition and structure of the molecule responsible for antibody activity emerged.

Several groups of immunochemists worked with the immunoglobulin molecule to provide the picture of antibody portrayed in Figure 11.1 (Putnam, 1969). This model illustrates the four chain structure of the molecule consisting of two identical heavy chains and two identical light chains. Based on functional studies, the molecule can be further divided into segments, labeled Fab (fragment antigen binding) and Fc (fragment crystallizable). Figure 11.1 also depicts the position of inter- and intrachain disulfide bonds, the location of enzymatic cleavage by pepsin and papain, and the location of the antigen binding site of the molecule.

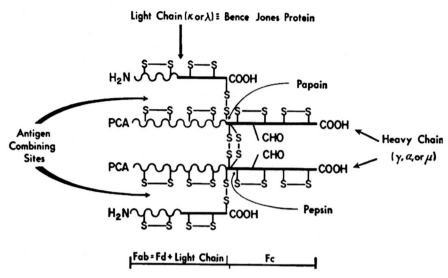

FIGURE 11.1 Diagram of the prototypical antibody molecule indicating the sites in the molecule sensitive to the action of the various enzymes used to decipher the molecular structure and the location of antigen binding. *From Putnam (1969).*

The studies important in unveiling this model are described in this chapter.

THE UNITARIAN HYPOTHESIS OF ANTIBODIES

Detection of antibody activity in the late 1800s relied on the observation that serum from immunized animals neutralized bacteria. Eventually, several different assay systems were developed to detect antibody activity: precipitation, agglutination, bacterial neutralization, and complement fixation (activation). The serum substances detected in these assays were referred to as precipitins, agglutinins, amboceptors (an antibody that activates complement and causes lysis), or opsonins (an antibody that enhanced phagocytosis).

Early in the twentieth century a debate developed about the number of functionally different antibodies that could be synthesized to an antigen. Initially each of the assay systems used for detection was thought to measure the effects of a distinct molecule. Studies performed between 1900 and the 1930s demonstrated that the various functions of antibody were performed by a single molecule. These studies led to the formulation of the unitarian hypothesis of antibody.

The unitarian hypothesis of antibody states that an antigen induces a single molecular form of antibody that can perform all of the in vitro functions attributed to antibody (i.e., agglutination, precipitation, fixing complement, opsonization, and neutralization). Hans Zinsser (1878–1940) was among the first to demonstrate that a single antibody molecule may be detected by different assay systems and thus perform several different functions.

Zinsser, received an MD degree from Columbia University in 1903. He studied the epidemiology of infectious diseases and in particular focused on the microorganisms responsible for typhus, *Rickettsia typhi* and *Rickettsia prowazeki*. He spent his academic career at Stanford, Columbia, and Harvard and developed the first vaccine against typhus in 1933. As a prolific author, he wrote *Rats, Lice and History*, the story of typhus that has been revised and reprinted for more than 70 years, and a *Textbook of Bacteriology* that was appreciated by students well into the 1990s.

In 1913, Zinsser studied two antibody-mediated phenomena—precipitation and complement fixation (Chapter 12)—and observed that the formation of a precipitate between a protein antigen and serum containing specific antibody removed complement from the serum.

Zinsser injected rabbits with sheep serum to induce precipitating antibody to serum proteins. He mixed serum from the immunized rabbits with various dilutions of sheep serum and separated the precipitates from the supernatants. He tested both precipitates and supernatants in an assay designed to detect complement activity by adding them separately to test tubes containing a mixture of sheep red blood cells (SRBC) and antibody specific for SRBC.

The degree of SRBC lysis provided a semiquantitative estimate of the amount of complement present in the precipitates and the supernatants. If precipitating antibodies did not fix complement, most or all of the complement activity would remain in the supernatant. Alternatively, if precipitating antibodies also fixed complement, most of the complement activity would be present in the tubes containing precipitation. Zinsser reports his results:

1. Antigen 1:10. Heavy precipitate; strong fixation by washed precipitate; slight fixation by supernatant fluid.

2. Antigen 1:100. Heavy precipitate; fixation by washed precipitate; none by supernatant fluid.

3 to 6. Antigen dilutions ranging from 1:200 to 1:5000. In all cases, although the precipitate is extremely slight in the last tubes, the fixing power resides entirely in the precipitate and not at all in the supernatant fluid.

In subsequent studies, serum from animals that had not been immunized was added to antigen–antibody precipitates. This serum contained complement. Following incubation, supernatants from these mixtures were added to antibody-sensitized red cells and the presence or absence of hemolysis noted. As in the previous experiment, lysis of the red cells would indicate that the antigen–antibody precipitates had no effect on the amount of complement in the serum, while the absence of lysis of the erythrocytes would signal that the antigen–antibody precipitate failed to remove complement. Results showed that the precipitate removed complement from the serum from unimmunized animals. Thus the same antibody both precipitated antigen and fixed complement.

From these results Zinsser reasoned that "the fixation of alexin (complement) by precipitates is not merely a mechanical adsorption, and in that it renders more likely the supposition that the so called precipitin is actually a protein sensitizer by which a foreign protein is rendered amenable to the proteolytic action of the alexin (complement)." As Zinsser concludes, "Carried to its logical conclusion, the acceptance of this view…leads to the conception that functionally there is but one variety of specific antibodies." In retrospect, this conclusion, while correct, was made on relatively meager data.

Other investigators reached similar conclusions. For example, Lloyd Fenton, working at Harvard Medical School (1931a), injected horses with polysaccharide from type I *S. pneumoniae*. He used the horse antibody to determine whether a correlation existed between the in vitro activity of antibody (precipitation, agglutination, and neutralization) and the in vivo activity measured as protecting mice against disease. The correlation coefficient between protection and precipitation was 0.93, between protection and agglutination 0.80, and between protection and neutralization 0.88. Fenton concluded from this study that the level of protection provided by an antibody could be measured by simple in vitro tests such as precipitation or neutralization rather than requiring the more expensive assay involving injecting groups of mice with the microbe and specific antibodies. Sera from which antipolysaccharide antibodies had been precipitated failed to protect mice in a passive transfer assay from lethal infection with *S. pneumoniae*. Fenton concluded that these results provide "further evidence…in support of the unitarian theory of antibodies," that is that antigen induces a single form of antibody that can perform all of the in vitro functions attributed to antibodies.

THE COMPOSITION AND STRUCTURE OF ANTIBODIES

The identification of antibodies as proteins in the gamma globulin fraction of serum occurred during the first three decades of the twentieth century. The investigations that led to these conclusions resulted from attempts to provide a better product for serotherapy for patients with infectious diseases.

In the 1890s, antibody treatment of infectious diseases was introduced, and by the first decades of the twentieth century, serum therapy became the treatment of choice for patients infected with microorganisms such as *C. diphtheriae*, *C. tetani*, *S. pneumoniae*, *Neisseria meningitidis*, *Haemophilus influenzae*, and group A *Streptococcus* (Casadevall, 1996). Chapter 3 recounts the development of serotherapy for diphtheria and tetanus. The antibodies used in these therapies were initially derived from horses injected with the target pathogens and/or their toxins. Today we know that the injection of foreign (horse) serum into a human may result in the production of antibodies directed against those foreign serum proteins. These newly formed antibodies can induce their own unique pathology characterized by fever, skin rash, joint pain, cardiac abnormalities, and kidney malfunction. This constellation of symptoms is termed serum sickness and is due to the formation of antigen (horse serum)–antibody (human antibodies) complexes (Chapter 33). These complexes are consequently trapped in small blood vessels where they activate an inflammatory response.

Attempts to enhance the potency of horse antibodies against *S. pneumoniae* while simultaneously decreasing the incidence or severity of serum sickness and other adverse reactions led to new information about the composition of antibodies. Specifically, Oswald Avery (1877–1955) demonstrated that the antibody activity to *S. pneumoniae* is contained in the globulin fraction of serum.

Avery, born in Halifax, Nova Scotia, moved with his family to New York at the age of 10. He received his MD from Columbia University and pursued a research career primarily at the Rockefeller Institute of Medical Research (later the Rockefeller University). Although he started his career as an immunochemist, Avery and his colleagues, Colin MacLeod and Maclyn McCarty, created the field of molecular biology when they demonstrated, in 1944, that genetic information is composed of DNA.

Avery fractionated horse serum by treatment with various concentrations of ammonium sulfate, a commonly used method for precipitating proteins from serum.

He evaluated these precipitates functionally by injecting them into mice that had been inoculated with a lethal dose of *S. pneumoniae*. The fractions that precipitated with 38–42% ammonium sulfate provided the greatest protection. This fraction was known to contain globulins and to exclude albumin and euglobulins. The globulin fraction also was the most active in agglutination and precipitation assays in vitro (Avery, 1915).

Results similar to Avery's were obtained by other investigators during the next 20 years (Chickering, 1915; Fenton, 1931b). These studies confirmed that antibodies are serum globulins with a molecular weight similar to other globulins. As a result, Michael Heidelberger concluded in 1937 that "it is generally accepted that antibodies are modified serum proteins" (Heidelberger and Pedersen, 1937).

Heidelberger (1888–1991), an organic chemist, was educated at Columbia University and the Federal Polytechnic Institute in Zurich. He focused his research on the isolation and characterization of the polysaccharides from *S. pneumoniae* and the development of techniques for the measurement of antigen–antibody interactions. Heidelberger performed extensive studies to determine optimal methods for precipitating antigen by antibody; these studies formed the basis for the quantitative precipitin test. Based on his studies of antibody binding, Heidelberger is often credited as the father of the field of quantitative immunochemistry.

In the mid-1930s, the identification and characterization of blood proteins was an exciting new field of study. Arne Tiselius (1902–1971) trained at the University of Uppsala, Sweden, in chemistry. He originally worked with Theodor Svedberg (1884–1971), who used ultracentrifugation to separate colloids, including proteins. Svedberg realized that proteins could also be separated by migration patterns in an electrical field, and he suggested that Tiselius focus on developing the technology for this new field. By 1930, Tiselius described electrophoretic separation of proteins and received his Doctor of Science degree based on this work.

Tiselius (1937a,b) separated serum by electrophoresis and demonstrated four components with different electrical charges. These components were identified as albumin and three globulin fractions: alpha, beta, and gamma (Figure 11.2). Based on this characterization of serum proteins, Tiselius received the Nobel Prize in Chemistry in 1948 "for his research on electrophoresis and adsorption analysis, especially for his discoveries concerning the complex nature of serum proteins."

Elvin Kabat (1914–2000) joined Tiselius' laboratory after earning his PhD for work performed in Heidelberger's lab. Kabat, received his undergraduate education at the City College of New York and completed his PhD at Columbia University. Kabat's doctoral dissertation

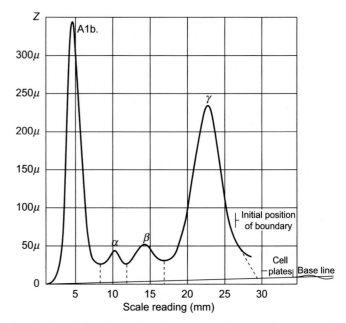

FIGURE 11.2 Electrophoretic patterns of serum from a rabbit injected with egg albumin containing ovalbumin-specific antibodies. Serum could be separated into four fractions based on electrophoretic mobility: albumin, alpha globulins, beta globulins, and gamma globulins. *From Tiselius and Kabat (1939).*

focused on the antibody response to pneumococcal polysaccharides. He demonstrated that antibody that agglutinated *S. pneumoniae* could also precipitate polysaccharide isolated from the bacterium (Heidelberger and Kabat, 1936). When he arrived in Uppsala, Sweden, to work in Tiselius' laboratory, Kabat brought a sample of the horse serum that contained antibodies to pneumococcal polysaccharides. Tiselius and Kabat analyzed this serum by electrophoresis and demonstrated that most of the antibody activity migrated with the gamma globulin fraction (Tiselius and Kabat, 1939).

During the next 15 years several other immunochemists characterized antibody molecules, and a general consensus was reached that they are a major component of the gamma globulin fraction of serum. This understanding set the stage for the next major advance in the field, leading to a detailed analysis of the molecular structure of antibodies and the development of the four chain model (Figure 11.1). These studies provided insights into the relationship between the structure and the biological functions of the molecule.

DEVELOPMENT OF THE FOUR CHAIN MODEL OF ANTIBODY

By the late 1950s, enzymatic cleavage and chemical modification led to detailed information about the structure of several proteins, including insulin, myoglobin, and hemoglobin. Three investigators, Rodney Porter in London and Gerald Edelman and Alfred Nisonoff in the United States, pursued studies modeled on these previous investigations that led to the current structural model of antibodies:

- Porter treated antibodies with the enzyme papain and obtained three fragments, two of which contained antigen binding sites and a third that crystallized spontaneously.
- Edelman treated antibody with a disulfide reducing agent and obtained data indicating that the molecule consists of two or more polypeptide chains.
- Nisonoff treated antibodies with the enzyme pepsin and obtained one fragment containing two antigen binding sites and several small peptides.

During the 1960s several models of antibody structure were proposed to explain these results, culminating in the four chain model depicted in Figure 11.1.

Papain Cleavage of Antibody

Rodney Porter (1917–1985) received his undergraduate education at the University of Liverpool England. He trained at Cambridge University with Frederick Sanger who was pursuing the primary structure (amino acid sequence) of insulin. Sanger eventually solved the molecular structure of insulin and received the Nobel Prize in Chemistry in 1958 "for his work on the structure of proteins, especially that of insulin." He was awarded a second Nobel Prize in Chemistry in 1980 along with Walter Gilbert "for their contributions concerning the determination of base sequences in nucleic acids."

Porter was influenced by the work being performed in Sanger's laboratory and earned his PhD in protein biochemistry in 1948. He accepted a position at the National Institute of Medical Research, London, to pursue studies on the structure of the antibody molecule. Porter injected rabbits with ovalbumin, bovine serum albumin, human serum albumin, or pneumococcal polysaccharide type III. Sera containing antibody to each of these antigens was fractionated and the gamma globulins treated with highly purified papain in the presence of a reducing agent, ethylenediamine-tetra-acetate (EDTA). Enzymatic treatment produced three large cleavage products that could be separated by column chromatography. He called these products fractions I, II, and III. None of the three fractions alone precipitated the original antigen. However, fractions I and II specifically inhibited precipitation of the antigen by the original antibody, thus suggesting that fractions I and II contained the antigen binding site of the original antibody. Fraction III crystallized spontaneously at neutral pH (Figure 11.3) and failed to bind antigen or to compete with whole antibody

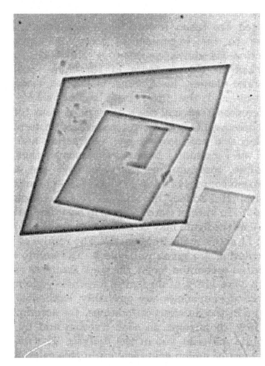

FIGURE 11.3 Crystals of fraction III of gamma globulin treated with papain. *From Porter (1959).*

in the precipitin assay. Further characterization demonstrated that fractions I and II had molecular weights of approximately 50,000 Da, while the molecular weight of fraction III was about 80,000 Da (Porter, 1959).

Analysis of the amino acid content of the three fractions revealed that fractions I and II are structurally similar to each other, while the amino acid content of fraction III is significantly different. Porter reacted each of the three fractions with an antibody prepared against whole rabbit gamma globulin; this antibody precipitated fraction III, indicating that fraction III contained most of the antigenic determinants recognized by a foreign species.

Porter proposed three possible arrangements of the fractions to explain the structure of antibody (Figure 11.4). A question was whether the antibody molecule contained one or multiple chains. While the structure labeled C in this figure proposes a two chain structure, the argument presented in the discussion of Porter's paper rejected this possibility and argued for a single chain molecule, as indicated by the structure labeled A.

Today immunologists agree that this conclusion that antibody is a single chain molecule is erroneous and that antibody is, in fact, composed of four polypeptide chains.

Treatment of Antibody with a Disulfide Reducing Agent

Gerald Edelman provided evidence that antibody molecules contain multiple polypeptide chains. Edelman

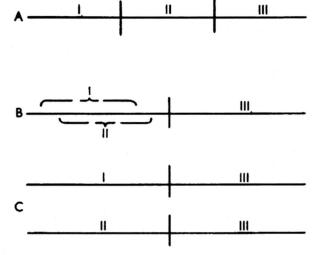

FIGURE 11.4 Diagram indicating how papain cleavage of immunoglobulin (antibody) could result in the three fractions described by Porter (1959). The author favored the structure shown in scheme A although subsequent studies would demonstrate that the immunoglobulin molecule was a multichain entity.

(1929–2014) received his MD from the University of Pennsylvania in 1954. He earned his PhD in 1960 from the Rockefeller Institute where he studied the structure of the antibody molecule. In addition to unraveling the multichain structure of antibody, he developed techniques for splitting the antibody molecule into smaller fragments, thus determining the entire amino acid sequence (Edelman et al., 1969).

Edelman treated human gamma globulin with β-mercaptoethylamine in 6M urea, a procedure that cleaves disulfide bonds. Breaking disulfide bonds in gamma globulin decreased the molecular weight of the molecule and suggested to Edelman "that human γ-globulin contains subunits linked at least in part by disulfide bonds" (Edelman, 1959). In follow-up studies, Edelman and Poulik (1961) reduced rabbit or human γ-globulin in the presence of high concentrations of urea. They separated the products of this treatment by column chromatography and electrophoresis and obtained two fractions. The antigenic determinants of these two fractions were different. Chemical analysis of these fractions revealed the presence of free sulfhydryl groups arguing for the presence of disulfide bonds in the intact molecule. These results prompted the development of the hypothesis that "7S γ-globulin molecules appear to consist of several polypeptide chains linked by disulfide bonds. Bivalent antibodies may contain two chains that are similar or identical in structure." Further analysis has shown that these two chains have different molecular weights and are called heavy (H) and light (L) chains.

In another series of experiments based on Porter's observations, Edelman et al. (1960) and Edelman and Poulik (1961) treated gamma globulin with the enzyme papain in the presence of a disulfide reducing agent. This treatment produced two major fragments that differed in their migration patterns on immunoelectrophoresis. One fragment, the fast (F) component, had a motility greater than the original gamma globulin (i.e., it migrated more toward the anode), while the other, the slow (S) fragment, was observed to migrate more toward the cathode. On further analysis, the S component corresponded to the Fab fragment (one L chain and the amino terminal half of one H chain), while the F component is composed of the Fc fragment (the carboxyl termini of the two H chains) (see Figure 11.1 above).

A difficulty with these studies is that the products obtained after treatment with urea are insoluble in aqueous solutions and therefore lose their biological activity. Consequently, it was difficult to determine which of the fractions contained the antigen binding site. To overcome this difficulty, Alfred Nisonoff and his group pursued a different path to determine the structure of gamma globulin.

Treatment of Antibody with Pepsin

Nisonoff (1923–2001) trained as a chemist at Rutgers University in New Jersey and Johns Hopkins University in Baltimore, Maryland, and became interested in immunochemistry after working with David Pressman at the State University of New York, Buffalo. Toward the end of his stay in Pressman's lab, Nisonoff initiated his studies on antibody structure by digesting rabbit gamma globulin with the enzyme pepsin followed by treatment with a reducing agent to split disulfide bonds (Nisonoff et al., 1960, 1961). The antibody used in these studies possessed antibody activity to ovalbumin.

Pepsin digestion of gamma globulin in the absence of the reducing agent produced a series of small peptides and a large fragment with a molecular weight of approximately 106,000 Da. The large fragment bound to two antigen molecules just as the whole antibody molecule did. Reduction of a single disulfide bond split the large component into two fragments, each of which had a molecular weight of 56,000 Da and a single antigen binding site. These results prompted Nisonoff et al. (1961) to speculate that "the univalent fragments formed by reduction of the peptic digest of rabbit antibody correspond to Porter's fractions I and II." While this speculation was almost correct, subsequent studies would reveal that papain and pepsin digest the gamma globulin molecule at slightly different sites (Figure 11.1).

The Four Chain Model

The final piece of evidence leading to the description of the four chain model depicted in Figure 11.4 resulted from studies carried out in Porter's laboratory

(Fleischman et al., 1962). Gamma globulin reduced with mercaptoethanol in the absence of urea resulted in splitting a number of disulfide bonds in the molecule. While the molecular weight (150,000 Da) at neutral pH was unaltered with this treatment, subsequent acidification yielded two products that could be separated by molecular weight sieving. One of the products (chain A—the H chain) had a molecular weight of approximately 50,000 Da, while the second product (chain B—the L chain) weighed 25,000 Da.

Porter's group extended these studies by enzymatically cleaving rabbit antibody to one of several antigens (human gamma globulin, bovine serum albumin, human serum albumin, ovalbumin, or pneumococcal polysaccharide type III) with papain followed by reduction of disulfide bonds. Papain fragments I, II, and III were isolated by column chromatography and treated with mercaptoethanol. Reduction of disulfide bonds in fractions I and II yielded two protein pieces that had equal molecular weights of 25,000 Da but were antigenically different. One piece was identical to the B chain, while the other contained the N-terminus of the A chain. These results led Julian Fleischman et al. (1963) to hypothesize that the intact antibody molecule was composed of two A or heavy (H) chains and two B or light (L) chains as is depicted in Figure 11.5.

The model depicted in Figure 11.1 accounts for the differences between the fragments produced by papain and pepsin cleavage. Treatment with papain produces three fragments: two Fab and one Fc. Pepsin cleavage results in the formation of a divalent fragment called $F(ab')_2$ to indicate the relationship with the Fab fragments and the fact that the fragment maintains its bivalent nature. Both Fab and $F(ab')_2$ fragments contain antigen binding sites.

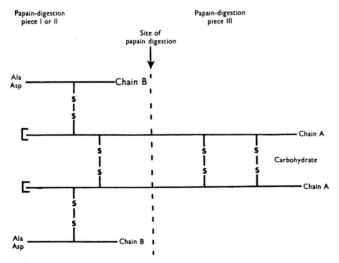

FIGURE 11.5 Proposed structure of the immunoglobulin molecule based on results of enzymatic degradation of the molecule. *From Fleischman et al. (1963).*

Numerous studies on antibody structure have confirmed the accuracy of this model as the basic structure for all five isotypes (classes) of immunoglobulin (IgM, IgG, IgA, IgE, and IgD). Determination of this four chain model culminated in the awarding of the Nobel Prize in Physiology or Medicine in 1972 jointly to Gerald M. Edelman and Rodney R. Porter "for their discoveries concerning the chemical structure of antibodies."

LOCATION OF THE ANTIGEN BINDING SITE

Publication of the Fleischman model of the antibody molecule led to speculation about the location of the antigen binding sites. Some clues came from the studies already reviewed in this chapter:

- In his original publication (1959), Porter showed that fragments I and II, but not fragment III, interfered with antigen–antibody reactions.
- Nisonoff et al. (1960, 1961) demonstrated that the large fragment obtained from pepsin digestion, the $F(ab')_2$, precipitated antigen and thus contained two antigen binding sites.
- Fleischman et al. (1963) showed that neither chain A nor chain B alone could precipitate antigen. They concluded that the antigen binding site is associated with the A (heavy) chain based on an experiment in which isolated chains were added to an antigen–antibody reaction. Chain A delayed the time of precipitation when added to antibody prior to the addition of antigen, while addition of chain B to antibody failed to alter precipitation.

These results suggested that the binding site is somewhere in the amino terminus of the immunoglobulin molecule. The next question was whether light chains, heavy chains, or a combination of the two chains were responsible for antigen binding. Edelman et al. (1963) first demonstrated that both heavy and light chains might be involved in forming the antigen binding site. Guinea pig antibodies specific for two different bacteriophages (f1 and f2) or the hapten dinitrophenol were dissociated into L and H chains. The individual chains had very little antibody activity, while mixtures of H and L chains partially restored the antigen binding capability. Although some antibody activity could be reconstituted by mixing H chains of one antibody with L chains of a different antibody molecule, reconstitution was greatest when the mixture contained H and L chains from the homologous antibodies. These results led the investigators to conclude that "both H and L chains contribute to immunologic specificity." Several years later X-ray crystallographic analysis of two different antibody combining sites demonstrated that antigen binding involved the combination of regions of both H and L chains (Amzel et al., 1974; Segal et al., 1974).

IMMUNOGLOBULIN ISOTYPES (CLASSES)

When first described, antibodies were referred to by names related to their function, including antitoxins, precipitins, agglutinins, hemolysins, hemagglutinins, bacteriolysins, and bacteriocidins. Paul Ehrlich initially used the term antibody (antikorper) to refer to antitoxins in 1891; however, this term was not widely used until over a decade later. Now, antibody is defined as a glyco-protein induced by antigenic challenge regardless of the in vitro or in vivo function of that molecule (reviewed in Lindenmann, 1976).

Today the terms antibody and immunoglobulin are often used interchangeably. Between the 1930s and 1966 several different classes, or isotypes, of immunoglobulin were identified. These isotypes are structurally similar but perform different functions in immune responses. The experiments reviewed in this section present the studies that were instrumental in the initial detection of the different immunoglobulin isotypes.

Discovery of Immunoglobulin Isotypes

In 1937, Elvin Kabat joined Arne Tiselius' laboratory in Sweden as a postdoctoral investigator. Together they identified two molecular forms (isotypes) of antibody. They injected rabbits with ovalbumin (OVA) to induce specific antibodies. They divided this rabbit serum into two aliquots, one of which was absorbed with OVA to remove antibodies and the other left untreated. They then separated the serum proteins of these two aliquots by electrophoresis. Comparison of the electrophoretic patterns of the absorbed and the nonabsorbed sera showed a decrease in the amount of protein in the gamma globulin region but not in the alpha or beta globulin regions (Tiselius and Kabat, 1939). Figure 11.6 illustrates the electrophoretic patterns produced by serum from a rabbit injected with ovalbumin before and after absorption with this antigen. This was the initial identification of an immunoglobulin isotype, now called IgG.

In this same paper, Tiselius and Kabat report that antibody to pneumococcal polysaccharide in serum from horses migrated primarily with the beta globulin fraction and consisted of a protein that had a molecular weight of close to 1 million Da by ultracentrifugation. Initially, the investigators erroneously concluded that antibodies formed in some species (monkey, human, rabbit) had a sedimentation coefficient of approximately 7S and a molecular weight of 150,000 Da, while antibodies from other species (horse, cow, pig) were much larger with a 19S sedimentation coefficient and a molecular weight of approximately 900,000 Da (Kabat and Pedersen, 1938; Kabat, 1939). While this distinction between high and low molecular weight antibodies defines the physical

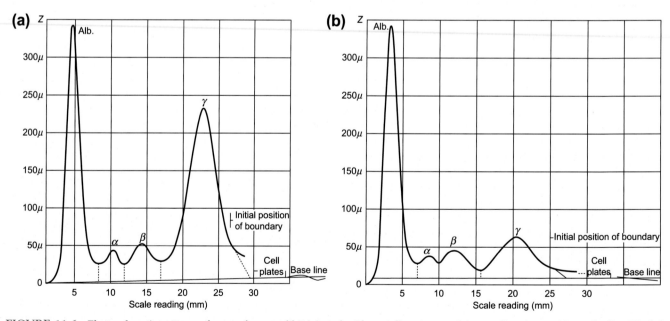

FIGURE 11.6   Electrophoretic patterns of serum from a rabbit injected with egg albumin containing ovalbumin-specific antibodies. The left panel illustrates the pattern of whole serum, while the right panel is the same serum following absorption with egg albumin to remove antibodies, most of which migrate with the gamma globulin fraction. *From Tiselius and Kabat (1939).*

chemical differentiation of IgG and IgM, several more years passed before investigators recognized IgM as a separate isotype.

In 1944, Jan Waldenstrom, working at the University of Uppsala in Sweden, described two patients presenting with anemia, bleeding from the mouth and nose, swollen lymph nodes, viscous serum, and an abnormal serum protein with a molecular weight of approximately 1 million Da. While unrecognized at the time, this is the initial description of the monoclonal gammopathie, now termed Waldenström macroglobulinemia. The abnormal serum protein is now classified as IgM and is secreted by a clone of malignant B lymphocytes. This protein is the pathologic counterpart of the high molecular weight antibodies originally described by Kabat and coworkers.

Upon returning to the United States, Kabat assumed a faculty position at the College of Physicians and Surgeons at Columbia University, New York. There he continued his work on the analysis of antibodies and demonstrated that the Wassermann antibody in humans (an antibody specific for cardiolipin extracted from bovine muscle or heart and used, at the time, to detect cases of syphilis) could exist as both gamma globulin (7S by ultracentrifugation with a molecular weight of 160,000–190,000 Da) and as a macroglobulin (19S by sedimentation with a molecular weight of almost 1 million daltons) (Davis et al., 1945). This represented an early indication that antibodies of the IgM isotype possessed antibody activity.

IgA was the next immunoglobulin isotype to be characterized (Heremans et al., 1959). Joseph Heremans and his colleagues, working at the University of Louvain in Belgium, designed studies to characterize the globulin that migrated in electrophoresis as β2A globulins. Some patients with multiple myeloma have an electrophoretic pattern characterized by increases in this serum fraction. Analysis of isolated β2A with antibodies to whole human serum depleted of antibodies to gamma globulin (IgG) and macroglobulins (IgM) demonstrated that the β2A molecule possessed unique antigenic markers. By ultracentrifugation most of the isolated β2A globulin had a sedimentation coefficient of 7S, while a minor fraction had a sedimentation coefficient of 10.5S.

Initially, antibody activity of the myeloma IgA was not detected. Antibody activity in IgA obtained from immunized individuals was demonstrated by Heremans et al. (1962) when they developed a method for isolating the three molecular forms of serum globulins (7Sγ-IgG, 19Sγ-IgM, and β2A-IgA). They used this method to study the distribution of antibody activity in human serum from an individual injected with diphtheria toxoid and from two individuals recovering from an infection with the gram negative bacteria, *Brucella*. Antibodies to both

diphtheria toxoid and to the bacteria were detected in all three globulin fractions.

Subsequent studies by Thomas Tomasi and S. Zigelbaum (1963), working at the University of Vermont College of Medicine, demonstrated that human saliva contained large quantities of gamma globulin, the vast majority of which is IgA. Similar findings were obtained when colostrum and urine were assayed (Chapter 30). Immunologists now realize that IgA is the main immunoglobulin isotype found in external secretions.

In 1965, a patient presented to David Rowe and John Fahey at the National Cancer Institute with an atypical myeloma protein. Physicochemical analysis of this protein showed that it shared light chains with the other known immunoglobulin isotypes but had a unique heavy chain. Antibodies to IgM, IgG, and IgA failed to react with this protein (Rowe and Fahey, 1965a). An antibody specific to this myeloma protein showed that human serum contained a molecule with similar immunochemical properties. This led Rowe and Fahey (1965b) to conclude that this represented a fourth immunoglobulin isotype, which they termed IgD.

The fifth and final isotype of immunoglobulin, IgE, was described almost simultaneously by Kimishige Ishizaka and his colleagues at the University of Colorado Medical School, Denver (1966), and by S. Gunnar O. Johansson and Hans Bennich, working at University Hospital, Uppsala, Sweden (1967). Johansson and Bennich described this immunoglobulin isotype when they studied a patient, identified as N.D., with a unique myeloma protein that did not react with any of the available antibodies directed against the heavy chains of IgA, IgD, IgG, or IgM. This protein possessed light chains identical to those found in other immunoglobulin isotypes. The protein had a molecular weight of approximately 200,000 Da and a sedimentation rate of 8S. Based on their inability to detect immunoglobulin ND in serum from nonmyeloma patients, they conclude that "if a normal counterpart to protein ND exists, it must be present in a concentration lower than 1–10 μg/ml serum."

Ishizaka and coworkers took a different approach and looked for the antibody responsible for allergic reactions. They initially purified antigens from ragweed pollen and determined which one was the most potent in a skin test for pollen allergy. They termed this antigen E. Working with individuals who were highly allergic to ragweed pollen they looked for antibodies that could bind this antigen. Once found, they characterized this antibody immunochemically and demonstrated that it was different from the other known isotypes of antibody. Since it bound to antigen E, they called it IgE.

Several characteristics suggested that protein ND and IgE were identical. In 1968, a meeting of investigators studying this new immunoglobulin isotype was held at the World Health Organization's International Reference Center for Immunoglobulins in Lausanne, Switzerland. Investigators compared their reagents (proteins and antibodies to these proteins) and concluded that a new immunoglobulin isotype had been discovered. A memorandum signed by the participants described this new immunoglobulin isotype and agreed to call it IgE (Bennich et al., 1968).

CONCLUSION

The composition and molecular structure of antibodies was unraveled by experiments performed over a period of 40 years by investigators working independently in laboratories in Europe and the United States. By the 1930s, immunologists understood that antibodies were glycoproteins found in the gamma globulin fraction of serum. During the 1930s and 1940s investigators demonstrated that the immune system produced antibodies to an astounding variety of esoteric antigens, including synthetic chemicals as well as some not directly related to potentially pathogenic microorganisms. Application of new techniques, such as electrophoresis and ultracentrifugation, led to an appreciation of the composition of antibody. Finally, in the late 1950s and early 1960s, a flurry of research solved the molecular organization of antibody and provided the now familiar four chain structure of a prototypical immunoglobulin. These experiments determined the relationship between antibody structure and function. Antibody molecules possess separate regions responsible for binding antigen and for initiating effector mechanisms such as complement activation, opsonization, and antibody dependent cell-mediated cytotoxicity (Chapter 26).

An important unresolved question was whether antibodies of different specificities were composed of the same or different amino acids. Determining the amino acid sequence of the H and L chains in different antibody molecules led to the answer. Instruction theories of antibody formation predicted that the primary sequence of antibodies would be identical regardless of the antibody specificity of the molecule. Selection theories of antibody formation, developed in the 1950s, predicted that antibodies of different specificities would have different primary amino acid sequences. In the mid-1960s, amino acid sequences of immunoglobulin heavy and light chains became available. Interpretation of these data showed that H and L chains from different antibody molecules possess unique sequences of amino acids, thus supporting the clonal selection theory (Chapter 6). Much of the variability between different antibodies is in the amino terminal region of

the chain where the antigen binding site is mapped. Chapter 18 provides additional information about these differences.

The realization that each lymphocyte produces antibody of a single specificity (Chapter 7) coupled with the knowledge that the amino acid sequences of antibodies of distinct specificities differ led to formulation of additional questions, including:

- How does a particular antibody-forming lymphocyte become committed to producing antibody of a unique specificity? (Chapter 18)
- What are the mechanisms by which potential antibody-forming lymphocytes interact with the environment and are signaled to synthesize and secrete their product? (Chapters 17 and 19)
- How does the immune system eliminate antibody-forming cells that might produce self-reactive antibodies? (Chapter 21)

References

Amzel, L.M., Poljak, R.J., Saul, F., Varga, J.M., Richards, F.F., 1974. The three dimensional structure of a combining region-ligand complex of immunoglobulin NEW at 3.5-Å resolution. Proc. Nat. Acad. Sci. U. S. A. 71, 1427–1430.

Avery, O., 1915. The distribution of the immune bodies occurring in antipneumococcus serum. J. Exp. Med. 21, 133–145.

Bennich, H.H., Ishizaka, K., Johansson, S.G.O., Rowe, D.S., Stanworth, D.R., Terry, W.D., 1968. Immunoglobulin E. A new class of human immunoglobulin. Immunochem. 5, 327–328.

Casadevall, A., 1996. Antibody-based therapies for emerging infectious diseases. Emerg. Inf. Dis. 2, 200–208.

Chickering, H.T., 1915. The concentration of the protective bodies in antipneumococcus serum. Specific precipitate extracts. J. Exp. Med. 22, 248–268.

Davis, B.D., Moore, D.H., Kabat, E.A., Harris, A., 1945. Electrophoretic, ultracentrifugal, and immunochemical studies on Wassermann antibody. J. Immunol. 50, 1–20.

Edelman, G.M., 1959. Dissociation of γ-globulin. J. Am. Chem. Soc. 81, 3155–3156.

Edelman, G.M., Cunningham, B.A., Gail, W.E., Gottlieb, P.D., Rutishauser, U., Waxdal, M.J., 1969. The covalent structure of an entire gamma G immunoglobulin molecule. Proc. Nat. Acad. Sci. U. S. A. 63, 78–85.

Edelman, G.M., Heremans, J.F., Heremans, M-Th, Kunkel, H.G., 1960. Immunological studies of human γ-globulin: relation of the precipitin lines of whole γ-globulin to the fragments produced by papain. J. Exp. Med. 112, 203–223.

Edelman, G.M., Olins, D.E., Gally, J.A., Zinder, N.D., 1963. Reconstitution of immunologic activity by interaction of polypeptide chains of antibodies. Proc. Nat. Acad. Sci. U. S. A. 50, 753–761.

Edelman, G.M., Poulik, M.D., 1961. Studies on structural units of the γ-globulins. J. Exp. Med. 113, 861–864.

Fenton, L.D., 1931a. The correlation of the protective value with the titers of other antibodies in type I antipneumococcus serum. J. Immunol. 21, 341–356.

Fenton, L.D., 1931b. The use of ethyl alcohol as precipitant in the concentration of antipneumococcus serum. J. Immunol. 21, 357–373.

Fleischman, J.B., Pain, R.H., Porter, R.R., 1962. Reduction of gammaglobulins. Arch. Biochem. Biophys. Acta (Suppl. 1), 174–180 .

Fleischman, J.B., Porter, R.R., Press, E.M., 1963. The arrangement of the peptide chains in γ-globulin. Biochem. J. 88, 220–228.

Heidelberger, M., Kabat, E.A., 1936. Chemical studies on bacterial agglutination. II. The identity of precipitin and agglutinin. J. Exp. Med. 63, 737–744.

Heidelberger, M., Pedersen, K.O., 1937. The molecular weight of antibodies. J. Exp. Med. 65, 393–414.

Heremans, J.F., Heremans, M-Th, Schultze, H.E., 1959. Isolation and description of a few properties of the β2A –globulin of human serum. Clin. Chim. Acta 4, 96–102.

Heremans, J.F., Vaerman, J.P., Vaerman, C., 1962. Studies on the immune globulins of human serum II. A study of the distribution of anti-Brucella and anti-diphtheria antibody activities among γSS-, γ1M- and γ1A-globulin fractions. J. Immunol. 91, 11–17.

Ishizaka, K., Ishizaka, T., Hornbrook, M., 1966. Physiochemical properties of reaginic antibody. IV. Presence of a unique immunoglobulin as a carrier of reaginic activity. J. Immunol. 97, 75–85.

Johansson, S.G.O., Bennich, H., 1967. Immunological studies of an atypical (myeloma) immunoglobulin. Immunology 13, 381–394.

Kabat, E.A., 1939. The molecular weight of antibodies. J. Exp. Med. 69, 103–118.

Kabat, E.A., Pedersen, K.O., 1938. The molecular weights of antibodies. Science 87, 372.

Lindenmann, J., 1976. Origin of the terms 'antibody' and 'antigen'. Scand. J. Immunol. 19, 281–285.

Nisonoff, A., Markus, G., Wissler, F.C., 1961. Separation of univalent fragments of rabbit antibody by reduction of a single, labile disulfide bond. Nature 189, 293–295.

Nisonoff, A., Wissler, F.C., Lipman, L.N., 1960. Properties of the major component of a peptic digest of a rabbit antibody. Science 132, 1770–1771.

Nuttall, G.H.F., 1888. Experimente über die bacterien feindlichen Einflüsse des thierischen Körpers. Zeitschr. F. Hyg. 4, 853–894.

Porter, R.R., 1959. The hydrolysis of rabbit γ-globulin and antibodies with crystalline papain. Biochem. J. 73, 119–126.

Putnam, F.W., 1969. Immunoglobulin structure: variability and homology. Science 163, 633–644.

Rowe, D.D., Fahey, J.L., 1965a. A new class of human immunoglobulin. I. A unique myeloma protein. J. Exp. Med. 121, 171–184.

Rowe, D.S., Fahey, J.L., 1965b. A new class of human immunoglobulin. II. Normal serum IgD. J. Exp. Med. 121, 185–199.

Schmalstieg, F.C., Goldman, A.S., 2009. Jules Bordet (1870-1961): a bridge between early and modern immunology. J. Med. Biog. 17, 217–224.

Segal, D.M., Padlan, E.O., Cohen, G.H., Rudikoff, S., Potter, M., Davies, D.R., 1974. The three-dimensional structure of a phosphorylcholine-binding mouse immunoglobulin Fab and the nature of the antigen binding site. Proc. Nat. Acad. Sci. U. S. A. 71, 4298–4302.

Tiselius, A., 1937a. A new apparatus for electrophoretic analysis of colloidal mixtures. Trans. Faraday Soc. 33, 524–531.

Tiselius, A., 1937b. Electrophoresis of serum globulin. Biochem. J. 31, 313–317.

Tiselius, A., Kabat, E.A., 1939. An electrophoretic study of immune serum and purified antibody preparations. J. Exp. Med. 69, 119–131.

Tomasi, T.B., Zigelbaum, S., 1963. The selective occurrence of γ1A globulins in certain body fluids. J. Clin. Invest. 42, 1552–1560.

Von Buchner, H., 1889. Über die bakterioentödtende wirkung des zellfreien blutserums. Zbl. Bakt. (Naturwiss) 5, 817–823.

Von Fodor, J., 1887. Die Fähigkeit des Bluts Bakterien zu vernichten. Dtsch. Med. Wochenschr. 13, 745–746.

Waldenström, J., 1944. Incipient myelomatosis or 'essential' hyperglobulinemia with fibrinogenopenia – a new syndrome? Acta Med. Scand. 67, 216–247.

Zinsser, H., 1913. Further studies on the identity of precipitins and protein sensitizers (albuminolysins). J. Exp. Med. 18, 219–227.

TIME LINE

1887–1889	von Fodor, Nuttall, and von Buchner independently describe a serum substance with antibacterial (antibody) activity
1913	Hans Zinsser shows that precipitins can fix complement in support of the Unitarian theory of antibody
1915	Oswald Avery demonstrates that antibody to *Streptococcus pneumoniae* is in the gamma globulin fraction of serum
1937	Michael Heidelberger and Kai Pedersen prove antibodies are serum proteins
1937	Arne Tiselius develops the technique of serum electrophoresis
1939	Arne Tiselius and Elvin Kabat show that antibody activity migrates in the gamma globulin fraction of serum
1939	Elvin Kabat separates antibodies of two different molecular weights
1948	Arne Tiselius awarded the Nobel Prize in Physiology or Medicine
1959	Joseph Heremans and colleagues identify serum IgA
1959	Rodney Porter fractionates IgG into three fragments with papain
1959	Gerald Edelman demonstrates that antibody has multiple polypeptide chains linked by disulfide bonds
1960–1961	Al Nisonoff shows that pepsin cleavage of antibody produces one large fragment and several small peptides
1962	Rodney Porter and coworkers separate heavy (H) and light (L) chains
1963	Julian Fleischman and colleagues propose a four chain structure of the IgG molecule
1963	Gerald Edelman and colleagues show both H and L chains are involved in forming the antigen binding site
1963	Thomas Tomasi and S. Ziegelbaum describe secretory IgA
1965	David Rowe and John Fahey report a patient with a unique paraprotein identified as IgD
1966	Kimishige Ishizaka and colleagues identify a unique immunoglobulin (IgE) associated with allergies
1967	S. Gunnar Johansson and Hans Bennich describe a patient with an atypical myeloma protein (IgE)
1969	Frank Putnam publishes a model of the prototypical antibody molecule
1972	Nobel Prize in Physiology or Medicine awarded to Edelman and Porter

12

Complement

INTRODUCTION

In the late 1880s several investigators injected experimental animals with bacteria (*Bacillus anthracis* or *Vibrio cholerae*) and induced the production of a serum substance that could kill the bacteria (von Fodor, 1887; Nuttall, 1888; von Buchner, 1889). This induced serum substance was called antibody shortly after its discovery. In addition to killing bacteria, antibody eliminates or controls potential pathogens by four mechanisms (Chapter 26):

- neutralization, a process in which antibody combines with antigen and inhibits it from binding to and invading susceptible cells of the body;
- opsonization, a process resulting in enhanced phagocytosis;
- antibody-dependent cell-mediated cytotoxicity; and
- activation of the complement system, resulting in cell lysis opsonization and the induction of an inflammatory response.

Both antibody and complement enhance phagocytosis and are considered opsonins. Phagocytic cells express receptors for the Fc portion of antibody, thus increasing the uptake of antigen–antibody complexes. Phagocytic cells also express receptors for the C3b component of complement and engulf foreign pathogens to which this factor is bound. The complement system consists of a series of 30 serum proteins. A primary group of 11 proteins act sequentially to trigger cell lysis and induce inflammation. The remaining proteins in the system modulate complement activation.

Complement is activated by three different pathways: the classical, the alternate, and the lectin. This nomenclature reflects the historical discovery of the three activation mechanisms. The classical pathway was originally described in the late 1800s and early 1900s and is the process initiated by antigen–antibody complexes. The second, alternate or properdin, pathway was described in the mid-twentieth century and does not require the presence of antibody. This properdin pathway evolutionarily predates the classical pathway and provides a method for the innate host defenses to eliminate potentially pathogenic microorganisms. The third pathway of complement activation, the lectin pathway, was first described in the 1970s. This method of complement activation, like the properdin pathway, proceeds in the absence of antibody. In this chapter the discovery of complement and the three mechanisms by which it can be triggered are presented from a historical viewpoint, starting with the classical pathway and ending with the lectin pathway.

EARLY EVIDENCE FOR COMPLEMENT

Observations made in the original description of antibody activity suggested two separate serum constituents that work together to eliminate bacteria:

1. George Henry Falkiner Nuttall (1862–1937) heated the serum containing antibody and destroyed the bactericidal activity; and

A Historical Perspective on Evidence-Based Immunology
http://dx.doi.org/10.1016/B978-0-12-398381-7.00012-5

2. Hans Ernst August Buchner (1850–1902) diluted the antibacterial serum with water and obtained two fractions: one that precipitated and a second that was soluble. Neither fraction alone possessed the bactericidal activity; however, if the two fractions were recombined, the bactericidal activity was restored. In addition, the soluble fraction of serum from animals that had not been injected with bacteria possessed a low level of naturally occurring bactericidal activity; he called this activity alexin.

Richard Friedrich Johannes Pfeiffer (1848–1945), working in Robert Koch's Institute of Hygiene at the University of Berlin, injected guinea pigs with cholera bacteria (*V. cholerae*) to induce specific antibodies (Pfeiffer, 1894; Pfeiffer and Issaeff, 1894). Serum taken from these injected animals inhibited the movement of the bacteria but did not lyse them. When a mixture of bacteria and antibody-containing serum was injected into the peritoneal cavity of another guinea pig, the bacteria disintegrated within a short time. The most likely explanation for this observation is that something in the peritoneal cavity provided help to the antibody in killing the bacteria. This initial observation of bacteriolysis was termed the Pfeiffer phenomenon and provided functional evidence that antibody requires a complementary system to effectively eliminate invading bacteria.

Within a year of Pfeiffer's observation, Jules Bordet demonstrated that normal serum could enhance (complement) the activity of specific antibodies to kill *V. cholerae* in vitro (Bordet, 1895, 1896). Jules Bordet (1870–1961) received his training as a physician in Brussels , Belgium. He worked at the Pasteur Institute (Paris) in the laboratory of Ilya Metchnikov until 1901 when he returned to Belgium to direct a newly formed Pasteur Institute in Brussels. In 1919, he was awarded the Nobel Prize in Physiology or Medicine "for his discoveries related to immunity."

Bordet showed that serum from an animal injected with a microbe contained two substances: one that existed prior to injection and a second that was induced by injecting the microbe. Serum from guinea pigs injected with *V. cholerae* killed the bacteria in vitro. Serum heated to 56 °C for 30 min failed to kill *V. cholerae*, but this activity could be regained by the addition of fresh serum from an uninjected animal (Bordet, 1895). The heat stable component, induced by injection of the bacteria, was termed sensibilatrices (antibody) while the heat labile component was called alexin (complement).

In 1898, Bordet described hemolytic sera—sera containing antibodies capable of lysing foreign red blood cells. He demonstrated that these sera also required alexin to lyse the cells (Bordet, 1898). Paul Ehrlich and Julius Morgenroth confirmed this observation in 1899 when they demonstrated that red blood cell lysis required the activity of a second serum component. Ehrlich and Morgenroth termed the serum component that assisted the lytic activity of antibody complement.

Further evidence that complement and antibody were separate entities derives from observations made by Simon Flexner (1863–1946) and Hideyo Noguchi (1876–1928) in 1902 at the University of Pennsylvania. They studied the effect of snake venom (cobra, moccasin, cottonmouth, and rattlesnake) on the bactericidal activity of serum from dog, rabbit, and mudpuppy (*Necturus maculosus*). Sera from these animals were variably bactericidal to *Salmonella typhi*, *Escherichia coli*, or *B. anthracis*. Treatment of these sera with snake venom depleted this bactericidal activity.

Flexner and Noguchi determined whether venom affected the antibody or complement by mixing serum from one animal that had been depleted of complement by heating to 56 °C with a serum from which antibody had been adsorbed by treatment with bacteria. Neither serum alone was bactericidal; however, mixing the two sera reconstituted the activity. Treating the individual serum with venom revealed that the action of the venoms was on the complement and not the antibody.

By the early 1900s, the existence of a substance in normal serum that helped specific antibody lyse bacteria and red blood cells was well established, and the term complement replaced other names given to the substance. Studies performed over the next 70 years demonstrated that complement consists of a number of serum proteins activated sequentially. As these individual proteins were discovered, investigators named them. Some of these names denoted the function of the proteins, while others referred to some physicochemical characteristic of the protein. Initially, the primary complement components were given numerical designation preceded by a C'. During the 1960s, the World Health Organization (WHO) arranged informal discussions among complement investigators and formalized complement nomenclature in a memorandum signed by the participants. The nomenclature suggested in this memorandum is used throughout this chapter (WHO, 1968).

Complement can be activated by three discrete pathways, only one of which requires the interaction of antigen with specific antibody. Activation of complement by antigen–antibody complexes is known as the classical pathway, while the two pathways occurring in the absence of antibody are termed the alternate pathway and the lectin pathway.

THE CLASSICAL PATHWAY

Activation of the complement system by the classical pathway occurs when antibody binds to its specific antigen (Figure 12.1). The antibodies in this complex display the Fc portion of the molecule to the environment. The

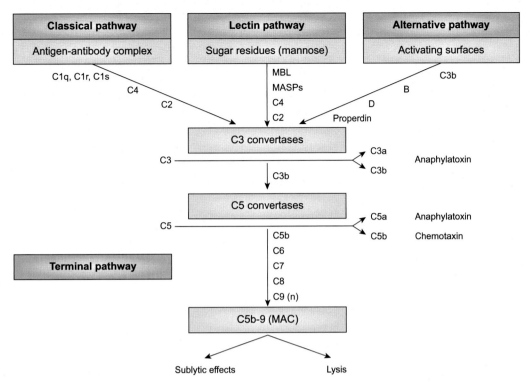

FIGURE 12.1 Diagram of the classical, alternate (properdin), and lectin pathways of complement activation. *From Cook and Botto, 2006:* http://www.nature.com/nrrheum/journal/v2/n6/fig_tab/ncprheum0191_F1.html.

first component of complement (C1q) binds two adjoining immunoglobulin Fc regions and initiates a sequence of enzymatic reactions that activates the remaining complement components. Complete activation of the system enhances several outcomes of both innate host defense mechanisms and adaptive immune responses, including

- phagocytosis of the pathogen,
- induction of an inflammatory response,
- release of chemotactic molecules that attract granulocytes and macrophages, and
- lysis of the pathogen.

Activation of complement by the classical pathway involves 11 complement proteins numbered C1—C9 (the C1 component includes three separate proteins: C1q, C1r, and C1s). The numbering of these components reflects the order in which they were discovered; however, the order of activation of these proteins is C1, C4, C2, C3, C5—C9. Several of the products resulting from enzymatic cleavage of these proteins possess biological activity, including chemotaxis (attracting inflammatory cells), vasodilation, and opsonization (enhancing phagocytosis). Completion of the enzymatic cascade leads to cell lysis.

By the mid-1920s investigators identified several individual complement components (Whitehead et al., 1925; Cooper, 2006; Lachmann, 2006). In 1907, A. Ferrata, working in Paul Ehrlich's laboratory in Germany, separated serum into two fractions by dialyzing against water. Such treatment caused some of the proteins to precipitate (termed euglobulins) while other proteins (the pseudoglobulins) remained soluble. Treating antibody-coated red blood cells with either euglobulin or pseudoglobulin failed to produce lysis of the red blood cells. However, if Ferrato treated the cells with a mixture of euglobulin and pseudoglobulin, the cells lysed.

In the same year, E. Brand demonstrated that the two fractions could be added sequentially to the antibody-coated red blood cells. He reported that the euglobulin interacted with the antibody and was required prior to the addition of the pseudoglobulin. Accordingly, he named the fractions the mid piece (euglobulin) and the end piece (pseudoglobulin) (Brand, 1907). These two fractions correspond to C1 and C2 in contemporary nomenclature.

A third component of complement (C3) was described by L. Omorokow in 1911 and by H. Ritz in 1912 using the lysis of antibody-treated erythrocytes as the assay system. C3 was removed from serum by treatment with cobra venom. In 1914, Arthur Coca, working at Cornell University in Ithaca, New York, showed that treatment of serum with yeast similarly removed this component of complement. This observation is important in subsequent investigations that led to the description of the alternate (properdin) path of complement activation.

The fourth component of complement (C4) was discovered in 1926 by John Gordon and colleagues, working in England. Gordon added guinea pig serum as a source of complement to ox or sheep erythrocytes coated with specific antibody, resulting in red blood cell lysis. Guinea pig serum treated with ammonia failed to lyse the antibody-coated red blood cells. Mixing ammonia-treated serum with serum heated to 56 °C restored erythrocyte lysis. These results suggested that ammonia inactivated some component of the complement system that was heat stable.

Although four components of complement were identified by the mid-1920s, the order of interaction of these components remained unknown until 1954. Manfred Mayer (1916–1984) and colleagues at Johns Hopkins University in Baltimore, Maryland, unraveled this information by studying the mechanism of antibody-mediated hemolysis of sheep erythrocytes. Techniques used to establish the sequence C1, C4, C2, C3 included

- preparation of reagents containing three of the four components and mixing them in various combinations (Bier et al., 1945);
- determination of the role of divalent cations Ca^{++} and Mg^{++} as enzymatic catalysts during the reaction of individual complement proteins (Levine et al., 1953); and
- quantitation of complement components and antibody in antigen–antibody complexes or in serum used as a complement source (Wallace et al., 1950).

By 1954, Mayer and his colleagues demonstrated that complexes of erythrocytes with antibody react initially with the C1 and C4 components in the presence of Ca^{++}. This complex then reacts with C2 in the presence of Mg^{++}. Finally, C3 reacts, resulting in a damaged cell that undergoes lysis and releases hemoglobin.

During the late 1950s into the 1960s several new techniques aided the separation and characterization of complement components: anion and cation exchange chromatography, gel filtration based on molecular size, zonal and gel electrophoresis, ultracentrifugation, radio-isotope labeling, immunodiffusion techniques, and preparation of antibodies specific for isolated proteins. Prior to the development of these techniques, studies on the components of complement depended on functional assays such as the lysis of antibody-treated erythrocytes; these evolving techniques enhanced the isolation and quantitation of additional complement components.

Irwin Lepow and colleagues at Western Reserve University in Cleveland, Ohio, separated the first component of complement using DEAE (diethylaminoethyl) chromatography into three fractions: C1q, C1r, and C1s (1963). C1q was identical to a serum protein (described previously) that is involved in a very early step in complement activation; C1q is now known to bind to the Fc portion of antibody molecules. C1r and C1s are activated by bound C1q and are responsible for forming an esterase essential to the continued enzymatic cleavage of distal complement components.

Studies identifying the terminal components of complement (C5–C9) were performed by three groups of investigators: Hans Müller-Eberhard and colleagues, initially in Uppsala, Sweden, and later in LaJolla, California; Robert A. Nelson and his group at the Howard Hughes Medical Institute in Miami, Florida; and Paul Klein and collaborators at the Johannes-Gutenberg University in Mainz, Germany. Müller-Eberhard and his group used human serum as the starting point while the other investigators studied guinea pig serum.

In 1960, Müller-Eberhard along with Ulf Nilsson, isolated a β_{1c}-globulin from fresh human serum using anion exchange chromatography. While this protein fraction failed to lyse sheep erythrocytes incubated with specific antibody, it did lyse antibody-coated red blood cells that had been incubated with complement components C1, C4, and C2. This suggested that the β_{1c} fraction of serum contains the C3 complement component; subsequent investigation revealed that this globulin comprised six components originally called C3a–C3f. During the ensuing 9 years these additional proteins (C3, C5, C6, C7, C8, and C9) were purified both in humans (C5—Nilsson and Müller-Eberhard, 1965; C6 and C7—Nilsson, 1967; C8—Manni and Müller-Eberhard, 1969; C9—Hadding and Müller-Eberhard, 1969) and guinea pigs (Nelson et al., 1966).

Complement activation by the classical pathway is the mechanism by which the adaptive immune response eliminates pathogenic microorganisms. However, since complement proteins are not specific for a particular pathogen, the system is classified as part of the innate host defenses. During the period between 1954 and 1972, investigators noted that in some situations the complement system could be triggered in the absence of antibody. Subsequent studies revealed two additional mechanisms of complement activation: the properdin or alternate pathway and the lectin pathway. All three pathways result in identical biological outcomes: opsonization, induction of an inflammatory response, and lysis of the invading microbe.

THE ALTERNATE (PROPERDIN) PATHWAY

Louis Pillemer (1908–1957) described the properdin pathway of complement activation in 1954. Pillemer, a biochemist/immunologist, earned his PhD in 1938 from Western Reserve University, now Case Western Reserve University, in Cleveland, Ohio. He spent most of his career in the Institute of Pathology at Case Western Reserve researching complement. Irwin Lepow, one of Pillemer's graduate students and colleagues, presented an overview of his scientific achievements in his Presidential Address to the American Association of

Immunologists in 1980. Among other accomplishments, Pillemer purified and characterized several of the complement components through the application of new and evolving methods of protein chemistry.

Discovery of the properdin pathway of complement activation resulted from an unsuccessful attempt at purifying C3. In 1900, Emil von Dungern showed that complement could be inactivated by adding yeast to serum (Fitzpatrick and DiCarlo, 1964). Pillemer and Ecker (1941) demonstrated that the inactivation of complement by yeast was due to the presence of a large polysaccharide, zymosan. Addition of zymosan to serum at 37°C results in the selective loss of C3 activity by the serum. Pillemer reasoned that zymosan adsorbs C3 from the serum and that purified C3 could be eluted from the zymosan–C3 complex.

In 1953, Pillemer and coworkers treated human serum with zymosan and subjected the resulting precipitate to a number of procedures designed to elute the adsorbed C3; these attempts failed. Further study showed that the interaction of zymosan with C3 required incubation at a temperature greater than 20°C in the presence of magnesium and other serum factors at pH 7.0 (Pillemer et al., 1953a,b) and suggested that the interaction between zymosan and C3 was not simple adsorption but rather involved an enzymatic reaction. Mixing zymosan with human serum at 37°C followed by centrifugation to remove the zymosan resulted in a supernatant containing decreased amounts of C3. When this experiment was performed at 17°C, the amount of C3 activity of the serum was not decreased. Moreover, increasing the temperature of the supernatant from this experiment to 37°C and adding more zymosan failed to decrease the amount of C3 activity.

Pillemer and his colleagues interpreted these results by proposing a previously undetected serum protein, properdin, which binds zymosan (Pillemer et al., 1954).

The complex of zymosan and properdin inactivates C3 at 37°C but not at 17°C. Figure 12.2 provides the results from experiments leading to this interpretation. Pillemer separated properdin from zymosan by treating the precipitate with high ionic strength medium. Characterization of properdin revealed that it is most likely a protein that constitutes approximately 0.03% of the total serum proteins. Properdin is not an antibody or a component of the coagulation or the classical complement systems.

Pillemer and colleagues proposed that properdin binds to pathogens and activates the C3 component of complement. Serum depleted of properdin failed to kill bacteria (Shigella dysenteriae), neutralize virus (influenza, mumps), or hemolyze sheep red blood cells.

Subsequent studies with properdin confirmed a separate system of complement activation that did not require antigen–antibody complexes. This system is now termed the properdin (alternate) complement pathway (Figure 12.1). Properdin does not serve as a link between a pathogen and the C3 component of complement as Pillemer suggested although it does play an important role in activation of the alternate system.

The publication of the original paper on the properdin pathway of complement activation was viewed as "a major breakthrough…in the understanding of and possible attack upon a broad array of diseases" (Lepow, 1980). Shortly, however, doubts were cast on the validity of Pillemer's interpretation of his data. Robert Nelson, working at Yale University in New Haven, Connecticut, reinvestigated this phenomenon and reported his results at two conferences in October 1956 and March 1957 as well as in a peer-reviewed publication (Nelson, 1958). Nelson's results contradicted Pillemer's conclusion, and Nelson proposed, erroneously, that serum contained a naturally occurring antibody to zymosan. Interaction of zymosan with this antibody inactivated complement by the classical pathway.

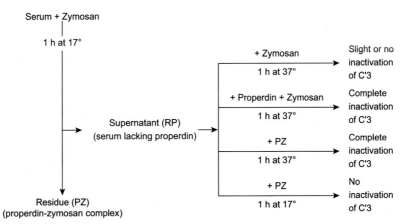

FIGURE 12.2 Interpretation of the experiment demonstrating the presence of a protein (properdin) involved in the activation of the C3 component of complement. Treatment of serum with zymosan at 17°C failed to decrease the amount of C3 in the serum (left side of figure). Treatment of the supernatant from this experiment with additional zymosan at 37°C did not decrease the amount of C3 while the addition of zymosan plus properdin at 37°C did decrease C3 activity. From Pillemer et al., 1954.

Despite being incorrect about the naturally occurring antibody, Nelson's interpretation was widely accepted by much of the immunological community at the time. The controversy may have contributed to Pillemer's death in 1957 due to an overdose of barbiturates at age 49.

Subsequent research has shown that an alternate (properdin) pathway of complement activation does exist and that Pillemer was essentially correct. Properdin has been purified and characterized and activates complement in the absence of antibody. The properdin complement pathway is initiated as a result of spontaneous hydrolysis of the C3 component of complement in serum. This produces a cleavage product, C3b, that binds to microbial surfaces, forming an enzyme, C3 convertase, which initiates the activation of the subsequent complement components (Figure 12.1). Properdin is not an antibody but rather is a stabilizer of this C3 convertase.

THE LECTIN PATHWAY

Several publications during the 1970s reported that serum binds and activates the C1 component of complement in the absence of antibody. In 1972, Pier Natali and Eng Tan, working at the Research Institute of the Scripps Clinic in LaJolla, California, showed that serum from an uninjected animal precipitates polyribonucleotides. The component of serum responsible for precipitating the polyribonucleotides is heat labile and resembles C1q (the complement component that interacts with antibody in the classical pathway of complement activation). Other investigators reported binding of C1 plus activation of the complement sequence by subcellular membranes of human heart (Pinkard et al., 1973), RNA tumor viruses (Cooper et al., 1976), the lipid A component of *Salmonella minnesota* lipopolysaccharide (Cooper and Morrison, 1978), and retrovirus membranes (Bartholomew and Esser, 1980). Complement activation requires interactions between pathogens and naturally occurring carbohydrate-binding proteins termed lectins. Two of these proteins, mannose-binding lectin (MBL) and ficolins (molecules with fibrinogen-like and collagen-like portions), recognize carbohydrates on the surface of pathogens. The binding of these lectins to their ligands initiates the complement system.

Initially activation appeared to be identical to that produced by the interaction of antigen–antibody complexes with C1q (the classical pathway) (Ikeda et al., 1987). In 1983, Kenneth Reid of Oxford University in England pointed out the structural similarities between MBL and C1q. This prompted Masayuki Ohta and coworkers at Kyoto University in Japan (1990) to revisit the mechanism of complement activation by the lectin pathway. They demonstrated that activation of complement by human MBL proceeded in the absence of C1q.

Cell-bound MBL binds to the complex of $C1r_2C1s_2$ and activates unique enzymes (serine proteases) that cleave the C4 and C2 components of complement. The cleaved C4-C2 complex then acts as a C3 convertase enzyme as in the classical pathway (Figure 12.1).

BIOLOGICAL ACTIVITY OF COMPLEMENT AND ITS FRAGMENTS

Enzymatic cleavage of many of the complement components produces fragments that participate in the biological functions of the system. These biological functions include vasodilation of blood vessels, attraction of inflammatory leukocytes, and opsonization and are most likely more important to the defense of the individual than the lysis of pathogens or infected cells.

Vasodilation (a widening of the blood vessels due to relaxation of smooth muscles in the vessel walls) results in increased local blood flow and an influx of inflammatory cells. In the mid-1960s, Irvin Lepow and his laboratory in Cleveland, Ohio, initiated a series of investigations on complement-induced vasodilation. In 1965, W. Dias de Silva and Lepow demonstrated that incubation of purified human C1 esterase (an enzyme formed by the cleavage of C1) with guinea pig or rat serum resulted in the formation of a substance that stimulated smooth muscle contraction. Smooth muscle activity was measured using isolated guinea pig ileum suspended in a tissue bath. Test samples were added to this preparation and the amount of contraction measured by a kymograph.

Because the substance produced in these studies mimicked the activity observed when mast cells are degranulated during an anaphylactic reaction, the authors termed the substance anaphylatoxin. During the next two years Lepow characterized anaphylatoxin and concluded that it derived from the cleavage of the C3 component of complement into C3a and C3b fragments. The smaller C3a fragment was the anaphylotoxin (Dias de Silva et al., 1967).

Joerg Jensen at the Howard Hughes Medical Institute in Miami, Florida, performed similar studies and reported in 1967 that one of the fractions produced by the cleavage of guinea pig C5 was also an anaphylatoxin. Jensen generated anaphylatoxin using four in vitro experimental designs:

1. treatment of guinea pig serum or fractions with cobra venom;
2. treatment of guinea pig serum or fractions with an antigen–antibody precipitate;
3. incubation of purified C5 with trypsin; or
4. reaction of erythrocyte-antibody C1, C4, C2, C3 complexes with C5.

Anaphylatoxin was assayed by measuring the contraction of guinea pig ileum in vitro; all four protocols resulted in smooth muscle contraction. Generation of anaphylatoxin by the first two protocols (positive controls) was expected since the entire complement system was present. Generation of anaphylatoxin by the treatment of C5 with trypsin (protocol #3) or the addition of C5 to red blood cells treated with antibodies and the first four components of complement (protocol #4) confirmed that activation of C5 serves as a source of anaphylatoxin. Jensen speculated that anaphylatoxin is released as a small fragment of the C5 molecule when it is cleaved by activated C3 or by serum enzymes. Subsequent studies showed that C5a, like C3a, has anaphylotoxic properties.

A second outcome of complement activation is opsonization or the enhancement of phagocytosis. In 1968, Waltraut Lay and Victor Nussenzweig, working at the New York University School of Medicine, showed that when complement is added to antigen–antibody complexes and the complexes are exposed to macrophages, phagocytosis is increased.

Lay and Nussenzweig used rosette formation to investigate complement-induced opsonization. During the late 1960s and early 1970s, three types of rosettes were described:

- E rosettes formed when human lymphocytes were mixed with sheep erythrocytes (SRBC). This phenomenon was used for several years as a clinical laboratory method to quantitate T lymphocytes in peripheral blood.
- EA rosettes formed by incubating peripheral blood leukocytes with antibody-coated SRBC were used to detect the presence of Fc receptors on cells.
- EAC rosettes formed when SRBC were mixed with antibody and complement detected cells that had complement receptors on their surface.

Lay and Nussenzweig investigated EAC rosette formation to determine the role of complement in phagocytosis.

SRBC mixed with IgM (19S) antibody failed to form rosettes when incubated with mouse macrophages. However, the addition of mouse complement to this mixture resulted in the formation of rosettes with most mouse macrophages and neutrophils as well as with a few monocytes. EAC rosettes also formed with between 10% and 25% of mature lymphocytes from mouse lymph nodes but not from immature thymus lymphocytes. The adherence of SRBC to phagocytic cells induced the formation of cytoplasmic extensions by the leukocytes, some of which appeared to surround the SRBC. Adherence between phagocytes and SRBC causes damage to the red cells, which become fragmented.

Serum deficient in C5 or C6 produced similar results and suggested to Lay and Nussenzweig that the leukocyte receptors bound one of the first four complement components. Subsequent investigations have demonstrated the expression of receptors on macrophages and other phagocytic cells specific for a breakdown product (C3b) of C3. C3b binds to the surface of a pathogen once the complement system is triggered and serves as an opsonin to enhance phagocytosis.

CONCLUSION

The complement system comprises over 30 different serum proteins that interact to enhance both innate host defense mechanisms and adaptive immune responses. Activation of this system results in the augmentation of phagocytosis, inflammation, cell movement (chemotaxis), and cell lysis. Three different pathways of complement activation have evolved:

- The alternate (properdin) pathway, described in the 1950s, involves the spontaneous cleavage of the C3 component of complement within serum and tissue fluids. If activated C3 finds a suitable substrate (i.e., bacterial cell wall, apoptotic or necrotic tissue) to bind, the subsequent complement components are activated.
- The lectin pathway, described in the 1970s and 1980s, involves the interaction of carbohydrate-binding proteins with ligands on the surface of pathogens. These lectins in turn interact with some of the components of the C1 complex to initiate the activation sequence.
- The classical pathway, described in 1895, requires the interaction of C1 with antibodies bound to antigen. This initiates the sequential activation of the other components of the system, leading to several biological functions.

Both the properdin and lectin pathways of complement activation appear to be evolutionarily older than the classical pathway, are integral parts of the innate host defense, and eliminate potential pathogens prior to initiation of the adaptive immune response. The proteins of the alternate and lectin pathways have been appropriated by the adaptive immune system and provide antimicrobial immunity following synthesis of specific antibodies.

References

Bartholomew, R.M., Esser, A.F., 1980. Mechanism of antibody-independent activation of the first component of complement (C1q) on retrovirus membranes. Biochem. 19, 2847–2853.

Bier, O.G., Leyton, G., Mayer, M.M., Heidelberger, M., 1945. A comparison of human and guinea pig complements and their component fractions. J. Exp. Med. 81, 449–468.

Bordet, J., 1895. Les leucocytes et les proprieties actives du serum chez les vaccines. Ann. Inst. Pasteur. 9, 462–506.

Bordet, J., 1896. Sur le mode d'action des serums preventives. Ann. Inst. Pasteur. 10, 193–219.

Bordet, J., 1898. Sur l'agglutination et la dissolution des globules rouges par le serum d'animaux injecties de sang defibriné. Ann. Inst. Pasteur. 12, 688–695.

Brand, E., 1907. Über das Verhalten der Komplemente bei der Dialyse. Berl. Klin. Wochsch. 44, 1075.

von Buchner, H., 1889. Über das bakterioentődtende wirkung des zellfreien blutserums. Zbl. Bakt. (Naturwiss) 5, 817–823.

Coca, A.F., 1914. A study of the anticomplementary action of yeast, of certain bacteria and of cobra venom. Z. Immunitätsforsch. 21, 604–610.

Cook, H.T., Botto, M., 2006. Mechanisms of disease: the complement system and the pathogenesis of systemic lupus erythematosus. Nat. Clin. Prac. Rheumatol. 2, 330–337.

Cooper, N.R., 2006. Complement: a nostalgic journey. The Hans J. Müller-Eberhard memorial lecture. Mol. Immunol. 43, 487–495.

Cooper, N.R., Jensen, F.C., Welsh, R.M., Oldstone, M.B., 1976. Lysis of RNA tumor viruses by human serum: direct antibody-independent triggering of the classical complement pathway. J. Exp. Med. 144, 970–984.

Cooper, N.R., Morrison, D.C., 1978. Binding and activation of the first component of human complement by the lipid A region of lipopolysaccharide. J. Immunol. 120, 1862–1868.

Dias de Silva, W., Eisele, J.W., Lepow, I.H., 1967. Complement as a mediator of inflammation. III. Purification of the activity with anaphylatoxin properties generated by interaction of the first four components or complement and its identification as a cleavage product of C3. J. Exp. Med. 126, 1027–1048.

Dias de Silva, W., Lepow, I.H., 1965. Anaphylatoxin formation by purified human C'1 esterase. J. Immunol. 95, 1080–1089.

Ehrlich, P., Morgenroth, J., 1899. Zür theorie der lysenwirkung. Berl. Klin. Wochenschr. 36, 6–9.

Ferrata, A., 1907. Die Unwirksamkeit der complexen Hämolysine in salzfreien Lösungen and ihre Unsache. Berl. Klin. Wochenschr. 44, 366.

Fitzpatrick, F.W., DiCarlo, F.J., 1964. Zymosan. Ann. N.Y. Acad. Sci. 118, 235–261.

Flexner, S., Noguchi, H., 1902. Snake venom in relation to haemolysis, bacteriolysis and toxicity. J. Exp. Med. 6, 277–301.

von Fodor, J., 1887. Die Fähigkeit des Bluts Bakterien zu vernichten. Dtsch. Med. Wochensch. 13, 745–746.

Gordon, J., Whitehead, H.R., Wormall, A., 1926. The action of ammonia on complement. The fourth component. Biochem. J. 20, 1028–1035.

Hadding, U., Müller-Eberhard, H.J., 1969. The ninth component of human complement: isolation, description and mode of action. Immunology 16, 719–735.

Ikeda, K., Sannoh, T., Kawasaki, N., Kawasaki, T., Yamashina, I., 1987. Serum lectin with known structure activates complement through the classical pathway. J. Biol. Chem. 262, 7451–7454.

Jensen, J., 1967. Anaphylatoxin in its relation to the complement system. Science 155, 1122–1123.

Lachmann, P., 2006. Complement before molecular biology. Mol. Immunol. 43, 496–508.

Lay, W.H., Nussenzweig, V., 1968. Receptors for complement on leukocytes. J. Exp. Med. 128, 991–1009.

Lepow, I.H., 1980. Louis Pillemer, properdin, and scientific controversy. J. Immunol. 125, 471–478.

Lepow, I.H., Naff, G.B., Todd, E.W., Pensky, J., Hinz, C.F., 1963. Chromatographic resolution of the first component of human complement into three activities. J. Exp. Med. 117, 983–1008.

Levine, L., Osler, A.G., Mayer, M.M., 1953. Studies on the role of Ca++ and Mg++ in complement fixation and immune hemolysis. III. The respective role of Ca++ and Mg++ in immune hemolysis. J. Immunol. 71, 374–379.

Manni, J.A., Müller-Eberhard, H.J., 1969. The eighth component of human complement (C8): isolation, characterization, and hemolytic efficiency. J. Exp. Med. 130, 1145–1160.

Mayer, M.M., Levine, L., Rapp, H.J., Marucci, A.A., 1954. Kinetic studies on immune hemolysis. VII. Decay of $EAC'_{1,4,2}$, fixation of C'_3 and other factors influencing the hemolytic action of complement. J. Immunol. 73, 443–454.

Müller-Eberhard, H.J., Nilsson, U., 1960. Relation of a β_1 glycoprotein of human serum to the complement system. J. Exp. Med. 111, 217–234.

Natali, P.G., Tan, E.M., 1972. Precipitin reactions between polyribonucleotides and heat labile serum factors. J. Immunol. 108, 318–324.

Nelson, R.A., 1958. An alternative mechanism for the properdin system. J. Exp. Med. 108, 515–535.

Nelson, R.A., Jensen, J., Gigli, I., Tamura, N., 1966. Methods for the separation, purification and measurement of nine components of hemolytic complement in guinea pig serum. Immunochem. 3, 111–135.

Nilsson, U., 1967. Separation and partial purification of the sixth, seventh and eighth components of human haemolytic complement. Acta Pathol. Microtiol. Scand. 70, 469–480.

Nilsson, U.R., Müller-Eberhard, H.J., 1965. Isolation of beta-$_{1F}$ from human serum and its characterization as the fifth component of the complement. J. Exp. Med. 122, 277–298.

Nuttall, G.H.F., 1888. Experimente über die bacterien feindlichen Einflüsse des thierischen Körpers. Zeitschr. für Hyg. 4, 853–894.

Ohta, M., Okada, M., Yamashina, I., Kawasaki, T., 1990. The mechanism of carbohydrate-mediated complement activation by the serum mannan-binding protein. J. Biol. Chem. 265, 1980–1984.

Omorokow, L., 1911. Über die Wirkung des Cobragiftes auf der Komplemente. Z. Immunitätsforsch. 10, 285.

Pfeiffer, R., 1894. Weitere Untersuchungen über das Wesen der Choleraimmunität und über specifische bactericide Processe. Z. Hyg. Infekt. 18, 1–16.

Pfeiffer, R., Issaeff, R., 1894. Über die specifische Bedeutung der Choleraimmunitat. Z. Hyg. Infect. 17, 355–400.

Pillemer, L., Blum, L., Lepow, I.H., Ross, O.A., Rodd, E.W., Wardlaw, A.C., 1954. The properdin system and immunity. I. Demonstration and isolation of a new serum protein, properdin, and its role in immune phenomenon. Science 120, 279–285.

Pillemer, L., Blum, L., Pensky, J., Lepow, I.H., 1953a. The requirement for magnesium ions in the inactivation of the third component of human complement (C'3) by insoluble residues of yeast cells (zymosan). J. Immunol. 71, 331–338.

Pillemer, L., Lepow, I.H., Blum, L., 1953b. The requirement for a hydrazine-sensitive serum factor and heat-labile serum factors in the inactivation of human C'3 by zymosan. J. Immunol. 71, 339–345.

Pillemer, L., Ecker, E.E., 1941. Anticomplementary factor in fresh yeast. J. Biol. Sci. 137, 139–142.

Pinkard, R.N., Olson, M.S., Kelley, R.E., DeHeer, D.H., Palmer, J.D., O'Rourke, R.A., Goldfein, S., 1973. Antibody-independent activation of human C1 after interaction with heart subcellular membranes. J. Immunol. 110, 1376–1382.

Reid, K.B., 1983. Proteins involved in the activation and control of the two pathways of human complement. Biochem. Soc. Tans. 11, 1–12.

Ritz, H., 1912. Über due Wirkung des Cobragiftes auf die Komplemente. Z. Immunitätsforsch 13, 62–63.

Wallace, A.L., Osler, A.G., Mayer, M.M., 1950. Quantitative studies of complement fixation. V. Estimation of complement-fixing potency of immune sera and its relation to antibody nitrogen content. J. Immunol. 65, 661–676.

Whitehead, H.R., Gordon, J., Wormall, A., 1925. The "third component" or heat-stable factor of complement. Biochem. J. 19, 618–625.

WHO, 1968. Nomenclature of complement. Bull. World Health Organ. 39, 935–938.

TIME LINE

1888	George Nuttall demonstrates that heating serum destroys its bactericidal activity
1889	Hans Buchener separates antibody from alexin (complement) by diluting antibacterial serum with water
1894	Richard Pfeiffer reports lysis of bacteria in vivo—the Pfeiffer phenomenon
1895	Jules Bordet differentiates complement and antibody based on sensitivity to heat
1899	Paul Ehrlich and Julius Morgenroth study complement-mediated lysis of red blood cells and coin the term complement
1900	Emil von Dungren shows that complement is activated by adding yeast to serum
1902	Simon Flexner and Hideyo Noguchi treat bactericidal serum with snake venom to inhibit complement
1907	A. Ferrata and E. Brand independently separate complement into two components
1911	L. Omorokow and H. Ritz isolate a third complement component
1914	Arthur Coca reports the removal of a component of complement by incubating serum with yeast cells
1919	Jules Bordet awarded the Nobel Prize in Physiology or Medicine
1926	John Gordon and colleagues discover C4

1954	Manfred Mayer and coworkers demonstrate the order of activation of the first four components of the complement system
1954	Louis Pillemer and colleagues isolate properdin, leading to the discovery of the alternate pathway of complement activation
1958	Robert Nelson presents data contradicting Pillemer's description of the alternate pathway of complement activation
1960	Hans Müller-Eberhard and Ulf Nilsson isolate β_{1c}-globulin and showed it contains C3
1963	Irvin Lepow and colleagues separate the first component of complement into three fractions
1965–1969	Hans Müller-Eberhard and colleagues characterize the final five components of the human complement system (C5–C9)
1967	Irvin Lepow and coworkers report the anaphylactic properties of C3a
1967	Joerg Jensen discovers the anaphylactic property of C5a
1972	Pier Natali and Eng Tan report the ability of C1q to bind polyribonucleotides in the absence of antibody, leading to the description of the lectin pathway of complement activation

13

Antibody Production Requires Thymus-Derived and Bone Marrow (Bursa)-Derived Lymphocyte Interactions

INTRODUCTION

Immunologists today agree that specific antibody synthesis to most antigens requires collaboration between T lymphocytes and B lymphocytes. The B lymphocyte is responsible for antibody production while the T lymphocyte plays a helper role. Help from T lymphocyte is required for isotype switching (from IgM to IgG, IgA, or IgE) and for the development of immunological memory.

Several observations made in the 1940s and 1950s provided the foundation for the experiments that resulted in these conclusions:

- Identity of the lymphocyte as the antigen-reactive cell by James Gowans and colleagues (Chapter 4). Studies on the "disappearing lymphocyte phenomenon" demonstrated that lymphocytes circulating from the thoracic duct through the circulatory system to peripheral lymphoid organs perform several immunological functions, including antibody production.
- Recognition by Astrid Fagraeus and others that the lymphocyte-derived plasma cell is the antibody-forming cell (Chapter 5).

- Independent discoveries by Rupert Billingham and Merrill Chase that cell-mediated immunity occurs in the absence of antibody (Chapter 3).
- Documentation by Gus Nossal that a single immunocompetent cell produces antibody of a single specificity (Chapter 7) as predicted by the clonal selection theory (Chapter 6).

These facts were well known in 1961 when Jacques Miller demonstrated that thymectomy of mice during the neonatal period led to an immunodeficient state (Chapter 9). The thymus is a lymphoepithelial organ that provides mature T lymphocytes to peripheral lymphoid organs. Miller observed that neonatally thymectomized mice had diminished antibody production although they could synthesize antibody to certain antigens. Other investigators also reported decreased antibody synthesis following neonatal thymectomy (Fichtelius et al., 1961; Jankovic et al., 1962; reviewed by Miller and Osoba, 1967).

The mechanism responsible for decreased antibody production in neonatally thymectomized animals remained unknown during most of the 1960s. At first the most plausible explanation was a decrease in the total number of lymphocytes. In 1964, Osoba and

Miller reconstituted neonatally thymectomized mice with thymus grafts. This procedure resulted in restoration of normal antibody production. These investigators interpreted their results and suggested that the thymus served as the source of antibody-forming lymphoid progenitors that subsequently migrated to other lymphoid organs such as the spleen and lymph nodes. In addition, both Niels Jerne (1955) and F. Macfarlane Burnet (1959) speculated that immunocompetent lymphocytes arose in the thymus and were exported to other peripheral lymphoid organs (Chapter 6).

Throughout the 1960s measurement of serum antibody remained the primary method to detect activation of the adaptive immune response. Several in vitro techniques, including precipitation, hemagglutination, and complement fixation had been developed and modified to provide semiquantitative estimates of the amount of serum antibody present. One problem with all these assays was the lack of information they provided about the cells involved in antibody synthesis and secretion in vivo. The hemolytic plaque assay provided a method of quantitating the number of antibody-forming cells active during an immune response.

THE HEMOLYTIC PLAQUE ASSAY

The hemolytic plaque assay (Jerne and Nordin, 1963) detects antibody formation by single lymphocytes. This assay quantifies the number of lymphocytes secreting antibodies to a particular antigen and permits visualization of the antibody-forming cell's morphology.

Jerne and Nordin injected mice with sheep erythrocytes (SRBC) as antigen. They prepared a single cell suspension of mouse lymphocytes and mixed them with SRBC and tissue culture medium containing agar. They placed this mixture in Petri dishes where it solidified. Following a short incubation, they flooded the petri dishes with a source of complement and returned to the incubator. Antibody-forming lymphocytes secrete specific antibodies that bind to the SRBC. Addition of complement results in lysis of those erythrocytes to which antibody has bound. At the end of the incubation the Petri dishes containing lymphocytes and SRBC are observed for clear areas or plaques (Figure 13.1).

Each plaque or clear area contains a single antibody-producing lymphocyte and therefore provides a method to quantitate the number of lymphocytes in a population actively secreting antibodies. These individual lymphocytes can be removed from the agar and characterized further. While the technique was originally designed to detect lymphocytes secreting antibodies to erythrocytes, modifications have been made, allowing the detection of antibody directed against other antigens,

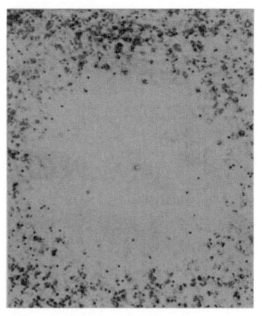

FIGURE 13.1   Photograph of the hemolytic plaque assay. Lymphocytes from a rabbit immunized with sheep erythrocytes were mixed with sheep erythrocytes and cultured in semi-solid tissue culture medium. During the first incubation, lymphocytes synthesizing antibodies specific for the sheep erythrocytes would secrete their products. Following the addition of a source of complement, the plates are reincubated, during which antibody bound to the erythrocytes activates complement and causes cell lysis. The clear area (plaque) in the lawn of red cells indicates the presence of an antibody-forming lymphocyte that can often be observed in the center of the plaque. *From Jerne and Nordin (1963).*

including many proteins such as bovine serum albumin and human gamma globulin. This assay became instrumental in several of the studies reviewed in this chapter.

T-B LYMPHOCYTE COLLABORATION IN ANTIBODY FORMATION

Three groups, working independently, contributed to the discovery that the production of a robust antibody response to most antigens requires the collaboration of T and B lymphocytes.

In 1966, Henry Claman and his colleagues at the University of Colorado Medical Center sublethally irradiated mice, reconstituted these irradiated mice using lymphoid cells from different anatomical sites (thymus, bone marrow, spleen), and injected them with SRBC. They quantified serum antibody with a hemolysis assay and measured antibody production by spleen fragments.

Results are presented in Table 13.1. Irradiated mice that received no lymphocytes or received only bone marrow cells produced minimal amounts of antibodies to SRBC. Injecting irradiated mice with adult thymus cells partially restored antibody production, while reconstituting irradiated mice with a mixture of thymocytes and

TABLE 13.1 Production of Antibodies in Irradiated Mice Reconstituted with Marrow Cells, Thymus Cells, or a Mixture of the Two. Group A is Extracted from a Larger Table Included in Claman et al., 1966; This Group Contains the Data Pooled From All the Groups Presented in This Publication

Group	Cells received	No. of animals	S.A. ± S.E.[a]	Hemolysins ±S.E.[b]
A	Adult thymus (5×10^7) + adult marrow (10^7)	20	53.7 ± 4.0	2.1 ± 0.5
	Adult thymus (5×10^7)	18	12.3 ± 3.4	0.2 ± 0.2
	Adult marrow (10^7)	4	1.3 ± 0.7	0
	No cells	19	0.8 ± 0.4	0
B	1-day Thymus (5×10^7) + adult marrow (10^7)	5	7.2 ± 3.4	0
	6-day Thymus (5×10^7) + adult marrow (10^7)	5	57.1 ± 12.8	3.2 ± 1.1
	1-day Thymus (5×10^7)	5	1.9 ± 1.2	0
C	Adult thymus (5×10^7) + adult spleen (10^6)	5	67.5 ± 12.9	2.6 ± 0.8
	Adult thymus (5×10^7) + 6-day spleen (10^7)	6	18.3 ± 3.4	1.8 ± 0.3
	Adult marrow (10^7) + adult spleen (10^6)	4	13.1 ± 12.1	0.2 ± 0.2
	Adult marrow (10^7) + 6-day spleen (10^7)	5	2.7 ± 1.7	2.6 ± 1.3
	Adult spleen (10^6)	4	10.0 ± 3.5	0.5 ± 0.3
	6-day spleen (10^7)	6	6.6 ± 2.4	1.8 ± 1.1
D	Normal thymus (3×10^7) + adult marrow (10^7)	5	47.8 ± 5.1	3.6 ± 0.6
	250-R thymus (3×10^7) + adult marrow (10^7)	5	17.9 ± 4.7	1.4 ± 0.9
	500-R Thymus (3×10^7) + adult marrow (10^7)	5	4.9 ± 3.5	0
	750-R Thymus (3×10^7) + adult marrow (10^7)	10	3.8 ± 1.7	0
E	Thymus graft + adult marrow (10^7)	5	1.3 ± 0.8	0

[a]Percentage of spleen fragments with hemolysis ± standard error.
[b]Log_2 hemolysin titers ± standard error.

adult marrow cells resulted in antibody production comparable to that observed in unmanipulated control mice (group A). Other results from these studies include

- marrow lymphocytes collaborate with thymocytes from six-day-old mice but not thymocytes from 1-day-old mice (group B);
- lymphocytes from adult spleen are not as efficient in restoring antibody production in irradiated mice as is a mixture of lymphocytes from adult spleen and adult thymus (group C); and
- irradiation of thymus lymphocytes destroys their collaboration with bone marrow cells in subsequent antibody production (group D).

The authors (Claman et al., 1966) conclude that "the data confirm the hypothesis of interaction between thymus and marrow cells (in the production of antibody), although the nature of this interaction is obscure".

Anthony Davies and his colleagues at the Chester Beatty Research Institute in London transferred lymphocytes to irradiated mice and demonstrated that bone marrow-derived cells and thymus-derived lymphocytes were both required for optimal antibody production

(Davies et al., 1967). They further showed that the bone marrow-derived cells, but not thymus-derived lymphocytes, synthesized and secreted antibody.

At the time of these studies, lymphocytes from the bone marrow and the thymus could not be differentiated morphologically or by phenotypic markers such as cell surface molecules. Davies and his coworkers used cells from two inbred strains of mice that could be distinguished based on the presence or absence of the T6 marker chromosome. The presence of this chromosome can be detected in stained cells arrested in metaphase due to its length (approximately one-half that of the shortest autosomal chromosome) and the presence of a constriction near the centromere. The chromosomal difference allowed the investigators to detect cells from each strain in a mixed population. Thus if bone marrow lymphocytes from one strain (i.e., strain A) are mixed with thymus lymphocytes from the second strain (A'), the investigators could identify the origin of the lymphocytes following injection into recipient mice. The two strains of mice used in these studies also possessed a minor histocompatibility difference that was exploited to prepare antibodies specific for each strain.

Davies' group thymectomized and irradiated strain A mice. They reconstituted these mice with bone marrow from strain A and thymus grafts from strain A'. They injected these mice with SRBC 30 and 44 days after cell transfer. The spleens from these intermediate host animals, which theoretically contained B and T lymphocytes from different strains, were subsequently used to reconstitute a second recipient that had been irradiated. Both A and A' mice were used as secondary recipients. Prior to irradiation, Davies and colleagues injected these second recipients with cells from the heterologous strain (strain A mice were injected with strain A' spleen cells, and strain A' mice were injected with strain A spleen cells). Previous studies had demonstrated that this immunization protocol was sufficient to eliminate lymphocytes of the relevant strain present in the reconstituting inoculum.

The investigators produced four experimental groups of secondary recipients using this protocol—all of the mice received a mixture of thymus and bone marrow cells that had been exposed to antigen (SRBC) in the intermediate host. Half of each group of secondary recipients was injected with SRBC to induce a secondary antibody response. Four to 6 days later blood was drawn and spleens were harvested. These samples were used in three assays:

- the number of lymphocytes derived from A or A' strains was measured by histological evaluation of spleen sections,
- the number of antibody-forming cells was detected by the hemolytic plaque assay, and
- the titer of antibody in individual sera was determined by hemolysin and hemagglutination analyses.

Secondary recipients that received both thymus-derived and bone marrow-derived lymphocytes synthesized more antibody to SRBC than did recipients that had been injected with only thymus lymphocytes or bone marrow lymphocytes. Lymphocytes expressing the chromosomal marker from the strain providing the thymus in the original transfer (T lymphocytes) responded mitotically to the antigenic challenge but failed to produce antibody. Alternatively, lymphocytes with the chromosomal marker indicating that they were originally from bone marrow (B lymphocytes) did not proliferate significantly in response to antigen but were the source for virtually all the antibody-forming cells in the secondary recipient.

The publications by Claman's group in 1966 and by Davies' group in 1967 failed to receive the attention they deserved. The observation that collaboration between lymphocytes from two different sources is required to produce an optimal antibody response was a major shift in thinking about the adaptive immune response. Investigations that would clarify the interpretation of these results were underway simultaneously in other

laboratories. For example, the separate maturation of lymphocytes in the thymus and in the bursa of Fabricius in chickens or bone marrow in mammals remained unappreciated until studies by Max Cooper and coworkers in Robert Good's laboratory (1965; 1966) (Chapter 10). Likewise, the description of T and B lymphocytes by Ivan Roitt and colleagues was not published until 1969.

Prior to identification of functionally distinct populations of lymphocytes, immunologists argued that all lymphocytes were identical and that the source of the cell was unimportant. It was not until the work of Jacques Miller and his group in 1968 that many, but not all, immunologists accepted the phenomenon of independent development of two types of lymphocytes, both of which are required for optimal antibody production.

Miller and his collaborators published a series of four papers back-to-back in the October 1968 issue of the *Journal of Experimental Medicine*. These studies supported the conclusions derived from previous work and provided definitive proof that both bone marrow-derived and thymus-derived lymphocytes are necessary to mount an antibody response. These papers also confirmed that lymphocytes derived from the bone marrow, but not from the thymus, synthesize and secrete antibodies.

Miller had previously reported that some mice thymectomized at birth failed to produce antibody when injected with antigen. This defect could be reversed by injecting thymectomized mice with thoracic duct lymphocytes (Miller et al., 1967). The studies published by Miller's group in 1968 were specifically designed to determine the relationship between the injected thoracic duct lymphocytes and the antibody-forming cells.

Graham Mitchell, a veterinarian, was Miller's first doctoral student in the late 1960s. He became interested in the thymus during his earlier training when he wrote a paper on the thymus at the urging of one of his professors. He joined the Walter and Eliza Hall Institute (WEHI) in Melbourne and earned his PhD in 1969. Following postdoctoral experiences in California, Switzerland, and England, he returned to the WEHI to establish a program in parasitology.

Miller and Mitchell (1968) identified the lymphocyte that reconstitutes antibody production to sheep erythrocytes in neonatally thymectomized mice. They thymectomized inbred mice within the first 36 h of life. Three to 5 weeks later they injected these mice with syngeneic lymphocytes derived from the thymus or thoracic duct along with an injection of SRBC. Some of the thymectomized animals served as controls and received only SRBC. Two to 10 days later, Miller and Mitchell harvested spleens from these mice and determined the number of lymphocytes secreting antibodies to SRBC using the hemolytic plaque assay.

Spleens from neonatally thymectomized mice injected with SRBC contain approximately one-tenth the number of antibody-forming cells as do spleens from mice with intact thymuses. Reconstitution of thymectomized mice with either thymus or thoracic duct lymphocytes restore the number of spleen cells producing antibodies specific for SRBC to that detected in intact unmanipulated mice. When lymphocytes from bone marrow are used for reconstitution the number of antibody-forming lymphocytes in the spleens did not return to normal. Injection of irradiated thymocytes or irradiated thoracic duct lymphocytes failed to restore the antibody response to SRBC.

Lymphocytes from the thymus or thoracic duct of semiallogeneic mice (F_1 hybrids) reconstituted the antibody response to SRBC in thymectomized animals to the same extent as did syngeneic lymphocytes. This model provided information about the source of the lymphocytes responsible for antibody production. Investigators treated spleen cells from reconstituted animals with antibodies specific for the histocompatibility antigens of either the recipient or the donor prior to measuring antibody formation. Treatment with complement lysed the cells expressing the relevant histocompatibility antigens.

Antibodies specific for the histocompatibility antigens of the neonatally thymectomized host decreased the number of antibody-forming lymphocytes detected in the hemolytic plaque assay. Since the thymectomized host was the source of bone marrow in this experimental design, the authors concluded that lymphocytes exist "in thymus or thoracic duct lymph, with capacities to react specifically with antigen and to induce the differentiation, to antibody-forming cells, of hemolysin-forming cell precursors derived from a separate cell line present in the neonatally thymectomized hosts." This confirmed the observations of Claman's group and of Davies' group that antibody-secreting lymphocytes are present in the bone marrow and not the thymus. Further studies by the Australian group verified this conclusion.

Mitchell and Miller presented information about the lymphocytes involved in the initiation of an antibody response in the second paper in this series (1968). They exposed mice to a dose of radiation sufficient to destroy the lymphoid tissue of the mouse and injected them with lymphocytes from thymus, bone marrow, or thoracic duct either individually or in combinations. These mice were subsequently injected with SRBC as antigen, and individual antibody-forming cells were detected using the hemolytic plaque assay.

Table 13.2 presents the results; neither syngeneic thymus nor syngeneic bone marrow alone restored a significant antibody response. However, reconstitution with thoracic duct lymphocytes, which we now know contains a mixture of B and T lymphocytes, resulted in the detection of a large number of plaque-forming cells.

The results in Table 13.3 extend these conclusions and show that irradiated mice reconstituted with thymocytes or bone marrow cells individually failed to mount a successful antibody response while a mixture of syngeneic bone marrow cells and thymocytes produced a response equivalent to that detected in irradiated mice injected with a mixture of bone marrow and thoracic duct lymphocytes.

Mitchell and Miller obtained conclusive evidence that antibody-forming lymphocytes are derived from bone marrow by injecting thymectomized, irradiated mice with syngeneic bone marrow. These mice subsequently received a second injection 2 weeks later of semiallogeneic thoracic duct lymphocytes plus SRBC. The investigators treated spleen cells from these reconstituted mice with antibody specific for the histocompatibility antigens of either the bone marrow donor or of the thoracic duct donor prior to measuring the number of plaque-forming cells. Treatment of lymphocytes from the bone marrow donor decreased the number of plaque-forming cells while similar treatment of lymphocytes from the thoracic duct had no effect on the number of antibody producers.

TABLE 13.2   Number of Antisheep Erythrocyte Antibody-Forming Cells Present in the Spleens of Irradiated Mice Reconstituted With Thymocytes, Bone Marrow Cells, or Thoracic Duct Cells and Immunized with Sheep Red Blood Cells. Optimal Antibody Responses Are Seen Only in Mice Reconstituted with Thoracic Duct Cells

Cells inoculated	No. of mice	Average PFC per spleen 8 days postirradiation (±SE)
SRBC only	16	15 ± 6.1
10×10^6 thymus cells + SRBC	14	15 ± 3.0
50×10^6 thymus cells + SRBC	8	45 ± 5.0
10×10^6 bone marrow cells + SRBC	16	27 ± 5.8
25×10^6 thoracic duct cells only	5	17 ± 4.4
10×10^6 thoracic duct cells + SRBC	23	1270 ± 338[a]

PFC, Plaque-forming cells.
[a]$P < 0.05 - < 0.01$ when this value is compared with those in all other groups.
From Mitchell and Miller (1968).

TABLE 13.3   Number of Antisheep Erythrocyte Antibody Forming Cells Present in the Spleens of Irradiated Mice Injected with Bone Marrow Alone or with Bone Marrow Mixed with Thymus or Thoracic Duct Cells. Optimal Antibody Responses Are Seen in Mice Reconstituted with Mixtures of Bone Marrow and Thymus or Bone Marrow and Thoracic Duct

Cells inoculated	No. of mice	Average PFC per spleen 8 days postirradiation (± SE)
SRBC	12	13 ± 1.8
10×10^6 bone marrow cells + SRBC	15	73 ± 23.5
50×10^6 thymus cells + SRBC	20	52 ± 19.3
50×10^6 thymus cells +10×10^6 bone marrow cells + SRBC	13	522 ± 341
10^6 Thoracic duct cells + SRBC	10	97 ± 34.7
10^6 Thoracic duct cells +10×10^6 bone marrow cells + SRBC	13	877 ± 218

PFC, Plaque-Forming Cells.
From Mitchell and Miller (1968).

Thus the antibody-forming lymphocytes are derived from the bone marrow donor rather than from the thoracic duct and confirmed that two types of lymphocytes exist in these reconstituted animals. The conclusion was that antigen-reactive, thymus-derived (T) lymphocytes interact with antibody-forming precursors (B lymphocytes).

Interaction of B and T lymphocytes stimulates the potential antibody-forming precursors to differentiate into antibody-producing lymphocytes that are detected in the plaque assay. Based on the evidence obtained from this series of experiments, Mitchell and Miller concluded that thymus contains antigen-reactive lymphocytes, the bone marrow contains antibody-forming precursors, and thoracic duct lymphocytes are a mixture of the two lymphocyte types.

The final two papers in this series corroborated the observations made in the first two. Nossal et al. (1968) reconstituted neonatally thymectomized mice with mixtures of bone marrow and thymus lymphocytes from mice that differ at a single chromosome. Chromosome analysis showed that the antibody-forming lymphocytes were all derived from the strain of mice donating the bone marrow rather than from the strain donating the thymocytes.

Finally, Martin and Miller injected mice with a rabbit antibody specific for mouse lymphocytes. Such treatment inhibited both the production of antibodies and cell-mediated immune responses. Since the investigators corrected both defects by injecting the treated mice with syngeneic thymocytes, the authors concluded "that, in vivo, anti-lymphocyte globulin acts selectively on the thymus-derived, antigen-reactive cells" (Martin and Miller, 1968).

T-INDEPENDENT ANTIGENS

Collaboration between B and T lymphocytes in antibody synthesis and secretion is necessary for the response to most antigens; however, several reports demonstrated that some foreign pathogens could induce an antibody response in the absence of T lymphocytes. These antigens are called T-independent antigens and are characterized by a polymeric structure that provides repeated antigenic determinants (epitopes). One example of such an antigen is lipopolysaccharide, a component of the outer membrane of gram negative bacteria. This unique structure allows the epitopes to cross-link the immunoglobulin receptors present on B lymphocytes and activate these lymphocytes to proliferate and synthesize antibody (Chapter 19).

B lymphocytes stimulated by T-independent antigens produce an IgM response with no switching of the antibody to other isotypes (classes) (Chapter 11). In addition, the response to T-independent antigens does not induce immunological memory, one of the hallmarks of the adaptive immune response (Chapter 2). Since IgM is very efficient in activating several of the effector mechanisms of the innate host defense mechanisms, including the complement system and phagocytosis, it is possible that this T-independent response represents an early evolutionary development of adaptive immunity.

CONCLUSION

The realization that two types of lymphocytes interact to induce an optimal antibody response to most antigens produced a rush of supporting experimental evidence. However, not all immunologists accepted these conclusions. Several anecdotes exist that even into the early 1970s, some senior immunologists remarked that the only thing connecting B and T were the letters _ULLSHI_. Other immunologists were known as late as 1972 to opine that "a lymphocyte is a lymphocyte is a lymphocyte."

Eventually, the preponderance of evidence overwhelmed these skeptics, and the reality of T and B lymphocyte collaboration in the antibody response was established. Subsequent investigation demonstrated a similar division of labor in the initiation of other effector mechanisms of the adaptive immune response, and immunologists now identify a plethora of subpopulations of T lymphocytes, each with individual functions (Chapters 23 and 24). Characterization of these subpopulations using monoclonal antibodies and identification of cytokines secreted provide methods for manipulating them in clinical situations, to reverse allograft rejection, to inhibit autoimmune disease, and to treat cancer (Chapters 33–38).

The studies reviewed here were performed prior to recognition of the differences between types of lymphocytes or the technology to characterize them based on cell surface phenotype. As described in Chapter 10, the designations T and B lymphocytes did not enter the immunologist's lexicon until 1969, and differentiation of lymphocyte types based on CD markers was still 10–15 years into the future. The studies reported by the Claman group (in Denver), the Davies group (in London), the Miller group (in Melbourne), and others opened the floodgates to our appreciation of the complexity of the lymphocytes of the immune response and their interactions required for optimal adaptive immunity, including antibody production.

References

Burnet, F.M., 1959. The Clonal Selection Theory of Acquired Immunity. Vanderbilt University Press, Nashville, TN.

Claman, H.N., Chaperon, E.A., Triplett, R.F., 1966. Immunocompetence of transferred thymus-marrow cell combinations. J. Immunol. 97, 828–832.

Cooper, M.D., Peterson, R.D.A., Good, R.A., 1965. Delineation of the thymic and bursal lymphoid systems in the chicken. Nature 205, 143–146.

Cooper, M.D., Peterson, R.D.A., South, M.A., Good, R.A., 1966. The functions of the thymus system and the bursa system in the chicken. J. Exp. Med. 123, 75–102.

Davies, A.J.S., Leuchars, E., Wallis, V., Marchant, R., Elliott, E.V., 1967. The failure of thymus-derived cells to produce antibody. Transplantation 5, 222–231.

Fichtelius, K.E., Laurell, G., Philipsson, I., 1961. The influence of thymectomy on antibody formation. Acta Pathol. Micrbiol. Scand. 51, 81–86.

Jankovic, B.C., Waksman, B.H., Arnason, B.G., 1962. Role of the thymus in immune reactions in rats I. The immunologic response to bovine serum albumin (antibody formation, Arthus reactivity, and delayed hypersensitivity) in rats thymectomized or splenectomized at various times after birth. J. Exp. Med. 116, 159–176.

Jerne, N.K., 1955. The natural-selection theory of antibody formation. Proc. Nat. Acad. Sci. U. S. A. 41, 849–857.

Jerne, N.K., Nordin, A.A., 1963. Plaque formation in agar by single antibody-producing cells. Science 140, 405.

Martin, W.J., Miller, J.F.A.P., 1968. Cell to cell interaction in the immune response IV. Site of action of antilymphocyte globulin. J. Exp. Med. 128, 855–874.

Miller, J.F.A.P., 1961. Immunological function of the thymus. Lancet 278, 748–749.

Miller, J.F.A.P., Mitchell, G.F., 1968. Cell to cell interaction in the immune response I. Hemolysin-forming cells in neonatally thymectomized mice reconstituted with thymus or thoracic duct lymphocytes. J. Exp. Med. 128, 801–820.

Miller, J.F.A.P., Mitchell, G.F., Weiss, N.S., 1967. Cellular basis of the immunological defects in thymectomized mice. Nature 214, 992–997.

Miller, J.F.A.P., Osoba, D., 1967. Current concepts of the immunological functions of the thymus. Physiol. Rev. 47, 437–520.

Mitchell, G.F., Miller, J.F.A.P., 1968. Cell to cell interaction in the immune response II. The source of hemolysin-forming cells in irradiated mice given bone marrow and thymus or thoracic duct lymphocytes. J. Exp. Med. 128, 821–837.

Nossal, G.J.V., Cunningham, A., Mitchell, G.F., Miller, J.F.A.P., 1968. Cell to cell interaction in the immune response III. Chromosomal marker analysis of single antibody-forming cells in reconstituted, irradiated or thymectomized mice. J. Exp. Med. 128, 839–853.

Osoba, D., Miller, J.F.A.P., 1964. The lymphoid tissues and immune responses of neonatally thymectomized mice bearing thymus tissue in millipore diffusion chambers. J. Exp. Med. 119, 177–194.

Roitt, I.M., Greaves, M.F., Torrigiani, G., Brostoff, J., Playfair, J.H.L., 1969. The cellular basis of immunological responses. A synthesis of some current views. Lancet 294, 367–371.

TIME LINE

1950	James Gowans identifies the lymphocyte as the antigen sensitive cell
	Niels Jerne and Macfarlane Burnet speculate that the thymus serves as a source for antibody-forming cells
1961	Jacques Miller describes the role of the thymus in the development of immune competence
1963	Niels Jerne and Albert Nordin develop the hemolytic plaque assay for the detection of antibody synthesis by single cells
1966	Henry Claman shows that a combination of thymus and bone marrow lymphocytes reconstitute a primary antibody response in irradiated mice better than either cell alone
1967	Anthony Davies demonstrates that a combination of thymus and bone marrow lymphocytes reconstitutes a secondary antibody response better than either cell alone; bone marrow-derived cells produce antibody while thymus-derived cells respond to antigen by proliferating
1968	Jacques Miller and Graham Mitchell describe the collaboration of thymus-derived and bone marrow-derived lymphocytes in antibody responses; bone marrow-derived cells produce antibody

14

Cell Collaboration in the Antibody Response: Role of Adherent Cells

INTRODUCTION

Optimal antibody production requires collaboration between B and T lymphocytes and an antigen-presenting cell (APC). APCs are defined as nonantigen-specific cells that express molecules coded for by the class II major histocompatibility complex (MHC) genes. The expression of these molecules allows the APC to present antigens to helper (CD4+) T lymphocytes (Chapter 20). Macrophages, B lymphocytes, and dendritic cells serve as APCs. The studies leading to these conclusions focused initially on macrophages; however, in 1973, Ralph Steinman and Zanvil Cohn described dendritic cells (Chapter 29). In this chapter many of the studies used cells described as macrophages based on separation methods such as adherence to plastic petri dishes or glass beads in vitro. In reality these cell preparations most likely included dendritic cells as well as macrophages, and therefore the results should be interpreted with this caveat.

The classic image of the macrophage engulfing and eliminating foreign material is central to the history of immunology. Ilya Metchnikov (1845–1916), working in Messina, Italy, initially described phagocytosis of foreign material as a mechanism for ridding the body of potentially dangerous invaders (Chapter 15; reviewed in Metchnikov, 1908). Phagocytosis by macrophages is a major component of the innate host defense mechanisms; however, the role of the macrophage in the adaptive immune response (IR) remained a mystery until the 1960s. Experiments dividing spleen cells into adherent and nonadherent populations demonstrated that synthesis of antibody to sheep erythrocytes required interactions of the two cell types.

Early in the history of immunology, instruction hypotheses of antibody formation erroneously ascribed antibody production to cells of the reticuloendothelial (RE) system. The RE system consists of several different cell types, including endothelial cells, fibrocytic cells, reticular cells, and cells with phagocytic capabilities (i.e., macrophages, monocytes, dendritic cells, Kupffer cells, and skin Langerhans cells). Instruction hypotheses proposed that the antigen served as a template upon which a complementary antibody molecule was formed; the information required to produce the antigen binding site of the antibody was originally thought to be imprinted on the cells of the RE system so that additional antibody molecules could be synthesized in the absence of antigen. Since the macrophage was the cell most intimately involved with the uptake of antigen, many immunologists mistakenly concluded that it must play a major role in antibody synthesis. Although several studies concluded that macrophages

A Historical Perspective on Evidence-Based Immunology
http://dx.doi.org/10.1016/B978-0-12-398381-7.00014-9

could synthesize antibodies (Sabin, 1939; Dixon et al., 1957), other competing studies revealed that antibody was not present in macrophages during an antibody response (Ehrich et al., 1946).

Experiments performed between 1942 and 1965 challenged the idea that macrophages and other phagocytic cells produced antibodies and conclusively established that the precursor cell for antibody formation is the small lymphocyte (Chapter 4) that transforms into plasma cells (Chapter 5). Studies performed in the late 1960s on the cells involved in antibody production provided evidence for the collaboration of two types of lymphocytes. These lymphocytes, originally defined as thymus-dependent and bursa (or bone marrow)-dependent, are now known as T and B lymphocytes (Chapter 13).

With the rejection of instruction hypotheses of antibody formation and the acceptance of F. Macfarlane Burnet's clonal selection theory, the function of phagocytic cells in antibody production required redefinition. Finally, in the late 1960s, several groups of investigators pursued studies on the role of macrophages in antibody synthesis. The experiments described in this chapter analyzed four major questions:

1. What morphological changes occur in lymphoid tissues following antigen activation?
2. Are antigen-activated phagocytic cells a source of information to antibody-forming lymphocytes?
3. Do phagocytes and lymphocytes collaborate in antibody formation?
4. What is the mechanism of phagocyte–lymphocyte interactions?

MORPHOLOGICAL CHANGES

Numerous histologists described the microscopic anatomy of various organs during the initiation of an adaptive immune response. Florence Sabin (1871–1953) published several studies on the cellular reactions to various antigens, including those of *Mycobacterium tuberculosis*. Sabin was born in Central City, Colorado, in 1871 and became one of the most prominent woman scientists of the early 1900s. She received her medical training at Johns Hopkins University in Baltimore, Maryland, and spent 25 years at her alma mater where she achieved several breakthroughs, including being the first woman to achieve the rank of professor. Her research focused on the development of blood and lymphatic vessels. In 1925, she joined the Rockefeller Institute for Medical Research in New York from which she retired in 1938.

Sabin studied the cellular changes in rabbits and guinea pigs injected with ovalbumin (OVA). Sabin traced OVA conjugated with a dark red dye through the body. Phagocytic cells in various organs, including liver, spleen,

and lymph nodes, engulfed the antigen–dye complex. Antibody to the antigen appeared in the serum when the dye–protein complexes disappeared from the phagocytes. Sabin thought she observed the cells that phagocytized the antigen lose some of their surface film when antibody appeared in the serum, and thus she "inferred that the cells of the reticulo-endothelial system normally produce globulin and that antibody globulin represents the synthesis of a new kind of protein under the influence of an antigen" (Sabin, 1939). This conclusion, which was made almost 20 years prior to the publication of Burnet's clonal selection theory, was consistent with the widely accepted instruction hypotheses of antibody formation.

Publication of Burnet's clonal selection theory (1957) and the realization that the lymphocyte is the antigen-reactive cell (Chapter 4) altered the interpretation of subsequent histological observations. Investigators during the 1960s reported observing physical interactions between phagocytes (macrophages) and lymphocytes involving intimate connections between the two cell types. This led to the suggestion that the macrophage may be providing an initial step in the process leading to antibody formation.

In 1960, J.A. Sharp and R.G. Burwell, working at the University of Leeds, England, injected rabbits with horse serum as antigen. Three to 12 days later they established cultures with the spleen cells from these rabbits and photographed them by time-lapse cinematography at 12 pictures per minute. Physical interactions between lymphocytes and macrophages were noted in the tissues derived from horse serum injected but not from control animals not exposed to the antigen. Lymphocytes migrated around the edges of the macrophages and established contact with the macrophage cell surface that lasted for up to 75 min. At times the lymphocytes moved away from the macrophage only to return to the same macrophage. Similar, prolonged interactions were not observed between lymphocytes and macrophages in cultures derived from control rabbits.

Sharp and Burwell offered several interpretations of these observations, including the possibility "that the macrophages, having taken up antigen from the extracellular fluid *in vivo*, are in the process of supplying an antigen-complex to the lymphocytes which then stimulates antibody production."

In 1964, Melvin Schoenberg and coworkers, working at Western Reserve University in Cleveland, used light and electron microscopy to demonstrate cytoplasmic connections between macrophages and lymphocytes. They injected rabbits with one of several antigens, including horse ferritin, diphtheria toxoid, or complete Freund's adjuvant and removed lymph nodes and spleens for observation. Control tissue was obtained from animals not injected with these antigens. Tissues observed with the light microscope revealed clusters of lymphocytes surrounding macrophages; these clusters were present in greater number in lymphoid tissue removed from injected rabbits than that from control animals. By electron microscopy, Schoenberg and coworkers described cytoplasmic connections (tubules) between some of the lymphocytes and the macrophages. They observed continuity between the two cell types with ribosome-like particles in the cytoplasmic connections. One or two lymphocytes per cluster were connected physically with the macrophage. Schoenberg and colleagues suggest that "there is a transfer of cytoplasmic content from the macrophage to lymphocytic cells" which may involve the transfer of ribosomes.

Progress in describing how macrophages activate antibody synthesis in an adaptive immune response depended on the establishment of an in vitro procedure for stimulating a primary antibody response. In 1966, Robert Mishell and Richard Dutton, working at the Scripps Clinic and Research Foundation in La Jolla, California, optimized the conditions necessary to induce an antibody response in vitro to foreign erythrocytes. Mouse spleen cells cultured in vitro with sheep erythrocytes synthesize and secrete detectable antibodies specific for the red blood cells 4–6 days later using the hemolytic plaque assay (Chapter 13).

Donald Mosier, an MD, PhD student at the University of Chicago, used this in vitro method in 1969 to demonstrate that cell clusters containing macrophages and lymphocytes are required during the early primary antibody response. Spleen cells from uninjected mice were established in Mishell-Dutton cell cultures with either sheep red blood cells (SRBC) or burro red blood cells (BRBC) as antigen to induce a primary antibody response. After 4 days of culture, the spleen cells associated in clusters. These clusters contained most of the cells that were proliferating and most, it not all, the cells that produced antibodies in the hemolytic plaque assay. Inhibition of cluster formation by mechanical means prevented cell proliferation and the formation of antibody. When both SRBC and BRBC were included in the cultures, Mosier observed separate cell clusters containing antibody-forming lymphocytes for each of the antigens.

INFORMATION EXCHANGE

Histological studies demonstrated a physical connection between macrophage and lymphocyte that resulted in an antibody response. These observations led investigators to hypothesize that information was transferred between the macrophage and the antibody-forming lymphocyte. To characterize the mechanism of information transfer, several investigators isolated soluble factors from macrophages exposed to antigen in vitro. These soluble factors stimulated antibody formation to the original antigen when added to lymphocytes in culture.

In 1959, Marvin Fishman, working at the Public Health Institute of the city of New York, demonstrated a role for a soluble factor produced by phagocytic cells in the initiation of an antibody response. Fishman exposed rat peritoneal exudate cells (consisting of mononuclear cells with phagocytic ability) to antigen (either bacteriophage T2 or hemocyanin) for 30 min in cell culture. He prepared a cell-free extract from these cells and added this to cultures of lymph node cells derived from immunologically naïve animals. He tested fluids from these lymph node cultures for antibody activity either by phage neutralization or by hemagglutination of red cells conjugated with hemocyanin. Fishman measured phage neutralization by incubating the culture media with T2 bacteriophage for 30 min followed by adding the phage to cultures of E. coli. Normally the addition of T2 bacteriophage to cultures of bacteria produced discrete plaques in the culture. Antibody present in the tissue culture media decreased the number of plaques observed on the bacterial cultures; this provided a semiquantitative estimate of the amount of antibody produced.

Five to 7 days after initiation of tissue cultures, specific antibody to T2 bacteriophage was detected; no antibody was produced in tissue cultures lacking the cell-free extract. Fishman obtained similar results using hemocyanin as the antigen in the cultures.

Treatment of the soluble factor with RNase (an enzyme that degrades RNA) prevented the factor from inducing an antibody response in cultures of lymph node cells. This suggested that the cell-free extract contained RNA (Fishman, 1961). Fishman added tritiated cytidine (a component of RNA) during the initial incubation of macrophages with antigen to determine the mechanism by which the RNA functioned. Fishman added a cell free extract from these macrophages to lymph node cells and located radiolabeled RNA by autoradiography. If in fact RNA is transferred from peritoneal cells to lymphocytes during stimulation of antibody synthesis, the radiolabel would be found in the lymphocytes.

Most of the label was incorporated into lymphocytes (Fishman et al., 1963). Although the process by which this immune-RNA functioned to induce lymphocytes to produce antibody remained unknown, Fishman and colleagues erroneously concluded that RNA isolated from macrophages that had processed antigen acted as messenger RNA to transfer genetic information to other cells to produce specific antibody (Biello et al., 1976). Other investigators reported the presence of antigenic fragments in the RNA preparations and speculated that the RNA merely served to transport the antigen to the lymphocytes (Askonas, 1965; Gottlieb et al., 1967)

These studies indicate that some interaction between phagocytic cells and lymphocytes is necessary to induce antibody synthesis. However, the suggestion that this interaction involved the transfer of genetic information from the phagocyte to the antibody-forming lymphocyte eluded confirmation by further research. The interaction between phagocytes and lymphocytes is essential in the stimulation of adaptive immunity; however, most immunologists today agree that this involves interaction of small intercellular signaling molecules (cytokines) produced by a variety of lymphoid and nonlymphoid cells as well as contact between cell surface proteins. Since the 1970s, numerous of cytokines involved in the initiation and regulation of the adaptive immune response have been isolated and characterized (Chapter 25). The main difference between cytokines and the factors described thus far in this chapter is that cytokines affect lymphocytes in a non-antigen-specific manner while immune-RNA appeared to induce lymphocytes to produce specific antibody.

Further understanding of phagocytic cells in the induction of antibody responses required insight into two areas of investigation:

1. evaluation of cells separated on the basis of adherence to plastic to collaborate in the induction of an antibody response in vitro; and
2. determination of the mechanism underlying the requirement for genetic compatibility of interacting cells in the adaptive immune response.

COLLABORATION BETWEEN ADHERENT AND NONADHERENT CELLS

One of the conclusions from the experiments described in the previous section is that antibody synthesis requires the interaction of two functionally different cells: one to phagocytize the antigen and the second to produce antibody. Investigators demonstrated the concept of cell interactions in antibody formation in the mid-1960s when they established that both thymus-derived and bone marrow-derived lymphocytes are necessary for the development of an antibody response to an array of antigens (Chapter 13). Further studies took advantage of in vitro separation techniques based on adherence to plastic.

Donald Mosier provided evidence that macrophage-like cells are essential in the induction of antibody synthesis when he separated spleen cells from unimmunized mice into two populations:

• plastic adherent, macrophage-rich (MR) cells; and
• plastic nonadherent, lymphocyte-rich (LR) cells.

Using the Mishell-Dutton culture technique Mosier induced a primary antibody response to sheep erythrocytes by MR and LR cells, either singly or in combination. Four days after culture initiation, antibody-forming cells were detected using the hemolytic plaque assay. Neither the adherent cells (MR) nor the nonadherent

(LR) populations alone resulted in lymphocytes secreting antibody specific for SRBC; however, mixtures of adherent and nonadherent cells produced an antibody response (Mosier, 1967). The results of these experiments are shown in Table 14.1.

Mosier asked if adherent cells that had phagocytized antigen could stimulate lymphocytes to synthesize antibody in the absence of additional antigen. He exposed MR cells to SRBC for 30 min after which the supernatant was removed and the cells were washed with tissue culture medium to remove SRBCs that had not been phagocytized. By histologic observation approximately 5% of the red cells originally added to the cultures remained within the adherent macrophages. Mosier added LR cell preparations to these cultures and determined antibody production 4 days later. The number of plaque-forming cells in these cultures equaled the number found in cultures in which the antigen was present continually.

In a further elaboration of this experimental protocol, Mosier, along with Lionel Coppleson (1968), separated mouse spleen cells into adherent (MR) and nonadherent (LR) cells. Three experimental groups were established:

• serial dilutions of MR cells with an excess of LR cells,
• serial dilutions of LR cells with an excess of MR cells, and
• serial dilutions of unseparated cells.

All cultures were stimulated with SRBC, and the number of plaque-forming cells was determined after 4 days of culture. Analysis of the slope of the regression curves obtained from plotting the quantity of cells in the serial dilutions against the number of cells producing antibody led Mosier and Coppleson to estimate the number of cell interactions required to obtain activated antibody-forming lymphocytes. Results suggested that "one adherent and two nonadherent cells interact during the primary immune response in vitro."

These investigations proved that production of antibody to sheep erythrocytes "involves both antigen phagocytosis by macrophages and macrophage lymphocyte interactions." The mechanism by which this interaction resulted in activation of lymphocytes remained unclear. The results are compatible with transfer of information between the macrophage and lymphocyte. Determination of the exact role of macrophages in the inducing an antibody production would require several additional years of basic research to answer three questions:

• Do macrophages interact directly with antibody-producing B lymphocytes or with helper T lymphocytes?
• What happens to antigen once phagocytized by a macrophage?
• How do macrophages enhance the activation of T and B lymphocytes?

TABLE 14.1 Requirement for the Presence of Both Macrophage Rich (MR) and Lymphocyte Rich (LR) Cells in Cell Culture to Induce an Antibody Response Against Sheep Erythrocytes. Neither MR nor LR Populations by Themselves Responded to the Antigen as Measured by the Number of Antibody-Forming Cells 4 Days Later

Cell populations	Day-4 response		
	Experiment 1	Experiment 2	Experiment 3
Normal spleen cells	1	2	1
Normal spleen cells + SRBC[a]	170	60	342
(MR 1 + SRBC) + normal cells	215	96	280
(MR 2 + SRBC) + normal cells	115	45	172
(MR 3 + SRBC) + normal cells	90	36	96
(MR 1 + SRBC) + LR 3	50	20	110
(MR 2 + SRBC) + LR 3	125	30	105
(MR 3 + SRBC) + LR 3	50	50	70
MR 1 + SRBC[b]	1	0	0
MR 2 + SRBC[b]	0	0	0
MR 3 + SRBC[b]	0	0	0
LR 1 + SRBC	6	2	4
LR 2 + SRBC	0	0	0
LR 3 + SRBC	0	0	0

SRBC, sheep red blood cells
[a]10^7 sheep red blood cells.
[b]Exposure to antigen either 30 min or throughout culture gave the same results.
From Mosier (1967).

GENETIC CONTROL OF MACROPHAGE–LYMPHOCYTE INTERACTIONS

Studies on the proliferative response of lymphocytes led to the next breakthrough in unraveling macrophage function. Several investigators used the induction of mitosis in lymphocytes as a surrogate for the stimulation of an adaptive immune response. In 1968, Evan Hersh and Jules Harris at the University of Texas, Houston, purified lymphocytes from human peripheral blood. Donors of these lymphocytes were known to have been exposed to one or more of the following antigens: streptolysin O, streptokinase-streptodornase, vaccinia, or purified protein derivative (PPD) (from *M. tuberculosis*). Lymphocytes or unseparated peripheral blood leukocytes (which contain both lymphocytes and macrophages) were cultured with these antigens. After several days in culture, a DNA precursor, ^{3}H-thymidine, was added to the cultures and the amount of radioactivity incorporated into the lymphocytes measured as an indicator of mitosis. Lymphocytes devoid of macrophages incorporated less than ^{3}H-thymidine in response to previously experienced antigens than did unseparated leukocytes. Culture of the purified lymphocytes on monolayers of macrophages from the same donor restored the proliferative response to the antigens.

Martin Cline and Virginia Swett at the University of California, San Francisco (1968), confirmed and extended these results. They separated monocytes from human peripheral blood, exposed them to PPD, removed soluble PPD, and cultured these monocytes with either autologous or allogeneic lymphocytes. The level of lymphocyte proliferation was determined by counting blast cells and by measuring the incorporation of ^{14}C-thymidine. Autologous but not allogeneic monocytes stimulated proliferation. Separation of the cells by a semipermeable membrane inhibited blast transformation, indicating that direct contact between the macrophage and lymphocyte was required for optimal proliferation.

Studies using inbred strains of animals revealed that the proliferative response of lymphocytes from both mice and guinea pigs to several antigens was controlled by autosomal dominant genes termed immune response (*IR*) genes. The concept of *IR* genes developed from studies using inbred strains of guinea pigs in the laboratory of Baruj Benacceraf at New York University in the early 1960s (Levine et al., 1963).

Guinea pigs have been used in scientific research for over 200 years. They were employed by Louis Pasteur and other nineteenth century investigators studying infectious diseases. Most of the studies used outbred strains of guinea pigs; however, two inbred strains (strain 2 and strain 13) have been developed and used in immunological research since the 1950s. These two strains differ from each other at the gene locus identified as the MHC.

Benacceraf and colleagues injected groups of inbred and outbred guinea pigs with two different synthetic antigens: dinitrophenyl-poly-L-lysine (DNP-PLL) and benzylpenicilloyl-poly-L-lysine (BPO-PLL). They measured adaptive immune responses using four different techniques:

- precipitation in vitro,
- transfer of serum to a naïve animal to induce an immediate hypersensitivity reaction (passive cutaneous anaphylaxis),
- injection of antigen subcutaneously to induce an Arthus reaction, and
- transfer of lymphocytes to induce a delayed hypersensitivity skin reaction.

Approximately 40% of outbred guinea pigs produced serum antibody and specifically sensitized lymphocytes to DNP-PLL and BPO-PLL. When two responder guinea pigs were mated, 82% of the offspring responded. None of the offspring from matings of two nonresponder guinea pigs responded to the antigens. When inbred guinea pigs were tested using these same antigens, 100% of strain 2 guinea pigs responded to both antigens while no strain 13 guinea pigs mounted a measurable response.

Levine et al. (1963) concluded that the response to PLL is under genetic control and suggested two explanations for this control based on the current understanding of the Ir gene:

- strain 2 but not strain 13 guinea pigs are capable of enzymatically degrading PLL, or
- genes expressed in strain 2 guinea pigs allow the coupling of PLL fragments to low molecular weight RNA.

Ten years later, B and T lymphocytes had been described as separate populations of immunocompetent cells, and many of the functions known to be under Ir gene control, such as delayed type hypersensitivity and lymphocyte proliferation, had been demonstrated to be mediated by T lymphocytes. In addition, nonresponder guinea pigs produced antibodies to DNP-PLL if this conjugate were itself conjugated to an immunogenic carrier. This indicated that the failure to produce specific antibody was due to a problem with T lymphocyte activation.

By the early 1970s, two additional antigens, DNP conjugated to a random polymer of glutamic acid and lysine (DNP-GL) and a random polymer of glutamic acid and tyrosine (GT), had been shown to be under Ir gene control:

- strain 2 but not strain 13 guinea pigs responded to DNP-GL,
- strain 13 but not strain 2 guinea pigs responded to GT, and

- F_1 hybrids of strain 2 and strain 13 responded to both antigens.

In a series of studies performed during the early 1970s, Ethan Shevach, William Paul, and Ira Green at the National Institutes of Health, Bethesda, Maryland, studied the response of inbred strains of guinea pigs to antigens known to be controlled by Ir genes. Their goal was to explain the relationship between Ir genes, histocompatibility antigens, and antigen recognition. Shevach and his colleagues (1972) used antibodies specific for histocompatibility antigens to interfere with induction of lymphocyte proliferation induced by antigens under Ir gene control. Lymphocytes purified from strain 2, strain 13, or (2×13) F_1 hybrids were incubated with antigen in the presence or absence of antibodies specific for either strain 2 or strain 13 histocompatibility antigens. Lymphocyte proliferation was measured 5 days later by quantitating the amount of ^{3}H-thymidine incorporated into the DNA of activated lymphocytes. Antibodies specific for histocompatibility antigens interfered with activation of lymphocytes specific for antigens known to be under Ir gene control. The authors concluded from these results "that immune response genes produce a cell surface-associated product and that this product plays a role in the mechanism of antigen recognition by the T lymphocyte."

Further studies on the role of Ir genes and histocompatibility antigens in the activation of T lymphocytes showed that recognition of antigens by T lymphocytes requires presentation of the antigen on macrophages histocompatible with the T lymphocytes (Rosenthal and Shevach, 1973; Shevach and Rosenthal, 1973). These investigators purified lymphocytes and macrophages individually from antigen-injected guinea pigs. Macrophages exposed to antigen for 60 min and washed were cultured with naïve lymphocytes for 24–48 h and ^{3}H-thymidine was added to detect lymphocyte proliferation.

Results indicated that the presentation of antigen by macrophages to lymphocytes requires that the two cell types be identical at the histocompatibility locus (MHC). Macrophages from (2×13) F_1 hybrids present antigen with equal efficiency to lymphocytes from either inbred strain. Macrophages from outbred guinea pigs present antigen to lymphocytes from one of the inbred strains only if the macrophages shared histocompatibility genes with the lymphocytes. Finally, macrophages incubated with antigen to induce lymphocyte proliferation were blocked by including antibodies to the proteins coded by the histocompatibility genes expressed by the macrophages.

These studies indicate that the first step in the initiation of an adaptive immune response involves the presentation of antigen by macrophages to lymphocytes. This led to the development of the concept of the APC. APCs are now defined by the expression of molecules coded for by class II MHC genes (Chapter 16) and include macrophages, dendritic cells, and B lymphocytes. Additional information about antigen presentation and the mechanism of T lymphocyte activation is covered in Chapter 20.

CONCLUSION

Unraveling the role of macrophages in the activation of an adaptive immune (antibody) response took several twists between the late 1800s and the 1970s. Based on instruction hypotheses of antibody formation, the macrophage was initially identified as one of the main antibody producers. With the introduction of the clonal selection theory, the macrophage was relegated to a supportive role. Investigators disagreed about whether macrophages provided information to lymphocytes in the form of messenger RNA or served as ancillary cells involved in maintaining lymphocyte homeostasis. Eventually the work performed in the early 1970s using a guinea pig model and synthetic antigens hinted at the true role of the macrophage as the APC.

One final twist in this story involved the discovery of another cell type, the dendritic cell, by Ralph Steinman (Chapter 29). These cells reside in all peripheral lymphoid tissues and express class II MHC-coded molecules. While not very efficient as phagocytic cells, these cells are extremely effective at presenting antigens to T lymphocytes to stimulate adaptive immune responses.

The discovery that APCs present antigen to T lymphocytes informed studies on the physiological role of the genes coding for molecules in the major histocompatibility complex (Chapter 16). This knowledge led to an understanding of

- T lymphocyte activation (Chapter 20);
- the mechanism by which potentially self-reactive T lymphocytes are eliminated during development (Chapter 22);
- the mechanism by which natural killer lymphocytes recognize their targets (Chapter 28); and
- the role of dendritic cells in the initiation of adaptive immune responses (Chapter 29).

APCs bridge the nonspecific innate host defense mechanisms with the adaptive immune response. This requires that APCs, particularly macrophages, possess a method for determining whether material with which they interact is potentially dangerous or benign. The experiments leading to the discovery of the cell surface receptors essential for this differentiation are presented in Chapter 15.

References

Askonas, B.A., Rhodes, J.M., 1965. Immunogenicity of antigen-containing ribonucleic acid preparations from macrophages. Nature 205, 470–474.

Biello, P., Fishman, M., Koch, G., 1976. Evidence that immune RNA is messenger RNA. Cell. Immunol. 23, 309–319.

Burnet, F.M., 1957. A modification of Jerne's theory of antibody production using the concept of clonal selection. Aust. J. Sci. 20, 67–68.

Cline, M.J., Swett, V.C., 1968. The interaction of human monocytes and lymphocytes. J. Exp. Med. 128, 1309–1325.

Dixon, F.J., Weigle, W.O., Roberts, J.C., 1957. Comparison of antibody responses associated with the transfer of rabbit lymph-node, peritoneal exudate, and thymus cells. J. Immunol. 78, 56–62.

Ehrich, W.E., Harris, T.N., Mertens, E., 1946. The absence of antibody in the macrophages during maximum antibody formation. J. Exp. Med. 83, 373–381.

Fishman, M., 1959. Antibody formation in tissue culture. Nature 183, 1200–1201.

Fishman, M., 1961. Antibody formation in vitro. J. Exp. Med. 114, 837–856.

Fishman, M., Hammerstrom, R.A., Bond, V.P., 1963. In vitro transfer of macrophage RNA to lymph node cells. Nature 198, 549–551.

Gottlieb, A.A., Glisin, V.R., Doty, P., 1967. Studies on macrophage RNA involved in antibody production. Proc. Nat. Acad. Sci. U.S.A. 57, 1849–1856.

Hersh, E.M., Harris, J.E., 1968. Macrophage-lymphocyte interaction in the antigen-induced blastogenic response of human peripheral blood leukocytes. J. Immunol. 100, 1184–1194.

Levine, B.B., Ojeda, A., Benacceraf, B., 1963. Studies on artificial antigens. III. The genetic control of the immune response to hapten poly-l-lysine conjugates in guinea pigs. J. Exp. Med. 118, 953–957.

Mechnikov, I., 1908. On the present state of the question of immunity in infectious diseases. In: Nobel Lectures, Physiology or Medicine 1901–1921. Elsevier Publishing Co, Amsterdam. 1967; accessed at http://nobelprize.org/nobel_prizes/medicine/laureates/1908/mechnikov-lecture.html.

Mishell, R.J., Dutton, R.W., 1966. Immunization of normal mouse spleen cell suspensions in vitro. Science 153, 1004–1006.

Mosier, D.E., 1967. A requirement for two cell types for antibody formation in vitro. Science 158, 1573–1575.

Mosier, D.E., 1969. Cell interactions in the primary immune response in vitro: a requirement for specific cell clusters. J. Exp. Med. 129, 351–362.

Mosier, D.E., Coppleson, L.W., 1968. A three-cell interaction required for the induction of the primary immune response in vitro. Proc. Nat. Acad. Sci. U.S.A. 61, 542–547.

Rosenthal, A.S., Shevach, E.M., 1973. Function of macrophages in antigen recognition by guinea pig T lymphocytes. I. Requirement for histocompatible macrophages and lymphocytes. J. Exp. Med. 138, 1194–1212.

Sabin, R.R., 1939. Cellular reactions to a dye-protein with a concept of the mechanism of antibody formation. J. Exp. Med. 68, 853–868.

Schoenberg, M.D., Mumaw, V.R., Moore, R.D., Weisberger, A.S., 1964. Cytoplasmic interaction between macrophages and lymphocytic cells in antibody synthesis. Science 143, 964–965.

Sharp, J.A., Burwell, R.G., 1960. Interaction ('peripolesis') of macrophages and lymphocytes after skin homografting or challenge with soluble antigens. Nature 188, 474–475.

Shevach, E.M., Paul, W.E., Green, I., 1972. Histocompatibility-linked immune response gene function in guinea pigs. Specific inhibition of antigen-induced lymphocyte proliferation by alloantiserum. J. Exp. Med. 136, 1207–1221.

Shevach, E.M., Rosenthal, A.S., 1973. Function of macrophages in antigen recognition by guinea pig T lymphocytes. II. Role of the macrophage in the regulation of genetic control of the immune response. J. Exp. Med. 138, 1213–1229.

Steinman, R.M., Cohn, Z.A., 1973. Identification of a novel cell type in peripheral lymphoid organs of mice. I. Morphology, quantitation, tissue distribution. J. Exp. Med. 137, 1142–1162.

TIME LINE

1908 — Ilya Metchnikov shares the Nobel Prize in Physiology or Medicine for his work on the immune response, including the development of his phagocyte theory

1900–1957 — Instruction hypotheses of antibody formation postulate that antibodies are synthesized by cells of the reticuloensdothelial system, including macrophages

1939 — Florence Sabin observes macrophages shedding surface film during an antibody response

1957 — Macfarlane Burnet publishes the clonal selection theory of antibody formation

1959 — Marvin Fishman describes immune RNA and suggests it is a macrophage product

1960 — J.A. Sharp and R.G. Burwell note associations between macrophages and lymphocytes in the tissue culture of cells from antigen-injected animals

1963 — Baruj Benacceraf and colleagues provide evidence that immune responses (IRs) in guinea pigs are under genetic control

1964 — Melvin Schoenberg and colleagues demonstrate cytoplasmic connections between macrophages and lymphocytes in lymphoid tissue from antigen-injected animals

1966 — Robert Mishell and Richard Dutton optimize conditions to induce a primary antibody response in vitro

1967 — Donald Mosier reports that plastic adherent cells (macrophages) collaborate with nonadherent cells (lymphocytes) in antibody responses

1969 — Donald Mosier demonstrates the requirement for macrophage–lymphocyte clusters during early primary antibody responses in vitro

1973 — Ethan Shevach and Alan Rosenthal provide evidence that the first step in initiating an IR involves the presentation of antigen by macrophages to histocompatible lymphocytes

1973 — Ralph Steinman and Melvin Cohn describe the dendritic cell in lymphoid tissue

1980 — Baruj Benacceraf shares the Nobel Prize in Physiology or Medicine with Jean-Baptiste Dausset and George Snell

2011 — Ralph Steinman shares the Nobel Prize for Physiology or Medicine with Bruce Beutler and Jules Hoffman

15

Recognition Structures on Cells of the Innate Host Defense Mechanisms

INTRODUCTION

Differentiation of self from foreign invaders is a hallmark of both innate host defense mechanisms and the adaptive immune response. Lymphocytes responsible for the adaptive immune response possess cell surface receptors specific for single antigens. The structure and genetic basis of these molecules are covered in Chapter 17. The mechanisms responsible for self–non-self recognition by cells of the innate defense system were discovered through a series of experiments employing animal models ranging from fruit flies to humans. The receptors revealed by these studies are expressed by phagocytic cells and illustrate the central role these cells play in innate host defense mechanisms and adaptive immune responses.

Ilya Metchnikov (1845–1916) trained in Russia and Germany prior to accepting a position at Odessa University. In 1882, he resigned this position due to political upheaval following the assassination of Czar Alexander II. He moved to Messina in Italy where he set up a laboratory in his home to pursue studies in comparative embryology, including the now classically recognized response of starfish larva to the injection of a foreign object. His description of the experiment has been related in a biography written by his daughter shortly after his death (Metchnikoff, 1921):

> One day when the whole family had gone to a circus to see some extraordinary performing apes, I remained alone with my microscope, observing the life in the mobile cells of a transparent star-fish larva, when a new thought suddenly flashed across my brain. It struck me that similar cells might serve in the defence of the organism against intruders. Feeling that there was in this something of surpassing interest, I felt so excited that I began striding up and down the room and even went to the seashore in order to collect my thoughts.
>
> I said to myself that, if my supposition was true, a splinter introduced into the body of a star-fish larva, devoid of blood-vessels or of a nervous system, should soon be surrounded by mobile cells as is to be observed in a man who runs a splinter into his finger. This was no sooner said than done.
>
> There was a small garden to our dwelling, in which we had a few days previously organised a 'Christmas tree' for the children on a little tangerine tree; I fetched from it a few rose thorns and introduced them at once under the skin of some beautiful star-fish larvae as transparent as water.
>
> I was too excited to sleep that night in the expectation of the result of my experiment, and very early the next morning I ascertained that it had fully succeeded.
>
> That experiment formed the basis of the phagocyte theory, to the development of which I devoted the next twenty-five years of my life.

The phagocyte theory proposed that defenses against foreign objects and invading microorganisms depend on mobile phagocytic cells to surround and engulf the foreign material (Metchnikoff, 1908). Metchnikov realized that the activation of these cells represents the initial steps in the inflammatory response. Metchnikov acknowledged the existence of antibodies; however, he was convinced that the primary mechanism by which the body protects against foreign microbes is through the action of phagocytes.

Immunologists now agree that protection of the host against foreign intruders involves activity of both cells and antibodies. Phagocytic cells and phagocytosis of foreign material play central roles in initiating both innate host defenses and adaptive immune responses. In the innate defenses, phagocytes engulf foreign material, including potential pathogens, destroy this foreign material, and initiate an inflammatory response. In the adaptive immune system, phagocytic cells engulf foreign antigens, process them to immunogenic peptides, and present these peptides to immunocompetent T lymphocytes to initiate a response. These stimulated T lymphocytes function as helper cells to assist B lymphocytes in producing antibody and to activate other T lymphocytes to lyse virally infected or malignantly transformed target cells. Once B lymphocytes synthesize and secrete antibody and cytotoxic T lymphocytes are activated, macrophages and other phagocytic cells are recruited to rid the body of the pathogenic insult.

When the phagocyte recognizes the pathogen, this sequence of events is initiated. Phagocytes express cell surface receptors coded for by germ line genes that recognize unique molecular patterns on the surfaces of microbes and other potentially dangerous invaders. Several investigators suggested the existence of these recognition receptors. For example, Peter Wilkinson of the University of Glasgow (1976), described mechanisms by which phagocytes might recognize foreign substances and suggested that phagocytes "may possess stereospecific receptors for all, or at least some, of the substances to which they respond." However, he concluded that "Clear evidence that phagocytic functions can be activated upon binding of extrinsic molecules to stereospecific integral cell-membrane receptors is still awaited."

In 1989, Charles Janeway (1943–2003), of Yale University, proposed the existence of similar receptors in his introductory lecture at the Cold Spring Harbor Symposium on Immunologic Recognition. Janeway termed these cell surface structures pattern recognition receptors (PRR) and predicted that they recognize molecular patterns associated with pathogens or other foreign substances.

Jules Hoffmann and Bruce Beutler validated this prediction in the 1980s and 1990s. Their studies included characterization of the response of mammals to bacterial toxins, determination of the genetic basis of insect defenses against fungi, and identification of the receptor for lipopolysaccharide (LPS). These investigations led to the awarding of the Nobel Prize in Physiology or Medicine in 2011 to Jules Hoffmann and Bruce Beutler. Unfortunately. Janeway died in 2003 and therefore was ineligible to share in this prize.

Prior to the identification of these receptors, however, several other proposed recognition mechanisms were tested and subsequently abandoned.

EARLY INVESTIGATIONS ON RECOGNITION BY PHAGOCYTIC CELLS

Molecules that Enhance Phagocytosis–Opsonization

Sir Almroth Wright (1861–1947) studied medicine at Trinity College in Dublin, receiving his MD in 1883. He studied at several other academic institutions before accepting an appointment at the Army Medical School in Netley in 1892. In the late 1890s, he successfully introduced typhoid vaccine to British troops in India. He was appointed professor of pathology at St Mary's Medical School in London in 1902 and worked there until shortly before his death. During the first decade of the twentieth century, he performed studies leading to the discovery of the phenomenon of opsonization. This work has been immortalized in the play *The Doctor's Dilemma* by George Bernard Shaw in which Wright appears as Sir Colenso Ridgeon.

Wright questioned "whether the blood fluids perform any role in connection with phagocytosis." He added human peripheral blood leukocytes to *Staphylococcus pyogenes* in the presence or absence of human serum. Following a short incubation, he counted the number of microbes associated with the leukocytes. Human serum contained a substance that enhanced phagocytosis of the bacteria; Wright termed the serum substance opsonin (from the Greek opsono—to prepare to eat) and the process opsonization (Wright and Douglas, 1903, 1904).

Wright demonstrated that serum contains two types of opsonins: one that is destroyed by heating the serum to between 50 and 60 °C and a second that is resistant to heating. The heat-labile component is not specific for the antigen and has subsequently been identified as complement, particularly the C3b component (Chapter 12). The heat-stable opsonin is immunologically specific and has been identified as antibody, particularly IgG1 and IgG3.

Although not recognized at the time, both complement and antibody function by forming a bridge between the invading bacteria (or other foreign substance) and cell surface receptors on the phagocytic cells. Antibody binds to the foreign invader to which it is specific and then to Fc receptors on phagocytes. Similarly, the C3b component of complement binds to complement receptors (CR1) on phagocytes after it binds to the foreign invader. The binding of these opsonin-containing complexes to their receptors triggers a series of events, starting with internalization of the foreign material by invagination of the phagocyte membrane. This phagosome merges with one or more lysosomes, cell organelles containing enzymes. Within the phagolysosome, the enzymes destroy the foreign substance, cleaving proteins into immunogenic peptides that are subsequently reexpressed on the surface of the phagocyte and presented to antigen-specific T lymphocytes.

Phagocytosis of the foreign material simultaneously induces the activation of several genes in the nucleus, resulting in the synthesis and secretion of cytokines, including IL-1, IL-6, and TNF-α, which initiates a local inflammatory response (Chapter 25).

Opsonization assists in phagocytosis of foreign material, but it is not the only mechanism by which phagocytes recognize potentially dangerous substances. Other recognition mechanisms proposed during the period between 1920 and 1980 included physical characteristics of the antigens and lectin-dependent interactions between pathogens and phagocytes.

Recognition Based on Physical Characteristics

Physical characteristics such as surface tension, amount of free energy, hydrophobicity, and net surface charge have all been proposed to play a role in the recognition of foreign material by phagocytes. Wallace O. Fenn (1922), from Harvard Medical School, Boston, Massachusetts, published a theoretical evaluation of the interaction between cells and solid surfaces and between cells and particles. He developed equations to calculate the surface energies between a hypothetical cell and a solid particle and proposed that ingestion of the particle depended on the surface tensions of the interacting components.

In 1933, Emily and Stuart Mudd at the University of Pennsylvania, evaluated the validity of these equations by characterizing interactions between rabbit or human phagocytes and foreign red cells or bacteria. Based on these observations they concluded that there is a "quantitative correlation…between phagocytosis and the surface properties of the particles ingested."

The role of physicochemical characteristics in the interaction between phagocytes and bacteria or between phagocytes and inert particles such as latex or styrene was investigated for several more decades. In 1978, C.J. van Oss working at the State University of New York, Buffalo, reviewed phagocytosis of various bacteria and concluded that "bacteria more hydrophobic than phagocytes readily become phagocytized; bacteria more hydrophilic than phagocytes resist phagocytosis." He also studied the role of serum in the phenomenon of phagocytosis and concluded that both specific antibody and complement, which had been demonstrated to enhance phagocytosis, increased the hydrophobicity of bacteria, thus explaining the opsonic activity of these substances.

Molecules that Enhance Phagocytosis: The Role of Lectins

Opsonization provided one explanation of how phagocytes recognized foreign invaders and destroyed them. While complement is a component of the innate host defense mechanisms and occurs naturally, antibody must be synthesized anew for each foreign substance. Other investigators studied the role of lectins (carbohydrate-binding proteins) in the interaction of foreign particles to phagocytes (reviewed by Sharon, 1984). These studies were inspired by observations on the effect plant lectins have on immunocompetent cells. Several plant products, such as phytohemagglutinin and concanavalin A, bind to and activate lymphocytes and macrophages. These lectins are specific for particular carbohydrates, suggesting mechanisms by which lectins may function in recognition.

Most cells, both microbial and mammalian, possess membrane glycoproteins and glycolipids. These molecules constitute a carbohydrate coating to the cell and enable interactions between foreign and host cells. Investigators proposed three ways by which these interactions occur:

- Carbohydrates on the surface of phagocytes bind to lectins expressed on the surface of foreign cells (bacteria).
- A lectin bridges the phagocyte and foreign cell by binding carbohydrates on both cells.
- Lectins on the surface of phagocytes bind to carbohydrates on the surface of foreign cells.

Subsequent studies identified a group of cell surface receptors expressed by phagocytes that bind both carbohydrates and other chemical structures on potential pathogens. A study of soluble lectins in recognition of foreign microbes by the innate host defenses has been replaced by experiments that focus on this group of immunologically nonspecific receptors known as PRR.

DISCOVERY OF PATTERN RECOGNITION RECEPTORS

PRR are proteins expressed by cells of the innate host defense system that bind to molecular patterns present on pathogens (pathogen-associated molecular patterns—PAMPs) or on other material that might pose a danger to the body (danger-associated molecular patterns). Charles Janeway predicted the existence of PRRs in 1989 based on the realization that the effector mechanisms for the elimination of potential pathogens are similar in both the innate host defense system and the adaptive immune response. These primitive effector mechanisms, which include phagocytosis and inflammation, evolved in invertebrates and were functional prior to the development of sophisticated gene rearrangement mechanisms involved in coding for antigen-specific receptors on lymphocytes (Chapter 18) and prior to the development of a mechanism for eliminating lymphocytes that are potentially self-reactive (Chapters 21 and 22). Janeway asked how these effector mechanisms were directed to the appropriate targets without injuring self. He proposed that "primitive effector cells bear receptors that allow recognition of certain pathogen-associated molecular patterns that are not found in the host."

Characterization of PRRs resulted from the convergence of three separate lines of investigation:

- evaluation of the response of mammals to bacterial toxins;
- determination of the genetic basis of innate host defenses of insects, particularly fruit flies; and
- identification of the mammalian cell surface receptor for endotoxin.

Response to Bacterial Toxins

The concept that bacteria induce pathology by the release of toxins developed early in the study of infectious diseases. By the late 1800s, the cause of pathology associated with the bacterial diseases diphtheria and tetanus was attributed to the action of toxins. In 1890, Emil von Behring and Shibasaturo Kitasato, working in Robert Koch's laboratory in Berlin, Germany, discovered antitoxins and used them successfully to treat these two diseases (Chapter 3).

Other bacteria, including *Staphylococcus aureus* and *Streptococcus pyogenes*, release exotoxins that interact with macrophages and lymphocytes, causing the activation of large numbers of both types of cells and the release of substantial amounts of inflammatory cytokines. These cytokines induce fever, hypotension, cardiovascular shock, seizures, and organ failure, particularly of the kidneys and liver. Even when treated, the mortality rate due to the action of these toxins (superantigens) is approximately 20%. Additional information about the mechanism by which these superantigens interact with the immune system is discussed in Chapter 33.

Gram negative bacteria such as *Escherichia coli* and *Salmonella typhimurium* contain toxins that can also induce pathology. Unlike exotoxins that are secreted by infecting bacteria, these toxins are structural components of the bacterial cell wall and are only released when the bacteria are lysed. As a result, these toxic molecules are called endotoxins. There are numerous endotoxins that consist of a lipid moiety covalently linked to a polysaccharide composed of O antigens; the generic term, LPS, refers to these molecules collectively.

Richard Pfeiffer (1858–1945), who studied the pathogenesis of *Vibrio cholerae* with Robert Koch in Berlin originally described the toxic nature of endotoxin. Pfeiffer attempted to protect guinea pigs against *V. cholerae* infection either by injecting them with the pathogen (active immunization) or by treating them with antibodies specific for *V. cholerae* (passive immunization—reviewed by Beutler and Rietschel, 2003). These immunized animals subsequently received an intraperitoneal injection of live *V. cholerae*. Several days later, no viable microorganisms were found in the abdominal cavity, yet the animals died. Pfeiffer (1892, 1894) hypothesized that the antibody destroyed the bacteria, causing the release of a toxin that proved lethal to the guinea pigs.

Confirmation of this hypothesis came from studies in which guinea pigs were injected with heat-killed *V. cholerae*: these animals also died. Based on these results, Pfeiffer proposed that the toxin (endotoxin) responsible for this phenomenon was in this case a component of the cell wall. He further theorized that endotoxins are constituents of the cell walls of many bacterial species, both gram negative and gram positive. Finally, he demonstrated the presence of endotoxin in *Salmonella typhi* and *Haemophillus influenza*.

For most of the twentieth century, the mechanism by which endotoxin interacted with mammalian cells and induced pathology remained unknown. Despite the availability of increasingly sophisticated techniques, two possible mechanisms for this interaction were entertained:

- endotoxin is inserted into the lipid bilayer of the cell membrane throughout the body, resulting in altered membrane function; or
- endotoxin interacts with a host cell receptor that transmits a signal to activate that cell.

Differentiation of these two alternatives evolved from studies performed on the host defense mechanisms of *Drosophila melanogaster*, the fruit fly.

Genetics of Fruit Fly Host Defense Mechanisms

Seminal discoveries in any given scientific field often emerge as a result of parallel investigations in complementary disciplines. Such is the case with the discovery of the cell surface receptors responsible for the detection of microorganisms and foreign material by macrophages and other cells of the mammalian innate host defense system.

This story involves several independent but related lines of research that developed in the 1980s and 1990s that include

- identification of a mutation in a gene (*Toll*) in fruit flies that affects embryological development;
- demonstration that fruit flies with a mutated *Toll* gene fail to control fungal infections;
- identification of the receptor coded for by the *Toll* gene termed the Toll receptor;
- characterization of the mammalian homologue of the *Drosophila* toll receptor;
- demonstration that endotoxin binds to a toll-like receptor (TLR); and
- recognition of the role TLRs play in the induction of mammalian host defense responses.

In 1985, Kathryn Anderson, Gerd Jürgens, and Christiane Nüsslein-Volhard, working at the Max Planck Institute in Tubingen, Germany, described mutations in fruit flies that are involved in the embryological development of the flies. One of the mutations disrupted the ventral–dorsal axis of the developing fly and resulted in flies with an underdeveloped ventral portion of their body. Upon seeing the first fly with this mutation, Nüsslein-Volhard exclaimed "Das war ja toll" (that was amazing/wild) and the gene thus was named *Toll* (Hansson and Edfeldt, 2005). During the course of these early studies, strains of flies with mutated *Toll* genes were isolated. In 1995, Christiane Nüsslein-Volhard was awarded the Nobel Prize in Physiology or Medicine along with Edward B. Lewis and Eric F. Weischaus "for their discoveries concerning the genetic control of early embryonic development."

In 1996, Jules Hoffmann and coworkers at the National Center for Scientific Research in Strasbourg, France, used these mutants to demonstrate that a functional, nonmutated *Toll* gene was required in order for adult *Drosophila* to control fungal infections. Hoffman (1941–present) received his education at the University of Strasbourg, earning a PhD in 1969. He became a member and eventually director of The French National Center for Scientific Research in Strasbourg, where he pursued basic research on the blood cells of grasshoppers and on the biochemistry of insect hormones. In the early 1990s, he developed a model system based on the fruit fly to study antimicrobial defense mechanisms.

Insect defenses to potential pathogens elicit three major responses (Hoffman, 1997):

- induction of coagulation and phenoloxidase systems,
- phagocytosis and encapsulation by blood cells, and
- synthesis and secretion of antibacterial and antifungal peptides.

The production of antimicrobial peptides is stimulated by products of the coagulation and phenoloxidase system and involves signaling through the NFκB (nuclear factor kappa-B) pathway. Significant similarities exist between the signaling cascades involved in induction of antimicrobial peptides in fruit flies and the induction of acute phase proteins in mammals (Lemaitre et al., 1996), including the activation of NFκB. Acute phase proteins are induced by proinflammatory cytokines such as IL-1 and TNF-α and are important in the vertebrate innate defense mechanisms against potential pathogens.

Strains of *Drosophila* carrying mutations in their *Toll* genes synthesize decreased quantities of antifungal peptides. Further study of the molecular pathways leading to the synthesis of these peptides revealed the expression of a cell surface receptor, coded for by the *Toll* gene, and termed the toll receptor. Stimulation of the toll receptor initiated a signaling cascade that resulted in the activation of NFκB.

Shortly after Hoffmann's group described the role of toll receptors in the antimicrobial defenses of fruit flies, Ruslan Medzhitov, working with Charles Janeway and Paula Preston-Hurlburt at Yale University School of Medicine, New Haven, Connecticut (Medzhitov et al., 1997), described the cloning and characterization of a mammalian homologue of the *Drosophila Toll* gene. They transfected this gene into human cell lines and demonstrated that the transfected cells expressed a cell surface molecule that they called a toll-like receptor (TLR). Stimulation of the TLR activated the NFκB pathway, leading to the synthesis and secretion of proinflammatory cytokines, including Il-1, IL-6, and IL-8. TLR stimulation also induced the transcription of other genes that are required for the activation of the adaptive immune response.

Discovery of the Receptor for Endotoxin (LPS)

Medzhitov and colleagues suggested that mammalian TLR might play a role in the initiation of host defenses. However, the natural ligand for TLR remained unknown until investigators identified the receptor for lipopolysacccharide (LPS).

Injecting most strains of mice with LPS leads to a potentially lethal syndrome characterized by fever, secretion of proinflammatory cytokines, leading to generalized inflammation, activation of the alternate complement pathway, and initiation of the coagulation cascade. In 1965, Gloria Heppner and David Weiss, working at the University of California, Berkeley, discovered a strain of mice resistant to the effects of LPS. These C3H/HeJ mice, derived from the C3H/HeN strain, possess a mutation in a gene locus responsible for the lethal effects of LPS. In the mid-1970s, James Watson and Roy Riblet (1974, 1975) of the Salk Institute of Biological Studies and Michael Glode and colleagues

(1977) at the National Institute of Dental Research characterized this gene locus (called *Lps*) and reported that LPS is not toxic to macrophages from C3H/HeJ mice while a similar dose of LPS killed macrophages from a closely related strain C3H/HeN.

In 1980, Suzanne Michalek and her colleagues at the National Institute of Dental Research in Bethesda, Maryland, showed that C3H/HeJ mice could be sensitized to LPS by irradiation with 850 rad followed by reconstitution with bone marrow cells from a C3H/HeN donor. Their results suggested that "lymphocytes and/or macrophages play a primary role in mediating a number of diverse and seemingly unrelated host responses to endotoxin." Subsequent studies by Masanobu Kawasaki and Anthony Cerami at The Rockefeller University, New York, in 1981 demonstrated that sensitization to LPS, as measured by a decrease in lipoprotein lipase, could be transferred by a culture supernatant from peritoneal exudate macrophages treated in vitro with LPS.

In 1986, Peter Tobias and colleagues at the Scripps Clinic and Research Foundation in LaJolla, California, isolated and purified a serum protein that bound LPS. Rabbits injected with LPS from *Salmonella minnesota* generated an inflammatory response characterized by the secretion of acute phase proteins into the serum. This serum also contained a protein that bound LPS specifically; the authors termed this protein LPS binding protein (LBP). Studies reported in 1990 by Samuel Wright of Rockefeller University in collaboration with the Tobias group identified a cell surface molecule, CD14, present on macrophages that bound LBP. The binding of LBP to CD14 activates macrophages. Investigators initially considered CD14 the receptor for LPS; however, structural studies of the molecule demonstrated that it lacked a cytoplasmic domain to transduce a signal to the nucleus.

While these studies were ongoing, Bruce Beutler (1957 to present), working in Cerami's laboratory at Rockefeller University, extended earlier observations and identified cachectin/tumor necrosis factor (TNF) as a primary mediator of LPS action (1985). Beutler received his MD from the University of Chicago and has held academic appointments at the University of Texas Southwestern Medical School, Dallas, and at Scripps Research Institute, La Jolla, California. He focused his immunological research on inflammation, particularly the role of the cytokine TNF in endotoxin-induced shock. He also performed studies on the mechanisms of LPS-induced cell activation and stimulation of the pro-inflammatory cytokine, TNF. Following a move to the University of Texas, Southwestern Medical School in Dallas, Beutler and colleagues focused their research on identifying the LPS receptor by mapping the *Lps* locus in two mouse strains (C3H/

HeJ and C57Bl/10ScCr) that are resistant to the action of LPS. In 1998, Alexander Poltorak and coworkers in Beutler's laboratory reported a mutation in a gene in the *Lps* locus. The gene they identified coded for the same receptor (TLR-4) that Medzhitov and his colleagues had reported the year before. Mice possessing a mutation in TLR-4 failed to respond to LPS and were therefore susceptible to lethal infection by gram negative bacteria. This was the first demonstration of the specificity of a TLR in vertebrates and of its role in the induction of a protective immune response.

Subsequent studies demonstrated that mammalian cells possess several different receptors that bind ligands on potential pathogens. Many of these have the basic structure of TLRs, but other molecular structures such as receptor kinases and C-type lectin receptors have also been described. In aggregate these receptors are termed PRR, and the pathogen-associated ligands that bind to them have been designated PAMPs. The binding of PAMPs to PRRs leads to phagocytosis of the pathogen and transcription of genes coding for inflammatory cytokines and other components of the host defense mechanisms. The phagocytized pathogen is relocated to lysosomes where pathogenic proteins are digested into peptides that associate with molecules coded for by the animals' major histocompatibility complex (MHC). Macrophages express these MHC-peptide complexes that are screened by antigen specific T lymphocytes. The studies performed to determine this sequence of events are described in Chapter 20.

This research identified the receptors on macrophages that detect foreign invaders. Based on their contributions, Jules Hoffmann and Bruce Beutler received one-half of the 2011 Nobel Prize for Physiology or Medicine for "their discoveries concerning the activation of innate immunity." This award was shared with Ralph Steinman, who discovered and characterized dendritic cells, another component of the innate host defenses (Chapter 29).

CONCLUSION

Over 100 years ago, Ilya Metchnikov observed phagocytic cells in the larva of sea stars and developed his phagocytic theory of immunity. While the role of the phagocyte in host defenses is essential, the study of antibodies in the adaptive immune response received the preponderance of attention by investigators during much of the twentieth century. The discovery of the mechanism by which phagocytic cells recognize foreign material renewed an appreciation for the contributions these cells make to the initiation of both innate host defenses and the adaptive immune response.

Several mechanisms of recognizing pathogens have evolved and are employed by both innate host defenses and adaptive immune responses. Lymphocytes interact with antigens through specialized receptors that require unique genetic rearrangements (Chapter 18) and unique selection mechanisms that protect the individual from pathology through the elimination of potentially self-reactive cells (Chapters 21 and 22). In addition, B and T lymphocytes recognize different forms of the antigens to which they react—B lymphocytes recognize conformational arrangements of foreign molecules while T lymphocytes recognize sequences of amino acids (peptides) that have been processed by specialized antigen-presenting cells and loaded onto molecules coded for by genes in the MHC (Chapter 20). Identification of these recognition mechanisms in the 1970s and 1980s convinced some immunologists that a more rapid, less specific method had to exist so that the innate host defense mechanisms could determine those invaders that are potentially harmful. The discovery of PRR provided an explanation by which host defenses interact with their environment.

The results presented in this chapter indicate that recognition by mammalian phagocytes evolved from mechanisms present in evolutionarily more distant species. The presence of homologous genes coding for receptors in both invertebrates and mammals demonstrates how important defenses against potential pathogens have been in the survival of vertebrates and invertebrates. The discovery of PRRs provides an explanation for the function of antigen-presenting cells in the adaptive immune response as well as the underlying pathophysiological mechanisms for a large number of autoinflammatory diseases such as familial Mediterranean fever, TNF receptor-associated periodic syndrome, and neonatal onset multisystem inflammatory disease (Chapter 31).

References

Anderson, K.V., Jürgens, G., Nüsslein-Volhard, C., 1985. Establishment of dorsal-ventral polarity in the *Drosophila* embryo: genetic studies on the role of the *Toll* gene product. Cell 42, 779–789.

Beutler, B., Greenswald, D., Hulmes, J.D., Chang, M., Pan, Y.-C.E., Mathison, J., Ulevitch, R., Cerami, A., 1985. Identity of tumor necrosis factor and the macrophage-secreted factor cachectin. Nature 316, 552–554.

Beutler, B., Rietschel, E.T., 2003. Innate immune sensing and its roots: the story of endotoxin. Nat. Rev. Immunol. 3, 169–176.

Fenn, W.O., 1922. The theoretical response of living cells to contact with solid bodies. J. Gen. Physiol. 4, 373–385.

Glode, L.M., Jacques, A., Mergenhagen, S.E., Rosenstreich, D.L., 1977. Resistance of macrophages from C3H/HeJ mice to the in vitro cytotoxic effects of endotoxin. J. Immunol. 119, 162–166.

Hansson, G.K., Edfeldt, K., 2005. Toll to be paid at the gateway to the vessel wall. Arterioscler. Thromb. Vasc. Biol. 25, 1085–1087.

Heppner, G., Weiss, D.W., 1965. High susceptibility of strain A mice to endotoxin and endotoxin-red blood cell mixtures. J. Bacteriol. 90, 696–703.

Hoffman, J.A., 1997. Immune responsiveness in vector insects. Proc. Nat. Acad. Sci. U. S. A. 94, 11152–11153.

Janeway, C.A., 1989. Approaching the asymptote? Evolution and revolution in immunology. Cold spring harbor symp. Quant. Biol. 54, 1–13.

Kawasaki, M., Cerami, A., 1981. Studies of endotoxin-induced decrease in lipoprotein lipase activity. J. Exp. Med. 154, 631–639.

Lemaitre, B., Nicolas, E., Michaut, L., Reichhart, J.-M., Hoffman, J.A., 1996. The dorsoventral regulatory gene cassette *spätzle/Toll/cactus* controls the potent antifungal response in *Drosophila* adults. Cell 86, 973–983.

Medzhitov, R., Preston-Hurlburt, P., Janeway, C.A., 1997. A human homologue of the *Drosophila Toll* protein signals activation of adaptive immunity. Nature 388, 394–397.

Metchnikoff, I., 1908. On the Present State of the Question of Immunity in Infectious Diseases. In: Nobel Lectures, Physiology or Medicine 1901-1921. Elsevier Publishing Co., Amsterdam, 1967; accessed at http://nobelprize.org/nobel_prizes/medicine/laureates/1908/mechnikov-lecture.html.

Metchnikoff, O., 1921. Life of Elie Metchnikoff 1845–1916. 116–117. http://todayinsci.com/M/Metchnikoff_Elie/MetchnikoffElie-Quotations.htm.

Michalek, S.M., Moore, R.N., McGhee, J.R., Rosenstreich, D.L., Mergenhagen, S.E., 1980. The primary role of lymphoreticular cells in the mediation of host responses to bacterial endotoxin. J. Infect. Dis. 141, 55–63.

Mudd, E.B.H., Mudd, S., 1933. The process of phagocytosis. The agreement between direct observation and deduction from theory. J. Gen. Physiol. 16, 625–636.

Pfeiffer, R., 1892. Untersuchungen über des Choleragift. Z. Hyg. 11, 393–411.

Pfeiffer, R., 1894. Untersuchungen über das Wesen der Choleraimmunität und über spezifisch bacterizide Prozesse. Z. Hyg. 18, 1–18.

Poltorak, A., He, X., Smirnova, I., Liu, M.-Y., Van Huffel, C., Du, X., Birdwell, D., Alejos, E., Silva, M., Galanos, C., Freundenberg, M., Riccardi-Castagnoll, P., Layton, B., Beutler, B., 1998. Defective LPS signaling in C3H/HeJ and C57BL/10ScCr mice: mutations in *Tlr4* gene. Science 282, 2085–2088.

Sharon, N., 1984. Surface carbohydrates and surface lectins are recognition determinants in phagocytosis. Immunol. Today 5, 143–147.

Tobias, P.S., Soldau, K., Ulevitch, R.J., 1986. Isolation of a lipopolysaccharide-binding acute phase reactant from rabbit serum. J. Exp. Med. 164, 777–793.

van Oss, C.J., 1978. Phagocytosis as a surface phenomenon. Ann. Rev. Microbiol. 32, 19–39.

von Behring, E.A., Kitasato, S., 1890. Über das Zustandekommen der Diphtheria-immunität und der Tetanus-immunität bei Thieren. Dtsch. Med. Wochenschr. 49, 1113–1114.

Watson, J., Riblet, R., 1974. Genetic control of responses to bacterial lipopolysaccharide in mice. I. Evidence for a single gene that influences mitogenic and immunogenic responses to lipopolysaccharide. J. Exp. Med. 140, 1147–1161.

Watson, J., Riblet, R., 1975. Genetic control of responses to bacterial lipopolysaccharide in mice. II. A gene that influences a membrane component involved in the activation of bone-marrow lymphocytes by lipopolysaccharide. J. Immunol. 114, 1462–1468.

Wilkinson, P.C., 1976. Recognition and response in mononuclear and granular phagocytes. A Rev. Clin. Exp. Immunol. 25, 355–366.

Wright, A.E., Douglas, S.R., 1903. An experimental investigation of the role of the blood fluids in connection with phagocytosis. Proc. Roy. Soc. Lond. 72, 357–370.

Wright, A.E., Douglas, S.R., 1904. Further observations on the role of the blood fluids in connection with phagocytosis. Proc. Roy. Soc. Lond. 73, 128–142.

Wright, S.D., Ramos, R.A., Tobias, P.S., Ulevitch, R.J., Mathison, J.C., 1990. CD14, a receptor for complexes of lipopolysaccharide (LPS) and LPS binding protein. Science 249, 1431–1433.

TIME LINE

1883   Ilya Metchnikov develops the phagocytic theory of immunity

1892   Richard Pfeiffer describes endotoxin as the agent of pathology during infection with *Vibrio cholerae*

1903   Almroth Wright demonstrates the presence of opsonins in human serum

1965   Gloria Heppner and David Weiss describe a strain of mice (C3H/HeJ) resistant to the toxic effects of LPS

1974–77   James Watson and Roy Riblet and Michael Glode, and coworkers identify the *Lps* gene

1985   Christiane Nüsslein-Volhard and colleagues describe a gene mutation in fruit flies that disrupts normal embryological development

1986   Peter Tobias and colleagues describe the appearance of an LPS-binding protein in the serum of rabbits injected with LPS

1989   Charles Janeway predicts the existence of pattern recognition receptors that recognize and bind pathogen-associated molecular patterns

1990   Samuel Wright and coworkers identify CD14 as a macrophage cell surface receptor that binds LPS-binding protein

1996   Jules Hoffmann and colleagues report on the role of *Toll* genes in controlling antifungal defense mechanisms in insects

1997   Ruslan Medzhitov and Charles Janeway identify a gene in humans analogous to *Toll* that is involved in activating adaptive immune responses

1998   Bruce Beutler and collaborators identify the receptor for endotoxin produced by gram-negative bacteria and demonstrate that it is coded for by a gene analogous to *Toll*

2011   Jules Hoffmann and Bruce Beutler awarded the Nobel Prize in Physiology or Medicine

The Adaptive Immune Response and Histocompatibility Genes

INTRODUCTION

The transplantation of spontaneously arising tumors between mice provided the initial clue that animals are immunologically unique. The fate of these transplants varied and included both successes and failures. Breeding mice that accepted a tumor with those that rejected the tumor suggested that success or failure of the transplanted tumor involved genetic differences between the animals. Initially, the genetic differences were thought to relate to the presence or absence in the recipients of tumor susceptibility genes.

We now appreciate that the success or failure of tumor transplants depends on the induction of an adaptive immune response by the recipient against cell surface proteins expressed by the donor. These proteins (histocompatibility antigens) are coded for by genes located in the major histocompatibility complex (MHC). Differences in the proteins expressed between the tumor donor and recipient lead to induction of an antitumor response; the failure of the tumors to grow is due to rejection by an adaptive immune response.

Advances in understanding histocompatibility proteins and the genes that encode them relied on the development of inbred strains of mice and other experimental animals through brother–sister mating. Inbred mice, which resemble monozygotic twins, provided the model for tumor transfer studies and, subsequently, tissue and organ transplantation experiments. Transplant studies confirmed the presence of a gene complex that controls the fate of transplanted tissue in a recipient. These investigations unraveled basic information about the histocompatibility gene complex and the proteins for which these genes code.

By the 1960s, investigators had described the existence of cell surface molecules in several vertebrate species coded for by genes in the MHC. However, the physiological function of these cell surface proteins remained unknown. Surgeons successfully transplanted healthy organs into patients with renal or cardiac failure only to lose the grafts due to the induction of an adaptive immune response directed against the proteins expressed on the cells of the graft coded for by the MHC. If organ transplants were to succeed, investigators would have to find methods to circumvent the adverse immune responses (Chapter 36).

Many immunologists rejected the idea that histocompatibility genes and proteins had evolved just to make

A Historical Perspective on Evidence-Based Immunology
http://dx.doi.org/10.1016/B978-0-12-398381-7.00016-2

organ transplants difficult. In the early 1970s investigators observed that several of the cell interactions involved in the adaptive immune response required that cells share histocompatibility genes. Experiments designed to study this phenomenon followed. The actual mechanism remained obscure until Rolf Zinkernagel and Paul Doherty demonstrated the role of MHC compatibility in the killing of virally infected cells by cytotoxic T lymphocytes in 1974. Publication of these results unleashed a plethora of investigations focused on T lymphocyte activation that culminated in the concepts of antigen-presenting cells (APCs) and MHC restriction (Chapter 20). Today immunologists agree that protein antigens are degraded into peptides that become associated with histocompatibility molecules on the surface of cells. This complex then presents the peptide to T lymphocytes to initiate the adaptive immune response.

DISCOVERY OF HISTOCOMPATIBILITY ANTIGENS AND GENES

Tumor Studies

As early as 5000 years ago, physicians reported spontaneously arising tumors in animals and humans. In the nineteenth century Rudolf Virchow described the pathological basis for cancer. Investigators in the first decade of the twentieth century asked whether spontaneously arising tumors could be transferred between animals of the same species. Rupert Billingham, a member of the Wistar Institute of Anatomy and Biology and the University of Pennsylvania in Philadelphia, published a review of transplantation in 1963. He reviewed several landmarks in the history of transplantation research, one of which was that C.O. Jensen transferred a tumor through 19 generations of random-bred mice in 1902. Approximately 50% of the tumors grew in the inoculated animals.

In 1909 Ernest Tyzzer studied the growth of spontaneously arising tumors transferred between Japanese waltzing mice and outbred albino mice. Japanese waltzing mice have a neurological disorder that results in circling behavior. This strain, developed by mouse fanciers, was at least partially inbred.

Tumors arising in Japanese waltzing mice could be transferred successfully to other Japanese waltzing mice but failed to grow when transplanted to albino mice. F_1 hybrids between Japanese waltzing mice and albino mice failed to reject the tumor. While some F_2 hybrid mice (produced by breeding two F_1 mice) accepted the tumor, others rejected it, suggesting that acceptance or rejection of tumors may be genetically determined, although the identification of the specific genes remained unknown.

Tyzzer (1875–1965) graduated from Brown University in Providence, Rhode Island, and received his MD from Harvard in 1902. From 1902 to 1905 he studied parasitology and the natural course of smallpox infection. In 1905 he became Director of Research for the Harvard Commission. Here he pursued studies on the occurrence of spontaneously arising tumors, the response to these tumors, and, with Clarence Little, the genetics of this response.

Clarence C. Little (1888–1971) received his undergraduate education and earned his PhD from Harvard. As an undergraduate he became interested in genetics and developed inbred strains of mice.

Little joined Tyzzer's laboratory and brought with him the highly inbred strains of mice he had developed; some of these, including the DBA and C57Bl strains, are still used today. These mice were used as recipients of a carcinoma that had arisen spontaneously in Japanese waltzing mice. The tumor failed to grow in mice of the inbred strains while it did grow in F_1 hybrids between Japanese waltzing mice and inbred mice. When the F_2 generation was tested, approximately 1.6% of these animals were susceptible to the transplanted tumor (Little and Tyzzer, 1916). At first the investigators proposed a non-Mendelian inheritance mechanism to explain these results. Eventually, Little realized that if a particular trait is determined by several genetic loci, inheritance could appear non-Mendelian (Little, 1914). Based on their results, Tyzzer and Little (1916) calculated that about 12 genes were involved in determining tumor rejection.

Between 1909 and 1924 Little provided experimental evidence that the rejection of tumors is an immunological phenomenon dependent on differences between donor and recipient. These observations presaged the laws of transplantation developed in 1948 by George Snell based on his studies using transplantation of tumors and nonmalignant tissue.

Transplantation Studies and Discovery of the MHC

Peter Gorer (1907–1961) identified and characterized a protein responsible for rejection of tumor transplants in the 1930s. Gorer (1907–1961), trained as a physician at Guy's Hospital in London, and pursued research at the Lister Institute for Preventive Medicine in London where he studied whether factors responsible for tumor rejection might be associated with blood group antigens. Gorer transplanted mice of one inbred strain with tumors from mice of a second inbred strain. Sera collected from the recipients were tested for antibodies specific for the red blood cells of the tumor donor; no antibodies were detected.

Gorer detected antigenic differences between erythrocytes of three inbred strains of mice using his own (human) serum as the source of antibodies (Gorer, 1936a). To study these differences, he injected rabbits with erythrocytes from three strains of mice to induce antibodies. These antibodies differentiated three antigens that he called I, II, and III and that are uniquely distributed in the strains (Gorer, 1936b). When Gorer transplanted tumors from mice expressing antigen II into mice whose red blood cells did not express antigen II, the tumor was rapidly rejected, and the recipient mice developed serum antibodies to antigen II (Gorer, 1937).

Gorer continued characterizing antigen II when he moved to the Jackson Laboratory, Bar Harbor, Maine, to collaborate with George D. Snell. Snell (1903–1996) received his undergraduate education at Dartmouth College in Hanover, New Hampshire. He earned his PhD in genetics from Harvard and joined the Jackson Laboratory to pursue research using inbred mouse strains available there. When Gorer joined the laboratory, Snell was searching for genes responsible for tumor rejection that he called histocompatibility genes. Gorer showed that the antigen II identified by his rabbit antibodies was coded for by one of the histocompatibility genes described by Snell.

Gorer and Snell renamed this gene and the protein it codes for H-2 (histocompatibility-2) (Gorer et al., 1948). Subsequent studies showed that cell surface proteins encoded by H-2 genes serve as targets for the rejection of tissue grafts from allogeneic animals. Other investigators defined the genetic region containing the H-2 gene and termed it the MHC.

Snell continued his studies on tumor transplantation and in 1948 concluded that a tumor

1. "grows progressively in 100% of the animals of the strain in which it originated,
2. fails to grow, or grows temporarily and then regresses in unrelated strains,
3. grows in 100% of F_1 animals where one parent is from the susceptible strain (strain of origin),
4. grows in a fraction of F_2 mice and mice from a backcross of F_1 and the resistant parent."

Snell concluded that "these results are satisfactorily explained by assuming that a tumour will grow progressively only in mice carrying certain dominant genes present in the stock of origin." This conclusion suggests that Snell considered the histocompatibility genes tumor susceptibility genes. Subsequent observations with transplants of healthy tissue led other investigators to develop similar "laws" of transplantation that include

- transplants from strain A animals to other stain A animals succeed;
- transplants from strain A animals to strain B animals fail;
- transplants from stain A animals to (A × B) F_1 recipients succeed;
- transplants from (A × B) F_1 animals to strain A recipients fail; and
- transplants from A animals to an F_2 recipient fail or succeed based on randomly inherited characteristics.

Based on these studies, George Snell was awarded the Nobel Prize for Physiology or Medicine in 1980. He shared the Prize with Jean Dausset and Baruch Benacceraf for "discoveries concerning genetically determined structures on the cell surface that regulate immunological reactions." Gorer died in 1961 and was therefore ineligible for the Prize awarded in 1980.

Jean Dausset (1916–2009) received much of his early education in Paris, France. He completed his medical training at the University of Paris and served as a physician in World War II. In 1958, Dausset identified the human MHC, analogous to the mouse H-2. Patients who received multiple blood transfusions had antibodies in their serum that agglutinated peripheral blood leukocytes from other individuals. Dausset reported agglutination of donor leukocytes using seven sera from multiply transfused donors. He termed the antigen detected by these antibody-containing sera MAC based on the first letter of the last names of three of the volunteers in this study; today this antigen is known as HLA-A2 (human leukocyte-associated antigen-A2). During the 1960s, Dausset and coworkers demonstrated that if donors and recipients of organ or tissue transplants both contained the same HLA antigens, the transplants were more likely to be accepted by the recipient.

Similar results were reported by two other groups in 1958. Jon van Rood and coworkers, working at the University Hospital in Leyden, the Netherlands, and Rose Payne and Mary Rolfs at Stanford University, Palo Alto, California, reported that some multiparous women possess serum antibodies that agglutinate leukocytes from their babies and from their spouses. In several of these women there was no history of previous blood transfusions, suggesting that the fetus was the source of the antigenic stimulus inducing antibody production. These maternally derived antibodies are identical to Dausset's antibodies to HLA proteins.

Baruj Benacceraf (1920–2011), born in Caracas, Venezuela, spent a significant portion of his early life in Paris. In 1940 he enrolled as an undergraduate student at Columbia University in New York. He pursued his medical training at the Medical College of Virginia in Richmond. Following service as a physician in postwar Europe, he started his research career in the laboratory of Elvin Kabat at Columbia. Benacceraf accepted positions in several institutes, including Broussais Hospital in Paris, New York University, the National Institute of

Allergy and Infectious Diseases, and finally Harvard Medical School. He contributed to the concept that MHC genes code for proteins that regulate immune responsiveness. He also developed the hypothesis of MHC restriction, the idea that antigen is presented to T cells "in the context" of molecules coded for by genes in the MHC gene complex.

Transplants of organs between two members of an outbred species are invariably rejected unless the adaptive immune response of the recipient is suppressed. In 1958, Peter Medawar, working at University College in London, reviewed the field of transplantation of healthy (as opposed to malignant) tissue. At that time Medawar and his colleagues demonstrated that transfer of lymphocytes from a mouse that had rejected a skin graft to a naïve mouse bearing a successful graft induced rejection of that graft. This result led to the conclusion that graft rejection is immunological in nature and involves induction of an adaptive immune response.

Additional studies focused on the stimulus responsible for inducing the transplant rejection and resulted in confirmation that the process of rejection of tissue grafts is identical to the destruction of transplanted tumors and that the target of both reactions is the proteins coded for by the MHC genes of the donor.

REGULATION OF THE ADAPTIVE IMMUNE RESPONSE BY MHC GENES

In 1963, Bernard Levine and Antonio Ojeda described the genetic control of immune responses in guinea pigs while working in Benacceraf's laboratory at New York University. Levine and Ojeda injected groups of inbred and outbred guinea pigs with the hapten-carrier conjugate dinitrophenyl-poly-L-lysine (DNP-PLL). They tested experimental and control animals for induction of an adaptive immune response by an intradermal injection of DNP-PLL. They observed the injection sites at 2–3 h and at 24 h. The early response detects the formation of antigen–antibody complexes in the skin (an Arthus reaction) while the delayed response is an indication of a T lymphocyte-mediated reaction.

The presence of serum antibody to DNP was also detected by the following:

* a passive hemolysis assay in which serum was mixed with sheep erythrocytes conjugated with DNP-bovine serum albumin (DNP-BSA); the addition of complement caused lysis of the red cells, indicating the presence of antibodies; and
* a passive cutaneous anaphylaxis assay in which serum was transferred to naïve guinea pigs that were challenged intradermally with DNP-BSA.

Approximately 40% of outbred guinea pigs produced antibody to DNP-PLL. When two responder guinea pigs were mated, 82% of the offspring synthesized antibody when injected with DNP-PLL. None of the offspring from matings of two nonresponder guinea pigs synthesized antibody to this antigen.

Similar results were obtained when outbred guinea pigs were injected with a second hapten-carrier conjugate, benzylpenicilloyl-PLL. However, when the investigators injected inbred guinea pigs with these same antigens, 100% of strain 2 guinea pigs produced antibody to both antigens while no strain 13 guinea pigs mounted a measurable antibody response.

Levine and colleagues (1963) postulated that the response to PLL is under genetic control and suggested two explanations that were later proved incorrect:

* guinea pigs that respond to PLL including strain 2 but not strain 13 animals possess a gene coding for an enzyme that degrades PLL, or
* genes expressed in responder guinea pigs allow the coupling of PLL fragments to low molecular weight RNA that provides an immunogenic signal to T lymphocytes.

This gene is the first specific immune response (*Ir*) gene identified. During the next several years, investigators identified a number of other *Ir* genes that controlled the immune response of experimental animals to

* other synthetic polypeptides (guinea pigs);
* weak antigens such as minor histocompatibility antigens and antigens on foreign erythrocytes (mice); and
* limiting doses of protein antigens, including bovine serum albumin, bovine gamma globulin, and ovalbumin (guinea pigs and mice).

In 1963, investigators proposed mechanisms by which *Ir* genes regulated the adaptive immune response; these hypotheses were developed prior to the functional separation of B and T lymphocytes. Once lymphocytes were categorized into discrete populations in the late 1960s, many functions known to be under *Ir* gene control, such as delayed type hypersensitivity and lymphocyte proliferation, were found to be mediated by T lymphocytes.

The requirement that cells of the adaptive immune response share histocompatibility genes and antigens was suggested by several additional observations made during the 1960s and early 1970s. Elizabeth Leuchars and colleagues at the Chester Beatty Research Institute, London, demonstrated in 1965 that allogeneic thymus grafts failed to restore "immune function" to thymectomized mice. Alan Aisenberg, working at

Harvard, confirmed this finding in 1970. These investigators speculated that the failure to restore immune function was due to rejection of the allogeneic thymus grafts by the recipient; however, they could not rule out the possibility that this reflected some positive effect of the histocompatibility genes on immune reactivity.

In 1967, Don Mosier, a student at the University of Chicago demonstrated that optimal antibody formation requires interaction between macrophages and lymphocytes (Chapter 14). One year later, Martin Cline and Virginia Swett (1968), working at the University of California, San Francisco, showed that macrophage–T lymphocyte interactions during induction of cell proliferation required compatibility at the MHC. Cline and Sweet exposed isolated human peripheral blood monocytes to purified protein derivative from *Mycobacterium tuberculosis*. They cultured these cells with autologous or allogeneic lymphocytes and measured the level of lymphocyte proliferation by counting blast cells and by detecting the incorporation of ^{14}C-thymidine into the cell's DNA. Monocytes stimulated proliferation of autologous but not allogeneic lymphocytes in this system.

In a 1972 review, Baruj Benacceraf of Harvard and Hugh McDevitt of Stanford concluded that most, if not all, genes responsible for regulating adaptive immune responses are linked to the MHC gene locus. By the early 1970s, the proliferative response of lymphocytes from both mice and guinea pigs to several antigens was shown to be under the control of autosomal dominant *Ir* genes. Investigations of the mechanism by which these genes regulated immune responsiveness showed that several of them functioned at the level of T lymphocyte activation.

In 1972, Berenice Kindred of the University of Konstanz in Germany collaborated with Donald Schreffler, working at the University of Michigan, to support the hypothesis that MHC-coded proteins play a role in immune responses in vivo. Nude mice lack a thymus due to a gene mutation, rendering them immunodeficient from birth, and are thus helpful in investigations to unravel the role of the thymus in maturation of T lymphocytes (Chapter 9). When reconstituted with thymocytes from mice sharing the MHC, nude mice can produce antibodies to sheep red blood cells (SRBC) and to bacteriophage T4; however, nude mice reconstituted with allogeneic thymus cells failed to produce any antibodies to these antigens. Kindred and Schreffler concluded that "H-2 compatibility alone is sufficient to allow the development of responsiveness to SRBC and T4."

The mechanism responsible for genetic control of T lymphocyte activation was investigated further in studies using guinea pigs. By the early 1970s, two additional antigens had been shown to be under *Ir* gene control:

- strain 2 but not strain 13 guinea pigs responded to DNP conjugated to a random polymer of glutamic acid and lysine (DNP-GL); and
- strain 13 but not strain 2 guinea pigs responded to a random polymer of glutamic acid and tyrosine (GT).

F1 hybrids of strain 2 and strain 13 responded to both antigens. Ethan Shevach, William Paul, and Ira Green at the National Institutes of Health, Bethesda, Maryland, used this experimental model to characterize the relationship between *Ir* genes, histocompatibility proteins on cell surfaces, and antigen recognition by the adaptive immune response. Shevach and colleagues (1972) designed experiments using antibodies specific for histocompatibility antigens to interfere with induction of lymphocyte proliferation induced by antigens under *Ir* gene control. They injected guinea pigs with antigen (strain 2 with DNP-GL, strain 13 with GT, and F$_1$ hybrids with both antigens) and incubated peritoneal exudate lymphocytes with antigen (DNP-GL or GT) in the presence or absence of antibodies specific for either strain 2 or strain 13 histocompatibility proteins (see Figure 16.1 for the experimental protocol). Five days later, they detected lymphocyte proliferation by measuring the amount of ^{3}H-thymidine incorporated into the DNA of the activated lymphocytes. Antibodies specific for histocompatibility antigens interfered with activation of lymphocytes to these antigens. The authors concluded from these results "that immune response genes produce a cell surface-associated product and that this product plays a role in the mechanism of antigen recognition by the T lymphocyte."

Shevach and his colleagues suggested that the antibody to proteins coded for by the MHC genes functioned by binding to a receptor on T lymphocytes and interfered with antigen recognition. Immunologists now agree that the proteins responsible for regulating immune responsiveness are located on macrophages or other antigen-presenting cells (APCs). Although the lymphocytes used in these studies were said to be purified, they actually contained between 10% and 15% macrophages and 5% neutrophils.

Further studies on the role of *Ir* genes and histocompatibility proteins in the activation of T lymphocytes showed that recognition of antigens by T lymphocytes requires the presentation of the antigen on macrophages histocompatible with the T lymphocytes (Rosenthal and Shevach, 1973; Shevach and Rosenthal, 1973). These investigators purified lymphocytes and macrophages from guinea pigs injected with DNP-GL or GT. Macrophages were incubated with either DNP-GL or with GT for 60 min after which

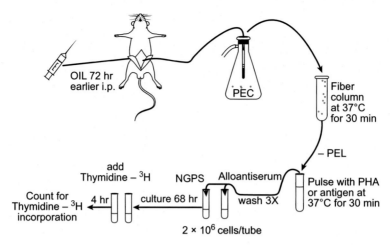

FIGURE 16.1   Protocol used by Shevach and colleagues to demonstrate that antibodies to proteins coded by genes in the MHC of guinea pigs specifically inhibited lymphocyte proliferation to antigens known to be under *Ir* gene control. *From Shevach et al. (1972).*

excess antigen was washed away. Rosenthal and She-vach added lymphocytes to the cultures and 24–48 h later detected lymphocyte proliferation by the incorporation of ^{3}H-thymidine.

Results indicated that presentation of antigen by macrophages to lymphocytes requires that the two cell types be identical at the histocompatibility complex. Macrophages from (2×13) F_1 hybrids presented antigen equally well to lymphocytes from either strain 2 or strain 13 animals. Macrophages from outbred guinea pigs presented antigen to lymphocytes from one of the inbred strains only if the macrophages shared MHC proteins with the lymphocytes. Finally, macrophages incubated with antigen failed to induce lymphocyte proliferation if serum containing antibodies to histocompatibility proteins was included in the assay system.

These studies showed that the first step in the initiation of an immune response requires presentation of antigen by macrophages to lymphocytes. From this information, investigators developed the concept of the APC. APCs, including macrophages, dendritic cells, and B lymphocytes, are covered in Chapter 20.

Requirement for MHC Compatibility in Killing Virally Infected Cells

Rolf Zinkernagel (1940 to present) and Peter Doherty (1944 to present), working in Canberra, Australia, performed a series of studies in mice demonstrating that cytotoxic T cells and virally infected fibroblasts must share at least one set of histocompatibility (H-2) proteins for efficient cell lysis. These investigators radiolabeled mouse fibroblasts infected with the lymphocytic choriomeningitis virus with ^{51}Cr. They overlaid these fibroblasts with spleen cells from mice injected with the same virus. After overnight incubation Zinkernagel and Doherty removed supernatants and measured the amount of radioactivity. Release of the chromium label from the virally infected fibroblasts provided a semi-quantitative measure of cytotoxicity.

As depicted in Table 16.1, optimal release of radioisotope required that the spleen cells and the virally infected fibroblasts share at least one set of H-2 proteins. In the table the infected fibroblasts were all from the C3H mouse strain that expresses H-2 proteins designated as H-2$^{k/k}$. Immune spleen cells from mice possessing at least one set of H-2^k proteins (CBA/H; CBA/H × C57Bl; AKR or C3H) lysed infected fibroblasts, resulting in the release of ^{51}Cr, while cells from strains lacking H-2$^{k/k}$ proteins failed to lyse the virally infected target cells (Zinkernagel and Doherty, 1974).

Zinkernagel and Doherty performed these experiments as postdoctoral fellows in the laboratory of Gordon Ada, chair of the Microbiology Department of the John Curtin School of Medical Research in Canberra, Australia. Ada (1922–2012) was trained at the Walter and Eliza Hall Institute in Melbourne with Sir MacFarlane Burnet. He received his DSc in 1959 and joined the John Curtin Medical School in 1968. As chair of the department, Ada cultivated an environment conducive to collaboration between immunologists and virologists interested in the immune response against infectious agents.

Rolf Zinkernagel received his medical education at the University of Basel in Switzerland. He studied for 2 years at the University of Lausanne, learning immunological techniques in infectious diseases, including methods for measuring the cytolytic activity of immune T lymphocytes against microbially infected cells.

TABLE 16.1   Cytotoxic Activity of LCM Immune Spleen Cells from Different Mouse Strains on Monolayers of LCM Infected or Normal (Noninfected) C3H Fibroblasts

			%[51]Cr release[a]	
Experiment	Mouse strain	H-2 type	Infected	Normal
1	CBA/H	k	65.1 ± 3.3	17.2 ± 0.7
	Balb/C	d	17.9 ± 0.9	17.2 ± 0.6
	C57B1	b	22.7 ± 1.4	19.8 ± 0.9
	CBA/H × C57B1	k/b	56.1 ± 0.5	16.7 ± 0.3
	C57B1 × Balb/C	b/d	24.8 ± 2.4	19.8 ± 0.9
	nu/+ or +/+		42.8 ± 2.0	21.9 ± 0.7
	nu/nu		23.3 ± 0.6	20.0 ± 1.4
2	CBA/H	k	85.5 ± 3.1	20.9 ± 1.2
	AKR	k	71.2 ± 1.6	18.6 ± 1.2
	DBA/2	d	24.5 ± 1.2	21.7 ± 1.7
3	CBA/H	k	77.9 ± 2.7	25.7 ± 1.3
	C3H/HeJ	k	77.8 ± 0.8	24.5 ± 1.5

LCM = lymphocytic choriomeningitis virus.

[a]%[51]Cr release by normal spleen cells on infected targets ranged from (experiment 1) 17.1 ± 0.3 to 20.0 ± 0.7; (experiment 2) 20.0 ± 1.4 to 25.3 ± 0.7; (experiment 3) 27.2 ± 2.0. From Zinkernagel and Doherty (1974).

He earned a PhD from the Australian National University in 1975. Peter Doherty was trained as a veterinarian in Australia before traveling to the University of Edinburgh for his PhD. He returned to Australia to assume a postdoctoral position at the University of Canberra and to collaborate on the work described. Based on these findings and subsequent expansion of the experimental system, Zinkernagel and Doherty shared the Nobel Prize in Physiology or Medicine in 1996 "for their discoveries concerning the specificity of the cell-mediated immune defence."

CORRELATION OF MHC GENE EXPRESSION WITH PATHOLOGY

Physicians observed anecdotally that many diseases occurred in greater frequency in families, suggesting that perhaps they were under some sort of genetic control. In 1953, Ian Aird and colleagues, working at the University of London, demonstrated a correlation between the ABO blood groups and gastric. Several similar observations were made during the next 15 years. However, the correlation proved weak, leading investigators to conclude that the genes coding for the blood groups did not provide a fine enough discrimination between healthy people and those with pathology.

Based on information about the role of histocompatibility genes in regulating immune responses, several investigators focused on the association between the expression of certain MHC proteins and the development of disease. In 1972, Hugh McDevitt and Walter

Bodmer at Stanford University School of Medicine published a review of the role of histocompatibility antigens in immune responsiveness and disease susceptibility in which they collated data suggesting "a statistical correlation between human histocompatibility antigens and certain forms of neoplastic and autoimmune diseases."

In 1973, two groups provided evidence that such an association occurred in individuals with the autoimmune, rheumatological disease, ankylosing spondylitis (AS). Maeve Caffrey and D.C.O. James with their colleagues (Brewerton et al., 1973; Caffrey and James, 1973), working at Westminster Hospital in London, used a lymphocytotoxicity assay to demonstrate that the lymphocytes from 48 of 50 patients with AS expressed HL-A 27, now named HLA-B27. Lee Scholsstein and colleagues at the University of California, Los Angeles, showed that peripheral blood cells from 35 of 40 patients with AS expressed the HLA-B27 protein. Between 4% and 8% of individuals without AS express this protein on their lymphocytes.

The original publications suggested two competing explanations for this association:

- close genetic linkage (linkage disequilibrium) of HLA-B27 with a gene involved in initiation of the disease, or
- an immunologic cross-reaction between the HLA-B27 antigen and the etiologic agent responsible for stimulating the autoimmune response.

At the time of these observations, the role of the HLA proteins in initiating adaptive immune responses had not yet been revealed. Once MHC compatibility between APCs and T lymphocytes was demonstrated, two additional possible hypotheses for the association of HLA-B27 with AS were presented:

- HLA-B27 presents a self-peptide to T lymphocytes (the arthritogenic peptide hypothesis); or
- abnormalities of the HLA-B27 molecules (dimerization, misfolding) induce inflammation, leading to the disease.

Numerous other associations between particular HLA genes and the development of pathology have been published. The relationship between the gene and disease is not absolute—not all patients who are diagnosed with a disease express the HLA molecule with which it has been associated, and not all individuals who express a particular HLA molecule are destined to develop the disease.

MOLECULAR STRUCTURE OF MHC-CODED PROTEINS

The structure of the proteins coded for by MHC genes provided clues to their function in the initiation of the adaptive immune response. Parallel studies with mouse and human proteins coded for by MHC genes were performed during the 1970s and 1980s. Peter Creswell and coworkers at Harvard demonstrated in 1973 that human class I histocompatibility proteins are composed of two chains, thus providing the initial step in this series of investigations that culminated in 1987 when Pamela Bjorkman and colleagues from Harvard published the three-dimensional structure of a human class I histocompatibility protein (Figure 16.1).

Creswell and coworkers stripped the surface HLA proteins from human lymphocytes and then radiolabeled these cells in vitro. Following a brief period of culture, these cells reexpressed the HLA proteins. The investigators treated the lymphocytes with the enzyme papain to solubilize the newly formed proteins that were subsequently purified by precipitation with specific antibodies to HLA and characterized by gel electrophoresis. Analysis of the resulting material showed the presence of two polypeptide chains: one with a molecular weight of approximately 11,000 Da and the other with a molecular weight of about 31,000 Da.

Howard Grey and colleagues at Harvard identified the smaller molecular weight peptide in 1973. Patients with renal tubular disease present with proteinuria due to the presence in the urine of an 11,700 Da polypeptide. This polypeptide, known as β2-microglobulin, is also expressed on human lymphocytes. Grey and coworkers posed the following question: Was the 11,000 Da peptide found in HLA proteins stripped from human lymphocytes related to β2-microglobulin?

Investigators radiolabeled human lymphocytes with ^{125}I or with ^3H amino acids, lysed these cells, and subjected them to immunoprecipitation with an antibody to β2-microglobulin. Characterization of the radioactive precipitates showed that virtually all of the cell-associated β2-microglobulin was bound to another larger polypeptide related to histocompatibility proteins. Based on these studies, the authors conclude "that the small subunits of HL-A antigens and β2-microglobulin are identical, or so closely related that they cannot be distinguished by immunological means" (Grey et al., 1973).

Subsequent studies demonstrated that the larger α-chain is coded by MHC genes. By 1987, when Bjorkman and her colleagues published their structure of the HLA class I proteins, several additional characteristics of these molecules had been identified:

- class I HLA proteins are expressed by virtually all somatic cells,
- several MHC gene loci code for α-chains of these proteins,
- any individual expresses several forms of these proteins coded by individual alleles,
- class I HLA proteins present viral and other antigens to CD^{8+} T lymphocytes, and
- the α-chain is composed of three domains, two of which (α1 and α2) are heterogeneous in amino acid sequence.

Bjorkman and her colleagues succeeded in crystallizing a human histocompatibility protein that was then subjected to X-ray crystallography. This provided a three-dimensional view in sufficient detail (Figure 16.2) to decipher the function of the molecule in presenting antigenic peptides. The structure of the class I HLA protein indicates that the two heterogeneous domains of the α chain are involved in forming a cleft that binds antigenic peptides for presentation to T lymphocytes.

Much of this work was performed in the laboratory of Jack Strominger (1925 to present) at Harvard. Strominger, educated at Harvard, received his MD from Yale. His academic career took him from the National Institutes of Health in Bethesda, Maryland, to Washington University in St. Louis, Missouri, and the University of Wisconsin before becoming a faculty member at Harvard. Strominger started his career investigating the mechanism by which penicillin interferes with bacteria cell wall synthesis. When he arrived at Harvard he changed direction and began working on the structural differences that account for HLA heterogeneity.

Strominger collaborated on many of his studies with Don Wiley (1944–2001), a virologist and structural biologist at Harvard. Wiley received his undergraduate training at Tufts University in Boston. After earning a PhD in

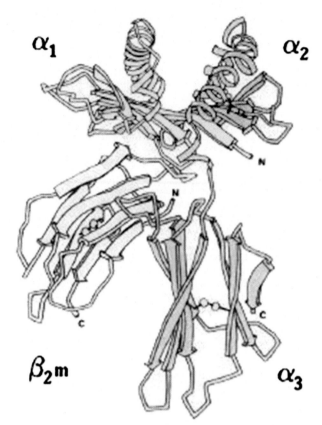

FIGURE 16.2 Three-dimensional structure of a human class I MHC molecule as revealed by X-ray crystallography. The three domains of the α-chain coded by the MHC gene are labeled, as is the β₂-microglobulin. The groove formed by the amino acids in the α_1 and α_2 domains constitutes the antigen binding site of the molecule. *From Bjorkman et al. (1987).*

biophysics from Harvard, he was appointed as a faculty member there. His early work involved determining the structure and related function of biologically important molecules, including the influenza hemagglutinin molecule. On November 15, 2001, Wiley disappeared while attending a meeting of the St Jude Children's Hospital Advisory Board in Memphis, Tennessee. His rental car was found on a bridge over the Mississippi River, and his body was recovered two months later several hundred miles downstream. His death was ruled an accident although at the time (before the body was recovered) there was some speculation that he may have been abducted by terrorists due to his expertise with several viruses that potentially could be used as bioweapons (Davis, 2014).

The structure of class II HLA proteins proved to be somewhat more difficult to determine, but by 1993, a three-dimensional view of one such molecule, HLA-DR1, was published (Brown et al., 1993). Once again this work was performed in the labs of Jack Strominger and Don Wiley. Class II HLA molecules are cell surface glycoproteins expressed on APCs, including macrophages, B lymphocytes, and dendritic cells. Class II

MHC molecules are heterodimers, consisting of one α and one β chain, both of which are coded for by genes in the MHC region on human chromosome 6. As with class I molecules, crystals were grown from the HLA-DR1 protein and subjected to X-ray crystallography. The picture obtained indicates that portions of both α and β chains are involved in binding antigenic peptides that are subsequently presented to T lymphocytes.

CONCLUSION

In the early 1900s, investigators described the rejection or acceptance of transplants of spontaneously arising tumors between individual experimental animals. These studies led eventually to the discovery of cell surface proteins that identified individuals of a species and that were involved in transplant rejection. The investigation of rejection of transplants of normal tissues and organs added credence to the existence of such histocompatibility proteins. However, the physiological function of these proteins emerged during the second half of the twentieth century. Studies during the 1960s and 1970s, demonstrated that several phenomena of the adaptive immune response are controlled by a genetic locus closely linked, or identical, to the locus coding for the proteins regulating tumor and tissue graft acceptance or rejection. The seminal studies of Peter Doherty and Rolf Zinkernagel, using T lymphocyte-mediated cytotoxicity of virally infected fibroblasts, recognized the requirement for the identity of genes at the MHC for several cellular reactions.

Proteins coded for by MHC genes are required for

- recognition of pathogens by T lymphocytes (Chapter 20);
- interaction of T lymphocytes with B lymphocytes in the initiation of optimal antibody synthesis and secretion (Chapters 13 and 19);
- maturation of T lymphocytes in the thymus (Chapter 22); and
- regulation of T lymphocyte-mediated effectors by T helper lymphocytes (Chapters 24 and 27).

In addition some of the complement components (Chapter 12) as well as some cytokines (Chapter 25) are coded for by genes in the MHC.

References

Aird, I., Bentall, H.M., Roberts, J.A.F., 1953. A relationship between cancer of stomach and the ABO blood groups. Brit. Med. J. I (#4814), 799–801.
Aisenberg, A.C., 1970. Allogeneic thymus grafts and the restoration of immune function in irradiated thymectomized mice. J. Exp. Med. 131, 275–286.

Benacceraf, B., McDevitt, H.O., 1972. Histocompatibility immune response genes. Science 175, 273–279.

Billingham, R.E., 1963. Transplantation: past, present and future. J. Invest. Derm. 41, 165–180.

Bjorkman, P.J., Saper, M.A., Samraoui, B., Bennett, W.S., Strominger, J.L., Wiley, D.C., 1987. Structure of the human class I histocompatibility antigen, HLA-A2. Nature 329, 506–512.

Brewerton, D.A., Cafrey, M., Hart, F.D., James, D.C.O., Nichols, A., Sturrock, R.D., 1973. Ankylosing spondylitis and HL-A 27. Lancet 301, 904–907.

Brown, J.H., Jardetzky, T.S., Gorga, J.C., Stern, L.J., Urban, R.G., Strominger, J.L., Wiley, D.C., 1993. Three-dimensional structure of the human class II histocompatibility antigen HLA-DR1. Nature 364, 33–39.

Caffrey, M.F.P., James, D.C.O., 1973. Human lymphocyte antigen association in ankylosing spondylitis. Nature 242, 121.

Cline, M.J., Swett, V.C., 1968. The interaction of human monocytes and lymphocytes. J. Exp. Med. 128, 1309–1325.

Creswell, P., Turner, M.J., Strominger, J.L., 1973. Papain solubilized HL-A antigens from cultured human lymphocytes contain two peptide fragments. Proc. Nat. Acad. Sci. U. S. A. 70, 1603–1607.

Dausset, J., 1958. Iso-leuco-anticorps. Acta Haematol. 20, 156–166.

Davis, D.M., 2014. The Compatibility Gene – How Our Bodies Fight Disease, Attract Others and Define Ourselves. Oxford University Press, USA.

Gorer, P., 1936a. The detection of hereditary genetic difference in the blood of mice by means of human blood group A serum. J. Genet. 32, 17–31.

Gorer, P., 1936b. The detection of antigenic differences in mouse erythrocytes by the employment of immune sera. Brit. J. Exp. Pathol. 17, 42–50.

Gorer, P., 1937. The genetic and antigenic basis of tumor transplantation. J. Pathol. Bacteriol. 44, 691–697.

Gorer, P., Lyman, S., Snell, G.D., 1948. Studies on the genetic and antigenic basis of tumor transplantation. Linkage between a histocompatibility gene and "fused" in mice. Proc. Roy. Soc. Lond. B Biol. Sci. 135, 499–505.

Grey, H.M., Kubo, R.T., Colon, S.M., Poulik, M.D., Cresswell, P., Springer, T., Turner, M., Strominger, J.L., 1973. The small subunit of HL-A antigens is β2-microglobulin. J. Exp. Med. 138, 1608–1612.

Kindred, B., Schreffler, D.C., 1972. H-2 dependence of co-operation between T and B cells in vivo. J. Immunol. 109, 940–943.

Leuchars, E., Cross, A.M., Dukor, P., 1965. The restoration of immunological function by thymus grafting in thymectomized irradiated mice. Transplantation 3, 28–35.

Levine, B.B., Ojeda, A., Benacceraf, B., 1963. Studies on artificial antigens. III. The genetic control of the immune response to hapten poly-L-lysine conjugates in guinea pigs. J. Exp. Med. 118, 953–957.

Little, C.C., 1914. A possible Mendelian explanation for a type of inheritance apparently non-Mendelian in nature. Science 40, 904–906.

Little, C.C., Tyzzer, E.E., 1916. Further experimental studies on the inheritance of susceptibility to a transplantable tumor, carcinoma (J.W.A.) of the Japanese waltzing mouse. J. Med. Res. 33, 393–453.

McDevitt, H.O., Bodmer, W.F., 1972. Histocompatibility antigens, immune responsiveness and susceptibility to disease. Am. J. Med. 52, 1–8.

Medawar, P.B., 1958. The croonian lecture. The homograft reaction. Proc. Roy. Soc. Lond. B 149, 145–166.

Mosier, D.E., 1967. A requirement for two cell types for antibody formation in vitro. Science 158, 1573–1575.

Payne, R., Rolfs, M.R., 1958. Fetomaternal leukocyte incompatibility. J. Clin. Invest. 37, 1756–1762.

Rosenthal, A.S., Shevach, E.M., 1973. Function of macrophages in antigen recognition by guinea pig T lymphocytes. I. Requirement for histocompatible macrophages and lymphocytes. J. Exp. Med. 138, 1194–1212.

Scholsstein, L., Teresaki, P.I., Bluestone, R., Pearson, C.M., 1973. High association of an HL-A antigen, W27, with ankylosing spondylitis. New. Eng. J. Med. 288, 704–706.

Shevach, E.M., Paul, W.E., Green, I., 1972. Histocompatibility-linked immune response gene function in guinea pigs. Specific inhibition of antigen-induced lymphocyte proliferation by alloantiserum. J. Exp. Med. 136, 1207–1221.

Shevach, E.M., Rosenthal, A.S., 1973. Function of macrophages in antigen recognition by guinea pig T lymphocytes. II. Role of the macrophage in the regulation of genetic control of the immune response. J. Exp. Med. 138, 1213–1229.

Snell, G.D., 1948. Methods for the study of histocompatibility genes. J. Genet. 49, 87–103.

Tyzzer, E.E., 1909. A study of inheritance in mice with reference to their susceptibility to transplantable tumors. J. Med. Res. 21, 519–573.

Tyzzer, E.E., Little, C.C., 1916. Studies on the inheritance of susceptibility to a transplantable sarcoma (J.w.B.) of Japanese waltzing mice. J. Cancer Res. 1, 387–389.

van Rood, J.J., Eernisse, J.G., van Leeuwen, A., 1958. Leucocyte antibodies in sera from pregnant women. Nature 181, 1735–1736.

Zinkernagel, R.M., Doherty, P.C., 1974. Restriction of in vitro T cell-mediated cytotoxicity in lymphocytic choriomeningitis within a syngeneic or semiallogeneic system. Nature 248, 701–702.

TIME LINE

1902	C.O. Jensen describes the resistance of mice to the transfer of tumors
1909	Ernest Tyzzer demonstrates that resistance to tumor transfers is genetic
1916	Clarence C. Little and Ernest Tyzzer estimate that about 12 genes are responsible for determining resistance or susceptibility to tumor transfers
1936	Peter Gorer reports antigenic difference on cells of different mouse strains
1937	Peter Gorer demonstrates a role for antigen II in rejection of tumors
1948	Peter Gorer and George D. Snell show that antigen coded for by the H-2 genes serves as a target for graft rejection
1958	Peter Medawar demonstrates that graft rejection is an immunological phenomenon
1958	Jean Dausset identifies the human MHC locus
1963	Baruj Benacceraf and colleagues report the genetic control of immune responses in the guinea pig
1972	Ethan Shevach and coworkers report that immune response genes (MHC) code for a cell surface molecule that is involved in antigen recognition by T lymphocytes
1973	D.A. Brewerton and colleagues and Lee Schlosstein and coworkers report an association between expression of HLA-B27 and ankylosing spondylitis

1974	Rolf Zinkernagel and Peter Doherty demonstrate that cytotoxic T lymphocytes killing of virally infected cells requires MHC compatibility	1987	Pamela Bjorkman and coworkers publish the three-dimensional structure of a human class I HLA molecule
1980	George Snell, Jean Dausset, and Baruj Benacceraf awarded the Nobel Prize in Physiology or Medicine "for their discoveries concerning genetically determined structures on the cell surface that regulate immunological reactions"	1993	Jerry H. Brown and colleagues decipher the three-dimensional structure of a human class I HLA molecule
		1996	Peter Doherty and Rolf Zinkernagel awarded the Nobel Prize in Physiology or Medicine

17

Interaction of Lymphocytes with Antigen: Identification of Antigen-Specific Receptors

INTRODUCTION

In 1957 F. Macfarlane Burnet presented the clonal selection theory of antibody formation (Chapter 6), postulating that antigen selects potential antibody-forming cells (lymphocytes) and activates those lymphocytes to synthesize and secrete specific antibody. Several predictions derive from this theory:

- lymphocytes capable of responding to a particular antigen exist prior to exposure to antigen,
- each lymphocyte is precommitted to respond to a single antigen,
- these precommitted lymphocytes possess a mechanism by which they recognize the particular antigen to which they will respond, and
- interaction of lymphocytes with the appropriate antigen results in cell activation and subsequent synthesis of antibody.

By contrast, instruction models of antibody formation hypothesized that antigen bound to a naturally occurring serum protein (globulin) either in the peripheral circulation or once the antigen had been phagocytized by cells of the reticuloendothelial system (i.e., macrophages and endothelial cells). Following phagocytosis, the antigen–globulin complex altered the configuration of the globulin and served as a template for the production of additional globulin molecules with the same binding capacity. The configuration of the binding site would be imposed on the molecule by the antigen, and this configuration would be incorporated into the synthesis mechanism of the cell.

The clonal selection theory postulates that lymphocytes are committed to produce one particular antibody prior to exposure to any antigen. These lymphocytes are activated when they interact with antigen for which they are specific. This specificity suggests that antigen-reactive lymphocytes express cell-surface receptors unique for the antigen to which they can respond. Antibodies possess immunological specificity and were a logical candidate for these cell-surface receptors.

At the time the clonal selection theory was proposed, researchers focused on antibody synthesis. Investigators in the 1950s and 1960s identified a second type of adaptive immune response, cell-mediated responses, that do not require antibodies. In addition, immunologists categorized immunocompetent lymphocytes into two functional populations: B and T lymphocytes, both of which are specific for unique antigens. This division

A Historical Perspective on Evidence-Based Immunology
http://dx.doi.org/10.1016/B978-0-12-398381-7.00017-4

required that antigen-specific receptors be identified for both types of lymphocytes. Immunologists initially predicted that both B and T lymphocytes would use the same molecule as their receptor; however, subsequent studies demonstrated that each lymphocyte population expresses structurally distinctive cell-surface receptors. In addition, B and T lymphocytes differ in the antigenic configurations they recognize. B lymphocytes distinguish antigens, which can be proteins, carbohydrates, lipids, or nucleic acids, based on structural conformation. T lymphocytes recognize peptides prepared from proteins and bind a linear sequence of amino acids.

Studies summarized in this chapter show that immunoglobulin serves as the receptor on antigen-reactive B lymphocytes while T lymphocytes express a unique receptor that recognizes antigens presented by cells bearing molecules coded for by genes in the major histocompatibility complex (MHC).

DISCOVERY OF THE B CELL RECEPTOR

The receptor on B lymphocytes that binds antigen is a membrane-associated immunoglobulin (mIg) that is called the B cell receptor (BCR). Early in the history of immunology, Paul Ehrlich (1900) predicted that antibody-forming cells expressed side chains to which antigen bound (Figure 17.1). This binding resulted in the shedding of the antibody–antigen complex and stimulated the cell to produce more molecules identical to the one that originally interacted with the antigen. In this proposal the antibody-forming cell possessed numerous receptors or side chains capable of binding to a variety of antigens. Ehrlich's side chain hypothesis fell out of favor with most immunologists when Karl Landsteiner and others demonstrated the large number of different antibody specificities to both natural and synthetic molecules the system could produce (Chapter 2). It was only in the 1960s that studies resurrected the idea that antibody-forming lymphocytes possess cell-surface molecules that bind antigen.

Methods Used to Detect mIg

Investigators designed two experimental models to demonstrate the presence of mIg on the surface of antigen-reactive cells: direct methods that involve visualizing cell-surface molecules and indirect methods that are based on the inhibition of cellular function by antibodies against cell-surface molecules. In 1961, Göran Möller, at the Karolinska Institute Medical School, Stockholm, Sweden, provided the first indication that antibody-forming lymphocytes possess immunoglobulin on their surface.

Möller sought optimal conditions for the detection of strain-specific antigens on the surface of cells from inbred mouse strains using the recently developed fluorescent antibody technique. He injected mice of strain A with tumor cells or lymphocytes from strain B to produce strain-specific antibodies. Strain A serum was mixed with strain B lymphocytes following which a fluorescein labeled rabbit antibody to mouse immunoglobulin was added. Staining was visualized by fluorescence microscopy. As a control, Möller added the fluorescein labeled rabbit antibody to untreated mouse lymphocytes with the expectation that no staining would occur. To his surprise, this process identified a small but reproducible number of lymphocytes from lymph nodes and bone marrow that apparently stained nonspecifically with rabbit antibody to mouse immunoglobulin. Further study ruled out the possibility that the staining observed in the control experiment was due to passively adsorbed serum immunoglobulin. Staining was not present in hematopoietic cells derived from fetal liver, and the level of staining increased in mice as they matured from birth to adult. Möller suggested that this nonspecific staining might be detecting cells involved in antibody production.

In 1965, Stewart Sell and P.G.H. Gell, working at the University of Birmingham Medical School in Birmingham, England, confirmed the presence of immunoglobulin on lymphocytes by measuring the induction of lymphocyte proliferation. These investigators hypothesized that interaction of lymphocyte surface receptors with their ligands would induce lymphocyte proliferation. While this phenomenon could theoretically be studied using antigen, the probability of obtaining a positive result was low since only a few cells would be activated. To enhance the detection of activated cells, Sell and Gell performed these experiments using antibodies against immunoglobulin. They predicted that such antibodies would induce proliferation in a large percentage of antigen-reactive lymphocytes.

Sell and Gell cultured rabbit peripheral blood lymphocytes with rabbit antibodies specific for allotypic markers on immunoglobulins. Allotypes are genetically determined differences in immunoglobulin molecules inherited according to Mendelian genetics. Antibodies to allotypes are produced in an animal lacking the allotype. For example, immunoglobulin from a rabbit of allotype A injected into a rabbit of allotype B will result in the production of antibodies to the antigenic determinants on the A immunoglobulin molecule.

Treatment of cells derived from a rabbit of allotype A with antibodies to allotype A induced activation of a significant number of lymphocytes and resulted in the initiation of DNA synthesis, as measured by the incorporation of ^{3}H-thymidine, and mitosis. Since this reaction was similar to that observed with other activators such as specific antigen and antibodies directed against lymphocytes, the investigators concluded that the antibodies specific for allotypes reacted with allotype containing immunoglobulin molecules on the surface of the lymphocytes to induce activation.

In 1970 Martin Raff and his coworkers, at the National Institute for Medical Research, London, used rabbit antibodies specific for mouse IgM labeled with fluorescein or with ^{125}I to detect the presence of immunoglobulins on the surface of lymphocytes. Raff and colleagues treated cell suspensions prepared from mouse spleen, lymph node, thoracic duct lymph, thymus, or bone marrow with labeled antibodies and the number of labeled cells was counted. Results presented in Table 17.1 show that a proportion of lymphocytes from all the organs tested, with the exception of the thymus, stained with the antibody to IgM. Control experiments suggested that the cells expressing the surface immunoglobulin most likely synthesized these molecules as opposed to absorbing them passively from serum.

Joseph Davie and William Paul (1971), working at the National Institute of Allergy and Infectious Diseases in Bethesda, Maryland, combined direct and indirect methods to further identify the molecules on lymphocytes that bind antigen. Lymphocytes from guinea pigs injected with dinitrophenylated-guinea pig albumin (DNP-GPA) were incubated with radiolabelled DNP. Davie and Paul identified and quantified lymphocytes that bound radiolabeled DNP. The number of antigen-binding lymphocytes from unimmunized animals initially was low but increased with immunization. Competition experiments in which the lymphocytes were first incubated with unlabeled DNP prior to the addition of radiolabeled DNP showed that the binding was antigen-specific, that is, the unlabeled antigen blocked binding of the labeled reagent.

Subsequent studies showed that the antigen (DNP) bound to immunoglobulin molecules on the cell surface. Lymphocytes were treated first with a fluoresceinated antibody to immunoglobulin followed by incubation with radiolabeled DNP. All antigen-binding lymphocytes also bound the antibody to immunoglobulin. Reversing the order of treatment, that is, incubating guinea pig lymphocytes with antibody to immunoglobulin prior to incubation with DNP, resulted in inhibition of antigen

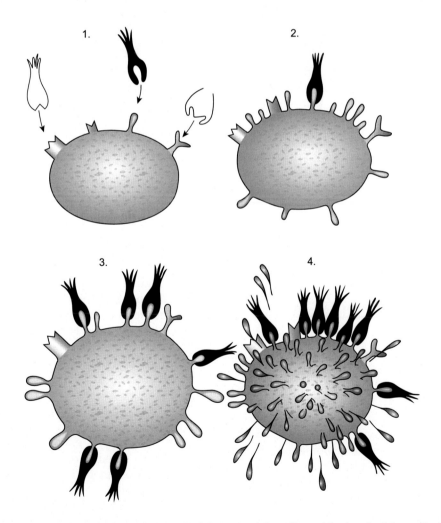

FIGURE 17.1 Ehrlich's side chain theory of antibody formation. Ehrlich proposed that cells capable of synthesizing antibodies possessed on their surface a number of different receptors, each of which could recognize a different antigen. Antigen would bind to one of these receptors and cause it to dissociate from the cell. This process in turn would result in the synthesis of additional antibody of the same specificity. *From Ehrlich (1900).*

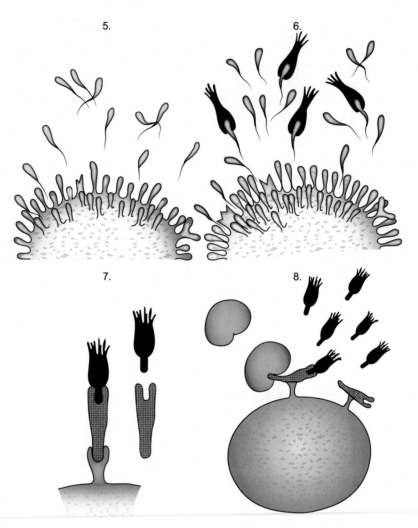

FIGURE 17.1 Continued.

binding. These results allowed Davie and Paul to conclude that the receptors on antigen-binding lymphocytes are, in fact, immunoglobulin in nature.

Immunoglobulin-Bearing Cells Are B Lymphocytes

By the early 1970s, the conclusion that lymphocytes interact with antigens using a membrane-associated immunoglobulin (mIg) had been confirmed in several species, including humans, mice, rabbits, chickens, rats, guinea pigs, and sheep. At the same time, functionally distinct populations of lymphocytes, B and T, had been characterized based on their developmental history. B and T lymphocytes could not be physically separated, leading to the question of which population possesses mIg. Two possibilities existed:

1. mIg is expressed only on B lymphocytes responsible for synthesizing antibodies, or

2. mIg is expressed on both B and T lymphocytes and used as a common antigen receptor.

Individuals with congenital immunodeficiencies and animal models of these diseases provided circumstantial evidence for a correlation between mIg-bearing cells and antibody-producing lymphocytes. For example, patients with X-linked agammaglobulinemia have decreased serum antibody levels and a greatly reduced number of lymphocytes in their peripheral lymphoid tissue that express mIg (Gray et al., 1971; Cooper and Lawton, 1972). Conversely, patients with deficient T lymphocyte function (i.e., thymic aplasia) have elevated numbers of peripheral blood lymphocytes expressing mIg, even though these individuals failed to demonstrate detectable elevation of serum immunoglobulin (Gajl-Peczalska et al., 1973).

Studies with experimental animals produced similar findings. Chickens surgically bursectomized and irradiated, or treated with antibodies to IgM and then bursectomized, had low serum antibody levels combined with

TABLE 17.1   Percentage of Cells Binding Immunoglobulin in Various Organs of Normal Mice. Lymphocytes Isolated from the Indicated Organs Were Incubated with Anti-Immunoglobulin Labeled Either with Fluorescein or a Radioactive Marker. Immunoglobulin-Bearing Cells Are Found in Every Organ Tested Except in the Thymus

Experiment no.	Spleen	Lymph node	Thoracic duct	Thymus	Bone marrow
A. Autoradiography					
1	41	17	14	0.31	15
2	36	–	–	–	–
3	43	16	–	0.14	–
4	44	18	–	0.21	–
Mean	41	17	14	0.22	15
B. Fluorescence					
1	38	13		0	
2	40	–		–	
3	39	13		–	
*4	36	23		0	
*5	–	16		–	
*6	33	22		0	
*7	–	15		–	
Mean	35	19		0	

*Experiments performed with BALB/c mice; all other experiments used CBA mice.
From Raff et al. (1970).

virtually no lymphocytes expressing mIg in their spleen or peripheral blood (Rabellino and Gray, 1971; Kincade et al., 1971).

Identity of the Isotype of mIg on B Lymphocytes

By the early 1970s, evidence that lymphocytes use cell-surface immunoglobulin to bind antigen included

- treatment of lymphocytes with antibody to immunoglobulin induces blast transformation,
- antibodies to light chains or to whole immunoglobulin inhibit antigen binding by lymphocytes, and
- antibodies specific for allotypic determinants bind lymphocytes.

These studies failed to identify the immunoglobulin isotype (class) of mIg. Five structurally different isotypes of immunoglobulin exist: IgG, IgA, IgM, IgD, and IgE. Several investigators initially concluded that the mIg on B lymphocytes was either IgM or IgG (Warner, 1974). Immunologists now agree that the mIg on naïve B lymphocytes consists of monomeric IgM and IgD.

The identification of monomeric IgM as the B lymphocyte receptor was demonstrated by Ellen Vitetta and her colleagues, working at the University of Texas Southwestern Medical School, Dallas. Vitetta et al. (1971)

labeled the surface of mouse splenic lymphocytes with radioactive iodine. They subsequently fractionated these lymphocytes into populations of large and small lymphocytes and isolated the mIg associated with each population. The radiolabelled immunoglobulin was reduced and alkylated and the heavy and light chains separated by electrophoresis. Results demonstrated that "95% of the radioactivity of the H chain from the small lymphocyte fraction and 90% from the large lymphocyte-plasma cell fraction were identified as μ by antigenicity and by molecular weight" (μ is the designation given to the IgM heavy chain).

David Rowe and his colleagues, working at the World Health Organization and the Basel Institute for Immunology in Switzerland identified IgD as a B lymphocyte-specific antigen receptor in 1973 using an experimental design that capitalized on the movement of cell-surface molecules in the plasma membrane. Rowe and coworkers treated human lymphocytes with antibodies specific for IgM labeled with fluorescein (a green emitting reagent) or antibodies specific for IgD labeled with rhodamine (a red emitting reagent). Antibody treatment of the cells occurred at either 37 °C or 4 °C. Treatment of lymphocytes with antibodies at 37 °C (capping conditions) causes movement of the membrane-associated molecules to one pole of the cell, resulting in the appearance of a "cap" containing the molecules and the fluorescent antibody. Conversely, treatment of lymphocytes at 4 °C (noncapping conditions) results in limited movement of the membrane-associated molecules and a cell that is stained uniformly around its entire circumference.

Treatment of peripheral blood lymphocytes with antibodies to IgM at 37 °C followed by treatment with antibodies to IgD at 4 °C resulted in a staining pattern in which IgM localized to a cap while IgD stained the entire cell surface. The investigators concluded that most B lymphocytes simultaneously express both isotypes. Similar results were presented in the mouse model (Melchers et al., 1974) using radiolabelled rather than fluorescein labeled antibodies.

Shortly after the discovery that B lymphocytes express both IgM and IgD, investigators questioned whether the two isotypes shared antigen-binding specificity. Although it was logical that the two mIgs on any one lymphocyte would bind the same antigen (based on the data supporting one cell: one antibody—Chapter 7), no information was available about the genetic mechanisms involved in coding for the large number of different antibody specificities. Some immunologists speculated that antibodies of different specificities were coded for by separate genes. If true, then how could a lymphocyte produce two different molecules (IgM and IgD), each binding the same antigen?

Investigators used two experimental approaches to address this question. In 1974 F. Salsano and colleagues, at the Institute of Immunology and Rheumatology of the Rikshospitalet in Oslo, Norway, reported that the IgM and IgD mIg on human lymphocytic leukemia cells have identical idiotypes. Immunoglobulin idiotypes refer to the unique antigen on immunoglobulin molecules formed by the amino acid sequence in and around the antigen-binding site of that immunoglobulin. Thus two antibodies that have identical idiotypes are thought to share antigen-binding sites. Shu Man Fu working in Henry Kunkel's laboratory at Rockefeller University in New York confirmed this observation in early 1975.

Patients with lymphocytic leukemia often present with a large amount of monoclonal immunoglobulin in their serum. In the patients studied by these two groups the monoclonal antibody was of the IgM class. Rabbits injected with this IgM produced antibodies specific for the idiotype of the IgM. These idiotypic antibodies reacted not only with the serum IgM but with both IgM and IgD expressed by the leukemic lymphocytes.

James Goding and Judith Layton provided independent evidence that the IgM and IgD receptors on B lymphocytes share antigenic specificity. Working at the Walter and Eliza Hall Institute of Medical Research in Melbourne, Australia in 1976, they compared the results when they capped mIg on mouse B lymphocytes with antibodies to IgM or IgD or with antigen. Using fluoresceinated antibodies specific for either IgM or IgD they demonstrated that the two mIgs on individual lymphocytes capped independently; this indicates that the antigenic determinants detected by the antibodies to IgM and IgD are on separate molecules. To determine if both IgM and IgD mIg have the same antigenic specificity, they injected mice with the hapten-carrier complex NIP-POL (4-hydroxyl-3-iodo-5-nitrophenylacetic acid conjugated to polymerized bacterial flagellin). Injected mice produced antibodies specific for NIP. Spleen cells from the injected mice were isolated by incubating them on plates of NIP-gelatin. When the temperature was elevated, the gelatin liquefied and the NIP-specific lymphocytes were harvested. Incubating these lymphocytes with NIP-POL at 37 °C led to the formation of a cap on the lymphocytes. When these lymphocytes were subsequently stained with fluoresceinated antibodies to IgM or IgD, all the fluorescence appeared in the caps. The authors conclude "that the two heavy chains on individual lymphocytes possess similar or identical antigen-combining sites."

Accessory Molecules of the BCR

Antigen selects B lymphocytes by virtue of the mIg (BCR) expressed on the lymphocyte surface. Once selected, the antigen cross-links the BCR, activating the lymphocyte and resulting in gene transcription, proliferation and antibody synthesis, and secretion. The molecular requirements for these actions include the receptor initiating a series of intracellular enzymatic reactions. The amino acid sequence of the BCR revealed relatively few intracellular amino acids insufficient to transduce signals to second messengers in the cytoplasm. Kerry Campbell and John Cambier (1990) at the University of Colorado Health Science Center searched for other molecules that might be associated with the BCR that might assist in transduction of the signal.

Many proteins responsible for signal transduction are phosphorylated. Campbell and Cambier hypothesized that B lymphocytes use a similar strategy. They tested this hypothesis by labeling B lymphocytes with [^{32}P] ATP. Campbell and Cambier lysing the lymphocytes and precipitating the immunoglobulin with antibodies. Analysis of the precipitate revealed the presence of three radiolabeled phospho-proteins that the investigators termed Ig-α, Ig-β, and Ig-γ. Isolation of the three chains, analysis of partial amino acid sequence, and relationship to known gene products expressed in B lymphocytes revealed that Ig-α is the product of the *mb*-1 gene while Ig-β and Ig-γ are products of the B29 gene (Campbell et al., 1991). These two genes are expressed early in the maturation of B lymphocytes. Further study demonstrated that the chain called Ig-γ is actually a truncated version of the Ig-β chain (Friedrich et al., 1993).

Monoclonal antibodies against the Ig-α and Ig-β chains were submitted to the Fifth Workshop on Leukocyte Differentiation Antigens in 1993 (IUIS/WHO, 1994). As a result, a cluster of differentiation (CD) designation was given to these accessory molecules: Ig-α is termed CD79a while Ig-β is CD79b.

Based on the data, a model in which surface IgM molecules are associated with one or more Ig-α chain and one or more Ig-β chains has been proposed. Transmission of signals initiated by the binding of antigen requires the activation of these two accessory molecules that initiate the sequence of intracellular signaling, leading to B lymphocyte activation.

DISCOVERY OF THE T CELL RECEPTOR

The receptor on T lymphocytes that binds antigen is composed of two polypeptide chains and is called the T cell receptor (TCR). The molecular identity of the TCR remained a mystery until 1982. Even though T lymphocytes interact with antigen and have the same degree of specificity as B lymphocytes, virtually nothing was known about the biochemical nature of their receptor molecules. Prior to identification of the structure of the TCR, several immunologists erroneously reported that thymocytes and thymus-derived lymphocytes expressed immunoglobulin molecules on their surface (Bankhurst et al., 1971; Lesley et al., 1971; Marchalonis et al., 1972).

Isolation of Glycoproteins from T Lymphocyte Clones and Lymphomas

B lymphocytes secrete antibodies, the molecular structure of which was described in the 1950s and early 1960s (Chapter 11). T lymphocytes do not secrete antigen-specific molecules. Thus when researchers started looking for the TCR they had no readily available molecule on which to base their search. However, tumor lines and clones derived from T lymphocytes were available, and several research groups hypothesized that these might possess antigen-specific receptors. The general approach was to develop antibodies specific for these cell lines and use the antibodies to isolate cell-surface molecules. Three research groups (Allison et al., 1982; Meuer et al., 1983; Haskins et al., 1983) used this approach and were successful in isolating glycoproteins from the tumors or T lymphocyte clones that were likely candidates for the TCR.

James Allison's group from the University of Texas System Cancer Center, Smithville, injected one inbred strain of mice (BALB/c) with a radiation-induced lymphoma from a second inbred strain (C57Bl). They used the spleen from injected BALB/c mice and developed hybridomas secreting monoclonal antibodies specific for the C57Bl lymphoma. The investigators postulated that the C57Bl lymphoma was derived from a single clone of T lymphocytes and, therefore, might express a unique cell-surface antigen. This unique molecule would represent the antigen-specific receptor on T lymphocytes that could be detected by antibody. Most antibodies from the resulting hybridomas bound to antigens found on the majority of lymphocytes from both fetal and adult mice. However, one of the monoclonal antibodies bound only to the C57Bl lymphoma cells used for the original injection. This antibody failed to bind adult lymphocytes from thymus, spleen, lymph nodes or bone marrow, or fetal lymphocytes from spleen or thymus. The antibody was also specific for the C57Bl lymphoma; it did not bind to other lymphomas.

Allison and colleagues isolated a glycoprotein from the surface of the lymphoma using the monoclonal antibody. The isolated glycoprotein contained two subunits with molecular weights of 39,000 and 41,000 daltons. A cell-surface glycoprotein of similar molecular structure was isolated from T lymphocytes but not from B lymphocytes. The authors conclude "that the apparently individually specific lymphoma antigen reactive with (monoclonal antibody 124-40) might be a clonally expressed epitope carried by a T cell surface component." While the paper published in the *Journal of Immunology* speculated briefly that the molecule identified in these studies might be the TCR, Lanier (2005) in an introduction to this paper in the Pillars of Immunology series in the *Journal of Immunology* recalls Allison identifying the molecule as the TCR during a poster presentation at the Keystone Symposium on B and T Cell Tumors: Biological and Clinical Aspects held in March of 1982.

Other investigators produced similar monoclonal antibodies that blocked antigen binding to T lymphocytes (Haskins et al., 1983) or interfered with the function of T lymphocytes (Meuer et al., 1983). Kathryn Haskins and her colleagues, at the University of Colorado Health Sciences Center, Denver, developed a hybridoma using lymphocytes from a mouse injected with a T lymphocyte clone specific for a peptide fragment of chicken ovalbumin. The monoclonal antibody secreted by this hybridoma bound to the T lymphocyte clone used for the original injections but not to other T lymphocyte clones and blocked the recognition of ovalbumin by the T lymphocytes.

Stefan Meuer working at the Sidney Farber Cancer Institute and Harvard Medical School in Boston, Massachusetts developed an antibody against a human cytotoxic T lymphocyte clone. The antibody blocked the effector function of this clone as well as antigen-induced proliferation. The antibody was used to isolate a cell-surface glycoprotein from the cytotoxic T lymphocyte clone that was composed of two polypeptide chains similar to the structure reported by Allison's group. Based on these structural studies, the two chains of the TCR were termed α and β.

Isolation of Genes Coding for the TCR

Early in 1984 two groups of investigators working independently reported the isolation of the genes coding for one of the chains of the TCR in humans (Yanagi et al., 1984) and in mice (Hedrick et al., 1984). The approach of both of these groups (Tak Mak's group at the University of Toronto and Mark Davis' group at Stanford University School of Medicine) was to clone DNA complementary to lymphocyte mRNA, isolate those clones that were specific for T lymphocytes, and deduce the proteins that could be coded. The gene isolated by this procedure codes for a protein of between 35,000 and 40,000 Da, the approximate molecular weight of the chains identified by structural studies. The cDNA clone reported by Hedrick and his colleagues hybridized to a region of the mouse genome that was rearranged in a T cell lymphoma and several T lymphocyte clones. The authors concluded that the gene codes one of the chains of the TCR. Based on deduced amino acid sequences, the consensus was that it codes for the β-chain as identified by the structural studies.

Further investigation led to the isolation of genes coding for two chains of the TCR from a murine cytotoxic T lymphocyte clone by a group led by Susumu Tonegawa (Saito et al., 1984a). Tonegawa (1939–present) received his undergraduate education at Kyoto University, earned a PhD at the University of California, San Diego, and became a member of the Basel Institute of Immunology in Switzerland. While in Basel, he determined the genetic mechanisms responsible for antibody diversity (Chapter 18). For this work he received the Nobel Prize in Physiology or Medicine in 1987 "for his discovery of the genetic principle for generation of antibody diversity." In 1981 he moved to the Massachusetts Institute of Technology where he and his group performed the genetic work resulting in the isolation of the genes coding for the chains of the TCR.

The Tonegawa group deduced the amino acid sequence of the two chains from a cDNA and demonstrated that the genes are expressed and rearranged in T lymphocytes but not in other cell types. Based on these data, plus information from other investigators, Tonegawa's group proposed the structure for the TCR shown in Figure 17.2. The receptor is composed of two chains (α and β) that are disulfide linked and are integral membrane proteins. When the amino acid sequences of the chains from several TCRs were compared, both chains possess variable and constant regions; the variable region contains the antigenbinding site and is coded for by a series of gene segments that rearrange in the T lymphocyte during maturation (Chapter 18).

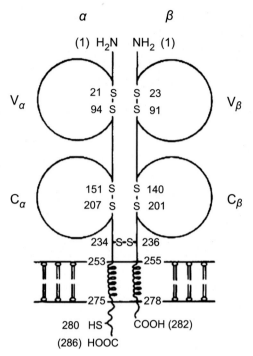

FIGURE 17.2 Diagram of the putative structure of the T cell receptor. This diagram indicated the involvement of two chains (α and β), both of which contain variable (V) and constant (C) regions. The antigenbinding site is located in the variable regions of the two chains. *From Saito et al. (1984a).*

Subsequent studies indicated that while one of the genes isolated by Tonegawa and his collaborators coded for the β-chain of the TCR, the other gene did not code for the α-chain as originally reported. The α-chain that had been isolated by Allison's group was N-glycosylated while the putative α-chain gene had no sequences that corresponded to sites for N-linked glycosylation. Additional T lymphocyte-specific genes were cloned and the gene coding for the α-chain was finally described (Chien et al., 1984; Saito et al., 1984b).

The gene originally thought to code for the α-chain of the TCR was eventually shown to code for a T lymphocyte-specific cell-surface molecule. This molecule is now termed the γ-chain, a component of a second type of TCR present on fewer than 10% of peripheral T lymphocytes. This γ-chain is paired with a δ-chain whose existence was reported by a group from the National Institutes of Health, Bethesda, Maryland, led by Ronald Schwartz (Pardoll et al., 1987).

Conclusive evidence that the TCR is the antigen-specific receptor came from gene transfer studies. In 1986 Zlatko Dembic and coworkers, at the Basel Institute for Immunology isolated genes coding for α and β chains of a cytotoxic T lymphocyte clone that had specificity for the hapten fluorescein. These genes were transferred (transfected) into another T lymphocyte clone that recognized a different hapten, SP (3-(*p*-sulphophenyldiazo)-4-hydroxyacetic acid). Analysis of the transfected lymphocytes revealed that the transferred genes were expressed and that the recipient lymphocytes were specific for fluorescein. The authors conclude that "these results provide the first definite proof that the T cell receptor α and β chain genes can transmit a functional specificity from one cytotoxic T cell to another." They further speculated that this model would provide information on the mechanism by which T lymphocytes recognize both antigen and cell-surface molecules coded for by the MHC (Chapter 20).

Accessory Molecules of the TCR

The TCR, like the BCR, has a relatively short intracytoplasmic tail that is most likely too short to engage the second messengers necessary to transduce a signal to the nucleus. The transduction function in T lymphocytes involves a series of *trans*-membrane glycoproteins that have been identified as the CD3 complex.

Prior to the description of the TCR, Jean Van Wauwe et al. treated human lymphocytes with a monoclonal antibody, OKT3, that possessed specificity for T lymphocytes. Working at the Janssen Pharmaceutical Research Laboratories in Beerse, Belgium, this group reported in 1980 that incubation of peripheral blood lymphocytes with OKT3 induced a mitogenic response in some lymphocytes. The responding lymphocytes were classified as T lymphocytes based on identification methods (rosette formation with sheep erythrocytes) available at the time. Additional study demonstrated that this monoclonal antibody bound to a cell-surface glycoprotein now known to be part of the CD3 complex.

Stefan Meuer and group, when they originally described the isolation of the human TCR (Meuer et al., 1983), reported that the TCR was noncovalently linked to the CD3 molecule on T lymphocytes. The CD3 complex is present on all peripheral T lymphocytes and consists of four membrane spanning polypeptides that are noncovalently linked to the α and β chains of the TCR. These four polypeptides (CD3γ, CD3δ, CD3ε, and CD3ζ) all have relatively long intracytoplasmic tails and amino acid sequences that can interact with signal transduction mechanisms within the cell.

CONCLUSION

The experiments performed to identify the antigen-specific receptors on B and T lymphocytes involved classical morphological approaches as well as molecular genetic investigations. The discovery of mIg as the BCR confirmed a long-held hypothesis that the antigen-specific receptor would mirror the main antigen-specific secretory product of the lymphocyte. This discovery led to the hypothesis that T lymphocytes would use a similar method of recognizing antigens in the environment even though T lymphocytes do not secrete an antigen-specific product. The identity of the TCR was revealed in the 1980s using the production of lymphocyte-specific antibodies and isolation of genes expressed only in T lymphocytes.

TCRs and BCRs recognize different antigenic determinants on pathogens. TCRs recognize a linear sequence of amino acids derived from (protein) antigens as a result of processing by an antigen presenting cell (APC). These peptides are bound by products of the MHC and displayed on the surface of the APC (Chapter 20). B lymphocytes by contrast recognize a three-dimensional configuration of an antigen; these configurations can be associated with proteins, carbohydrates, lipids, or nucleic acids. The structure of the binding site of the BCR is thus different than the binding site of the TCR.

Identification of the antigen-specific receptors on B and T lymphocytes allowed the design of experiments to determine the process responsible for the generation of diversity in the adaptive immune response (Chapter 18) as well as the mechanism by which B and T lymphocytes are activated (Chapters 19 and 20). The description of the structure of the TCR and the BCR provided information on the regulation of the cells of the adaptive immune response since antigen-specific receptors are necessary to explain the induction of unresponsiveness (tolerance) in both B lymphocytes (Chapter 21) and T lymphocytes (Chapter 22).

References

Allison, J.P., McIntyre, B.W., Bloch, D., 1982. Tumor specific antigens of murine T-lymphoma defined with monoclonal antibody. J. Immunol. 129, 2293–2300.

Bankhurst, A.D., Warner, N.L., Sprent, J., 1971. Surface immunoglobulins on thymus and thymus-derived lymphoid cells. J. Exp. Med. 134, 1005–1015.

Burnet, F.M., 1957. A modification of Jerne's theory of antibody production using the concept of clonal selection. Aust. J. Sci. 20, 67–68.

Campbell, K.S., Cambier, J.C., 1990. B lymphocyte antigen receptors (mIg) are non-covalently associated with a disulfide linked, inducibly phosphorylated glycoprotein complex. EMBO J. 9, 441–448.

Campbell, K.S., Hager, E.J., Friedrich, J., Cambier, J.C., 1991. IgM antigen receptor complex contains phosphoprotein products of B29 and *mb*-1 genes. Proc. Nat. Acad. Sci. USA 88, 3982–3986.

Chien, Y-H., Becker, D.M., Lindsten, T., Okamura, M., Cohen, D.I., Davis, M.M., 1984. A third type of murine T-cell receptor gene. Nature 312, 31–35.

Cooper, M.D., Lawton, A.R., 1972. Circulating B cells in patients with immunodeficiency. Am. J. Pathol. 69, 513–528.

Davie, J.M., Paul, W.E., 1971. Receptors on immunocompetent cells II. Specificity and nature of receptors of dinitrophenylated guinea pig albumin 125I-binding lymphocytes of normal guinea pigs. J. Exp. Med. 134, 495–516.

Dembic, Z., Haas, W., Weiss, S., McCubrey, J., Kiefer, H., von Boehmer, H., Steinmetz, M., 1986. Transfer of specificity by murine α and β T-cell receptor genes. Nature 320, 232–238.

Ehrlich, P., 1900. On immunity with special reference to cell life. Proc. R. Soc. 66, 424–428.

Friedrich, J., Campbell, K.S., Cambier, J.C., 1993. The γ subunit of the B cell antigen-receptor complex is a C-terminally truncated produce of the B29 gene. J. Immunol. 150, 2814–2822.

Fu, S.M., Winchester, R.J., Kunkel, H.G., 1975. Similar idiotypic specificity for the membrane IgD and IgM of human B lymphocytes. J. Immunol. 114, 250–252.

Gajl-Peczalska, K.J., Park, B.Y., Biggar, W.D., Good, R.A., 1973. B and T lymphocytes in primary immunodeficiency disease in man. J. Clin. Invest. 52, 919–928.

Goding, J.W., Layton, J.E., 1976. Antigen-induced co-capping of IgM and IgD-like receptors on murine B cells. J. Exp. Med. 144, 852–857.

Grey, H.M., Rabellino, E., Pirofsky, B., 1971. Immunoglobulins on the surface of lymphocytes. IV. Distribution in hypogammaglobulinemia, cellular immune deficiency, and chronic lymphatic leukemia. J. Clin. Invest. 50, 2368–2375.

Haskins, K., Kubo, R., White, J., Pigeon, M., Kappler, J., Marrack, P., 1983. The major histocompatibility complex restricted antigen receptor on T cells. I. Isolation with a monoclonal antibody. J. Exp. Med. 157, 1149–1169.

Hedrick, S.M., Cohen, D.I., Nielsen, E.A., Davis, M.M., 1984. Isolation of cDNA clones encoding T cell-specific membrane-associated proteins. Nature 308, 149–153.

IUIS/WHO Subcommittee on CD Nomenclature, 1994. CD antigens 1993: an updated nomenclature for clusters of differentiation on human cells. Bull. WHO 72, 807–808.

Kincade, P.W., Lawton, A.R., Cooper, M.D., 1971. Restriction of surface immunoglobulin determinants to lymphocytes of the plasma cell line. J. Immunol. 106, 1421–1423.

Lanier, L.L., 2005. First sighting of the elusive T cell antigen receptor. J. Immunol. 174, 1173.

Lesley, J.F., Kettman, J.R., Dutton, R.W., 1971. Immunoglobulins on the surface of thymus-derived cells engaged in the initiation of a humoral immune response. J. Exp. Med. 134, 618–629.

Marchalonis, J.J., Cone, R.E., Atwell, J.L., 1972. Isolation and partial characterization of lymphocyte surface immunoglobulins. J. Exp. Med. 135, 956–971.

Melchers, U., Vitetta, E.S., McWilliams, M., Lamm, M.E., Phillips-Quagliata, J.M., Uhr, J.W., 1974. Cell-surface immunoglobulin. X. Identification of an IgD-like molecule on the surface of murine splenocytes. J. Exp. Med. 140, 1427–1431.

Meuer, S.C., Fitzgerald, K.A., Hussey, R.E., Hodgkin, J.C., Schlossman, S.F., Reinherz, E.I., 1983. Clonotypic structures involved in antigen-specific human T cell function: relationship to the T3 molecular complex. J. Exp. Med. 157, 705–719.

Möller, G., 1961. Demonstration of mouse isoantigens at the cellular level by the fluorescent antibody technique. J. Exp. Med. 114, 415–434.

Pardoll, D.M., Fowlkes, B.J., Bluestone, J.A., Kruisbeek, A., Maloy, W.L., Coligan, J.E., Schwartz, R.H., 1987. Differential expression of two distinct T-cell receptors during thymocyte development. Nature 326, 79–81.

Rabellino, E., Grey, M.M., 1971. Immunoglobulins on the surface of lymphocytes. III. Bursal origin of surface immunoglobulins on chicken lymphocytes. J. Immunol. 106, 1418–1420.

Raff, M.C., Sternberg, M., Taylor, R.B., 1970. Immunoglobulin determinants on the surface of mouse lymphoid cells. Nature 225, 553–554.

Rowe, D.S., Hug, K., Forni, L., Pernis, B., 1973. Immunoglobulin D as a lymphocyte receptor. J. Exp. Med. 138, 965–972.

Saito, H., Kranz, D.M., Takagaki, Y., Hayday, A.C., Eisen, H.N., Tonegawa, S., 1984a. Complete primary structure of a heterodimeric T-cell receptor deduced from cDNA sequences. Nature 309, 757–762.

Saito, H., Kranz, D.M., Takagaki, Y., Hayday, A.C., Eisen, H.N., Tonegawa, S., 1984b. A third rearranged and expressed gene in a clone of cytotoxic T lymphocytes. Nature 312, 36–40.

Salsano, F., Froland, S.S., Natvig, J.B., Michaelsen, T.E., 1974. Same idiotype of B-lymphocyte membrane IgD and IgM. Formal evidence

for monoclonality of chronic lymphocytic leukaemia cells. Scand. J. Immunol. 3, 841–846.

Sell, S., Gell, P.G.H., 1965. Studies on rabbit lymphocytes in vitro. I. Stimulation of blast transformation with an antiallotype serum. J. Exp. Med. 122, 423–440.

Van Wauwe, J.P., De Mey, J.R., Goossens, J.G., 1980. OKT3: a monoclonal anti-human T lymphocyte antibody with potent mitogenic properties. J. Immunol. 124, 2708–2713.

Vitetta, E., Baur, S., Uhr, J.W., 1971. Cell surface immunoglobulin. II. Isolation and characterization of immunoglobulin from mouse splenic lymphocytes. J. Exp. Med. 134, 242–264.

Warner, N.L., 1974. Membrane immunoglobulins and antigen receptors on B and T lymphocytes. Adv. Immunol. 19, 67–216.

Yanagi, Y., Yoshikai, Y., Leggett, K., Clark, S.P., Aleksander, I., Mak, M., 1984. A human T cell-specific cDNA clone encodes a protein having extensive homology to immunoglobulin chains. Nature 308, 145–149.

TIME LINE

1901	Paul Ehrlich publishes his side-chain theory postulating that antibody-forming cells possess receptors by which they identify antigens
1957	F. Macfarlane Burnet proposes the clonal selection theory of antibody formation
1961	Göran Möller demonstrates that a small proportion of normal, mouse lymphocytes bind rabbit antibody to mouse immunoglobulin
1970	Martin Raff et al. show that lymphocytes from all organs except the thymus can be stained with anti-IgM antibodies
1971	Joseph Davie and William Paul demonstrate that antigen and antibody to immunoglobulin compete for binding sites on antibody-forming lymphocytes
1971	Ellen Vitetta identifies the BCR as IgM molecules
1973	David Rowe and collaborators identify IgD on the surface of human B lymphocytes
1980	Jean Van Wauwe and others use a monoclonal antibody to identify a cell-surface molecule on T lymphocytes that induces proliferation when stimulated (CD3)
1982	James Allison isolates the β-chain of the TCR
1983	Kathryn Haskin's group and Stefan Meuer's group report the isolation and function of polypeptide chains making up the TCR
1983	Stefan Meuer et al. demonstrate that the TCR is noncovalently linked to the CD3 complex
1984	Susumu Tonegawa et al. isolate the genes coding for the TCR
1990	John Cambier and Kerry Campbell identify the accessory molecules involved in signal transduction following engagement of the BCR

18

Generation of Diversity in the Adaptive Immune Response

INTRODUCTION

B lymphocytes interact with antigen in their environment through cell surface immunoglobulins that, when bound, provide a signal to activate the lymphocyte to proliferate and to synthesize and secrete antibody. All the immunoglobulin receptors present on any given B lymphocyte are identical with respect to their antigenic specificity. An individual possesses several million different B lymphocytes that synthesize unique antibodies. The process responsible for B lymphocyte diversity generated strenuous debate during the late 1960s and early 1970s. For example, Lee Hood and David Talmage argued in 1970 that the germline DNA contained a separate gene for every possible polypeptide chain (H and L) in an immunoglobulin molecule. Alternatively, Niels Jerne (1971) argued that only a limited number of genes encoding antibody molecules existed in the germ line and that these diversified somatically as the B lymphocytes matured.

Susumu Tonegawa solved the conundrum raised by these conflicting arguments and was awarded the Nobel Prize in Physiology or Medicine in 1987. In his Nobel Address, he noted difficulties with both proposals (Tonegawa, 1988). The germline hypothesis advanced by Hood and Talmage required a very large number of genes coding for individual heavy and light chains and implied that almost the entire human genome be involved in coding for antibodies. Additionally, this hypothesis failed to explain the inheritance of immunoglobulin allotypes, which are genetic markers on immunoglobulin heavy and light chains present in some members of a species but absent in others. These markers segregate as a single Mendelian trait. If the germline hypothesis were correct, a large number of individual genes would all need to maintain the nucleotide sequence coding for these markers.

The somatic diversification hypothesis championed by Jerne required a unique genetic mechanism with no precedence for the generation of diversity. The developmental history of B lymphocytes and the molecular genetics of immunoglobulin synthesis provided evidence for rearrangement of several gene segments to code for a single antibody.

While this debate raged, the antigen-specific receptor on T lymphocytes remained unidentified. Some immunologists postulated that the T cell receptor (TCR) was a unique class of immunoglobulin (Chapter 17), leading to the erroneous conclusion that the solution to the problem of the generation of diversity in B and T lymphocytes would be identical. While the structure of the TCR differed from the structure of the B cell receptor (BCR), the mechanisms responsible for the generation of diversity in the two lymphocyte populations are strikingly similar. This chapter provides a review of how information about the mechanism of diversity generation in B lymphocytes provided important clues to deciphering the mechanism of diversity generation in T lymphocytes.

GENERATION OF DIVERSITY IN B LYMPHOCYTES

The B lymphocyte repertoire, the total number of different antigens to which an individual can produce antibodies, exceeds one million. Assuming that the clonal selection theory is valid, then the total number of B lymphocytes each expressing a unique BCR must also exceed one million. Given that the genetic material of an individual is composed of fewer than 30,000 genes, how could the genome code for this large number of antibody specificities?

Initial studies focused on calculations of the number of genes required to code for such a large number of specificities. Some calculations concluded that, if every antibody was coded by a separate gene, a large proportion of the human genome would be committed to immunoglobulin synthesis. While the immune system is essential to life, even the most ardent supporters of the discipline found this position untenable.

Unraveling the mechanism by which the antibody repertoire reaches the level of diversity seen in vertebrates depended on three types of experimental data:

1. amino acid sequences of antibody molecules,
2. analysis of the number of germline genes available to code for antibody, and
3. organization of the genes coding for antibodies in the germ line and in mature lymphocytes.

Amino Acid Sequences

Techniques such as Edman degradation to determine the amino acid sequence of proteins were developed during the 1950s and 1960s. When investigators applied these techniques to H and L chains of antibody molecules, sequence data revealed that the amino acids from different antibodies are similar and that differences between antibodies are localized to the amino terminus of the molecule. Differences in amino acid sequence could explain individual antibody specificity. Thus investigators concluded that the specificity of immunoglobulin is restricted to the amino terminus of the molecule. Experimental protocols addressing unique genetic mechanisms focused on the amino terminus of the molecule.

At the time of these studies, researchers required a relatively large quantity of purified protein to unravel amino acid sequences. Antibodies derived from an induced immune response are heterogeneous, consisting of a number of different molecules, none of which are present in sufficient quantity to provide enough material to determine a single sequence. To overcome this problem, investigators studied serum from patients presenting with multiple myeloma, a disease characterized by a clone of malignant B lymphocytes that produce a large quantity of homogeneous immunoglobulin. Many of these patients also secrete Bence Jones proteins, immunoglobulin light chains found in the urine. Each patient secretes a unique Bence Jones protein. Since these light chains are the product of the malignant B lymphocytes, they provide a source of homogeneous proteins (Chapter 35).

Analysis of the amino acid sequences of Bence Jones proteins from several patients showed that these chains consist of an amino terminal region containing amino acid variation (the variable (V) regions) and a carboxyl terminal containing identical amino acids from chain to chain (the constant (C) regions) (Hilschmann and Craig, 1965; Titani et al., 1965). Figure 18.1 compares the order of amino acids of the three Bence Jones proteins sequenced by the late 1960s. Approximately 110 amino acid residues in the amino terminus of the molecule demonstrated significant variation, while the remaining amino acids were identical in all three chains studied.

The amino acid sequences of heavy chains from patients with multiple myeloma demonstrated a similar division into V and C regions (Press and Hogg, 1969; Edelman et al., 1969). Based on these data as well as emerging information obtained on the chemical structure of antibodies (Chapter 11) investigators focused on the V regions of the heavy and light chains as the site of antigen binding and hence of the specificity of the BCR.

Determination of the Number of Germline Light Chain Genes

Starting in the early 1970s, molecular biology techniques were developed that permitted investigation of DNA and RNA in detail. These techniques included isolation of specific messenger RNA (mRNA), hybridization of RNA with DNA, and cleavage of DNA and RNA with restriction endonucleases. Molecular immunologists enthusiastically adapted this new technology to address questions about the generation of diversity of antibody and B lymphocytes.

Susumu Tonegawa, a leader in the emerging field of molecular immunology, received his undergraduate education at the University of Kyoto, Japan. He earned his PhD in molecular biology from the University of California, San Diego, and completed postdoctoral training in Renato

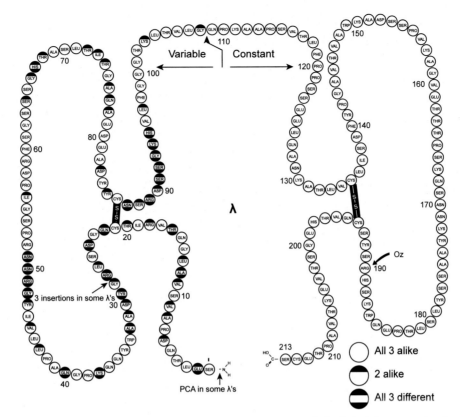

FIGURE 18.1 Comparison of the amino acid sequences of three Bence Jones proteins (light chains) demonstrating that the amino terminus of the three proteins are variable at a number of positions while the amino acids making up the carboxy terminus are invariant. *From Putnam, 1969.*

Dulbecco's laboratory at the Salk Institute in San Diego, California. In 1970, Tonegawa joined the Basel Institute for Immunology in Switzerland where he applied the molecular biology techniques he had learned during his training, including use of restriction enzymes and recombinant DNA, to immunological questions such as the genetic mechanisms responsible for antibody diversity.

When Tonegawa started his research in Basel, immunologists still debated whether antibody diversity was due to the inheritance of a large number of genes (the germline hypothesis) or if a few inherited genes underwent a unique process of somatic diversification. Tonegawa reasoned that mRNA isolated from myeloma cells represented the genes used to code for the myeloma proteins being synthesized and secreted. This message would contain information to produce both V and C regions and should hybridize with all DNA that contains the C region gene. Hybridization of this mRNA to liver (germline) DNA would result in two possible outcomes:

1. If the germline hypothesis is correct, the mRNA would bind to many genes, all containing the C region genetic code.
2. If the somatic diversification hypothesis is correct, the mRNA would bind to one or a few C region genes.

In 1974, Tonegawa and colleagues hybridized mRNA specific for kappa (κ) light chains isolated from mouse myeloma cells to liver DNA. Based on reiteration frequency and competition hybridization experiments, the authors conclude that "the number of germ line genes seems to be too small to account for the observed variability of antibody V regions." They speculate that "there must exist a mechanism for extensive somatic generation of antibody diversity."

Continuing this research, Tonegawa in 1976, hybridized mRNA specific for λ light chains isolated from mouse myeloma cells to liver DNA. Amino acid sequence data for the V regions of λ chains suggested a minimum of 25 different λ chains represented in the myelomas available at the time. Tonegawa predicted that if all antibody variability were due to inheritance of different genes for these chains, one would expect that mRNA for one λ chain would hybridize with at least 25 different genes, all of which would cross-react.

mRNA coding for an antibody light chain, hybridized with germline DNA with a reiteration frequency similar to that seen with mRNA specific for α- or β-globin genes. Since globin genes code for a single protein and not multiple proteins, as is the case with immunoglobulin genes, Tonegawa concluded that a limited number of light chain genes existed in the germ line and that variability in antibody genes resulted from some somatic diversification mechanism. Over the next several years, Tonegawa and his coworkers extended these studies to immunoglobulin heavy chains and concluded that genes coding for both light and heavy chains undergo somatic diversification.

Organization of the Genes Coding for Immunoglobulin Molecules

Results supporting the inheritance of one or a few immunoglobulin genes that undergo somatic diversification led to further questions. If the immunoglobulin chains were inherited as a single gene, the mechanism responsible for introducing variability into some nucleotides (the amino terminus) while sparing nucleotides in the carboxyl terminus begged for an explanation. Speculation that an immunoglobulin polypeptide may be coded by two separate DNA sequences was initially presented by William J. Dreyer (1928–2004) and J. Claude Bennett (1933–present) in 1965. Working at the California Institute of Technology in Pasadena, California, they hypothesized that the variable portion of light chains is coded for by germline genes that are combined with the gene coding for the C region during the differentiation of the antibody-forming lymphocyte. This combination became fixed by some unknown mechanism for the life of that lymphocyte. This hypothesis explained data emerging about the inheritance of allotypes but still required the inheritance of a large number of genes coding for the V regions of the chains.

The Dreyer–Bennett hypothesis that V and C regions of the immunoglobulin chains were coded for by separate genes was questioned by many immunologists and geneticists. At the time, most molecular biologists agreed that a single gene coded a single polypeptide chain. Additionally, genetic material in eukaryotic cells was considered stable throughout development and cell differentiation. Research during the late 1970s supported the Dreyer–Bennett hypothesis and resulted in three conclusions:

- V and C regions of the immunoglobulin chains are coded for by two genes;
- a third gene segment, a joining (J) gene, exists that codes for 10–15 amino acids located between the V and C regions; and
- in the genes coding for some immunoglobulin chains, a separate diversity (D) gene exists that codes for a short segment of amino acids located between the V and J regions.

In the mid-1970s, Susumu Tonegawa and colleagues devised an experimental approach to test the Dreyer–Bennett hypothesis using restriction enzymes to analyze the DNA coding for immunoglobulin chains. Restriction enzymes are DNA-cutting enzymes that recognize and cleave a specific sequence of nucleotides. For

example, the *Bam*H1 enzyme will cleave DNA between the two guanines in the sequence GGATCC. This provides shorter DNA fragments that prove useful for hybridization experiments.

If an immunoglobulin light chain is coded for by separate V and C genes, coding for V and C regions of the protein, treatment of embryonic DNA with restriction enzymes would hypothetically produce DNA fragments that differ from those generated by treating DNA derived from immunoglobulin-secreting myeloma cells. To test this hypothesis, Tonegawa and colleagues isolated DNA from mouse embryos and from myeloma cell lines and digested this DNA with the *Bam*H1 restriction enzyme. They separated the DNA fragments by electrophoresis on agarose gel and hybridized them with iodinated mRNA probes specific for the entire κ light chain or for the C region of the κ chain.

As reported by Nobumichi Hozumi and Susumu Tonegawa in 1976, "the pattern of hybridization was completely different in the genomes of embryo cells and of the plasmacytoma." The DNA from the embryo had two components selected by the probes: one that hybridized with C gene sequences and the other that hybridized with V gene sequences. The DNA from the myeloma cells had only a single component that hybridized with both V- and C-gene probes. The authors interpreted the results "to mean that the V_κ and C_κ genes...are joined to form a contiguous polynucleotide stretch during differentiation of lymphocytes."

The finding that a single polypeptide chain could be coded for by the combination of two separate genes provided a theoretical mechanism for B lymphocytes to generate a large number of different antigen binding specificities. Immunologists agree that as B lymphocytes differentiate the V and C genes randomly recombine to form a single DNA sequence.

Advances in this field required an enhanced determination of DNA sequences. The development of recombinant DNA technology permitted molecular immunologists to clone V and C genes from embryonic cells and from myeloma cells and to compare their nucleotide sequences.

Tonegawa isolated a DNA clone from embryonic cells that specifically hybridized with mRNA coding for λ chains. Electron microscopy as well as DNA sequencing showed that the isolated clone coded for the V gene (Tonegawa et al., 1977, 1978). Subsequent DNA sequences were isolated using other DNA clones that allowed the study of a number of sequences specific for both κ and λ chains. Studies using DNA fragments isolated from embryonic cells and from myeloma cells proved that the V and C genes are physically separate in the germ line and rearranged in the antibody-forming lymphocytes (Brack et al., 1978; Lenhard-Schuller et al., 1978). Analyses of these clones demonstrated that while the V gene and the C gene are closer together in the myeloma cell than they are in the germline configuration, they are still separated by a few kilobases of DNA that are not translated in the final polypeptide chain. The DNA is thus transcribed into an mRNA and the extraneous RNA spliced out during RNA processing (Figure 18.2).

Additional evidence that immunoglobulin chains are coded for by multiple genes came from studies performed in Leroy Hood's laboratory at the California Institute of Technology (Barstad et al., 1974). These investigators compared the sequences of the N-terminal 20 amino acid residues of 13 heavy chains from BALB/c mice with published sequences of the same residues from 15 other heavy chains. They divided these sequences into sets and subsets based on similarities of the residues and concluded that "there are at least eight germ line genes coding for the variable regions of mouse heavy chain."

In 1978, Martin Weigert and colleagues, working at the Fox Chase Cancer Center in Philadelphia, Pennsylvania, in collaboration with Leroy Hood at the California Institute of Technology in Pasedena, compared the complete amino acid sequences of 22 κ chain V regions. This evaluation showed that these V regions are coded for by a minimum of six germline genes. Further assessment of these light chains suggested to the authors that

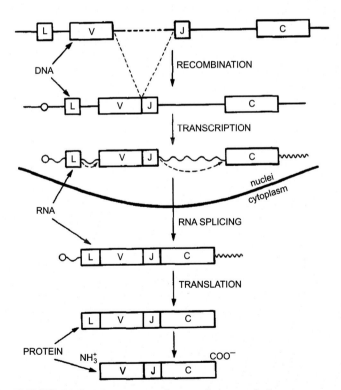

FIGURE 18.2 The sequence of events that occur during rearrangement and expression of an immunoglobulin light chain gene. The top drawing illustrates the DNA as it exists in the germ line. As the B cell differentiates, the J gene is rearranged and transcribed to an mRNA that contains an intron (DNA sequence that is not translated). The mRNA is processed and the spliced RNA is translated to form the light chain. *From Tonegawa, 1988.*

approximately the last 12 amino acids are coded for by a separate germline gene that they term the J gene.

This conclusion was confirmed by J.G. Seidman and Phillip Leder (1978), working at the National Institute of Child Health and Human Development, Bethesda, Maryland, who studied the genes coding for κ chains. Seidman and Leder cloned the V genes and showed that they failed "to code for the final 10 or so amino acids that had, by sequence analysis, always been associated with the variable region" of the protein. Speculation that this J region gene is rearranged to the V gene during B lymphocyte differentiation provides a partial answer to the generation of antibody diversity with a minimal amount of genetic material.

When investigators turned their attention to heavy chains, they unraveled a similar organization of the genes encoding these polypeptides. By amino acid sequence analysis, heavy chains are composed of discrete V, J, and C regions. Genes coding for these regions are rearranged in the differentiating B lymphocyte. Similar to light chains, a relatively large number of V region and J region genes are present in the germ line.

A third gene segment coding for a portion of the heavy chain V region was discovered in 1980 by Hitoshi Sakano, working with Susumu Tonegawa and coworkers at the Basel Institute for Immunology. This group studied the structure of the gene coding for a mouse myeloma protein. The light chain gene was composed of recombined V and J regions making up the V gene. The heavy chain V gene by contrast is composed of an additional gene segment since "a 14 residue peptide comprising the third hypervariable region...is encoded in neither the germline V gene nor the J DNA segment." The authors suggest that this portion of the heavy chain is coded in a separate gene segment termed the D gene. Thus the formation of a complete gene for the heavy chain requires two DNA recombination events (V-D and D-J) that determine the amino acid sequence forming the antigen binding site (Sakano et al., 1980). VDJ rearrangement is mediated by recombinases, including enzymes codie for by recombination activating genes 1 and 2 (RAG 1 and 2), terminal deoxynucleotidyl transferase, and Artemis nuclease.

These studies of the genetic control of immunoglobulin structure resulted in the awarding of the Nobel Prize in Physiology or Medicine in 1987 to Susumu Tonegawa "for his discovery of the genetic principle for generation of antibody diversity."

GENERATION OF DIVERSITY IN T LYMPHOCYTES

The genetic mechanisms involved in the gene rearrangement and other molecular events that occur in B lymphocytes leading to antibody diversity are also seen in the differentiation of T lymphocytes and the formation of the TCR.

T lymphocytes, like B lymphocytes, interact with antigens in their environment via cell surface receptors. Unlike B lymphocytes, which recognize three-dimensional shapes of antigens, T lymphocytes recognize short peptide sequences along with a portion of a molecule coded by the major histocompatibility gene complex (MHC) of the species (Chapter 20). This phenomenon, termed MHC restriction, requires that foreign epitopes are presented by other cells of the organism. CD4$^+$ T lymphocytes recognize antigen presented by specialized antigen-presenting cells (macrophages, dendritic cells, B cells) that express class II MHC molecules, while CD8$^+$ T lymphocytes recognize antigen presented by virtually every cell of the body expressing class I MHC molecules (Chapter 20).

An individual T lymphocyte possesses numerous, identical TCRs, all of which bind to the same antigen-MHC. Based on the tenets of the clonal selection theory, the determination of which T lymphocytes will respond to a given antigen depends on the interaction of antigen with a matching TCR on the lymphocyte.

Once the structure of the TCR was identified a major question remained: what is the mechanism responsible for the generation of the large number of specificities in the T lymphocyte repertoire? Some clues were derived from the evidence generated during the study of the ontogeny of B lymphocyte as described in the first part of this chapter.

Structure of the TCR and Its Genetic Organization

The TCR was initially characterized in the early 1980s by groups of investigators led by James Allison at the University of Texas System Cancer Center, Smithville, Kathryn Haskins at the University of Colorado, Denver, and Stefan Meuer at Harvard using monoclonal antibodies specific for individual clones of T lymphocytes. The studies performed with these cell lines and monoclonal antibodies are presented in Chapter 17. Results from these investigations demonstrated that the TCR comprises two polypeptide chains (α and β), each of approximately 40 kDa. Similar to the BCR, comparison of the amino acid structure of TCRs isolated from different clones of T lymphocytes showed that the chains could be divided into V and C regions.

Within 6 months of the identification of the TCR, DNA clones for one of the chains of the TCR were isolated from both human and mouse T lymphocytes by two groups of investigators: Tak Mak and colleagues at the University of Toronto, Canada (Yanagi et al., 1984), and Mark Davis and coworkers, working at the National Institute of Allergy and Infectious Diseases in Bethesda, Maryland, and Stanford University in Palo Alto, California (Hedrick et al.,

1984). These investigators hybridized complementary DNAs (cDNAs) with mRNA expressed in T lymphocytes but not in B lymphocytes. Analysis of the cDNA clones indicated that the mRNA from which they were hybridized were T lymphocyte-specific, came from genes that had rearranged during T lymphocyte differentiation, and had a sequence similar to, but not identical to, mRNA coding for immunoglobulin chains.

Comparison of the nucleotide sequences of these cDNA clones with other DNA clones isolated from thymocytes demonstrated the presence of V, J, and C regions similar to those found in the genes coding for the light chains of the BCR. Further analysis of β-chain genes revealed the existence of a segment of the rearranged gene located between the V and J regions but coded for by neither (Chien et al., 1984; Kavaler et al., 1984; Siu et al., 1984). This region is called the D region, similar to the D region in the gene coding for the heavy chain of the BCR.

The rearrangement of the genes coding for TCRs occurs while the T lymphocytes are maturing in the thymus (Chapter 9) prior to exposure to antigen. This is an apparently random process that results in the formation of a large number of T lymphocytes, each of which possesses a single binding capability. By chance, some of these receptors possess specificity for foreign antigens, while others possess specificity for self-antigens. Mechanisms exist to eliminate these maturing lymphocytes and to censor the total T lymphocyte repertoire to provide only lymphocytes capable of reacting to foreign antigens. The mechanisms involved in this censoring are presented in Chapter 22.

CONCLUSION

Both B and T lymphocytes interact with antigens in their immediate environment through antigen-specific cell surface receptors. As presented in Chapter 17, the BCR is a membrane-associated immunoglobulin, while the TCR is a heterodimer comprised of α and β chains. Since each lymphocyte responds to a single antigen and the total number of antigens to which an individual can respond exceeds one million, the mechanism of diversity generation was hotly debated in the 1960s and 1970s. Two competing hypotheses were argued:

- the germ line contained individual genes coding for each of the antibodies (and TCRs) the individual could synthesize; or
- the germ line contained a few genes coding for antibodies (and TCRs) that were subjected to somatic diversification during lymphocyte maturation.

The experiments reviewed in this chapter demonstrate that the second hypothesis is essentially correct and that both B and T lymphocytes proceed through a differentiation process, resulting in the expression of unique antigen-specific cell surface receptors. In summary, these experiments showed that

- amino acid sequence data divide BCR and TCR chains into V and C regions;
- antigen specificity of the BCR and TCR is located in the V regions of the chains;
- the germ line contains a relatively small number of genes coding for BCR and TCR chains;
- each BCR or TCR chain is coded for by three or four gene segments that are rearranged during lymphocyte differentiation;
- these gene segments code for V, (D), J, and C regions of the BCR and TCR;
- each genome contains multiple different genes coding for the V, D, and J segments; and
- rearrangement of these genes is random, leads to the transcription of a single mRNA coding for the BCR or TCR chain, and ensures diversity.

The mechanism by which these gene segments are rearranged involves the activation of several nuclear enzymes. The rearrangement of gene segments in B and T lymphocytes has provided a unique base for answering a host of other questions, including

- the process by which B and T lymphocytes are activated (Chapters 19 and 20);
- the processes responsible for the elimination of potentially autoreactive lymphocytes (Chapters 21 and 22); and
- the regulatory mechanisms available for maintaining homeostasis in the adaptive immune response (Chapter 24).

The results presented in this chapter relied on new technologies, particularly in the field of molecular biology and genetics. These techniques are used in studies on the different populations of lymphocytes (Chapter 23), intercellular communication in the immune response (Chapter 25), and the development of therapies for immunopathologies, including autoimmune diseases (i.e., rheumatoid arthritis, systemic lupus erythematosus—Chapter 34), hypersensitivities (i.e., asthma, toxic shock syndrome—Chapter 33), immunodeficiencies (i.e., agammaglobulinemia, AIDS—Chapter 32), and immunoproliferative diseases (i.e., multiple myeloma, Waldenstrom macroglobulinemia—Chapter 35).

References

Barstad, P., Farnsworth, V., Weigert, M., Cohn, M., Hood, L., 1974. Mouse immunoglobulin heavy chains are coded by multiple germ line variable region genes. Proc. Nat. Acad. Sci. U.S.A. 71, 4096–4100.

Brack, C., Hirama, M., Lenhard-Schuller, R., Tonegawa, S., 1978. A complete immunoglobulin gene is created by somatic recombination. Cell 15, 1–14.

Chien, Y.-H., Gascoigne, N.R.J., Kavaler, J., Lee, N.E., Davis, M.M., 1984. Somatic recombination in a murine T-cell receptor gene. Nature 309, 322–326.

Dreyer, W.J., Bennett, J.C., 1965. The molecular basis of antibody formation: a paradox. Proc. Nat. Acad. Sci. U.S.A. 54, 864–869.

Edelman, G.M., Cunningham, B.A., Gall, W.E., Gottlieb, P.D., Rutishauser, U., Waxdal, M.J., 1969. The covalent structure of an entire γG immunoglobulin molecule. Proc. Nat. Acad. Sci. U.S.A. 63, 78–85.

Hedrick, S.M., Cohen, D.I., Nielsen, E.A., Davis, M.M., 1984. Isolation of cDNA clones encoding T cell-specific membrane-associated proteins. Nature 308, 149–153.

Hilschmann, N., Craig, L.C., 1965. Amino acid sequence studies with Bence-Jones proteins. Proc. Nat. Acad. Sci. U.S.A. 53, 1403–1409.

Hood, L., Talmage, D.W., 1970. Mechanism of antibody diversity: germ line basis for variability. Science 168, 325–334.

Hozumi, N., Tonegawa, S., 1976. Evidence for somatic rearrangement of immunoglobulin genes coding for variable and constant regions. Proc. Nat. Acad. Sci. U.S.A. 73, 3628–3632.

Jerne, N.K., 1971. The somatic generation of immune recognition. Eur. J. Immunol. 1, 1–9.

Kavaler, J., Davis, M.M., Chien, Y-H, 1984. Localization of a T-cell receptor diversity-region element. Nature 310, 421–423.

Lenhard-Schuller, R., Holm, B., Brack, C., Hirama, M., Tonegawa, S., 1978. DNA clones containing mouse immunoglobulin kappa chain genes isolated by in vitro packaging into phage lambda coats. Proc. Nat. Acad. Sci. U.S.A. 75, 4709–4713.

Press, E.M., Hogg, N.M., 1969. Comparative study of two immunoglobulin G Fd-fragments. Nature 223, 807–810.

Putnam, F.W., 1969. Immunoglobulin structure: variability and homology. Science 163, 633–644.

Sakano, H., Maki, R., Kurosawa, Y., Roeder, W., Tonegawa, S., 1980. Two types of somatic recombination are necessary for the generation of complete immunoglobulin heavy-chain genes. Nature 286, 676–683.

Seidman, J.G., Leder, P., 1978. The arrangement and rearrangement of antibody genes. Nature 276, 790–795.

Siu, G., Clark, S.P., Yoshikai, Y., Malissen, M., Yanagi, Y., Strauss, E., Mak, W.T., Hood, L., 1984. The human T cell antigen receptor is encoded by variable, diversity and joining segments that rearrange to generate a complete V gene. Cell 37, 393–401.

Titani, K., Whitley Jr., E., Avogardo, L., Putnam, F., 1965. Immunoglobulin structure: partial amino acid sequence of a Bence Jones protein. Science 149, 1090–1092.

Tonegawa, S., 1976. Reiteration frequency of immunoglobulin light chain genes: further evidence for somatic generation of antibody diversity. Proc. Nat. Acad. Sci. U.S.A. 73, 203–207.

Tonegawa, S., 1988. Somatic generation of immune diversity. Biosci. Reports 8, 3–26.

Tonegawa, S., Brack, C., Hozumi, N., Schuller, R., 1977. Cloning of an immunoglobulin variable region gene from mouse embryo. Proc. Nat. Acad. Sci. U.S.A. 74, 3518–3522.

Tonegawa, S., Maxam, A.M., Tizard, R., Bernard, O., Gilbert, W., 1978. Sequence of a mouse germ-line gene for a variable region of an immunoglobulin light chain. Proc. Nat. Acad. Sci. U.S.A. 75, 1485–1489.

Tonegawa, S., Steinberg, C., Dube, S., Bernardini, A., 1974. Evidence for somatic generation of antibody diversity. Proc. Nat. Acad. Sci. U.S.A. 71, 4027–4031.

Weigert, M., Gatmaitan, L., Loh, E., Schilling, J., Hood, L., 1978. Rearrangement of genetic information may produce immunoglobulin diversity. Nature 276, 785–790.

Yanagi, Y., Yoshikai, Y., Leggett, K., Clark, S.P., Aleksander, I., Mak, T.W., 1984. A human T cell-specific cDNA clone encodes a protein having extensive homology to immunoglobulin chains. Nature 308, 145–149.

TIME LINE

1965   William Dreyer and J. Claude Bennett hypothesize that immunoglobulin polypeptides are coded for by two separate genes (DNA sequences)

1965   Norbert Hilschman and Lyman Craig and Frank Putnam and colleagues report partial amino acid sequences of light chains and divide the molecules into variable (V) and constant (C) regions

1969   Elizabeth Press and Nancy Hogg and Gerald Edelman and colleagues provide evidence that heavy chains have V and C regions

1976   Susumu Tonegawa publishes hybridization data supporting the presence of a limited number of germline light chain genes that undergo somatic diversification

1976   Nobumichi Hozumi and Susumu Tonegawa report that immunoglobulin genes in the germ line are organized differently than they are in plasma cells

1978   Martin Weigert and colleagues and J.G. Seidman and Phillip Leder present evidence that light chain V and C regions are separate in the germ line; identification of a gene coding for the J region

1980   Mark Davis and colleagues demonstrate that genes coding for heavy chain rearrange during B cell differentiation; identification of a gene coding for the D region

1984   Tak Mak and colleagues and Mark Davis and coworkers provide evidence that the T cell receptor is coded for by genes that rearrange during differentiation

1987   Susumu Tonegawa is awarded the Nobel Prize in Physiology or Medicine

19

B Lymphocyte Activation

INTRODUCTION

B lymphocytes recognize antigens/pathogens, transform to plasma cells, and synthesize and secrete antibodies specific for that antigen. This simple statement represents experimental data collected by many immunologists working around the world over several decades. The conclusions drawn from these experiments were reviewed in previous chapters:

- Antibody-forming plasma cells mature from small lymphocytes (Chapter 5) that differentiate in a central lymphoid organ represented by the bursa of Fabricius in birds or the bone marrow in mammals (Chapter 10).
- Optimal antibody synthesis by activated B lymphocytes requires help from T lymphocytes (Chapter 13).
- Plasma cells are monospecific; that is, all the antibodies produced by a single cell have the identical antigenic binding specificity (Chapter 7).
- B lymphocytes interact with antigens in the environment by receptors (B cell receptors (BCRs)) expressed on their surface—these receptors are structurally similar to the antibodies that the plasma cell will synthesize once activated (Chapter 17).

These data spurred the question of how B lymphocytes are activated by the antigens they bind. F. Macfarlane Burnet's clonal selection theory (1957) focused on the interaction of antigen with antigen-sensitive cells, resulting eventually in the synthesis of antibodies. In 1959, *Science* published two papers reviewing the question of immunologic specificity and how Burnet's theory changed contemporary immunologic concepts. In one article, David Talmage, from the University of Chicago, Illinois, argued that the classical instruction theories of antibody formation were no longer tenable and that "immunological specificity (is) based on a unique combination of natural globulins." However, Talmage did not embrace the concept that antibody specificity was dictated by a unique arrangement of DNA. In an accompanying essay, Joshua Lederberg, who worked with Gus Nossal to demonstrate that an antibody-synthesizing cell produces antibodies of a single specificity (Chapter 7), proposed that antibody-forming cells lymphocytes possess a "unique sequence of nucleotides in a segment of their chromosomal DNA" that is subject to a high rate of spontaneous mutation. Lederberg, a professor at Stanford University Medical School, Palo Alto, California, argued that interaction of antigen with the BCR on an immature lymphocyte leads to suppression whereas the identical interaction when the cell is mature leads to stimulation, including increased antibody synthesis.

Lederberg's proposed mechanism explaining the activation of antibody-forming cells initiated a series of studies focused on detailing this process. While his initial hypothesis that B lymphocytes could be activated following a single interaction of antigen with the cell surface receptor has proven erroneous, several of the propositions he expounded in 1959 remain tenable today (Table 19.1).

This chapter emphasizes the experiments performed to determine the molecular mechanisms of B lymphocyte activation, highlighting the events that occur during interactions between B and T lymphocytes, the action of soluble factors (cytokines) to enhance and mimic these interactions, and the mechanisms by which the B lymphocytes switch from synthesizing IgM to other immunoglobulin isotypes.

TABLE 19.1   The Nine Proposals Presented by Joshua Lederberg in His Defense of Burnet's Clonal Selection Theory

A1	The stereospecific segment of each antibody globulin is determined by a unique sequence of amino acids.
A2	The cell making of a given antibody has a correspondingly unique sequence of nucleotides in a segment of its chromosomal DNA: its "gene for globulin synthesis."
A3	The genic diversity of the precursors of antibody-forming cells arises from a high rate of spontaneous mutation during their lifelong proliferation.
A4	This hypermutability consists of the random assembly of the DNA of the globulin gene during certain stages of cellular proliferation.
A5	Each cell, as it begins to mature, spontaneously produces small amounts of the antibody corresponding to its own genotype.
A6	The immature antibody-forming cell is hypersensitive to an antigen–antibody combination: it will be suppressed if it encounters the homologous antigen at this time.
A7	The mature antibody-forming cell is reactive to an antigen–antibody combination: it will be stimulated if it first encounters the homologous antigen at this time. The stimulation comprises the acceleration of protein synthesis and the cytological maturation, which marks a "plasma cell."
A8	Mature cells proliferate extensively under antigenic stimulation but are genetically stable and therefore generate large clones genotypically preadapted to produce the homologous antibody.
A9	These clones tend to persist after the disappearance of the antigen, retaining their capacity to react promptly to its later reintroduction.

From Lederberg, 1959.

TWO-SIGNAL MODEL OF B LYMPHOCYTE ACTIVATION

In 1968, Peter Bretscher and Melvin Cohn at the Salk Institute for Biological Studies in San Diego, California, proposed that B lymphocytes are paralyzed (inactivated) if a single antigenic determinant binds to BCR and activated if the BCR is stretched and receives signals from two identical antigenic determinants. In the model, depicted in Figure 19.1, Bretscher and Cohn hypothesized that the carrier antibody is directed to an antigenic determinant (epitope) different than the one bound to the cell surface immunoglobulin receptor.

Two years later, Bretscher and Cohn (1970) refined their model and proposed that the carrier antibody delivers a signal to the B lymphocyte different from that provided by cross-linking the antigen. This revised model depicted in Figure 19.2 was compared to the one proposed by Joshua Lederberg in 1959. Lederberg argued that the outcome of the interaction between antigen- and antibody-forming lymphocyte depended on the differentiation state of the lymphocyte. Bretscher and Cohn by contrast proposed that activation requires interaction with the antigen plus a second stimulus, here represented by carrier antibody, while the outcome of a B lymphocyte interacting with antigen in the absence of the second signal resulted in the induction of tolerance.

The two-signal hypothesis, thus, included a mechanism for the induction of immunologic tolerance in new lymphocytes arising throughout the life of the individual. In addition it was consistent with the data indicating that an optimal antibody response required collaboration of B and T lymphocytes.

The Bretscher–Cohn hypothesis, however, failed to explain the origin of the carrier antibody. If the carrier

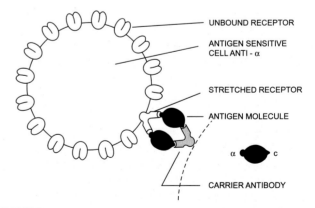

FIGURE 19.1   Original depiction of the Bretscher and Cohn model of B lymphocyte activation depicting the presence of a carrier antibody that helped cross-link the antigen molecules as they bound immunoglobulin surface receptors. In this model, the carrier antibody is directed at an antigenic determinant different than the one that interacts with the B cell. *From Bretscher and Cohn, 1968.*

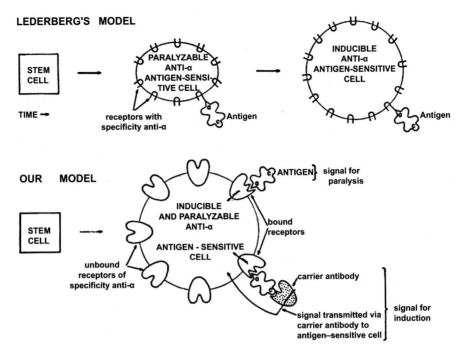

FIGURE 19.2 Updated version of the Bretscher–Cohn two-signal model, including a comparison of Lederberg's model based on a single interaction with antigen. *From Bretscher and Cohn, 1970.*

antibody was produced by B lymphocytes, these cells would also require stimulation by two signals. At least two explanations were proposed to solve this conundrum: either the carrier antibody was a unique class of antibody that could be produced without a second signal, or the original carrier antibodies were acquired via passage across the placenta from the mother. Neither explanation has stood the test of time and investigators performed additional experiments to determine the validity of the two-signal hypothesis.

SIGNAL 1: THE B CELL RECEPTOR

The BCR is a membrane-associated immunoglobulin (—Chapter 17) structurally similar to the antibody molecule the B lymphocyte is genetically committed to synthesize and secrete (Chapter 18). The antigen binding site of this BCR is dictated by the instructions carried in the variable region of the DNA coding for the heavy and light chains. As a result, the BCR recognizes antigen in its native form without processing by antigen-presenting cells such as macrophages or dendritic cells, as is required by T lymphocytes (Chapter 20). The antigen that is recognized may be soluble, for example, tetanus toxoid or foreign proteins, or a component of a cell surface such as bacteria, viruses, fungi, and protozoal parasites. BCRs recognize antigens composed of any chemical class, including proteins, carbohydrates, lipids, or nucleic acids.

By the early 1970s, immunologists divided antigens into two classes: thymus-dependent or thymus-independent,

based on the requirement for help from T lymphocytes in induction of antibody synthesis. In 1971, Marc Feldman and Antony Basten at the Walter and Eliza Hall Institute of Medical Research in Melbourne, Australia, studied the differences between thymus-dependent and thymus-independent antigens using mice assigned to one of three experimental groups:

- lethally irradiated mice rescued by an injection of syngeneic bone marrow,
- lethally irradiate, thymectomized mice rescued by an injection of syngeneic bone marrow, and
- unmanipulated mice.

Lymphocytes derived from the spleens of each of these three groups of mice were placed in tissue culture with either a thymus-dependent antigen (sheep erythrocytes (SRBC)) or a thymus-independent antigen (polymerized flagellin (POL) from *Salmonella adelaide*). Basten and Feldman quantified IgM antibodies to these antigens 4 days later. Lymphocytes from groups 1 and 3 secreted antibodies to both SRBC and POL while lymphocytes from group 2 secreted antibodies only to POL.

When the investigators dissociated antigenic determinants from the POL and presented them in a monomeric form, spleen cells from the thymectomized, irradiated, reconstituted animals (group 2) failed to produce antibodies even when the antigen was present in high concentrations. Similar results were seen when these studies were repeated with two different antigens: dinitrophenyl (DNP) coupled to POL (a thymus-independent antigen) or DNP coupled to donkey red blood cells (a thymus-dependent antigen). Spleen cells from irradiated, bone marrow-rescued mice produced comparable antibody responses to both forms of DNP while spleen cells from thymectomized, irradiated, bone marrow-rescued animals synthesized antibodies to DNP-POL but failed to respond to DNP conjugated to donkey erythrocytes.

Feldman and Basten concluded that the "requirement for T cells in antibody production is not a property of specific antigenic determinants, but depends on the mode of antigenic presentation." Other investigators (i.e., Coutinho and Möller, 1973) argued that T-independent antigens possessed an intrinsic, mitogenic property that helped them stimulate B lymphocytes to divide and synthesize antibody. While several thymus-independent antigens are B lymphocyte mitogens, not all T-independent antigens are mitogenic to B lymphocytes and investigators concluded that the mechanism by which these antigens stimulate B lymphocytes requires the antigens to cross-link the BCRs of the antigen-specific lymphocytes. Cross-linking of BCR in turn requires that T-independent antigens contain several identical antigenic determinants.

Subsequent studies showed that the antibody produced in response to T-independent antigens is exclusively of the IgM class, never switching to IgG or any other isotype. Likewise, responses to T-independent antigens fail to generate memory, and subsequent responses to these antigens are identical to the primary response.

Role of CD79 in B Lymphocyte Activation

Interaction of the BCR with its specific antigen is a necessary first step in the activation of B lymphocytes. Investigators noted that the BCR includes a short intracytoplasmic tail, consisting of three amino acid residues that is too short to interact with second messengers in the cytoplasm involved in transmitting a signal to the nucleus. As described in Chapter 17, in 1990, Kerry Campbell and John Cambier at the University of Colorado Medical School sought and found accessory molecules associated with the BCR that serve this transduction function. Two other groups of investigators, one led by Joachim Hombach in Freiburg, Germany (Hombach et al., 1990), and a second headed up by Carel van Noesel in the Netherlands, reported independently in 1990 the isolation of these same molecules. Originally termed Ig-α and Ig-β, these chains have been characterized by monoclonal antibodies and are now called, respectively, CD79a and CD79b.

CD79a and CD79b are noncovalently linked to the BCR. These accessory molecules contain an amino acid sequence that activates tyrosine kinase, an essential enzyme in the sequence of intracellular signals leading to gene transcription. While this signal may be sufficient to induce the production of IgM antibodies following cross-linking of the BCR, optimal antibody responses to most antigens require a second signal provided either by soluble factors or cell-to-cell interactions.

SIGNAL 2: SOLUBLE FACTORS AND CELL-TO-CELL INTERACTIONS

At the time the original two-signal hypothesis was published, studies differentiating thymus-dependent T lymphocytes and bursa (or bone marrow)-dependent B lymphocytes were also published. Moreover, as presented in Chapter 13, immunologists agreed that activation of an optimal antibody response to most antigens required synergy between these two lymphocyte populations. To accommodate these emerging findings, Bretscher and Cohn (1970) speculated that thymus-derived lymphocytes provided carrier antibodies that served as antigen-specific receptors on these helper T lymphocytes. Although the TCR is not an antibody, subsequent investigations revealed the requirement that both B and T lymphocytes need to bind antigenic determinants to induce optimal antibody synthesis. Initial support for this proposal came from experiments performed in the early 1970s by Avrion Mitchison and colleagues.

Mitchison (1928 to present), trained at Oxford in the laboratory of Sir Peter Medawar, worked as Professor of Zoology at University College, London, and at the National Institute of Medical Research at Mill Hill. His contributions to immunology include seminal experiments on T–B lymphocyte collaboration and immunologic tolerance.

The conclusion that optimal antibody synthesis required collaboration between T and B lymphocytes relied on studies that employed relatively complex antigens such as erythrocytes from a foreign species. This complexity hindered determination of the mechanism of T–B lymphocyte interaction.

Starting in the late 1960s, several investigators employed simple haptens (antigenic determinants) coupled to carrier proteins as antigenic stimuli. Animals injected with hapten alone fail to produce antibodies while animals injected with haptens conjugated to a protein carrier synthesize hapten-specific antibody. If an animal is injected twice with the same hapten-carrier conjugate, a secondary, IgG, antibody response results. However, if the hapten is conjugated to a different carrier protein for the second injection, a primary, IgM, antihapten response occurs. This phenomenon is known as the carrier effect.

Mitchison and his laboratory (Boak et al., 1971; Mitchison, 1971a,b) relied on the carrier effect to investigate the role of T and B lymphocytes in the initiation of an antibody response. These investigators transferred lymphocytes from mice injected with the hapten 4-hydroxy-5-iodo-3-nitrophenacetyl (NIP) conjugated to ovalbumin (OVA) provided lymphocytes to irradiated, syngeneic mice. Some of the donor mice were also injected with the unrelated proteins chicken gamma globulin (CGG) or bovine serum albumin (BSA). Mitchison and coworkers injected irradiated recipient mice with one of the following hapten-carrier conjugates: NIP-OVA, NIP-CGG, or NIP-BSA and quantitated serum IgM and IgG antibodies specific for NIP.

Irradiated mice reconstituted with lymphocytes from mice primed with NIP-OVA synthesized an IgG antibody response when injected with NIP-OVA. Reconstitution of irradiated mice with lymphocytes derived from donors primed with NIP-OVA synthesized IgM antibodies to NIP when injected with NIP-CGG or NIP-BSA. Mice reconstituted with lymphocytes from donors primed with NIP-OVA and either CGG or BSA produced an intermediate (some IgG but primarily IgM) antibody response to NIP when subsequently injected with NIP-CGG or NIP-BSA.

These results confirmed cooperation between two types of lymphocytes: one specific for the hapten and the other specific for the carrier. Other observations identified the cells that bound the carrier determinants as thymus-derived helper T lymphocytes while B lymphocytes bound hapten and synthesized specific antibody. Finally, these results demonstrated a requirement that the hapten and carrier be physically linked to induce an optimal memory (IgG) antibody response.

Investigators now agree that both T and B lymphocytes are required to bind antigenic determinants and interact in order to induce an antibody response to T-dependent antigens. Several mechanisms to explain this requirement have been proposed:

- T lymphocytes provide a surface to which antigen binds, thus providing an increased concentration for B lymphocytes. In this view, antigen serves as a bridge linking receptors on the two lymphocytes.
- T lymphocytes secrete a factor that activates B lymphocytes.

- T and B lymphocytes physically interact, thus triggering activation of antibody synthesis and secretion.

All three mechanisms play a role in inducing antibody synthesis. Research during the 1970s and 1980s focused on isolation and characterization of soluble mediators secreted by T lymphocytes and other cells that activate B lymphocytes. Studies in the 1980s and 1990s demonstrated that interactions between cell surface molecules on T and B lymphocytes provide activation signals for B lymphocytes.

Soluble Factors (Cytokines) in B Lymphocyte Activation

In 1971, Richard Dutton and his colleagues at the University of California, San Diego, hypothesized that the requirement for T lymphocytes in the activation of antibody secretion by B lymphocytes could be replaced by a soluble factor. The results of two experiments published in the early 1970s proved this proposal correct.

In 1972, Marc Feldman and Antony Basten, working at the Walter and Eliza Hall Institute in Melbourne, Australia, cultured T and B lymphocytes in chambers separated by a cell impermeable membrane. Chamber 1 contained spleen cells derived from mice injected with dinitrophenylated flagella (DNP-Fla) from *S. adelaide* and served as a source of DNP-primed B lymphocytes. The second chamber contained activated T lymphocytes specific for the antigen keyhole limpet hemocyanin (KLH). Mice irradiated with a lethal dose of radiation and rescued by an injection of thymocytes were stimulated with KLH to produce a population of activated T lymphocytes.

Table 19.2 presents the results of this experiment. If DNP-Fla-stimulated spleen cells are cultured with

TABLE 19.2   Interaction of T and B Lymphocytes Across a Cell Impermeable Membrane

Lower compartment		Upper compartment		Anti-DNP response (AFC/culture ± s.e.)	
Cells	Antigen	Cells	Antigen	Experiment 1	Experiment 2
DNP-Fla-primed spleen cells	DNP-KLH	Nil	DNP-KLH	113 ± 16	0
DNP-Fla-primed spleen cells + ATC$_{KLH}$	DNP-KLH	Nil	DNP-KLH	1620 + 248	1474 ± 553
DNP-Fla-primed spleen cells	DNP-KLH	ATC$_{KLH}$	DNP-KLH	1260 ± 495	1090 ± 188
DNP-Fla-primed spleen cells	DNP-KLH	ATC$_{SRBC}$	SRBC + DNP-KLH	330 ± 179	186 ± 66

40×10^6 spleen cells from DNP-Fla-primed mice were cultured in the lower compartment of double flasks for 4 days. Ten micrograms per milliliter of DNP-KLH and 3×10^6 SRBC/ml was used as antigen. The volume of the cultures was 3 ml. 3×10^6 thymus cells activated to KLH (ATC$_{KLH}$) or SRBC (ATC$_{srbc}$) were added to either the top or the bottom compartment of double chambers. ATC$_{KLH}$ significantly restored the anti-DNP response. There was no significant difference between the responses with ATC present in the top or the bottom compartment. Each value represents the arithmetic mean ± the standard error (s.e.) of the mean of three cultures. Four other experiments have yielded similar results, whether these were performed in SERF positive or negative media. DNP, dinitrophenyl; DNP-Fla, dinitrophenylated flagella; DNP-KLH, dinitrophenylated keyhole limpet hemocyanin; SRBC, sheep erythrocytes; AFC, antibody-forming cells.
From Feldman and Basten, 1972.

DNP-KLH in the absence of activated T lymphocytes, only minimal numbers of antibody-forming lymphocytes to DNP are detected in the cultures (line 1). When both T and B lymphocytes are incubated with DNP-KLH, the number of antibody-forming cells increased greater than 10-fold whether the two cell types were separated by a cell impermeable membrane (line 3) or allowed to physically interact (line 2). A minimal number of antibody-forming cells were detected if the B lymphocytes were incubated with DNP-KLH in the presence of T lymphocytes that had been activated to an unrelated antigen such as SRBC (line 4). These results support a T lymphocyte-derived soluble factor that is involved in stimulating B lymphocytes.

Anneliese Schimpl and Eberhard Wecker, working at the University of Würzberg, Germany, provided additional evidence of a factor that could replace T lymphocytes in the activation of antibody synthesis (1972). Mouse spleen cells cultured with SRBC develop antibody-forming lymphocytes detectable by a hemolytic plaque assay. Treatment of these cultures with an antibody to T lymphocytes decreases the number of these antibody-forming B lymphocytes. Schimpl and Wecker corrected this decrease by adding a supernatant from mixed lymphocyte cultures. The active factor in the supernatant was produced by T lymphocytes since treatment of the allogeneic lymphocytes with an antibody to T lymphocytes plus complement decreased the activity of the supernatant. This T lymphocyte replacing factor could also help B lymphocytes from athymic, nude mice develop an anti-SRBC response.

The T lymphocyte replacing factors described in these studies were most likely a mixture of a number of molecules derived from both T lymphocytes and macrophages. Identification of unique T lymphocyte-derived factors that could activate B lymphocytes was reported in 1982. Maureen Howard and her colleagues at the National Institute of Allergy and Infectious Diseases in Bethesda, Maryland, as well as Susan Swain and Richard Dutton (Swain and Dutton, 1982) at the University of California, San Diego, isolated and partially characterized supernatants from cultures of T lymphocytes. These factors, termed B cell growth factor (BCGF), serve as activators of B lymphocyte proliferation.

The general design of the experiments performed by the two groups was similar. Howard and her colleagues stimulated cultures of a thymoma with phorbol myristate acetate, a substance known to stimulate T lymphocytes. Swain and Dutton used a T lymphocyte line that was specific for a foreign histocompatibility antigen. In both cases, these culture supernatants were added to cultures of B lymphocytes. Activity of the factors was measured by synthesis of DNA and proliferation of the B lymphocytes.

During the ensuing years, investigators described a large number of additional factors that are now termed cytokines involved in B lymphocyte activation. The cytokines displayed a variety of functions, including B cell differentiation (BCDF), B cell stimulation (BSF), and BCGF. Several cytokines have been cloned to purity. Most immunology resources contain tables listing the various cytokines (interleukins-IL) and their activity. Those that significantly activate B lymphocytes and activate antibody production include IL-4 (originally known as BCGF-1 and BSF-1), IL-5 (BCGF-2), IL-6 (BSF-2 and BCDF), and IL-13. Additional information on the discovery of these and other cytokines is presented in Chapter 25.

Cytokines function by binding cell surface receptors that transmit an intracellular signal to the nucleus. One method to detect these receptors is to produce antibodies to cell surface molecules and determine whether the antibodies block the binding of the cytokine to that cell. A second method is to determine whether antibody bound to the receptor alters the functioning of the cell. In the case of B lymphocytes, these studies measured the initiation of mitosis and/or the synthesis of antibody.

Hidetaka Yakura and colleagues, working at the Asahikawa Medical College in Japan and the Memorial Sloan Kettering Cancer Center in New York, developed a monoclonal antibody that bound a cell surface antigen (Lyb-2) found on mouse B lymphocytes but not on T lymphocytes (1986). Yakura and colleagues concluded that this antibody identified the receptor for BSF based on three observations:

- addition of the monoclonal antibody to cultures of mouse B lymphocytes along with BCGF or interleukin-1 activated the cells to proliferate,
- addition of the monoclonal antibody to B lymphocytes along with BSF failed to induce proliferation, and
- treatment of B lymphocytes with the monoclonal antibody blocked the adsorption of BSF activity from T lymphocyte supernatants.

Using a similar strategy, Edward Clark and Jeffrey Ledbetter (1986) at the University of Washington and Oncogen Corporation, Seattle, Washington, developed two monoclonal antibodies that reacted only against human B lymphocytes. One monoclonal antibody identified a 50-kDa, B lymphocyte-specific molecule (Bp50) while the second identified a 35-kDa molecule (Bp35). They used these two antibodies to stimulate resting B lymphocytes from human tonsils or peripheral blood and compared their results to the treatment of B lymphocyte with an antibody to the BCR.

Treatment of resting B lymphocytes with the antibody to Bp35 activated these cells to enlarge and to synthesize RNA but failed to stimulate the synthesis of DNA. This result is similar to that seen when these B lymphocytes are stimulated with antibody to the BCR or with

BSF. Treatment of resting B lymphocytes with antibody to Bp50 failed to activate the cells; however, treatment of activated B lymphocytes (i.e., ones that had been treated with BSF, antibody to Bp35, or antibody to the BCR) with antibody to Bp50 stimulated these lymphocytes to finish the cell cycle. This latter action is similar to what is observed when activated B lymphocytes are stimulated with BCGF.

Clark and Ledbetter concluded that "the Bp35 and Bp50 surface molecules function in the regulatory control of B-cell activation and progression through the cell cycle." They postulate that this control may involve interaction of B lymphocytes with soluble factors (cytokines) or through cell-to-cell contacts with T lymphocytes.

Cell-to-Cell Interaction in Activation of Antibody Formation

Morphological observations of lymphoid tissue during the initiation of an antibody response revealed physical interactions between different lymphocytes. Both T and B lymphocytes have been identified in these conjugates. The appearance of these interactions led some immunologists to describe them as synapses similar to those seen in the central nervous system (Figure 19.3).

The 50-kDa molecule present on B lymphocytes but not on T lymphocytes identified by the monoclonal antibody produced by Clark and Ledbetter has been further characterized. By the late 1980s, the molecule identified by this monoclonal antibody (Bp50) had been renamed CD40, and several groups demonstrated that this molecule was involved in B lymphocyte activation. Antibodies specific for CD40 fail to stimulate proliferation of B lymphocytes when used alone but cooperate with other B lymphocyte-specific stimuli, including antibodies to the BCR or to another B lymphocyte-specific molecule, CD20, to induce mitosis. Optimal activation occurred in these studies when lymphocytes were first treated with antibody to the BCR followed by treatment with antibody to CD40. This sequence suggested that signals received through the CD40 molecule might be important in clonal expansion, antibody production, isotype switching, and the development of memory B lymphocytes.

The identification of CD40 as an essential molecule in the stimulation of B lymphocytes allowed studies of the ligand on T lymphocytes that might bind CD40. Randolph Noelle and coworkers at Dartmouth Medical School, Hanover, New Hampshire, solubilized T helper lymphocyte membranes and identified a 39-kDa glycoprotein that bound CD40 on B lymphocytes and transduced a signal for antibody synthesis (Noelle et al., 1992). For several years this ligand was known only as CD40L; it is now named CD154.

Patients with a rare congenital immunodeficiency disease, hyper-IgM syndrome, provided proof that the interaction between CD40 and CD154 is required for the typical antibody response. Alejandro Aruffo, working at the Bristol-Myers Squibb Pharmaceutical Research Institute and the University of Washington in Seattle, collaborated with other investigators to study patients with this rare immunodeficiency disease (Aruffo et al., 1993). Patients with hyper-IgM syndrome possess B and T lymphocytes within normally established reference ranges. Serum IgM levels in these individuals are often elevated while the concentrations of other classes of immunoglobulin, particularly IgG and IgA, are severely depressed. B lymphocytes from patients with hyper-IgM syndrome express functional CD40; however, T lymphocytes from these same individuals fail to bind CD40 in vitro. Genetic analysis of T lymphocytes from patients with this syndrome demonstrates a mutation in the gene coding for a T lymphocyte-specific molecule, gp39. This molecule is the ligand for CD40 and is now named CD154. These data suggest that the defect in hyper-IgM syndrome is the failure of T lymphocytes to provide a signal to activated B lymphocytes.

These data confirm that B lymphocyte activation requires interactions with a T lymphocyte and follows a specific sequence of events. Initially, antigen binds specific BCRs, which is followed by interaction of CD40 on B lymphocytes with its ligand, CD154 on T lymphocytes. This two-signal sequence elicits an optimal antibody response but also provides a pathway by which the response can be regulated in situations where it might become pathogenic such as in autoimmune diseases.

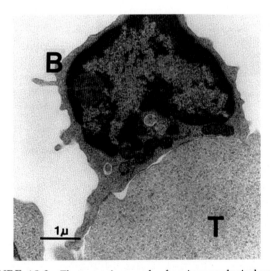

FIGURE 19.3 Electron micrograph of an immunological synapse between a B and T lymphocyte (http://users.rcn.com/jkimball.ma.ult ranet/BiologyPages/U/Uhr.gif).

ISOTYPE SWITCHING

A Single B Lymphocyte Produces Multiple Isotypes

The discovery of the five isotypes of antibody (Chapter 11) led to questions about the cellular source of these molecules. While immunologists agree on the structural relationship of the isotypes, the genetics of immunoglobulin production was yet to be discovered. Investigators proposed two competing hypotheses:

1. each isotype is synthesized by separate B lymphocytes, or
2. a single B lymphocyte changes or switches the isotype it produces at different times during the response.

The initial question was whether the plasma cells that produced IgG antibodies also were responsible for IgM production. To answer this question Gus Nossal and his colleagues (1964) determined if isolated lymphocytes in microdrops produced antibody of more than one isotype. They used this technique previously to determine that a given cell produced antibodies of only one specificity (Chapter 7).

Nossal's group injected rats with *S. adelaide* flagella to induce both primary and secondary antibody responses. At intervals, they isolated lymphocytes from the popliteal lymph nodes and separated antibody-forming lymphocytes by agglutination with flagella. Solitary lymphocytes in microdrops were mechanically disrupted to release their antibody. The identification of the isotype of this antibody was determined by its sensitivity to a rabbit antibody specific for rat IgG immunoglobulin or to 2-mercaptoethanol (2-ME), a disulfide reducing agent. IgM antibody is sensitive to treatment with 2-ME while IgG antibody is resistant to 2-ME treatment. The results demonstrated that most cells produce only one isotype of antibodies; however, 17 of 144 cells tested produced both IgM and IgG. The authors concluded that "the results suggested that many cells or cell clones go through a sequence whereby each forms first 19S (IgM) and later 7S (IgG) antibody with identical combining sites."

The sequential synthesis of IgM followed by IgG by the same B lymphocyte was demonstrated by experiments performed by Max Cooper's group at the University of Alabama, Birmingham (Kincade et al., 1970). Chickens possess a bursa of Fabricius, a lymphoepithelial organ responsible for the development of B lymphocytes (Chapter 10). The bursa can be surgically removed, resulting in a deficiency of B lymphocytes that is reflected by decreased levels of immunoglobulin. Previous studies had shown a sequential development of IgM and IgG synthesis; that is, chickens bursectomized at hatching produced IgM antibodies but no IgG when injected with antigen as adults while bursectomy performed on day

19 of incubation (2 days before hatching) eliminated the subsequent production of both IgM and IgG antibodies.

Injection of chicken embryos on the 13th day of incubation with antibodies to IgM inhibits the maturation of B lymphocytes and results in the elimination of IgM-containing lymphocytes in the bursa on days 16 and 19 of incubation. Treatment of chicken embryos with antibody to IgM on day 13 of incubation followed by bursectomy at hatching resulted in suppressed synthesis of both IgG and IgM. These results suggest that "IgG-producing cells arise exclusively from cells that previously synthesized IgM."

Structural studies of antibodies showed that the isotype of an immunoglobulin molecule is determined by the amino acid sequence in the constant region of the heavy chain (Chapter 11). This diversity is reflected in the organization of the gene segments responsible for coding for the immunoglobulins (Chapter 18). Immunologists now agree that an individual B lymphocyte may produce any of the immunoglobulin isotypes, thus allowing the adaptive immune system to produce antibodies possessing different effector functions, all of which have the identical antigenic specificity. These results led to the question: What triggers the B lymphocyte to switch from synthesizing one isotype to another?

Signals for Isotype Switching

B lymphocytes express BCRs on their membranes prior to interaction with antigen; these receptors are IgM and IgD. On any given B lymphocyte, the binding sites (V regions) of these receptors are identical while the constant regions are different. Upon activation by antigen, the B lymphocyte synthesizes and secretes specific antibody of the IgM isotype during the primary response. Secondary responses are characterized by a genetic switch, leading to the synthesis and secretion of antibodies of one or more of the other isotypes, IgG, IgA, or IgE. The signal for this switch involves interaction of the B lymphocyte with an activated T lymphocyte (most likely through binding of CD40 with CD154) as well as binding of cytokines. The final product of any B lymphocyte is a balance of positive and negative signals received from environmental cytokines and from subpopulations of CD4[+] T lymphocytes.

Peter Isakson and coworkers at the University of Texas Health Science Center at Dallas provided one of the initial reports of the role of a soluble factor (cytokine) in isotype switching in 1982. These investigators stimulated mouse B lymphocytes with lipopolysaccharide (LPS) from *Salmonella typhosa*. LPS induces B lymphocytes to proliferate and to secrete immunoglobulin primarily of the IgM isotype. Addition of supernatants from T lymphocyte cultures to these B lymphocytes induced a switch to IgG immunoglobulin. The factor present in the T lymphocyte supernatants was different from other T lymphocyte factors, including Il-1, Il-2, T cell-replacing factor, colony-stimulating factor, macrophage-activating factor, or immune interferon. The authors term the factor B cell differentiation factor; subsequent studies have shown this factor to be Il-4.

Il-4 also enhances the synthesis and secretion of IgE immunoglobulin from both mouse and human B lymphocytes. The stimulus to switch to IgG or IgE most likely involves the presence of other cytokines in the environment (interferon-γ inhibits IgE production in cultures of mouse lymphocytes) as well as the presence of subpopulations of CD4+ T lymphocytes (Chapter 23).

Similar studies using in vitro systems provided evidence for other cytokines in the switch from IgM to synthesis and secretion of other isotypes (Chapter 25). Robert Coffman and colleagues at the DNAX Research Institute in Palo Alto, California, reported in 1989 that transforming growth factor β (TGF-β) enhanced the production of IgA by mouse lymphocytes stimulated in vitro by LPS from *S. typhosa*. The addition of Il-2 and Il-5 to these cultures with TGF-β enhanced IgA production to an even greater extent. Simultaneously, TGF-β inhibited the secretion of other immunoglobulin isotypes in these cultures, including IgG and IgM.

CONCLUSION

Many immunologists working around the world confirmed that the activation of B lymphocytes resulted in the production of antibodies. Prior to the characterization of lymphoid cells into discrete B and T populations, several immunochemists identified the presence of different isotypes of antibody. The cellular source of these different antibodies and their relationship to each other remained unknown until immunoglobulins were sequenced and their structure was unveiled (Chapter 11).

In the mid-1960s, several groups revealed that two major types of lymphocytes existed: antibody-forming B lymphocytes and T lymphocytes that did not synthesize antibodies but proved prominent in cell-mediated immunity. Investigators assigned a helper function for antibody production to T lymphocytes (Chapter 12). Realization that antibody formation requires lymphocyte-to-lymphocyte interaction led to the development of the two-signal hypothesis of B lymphocyte activation by Bretscher and Cohn. This hypothesis was supported by the identification of receptors on B and T lymphocytes that interacted during B lymphocyte proliferation and antibody synthesis and by the isolation and characterization of T lymphocyte-derived soluble factors (cytokines) that stimulate B lymphocyte proliferation and gene expression (Chapter 25).

A third line of investigation supported that B lymphocyte activation resulted in the synthesis and secretion of antibodies of different isotypes. Compelling evidence to confirm the two-signal hypothesis derived from

- the unraveling of the genetic mechanisms involved in the generation of antibody diversity during B lymphocyte maturation (Chapter 17); and
- observations from studies of experimentally induced and naturally occurring immunodeficiency states.

The experiments that illuminated B lymphocyte activation and subsequent isotype switching led to the development of monoclonal antibodies that serve as experimental reagents and as potential immunotherapeutics.

References

Aruffo, A., Farrington, M., Hollenbaugh, D., Li, X., Milstovich, A., Nonoyama, D., Bajorath, J., Grosmaire, L.S., Stenkamp, R., Neubauer, M., Roberts, R.L., Noelle, R.J., Ledbetter, J.A., Francke, U., Ochs, H., 1993. The CD40 ligand, gp39, is defective in activated T cells from patients with X-linked hyper-IgM syndrome. Cell 72, 291–300.

Boak, J.L., Mitchison, N.A., Pattisson, P.H., 1971. The carrier effect in the secondary response to hapten-protein conjugates. III. The anatomical distribution of helper cells and antibody-forming-cell-precursors. Eur. J. Immunol. 1, 63–65.

Bretscher, P.A., Cohn, M., 1968. Minimal model for the mechanism of antibody induction and paralysis by antigen. Nature 220, 444–448.

Bretscher, P.A., Cohn, M., 1970. A theory of self-nonself discrimination. Science 169, 1042–1049.

Campbell, K.S., Cambier, J.C., 1990. B lymphocyte antigen receptors (mIg) are non-covalently associated with a disulfide linked, inducibly phosphorylated glycoprotein complex. EMBO J. 9, 441–448.

Clark, E.A., Ledbetter, J.A., 1986. Activation of human B cells mediated through two distinct cell surface differentiation antigens, Bp35 and Bp50. Proc. Nat. Acad. Sci. U.S.A. 83, 4494–4498.

Coffman, R.L., Lebman, D.A., Shrader, B., 1989. Transforming growth factor β specifically enhances IgA production by lipopolysaccharide-stimulated murine B lymphocytes. J. Exp. Med. 170, 1039–1044.

Coutinho, A., Möller, G., 1973. B cell mitogenic properties of thymus-independent antigens. Nat. New. Biol. 245, 12–14.

Dutton, R.W., Falkoff, R., Hirst, J.A., Hoffman, M., Kappler, J.W., Kettman, J.R., Lesley, J.F., Vann, D., 1971. Is there evidence for a non-antigen specific diffusible chemical mediator from the thymus-derived cell in the initiation of the immune response? Prog. Immunol. 1, 355–368.

Feldmann, M., Basten, A., 1971. The relationship between antigenic structure and the requirement for thymus-derived cells in the immune response. J. Exp. Med. 134, 103–119.

Feldmann, M., Basten, A., 1972. Specific collaboration between T and B lymphocytes across a cell impermeable membrane in vitro. Nat. New. Biol. 237, 13–15.

Hombach, J., Lottspeich, F., Reth, M., 1990. Identification of the genes encoding the IgM-α and Ig-β components of the IgM antigen receptor complex by amino-terminal sequencing. Eur. J. Immunol. 20, 2795–2799.

Howard, M., Farrar, J., Hilfiker, M., Johnson, B., Takatsu, K., Hamaoka, T., Paul, W.E., 1982. Identification of a T cell derived B cell growth factor distinct from interleukin 2. J. Exp. Med. 155, 914–923.

Isakson, P.C., Puré, E., Vitetta, E.S., Krammer, P.H., 1982. T cell-derived B cell differentiation factor(s). Effect on the isotype switch of murine B cells. J. Exp. Med. 155, 734–738.

Kincade, P.W., Lawton, A.R., Bockman, D.E., Cooper, M.D., 1970. Suppression of immunoglobulin G synthesis as a result of antibody-mediated suppression of immunoglobulin M synthesis in chickens. Proc. Nat. Acad. Sci. U.S.A. 67, 1918–1925.

Lederberg, J., 1959. Genes and antibodies. Science 129, 1649–1653.

Mitchison, N.A., 1971a. The carrier effect in the secondary response to hapten-carrier conjugates. I. Measurement of the effect with transferred cells and objections to the local environment hypothesis. Eur. J. Immunol. 1, 10–17.

Mitchison, N.A., 1971b. The carrier effect in the secondary response to hapten-carrier conjugates. II. Cellular cooperation. Eur. J. Immunol. 1, 18–27.

Noelle, R.J., Roy, M., Shepherd, D.M., Stamenkovic, I., Ledbetter, J.A., Aruffio, A., 1992. A 39-kDa protein on activated helper T cells binds CD40 and transduces the signal for cognate activation of B cells. Proc. Nat. Acad. Sci. U.S.A. 89, 6550–6554.

Nossal, G.J.V., Szenberg, A., Ada, G.L., Austin, C.M., 1964. Single cell studies on 19S antibody production. J. Exp. Med. 119, 485–502.

Schimpl, A., Wecker, E., 1972. Replacement of T-cell function by a T-cell product. Nat. New. Biol. 237, 15–17.

Swain, S.L., Dutton, R.W., 1982. Production of a B cell growth-promoting activity, (DL) BCGF, from a cloned T cell line and its assay on the BCL1 B cell tumor. J. Exp. Med. 156, 1821–1834.

Talmage, D.W., 1959. Immunological specificity. Science 129, 1643–1648.

van Noesel, C.J.M., Borst, J., De Vries, E.F.R., van Lier, R.A.W., 1990. Identification of two distinct phosphoproteins as components of the human B cell antigen receptor complex. Eur. J. Immunol. 20, 2789–2793.

Yakura, H., Kawabata, I., Ashida, T., Shen, F.W., Katagiri, M., 1986. A role for Lyb-2 in B cell activation mediated by a B cell stimulatory factor. J. Immunol. 137, 1475–1481.

TIME LINE

1957	F. Macfarlane Burnet presents the clonal selection theory of antibody formation
1959	Joshua Lederberg proposes that antigen activates antibody-forming cells by binding to cell surface receptors
1964	Gus Nossal and colleagues demonstrate that a single cell can produce both IgM and IgG
1968	Peter Bretscher and Melvin Cohn propose a two-signal model for B cell activation
1970	Max Cooper's group reports that B cells produce IgM prior to producing IgG
1971	Avrion Mitchison investigates the carrier effect and publishes results supporting the two-signal model of B cell activation
1971	Marc Feldman and Antony Basten conclude that both T and B lymphocytes bind antigenic determinants during induction of antibody responses
1973	Marc Feldman and Antony Basten and Anneliese Schimpl and Eberhard Wecker demonstrate that soluble factors can replace T lymphocytes in B lymphocyte activation
1982	Maureen Howard and colleagues isolate B cell stimulating factor
1982	Susan Swain and Richard Dutton isolate B cell growth factor
1986	Hidetaka Yakura and colleagues and Edward Clark and Jeffrey Ledbetter develop monoclonal antibodies for B cell antigen-specific receptors identifying CD40
1990	Kerry Campbell and John Cambier describe the B cell-specific signaling molecules, CD79a and CD79b
1992	Randolph Noell and colleagues identify the CD40 ligand (CD154)

20

Activation of T Lymphocytes
and MHC Restriction

INTRODUCTION

T lymphocytes express a cell surface receptor, the T cell receptor (TCR), that binds a single antigen. TCRs recognize short linear peptides, 8 to 12 amino acids, that are derived from protein antigens. By contrast, antigen-specific receptors on B lymphocytes recognize three-dimensional configurations of antigens. Peptides are presented to T lymphocytes by cells expressing molecules coded for by the major histocompatibility complex (MHC) of the animal. Two mechanisms of antigen presentation have evolved. Peptides such as those produced by malignantly transformed or virally infected cells associate with class I histocompatibility molecules and are recognized by CD8+ T lymphocytes while peptides, including those from extracellular bacteria, fungi, and protozoal parasites, associate with class II histocompatibility molecules and are recognized by CD4+ T lymphocytes.

T lymphocytes, like B lymphocytes, require two signals to be activated. Activation is initiated when a T lymphocyte recognizes and binds antigen through its TCR. Binding of antigen is necessary but insufficient to initiate the sequence of intracellular events resulting in an activated lymphocyte. A second, costimulatory signal provided by the interaction of cell-surface molecules on T lymphocytes and the antigen-presenting cell (APC) is required for full activation. Once activated, T lymphocytes proliferate to produce a clone of identical antigen-specific T lymphocytes. In addition, the signals provided by binding antigen and costimulatory molecules induce gene transcription, leading to synthesis and secretion of cytokines and chemokines.

T lymphocytes are divided into two populations based on the expression of cell surface markers defined as CD4 and CD8 (Chapter 23). CD8+ T lymphocytes are classically referred to as cytotoxic cells and are responsible for killing virally infected and malignantly transformed somatic cells. CD4+ T lymphocytes are considered helper cells; immunologists currently divide them into at least five subpopulations (T_H1, T_H2, T_H17, T_{FH}, and T_{REG}) that perform an array of different

A Historical Perspective on Evidence-Based Immunology
http://dx.doi.org/10.1016/B978-0-12-398381-7.00020-4

functions (Chapters 23, 24, and 27) in the adaptive immune response, including

- synthesis and secretion of cytokines and chemokines that induce inflammation (T_H17);
- provision of second signals (help) to antibody-producing B lymphocytes (T_H2 and T_{FH});
- provision of second signals (help) to cytotoxic T lymphocytes (T_H1); and
- regulation of B lymphocytes and other T lymphocytes (T_{REG}).

Kevin Lafferty and A.J. Cunningham, working at the John Curtin School of Medical Research in Canberra, Australia, proposed in 1975 that two signals are required to activate T lymphocytes. Studies presented in this chapter confirm the validity of this hypothesis and identify the cell surface molecules responsible for these activation signals. During the course of these investigations, Rolf Zinkernagel and Peter Doherty, also of the John Curtin School of Medical Research, demonstrated that T lymphocytes recognize antigen associated with molecules coded for by an individual's MHC genes. The story presented in this chapter depends on information found in other parts of this book, including the structure and function of histocompatibility molecules (Chapter 16), the molecular makeup of the TCR (Chapter 17), and the genetic mechanisms involved in generating immunological diversity (Chapter 18). Mechanisms that prevent T lymphocytes from being activated by self are covered in Chapter 22.

EXPERIMENTAL APPROACHES TO MEASURE T LYMPHOCYTE ACTIVATION

Several in vitro procedures are used to determine T lymphocyte activation, including cell proliferation, provision of help for B and T lymphocytes, synthesis and secretion of soluble factors (cytokines and chemokines), and generation of cellular cytotoxicity.

Proliferation of T lymphocytes is measured following stimulation by either specific antigen or a nonspecific mitogen such as phytohemagglutinin. Investigators culture T lymphocytes with one of these stimuli for 3–5 days. After this culture period lymphocytes can be evaluated histologically for the presence of mitotic figures. Alternatively, 18–24 h prior to culture termination, a radiolabeled precursor of DNA, usually ^{3}H-thymidine, is added to the experiment. Cells are harvested, and the amount of radioisotope is incorporated by the lymphocytes quantitated.

To determine T lymphocyte helper function, investigators designed in vitro assays in which different lymphocyte populations could be cocultured. One experimental design to detect T helper activity for

antibody synthesis involves adding various numbers of T lymphocytes to cultures of B lymphocytes plus antigen. Several days later the amount of antibody in the culture supernatants is measured. For most antigens, B lymphocytes stimulated by antigen in the absence of T lymphocytes fail to secrete any antibody. The amount of antibody present in cultures supplemented with T lymphocytes provides a measure of the helper activity of those lymphocytes.

T lymphocytes stimulated in vitro by specific antigens or mitogens release cytokines and/or chemokines into the tissue culture medium. The amount of these soluble factors can be quantitated using several different assay systems, including immunodiffusion, radioimmunoassay, and enzyme-linked immunosorbent assay (ELISA). Comparison of stimulated and control cultures provides a measure of activation of the T lymphocytes.

Generation of cytotoxic T lymphocytes requires in vitro culture of lymphocytes from one animal (the responder) with inactivated lymphocytes or other cells from a genetically dissimilar animal (the target). Following culture for several days, the viable lymphocytes are harvested and recultured with target cells that have been radiolabeled with ^{51}Cr. Interaction of the responder lymphocytes with target cells causes release of the radioisotope, thus providing a semiquantitative measure of the amount of cytotoxicity generated.

THE TWO-SIGNAL HYPOTHESIS OF T LYMPHOCYTE ACTIVATION

As presented in Chapter 19, Peter Bretscher and Melvin Cohn at the Salk Institute for Biological Studies in San Diego, California (1968, 1970), initially theorized that activation of antigen-sensitive cells required two signals. While they focused on activation of antibody-forming B lymphocytes, Lafferty and Cunningham extended this concept to T lymphocytes in 1975, during their studies of allogeneic interactions, including

- host versus graft reactions as exemplified by rejection of foreign (allogeneic) grafts;
- graft versus host reactions (a response induced by injecting viable lymphocytes into an immunoincompetent allogeneic host); and
- mixed lymphocyte responses (an in vitro response involving the culturing of lymphocytes from two individuals or strains that express different genes coding for histocompatibility antigens).

The cells responsible for all three of these responses are thymus-dependent and hence T lymphocytes. Initially, it was thought that T lymphocytes could be activated in these responses by interacting with a foreign

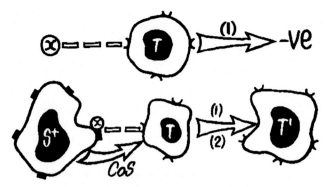

FIGURE 20.1 Diagrammatic representation of the two-signal model of T cell activation. Binding of antigen to the T cell receptor (top) fails to activate the cell. In the bottom diagram, a stimulator (S) cell is required to present the antigen to the potentially responsive T cell. This stimulator cell also produces costimulator factors that enhance activation of the T cell. *From Lafferty et al. (1983).*

(histocompatibility) antigen. However, two observations made this one-signal hypothesis untenable:

- Activation of T lymphocytes failed to occur if the cells possessing the foreign antigen were nonviable, even though the dead cells still expressed histocompatibility antigen on their surface.
- Not all foreign cells induced a response. Fibroblasts, erythrocytes, and platelets failed to stimulate a proliferative response when cultured with foreign lymphocytes.

The conclusion from these observations was that the foreign stimulating cell provided some sort of information in addition to the antigen. The original representation of the two-signal hypothesis is presented in Figure 20.1. In this model antigen alone cannot activate the T lymphocyte. A stimulator (S) cell is required to present the antigen to the potentially responsive T lymphocyte. This stimulator cell also produces costimulator factors that enhance this activation.

While flawed, this model provided a concept that guided further experimentation.

SIGNAL 1: TCR RECOGNITION

Paul Ehrlich proposed in 1900 that antibody-forming cells expressed "side chains" by which antigen was recognized. The validity of this proposal was not fully appreciated for more than 60 years. By then two functional populations of antigen-reactive lymphocytes had been described. As reviewed in Chapter 17, the antigen-specific receptor for B lymphocytes is an immunoglobulin, as demonstrated by

- staining of the surface of B lymphocytes with fluorescein-labeled antibodies to immunoglobulin; and
- induction of B lymphocyte proliferation by treatment with antibody specific for IgM.

These results were obtained simultaneously with characterization of separate B and T lymphocyte populations. Several investigators presented parallel data showing that T lymphocytes also possessed cell surface immunoglobulins that acted as antigen-specific receptors. Some of these reports described a new isotype of T lymphocyte-associated immunoglobulin named IgT or IgX.

The presence of immunoglobulin as the TCR made sense in a certain parsimonious way. However, two experiments argued against the presence of immunoglobulin on T lymphocytes:

- immunoglobulin-like molecules could not be detected on the surface of T lymphocytes following stringent purification methods to exclude B lymphocytes; and
- antibodies to immunoglobulin failed to block the interaction between antigen and T lymphocytes.

In the early 1970s, investigators observed that interactions between T lymphocytes and other cells in the adaptive immune response require that the two cells be from animals that shared histocompatibility antigens. Berenice Kindred at the University of Konstanz, Germany, and Donald Shreffler from the University of Michigan collaborated to demonstrate in 1972 that interactions between T and B lymphocytes during the initiation of antibody production are only successful if the lymphocytes are histocompatible. Similarly, Rolf Zinkernagel and Peter Doherty demonstrated in 1974 that the interaction between cytotoxic T lymphocytes and virally infected fibroblasts required that the lymphocytes and fibroblasts be histocompatible. These results suggested that T lymphocytes, unlike B lymphocytes, recognize antigen along with another cell surface protein and led to the concept of MHC restriction—T lymphocytes only recognize antigen presented to them by molecules coded for by the histocompatibility genes of that organism.

MHC RESTRICTION

In 1965, Elizabeth Leuchars and coworkers at the Chester Beatty Research Institute in London demonstrated that grafts of thymus tissues restored immune function to thymectomized mice only if the donor and recipient shared some or all histocompatibility antigens. Similar results were presented by Alan Aisenberg from Harvard University Boston, Massachusetts, in 1970. These investigators hypothesized that the failure to reconstitute thymectomized mice was due to rejection of the allogeneic grafts by the host although subsequent interpretation of these results points to a requirement for histocompatibility even during T lymphocyte maturation.

Peter Gorer (1907–1961) initially described histocompatibility antigens in inbred mice in the 1930s. Gorer received his medical degree from Guy's Hospital in London and pursued a career that focused on the role of histocompatibility antigens in the rejection of tumor transplants (Chapter 36). In 1936, Gorer injected rabbits with erythrocytes from several inbred strains of mice; the resulting antibodies identified three antigens, termed I, II, and III, which were differentially distributed in the strains. When Gorer transplanted tumors from mice expressing antigen II into mice lacking this antigen, the tumor was rapidly rejected, and the serum of the recipient mouse possessed antibodies to antigen II (Gorer, 1937).

At the same time that Gorer identified antigen II, George D. Snell at the Jackson Memorial Laboratory, Bar Harbor, Maine, investigated tumor resistance genes that he termed histocompatibility genes. In 1948, Gorer and Snell collaborated to characterize the gene coding for antigen II; they named this gene and the antigen for which it codes H-2 (histocompatibility-2).

Gorer demonstrated that antitumor responses are specific for H-2 antigens, thereby concluding that H-2 antigens are involved in inducing tumor rejection (Gorer, 1937). Subsequent studies showed that antigens coded for by H-2 genes also serve as targets for the rejection of foreign tissue grafts. Other investigators defined the genetic region containing the H-2 gene and termed it the MHC.

Kindred and Schreffler in 1972 performed experiments that indicated that MHC-coded molecules play a role in immune responses other than graft and tumor rejection. Nude mice lack a thymus due to a gene mutation and therefore are immunodeficient from birth. They consequently serve as an experimental model in investigations on the role of the thymus in the development of T lymphocytes (Chapter 9). Nude mice reconstituted with syngeneic thymocytes and injected with sheep erythrocytes or bacteriophage T4 produce antibodies. However, nude mice reconstituted with allogeneic thymus cells failed to produce any antibodies when injected. A conclusion of these studies was that "the H-2 complex must play an active role in an enduring cooperation between bone marrow-derived (B) cells and thymus-derived (T) cells."

APCs and T Lymphocytes

Optimal antibody responses against many antigens require collaboration between a minimum of three cell types: T lymphocytes, B lymphocytes, and an APC. The APC is usually represented as a macrophage (see Chapter 14) or a dendritic cell (Chapter 29). At the time Kindred and Shreffler reported their observations, the mechanism underlying this collaboration was unknown. Some investigators hypothesized the lymphocytes that interact in the initiation of the antibody response recognize both antigen and self-histocompatibility molecules.

David Katz, working in the laboratory of Baruj Benacceraf at Harvard Medical School, confirmed that cellular interactions in the immune response require histocompatible lymphocytes (Katz et al., 1973). Katz and his colleagues studied T–B lymphocyte cooperation both in vivo, using an adoptive transfer system, and in vitro, using a culture system permitting the initiation of a primary antibody response (Chapter 13). Figure 20.2 presents the experimental protocol used in these in vivo studies.

This experimental protocol is based on the carrier-hapten effect where T lymphocytes respond to carrier (BGG or KLH) while B lymphocytes respond to hapten (DNP). Katz and coworkers injected mice of one inbred strain (strain A) with bovine gamma globulin (BGG) to induce a primary response. Two to 4 months later lymphocytes from the spleens of these mice, which contain T lymphocytes specific for BGG, were transferred to $(A \times B)$ F_1 hybrids. Twenty-four hours later recipient mice received a sublethal dose of irradiation followed by an injection of B lymphocytes derived from the spleens of strain A or strain B mice. The donors of the B lymphocytes had been injected with the hapten-carrier conjugate DNP-KLH (dinitrophenol linked to keyhole limpet hemocyanin).

In this protocol, the F_1 hybrids serve as in vivo "test tubes" containing T lymphocytes from A strain mice specific for BGG and B lymphocytes from either A or B strain mice that are specific for DNP. The recipients were injected with DNP-BGG and bled 7 days later to measure antibodies specific for DNP.

In control experiments, mixing strain A BGG primed cells (source of T lymphocytes) with strain A DNP-KLH primed B lymphocytes in a strain A recipient produced a significant antibody response to DNP. When $(A \times B)$ F_1 hybrids were used as the recipient, optimal antibody to DNP was formed only when the B and T lymphocytes were from the same parental strain (either A or B). As described by the authors, "very good T–B cell cooperative interactions were observed to occur between T and B lymphocyte populations derived from syngeneic donors, whereas no cooperative response was obtained when T cells were derived from one parental strain and B cells from the other."

Parallel in vitro studies employed T lymphocytes from mice injected with BGG or KLH and B lymphocytes from mice injected with DNP. Katz and his colleagues incubated these lymphocytes with DNP-BGG in vitro. Several days later they quantitated the number of lymphocytes producing antibody specific for DNP using a hemolytic plaque assay. Optimal antibody responses required the T and B lymphocytes be syngeneic. Allogeneic lymphocytes did not efficiently cooperate in the production of antibodies. The authors conclude that "the

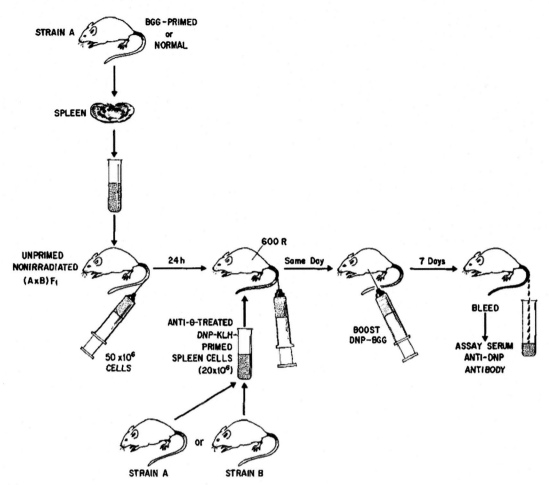

FIGURE 20.2 Protocol used by Katz et al. (1973) to study the requirement for histocompatibility of T cells and B cells in an antibody response.

gene(s) that conditions the capability for physiologic T–B cell cooperation must be shared in common by the respective cell types" and "this gene (or genes) belongs to the major histocompatibility system of the mouse."

Alan Rosenthal and Ethan Shevach from the National Institute of Allergy and Infectious Diseases, Bethesda, Maryland, demonstrated in 1973 a requirement for histocompatibility between T lymphocytes and macrophages based on an antigen-induced proliferation assay. These investigators isolated lymphocytes from strain 2 and strain 13 guinea pigs (which differ at the MHC) that had been injected with antigen (either 2,4-dinitrophenylated guinea pig albumin (DNP-GPA) or purified protein derivative (PPD) from *Mycobacterium tuberculosis*). Macrophages, isolated from peritoneal exudates induced in strain 2 or 13 guinea pigs by the injection of sterile mineral oil, were incubated with either DNP-GPA or PPD for an hour, washed, and then mixed with immune T lymphocytes. Forty-eight to 70 hours later Rosenthal and Shevach measured lymphocyte proliferation in vitro by determining the uptake of ^{3}H-thymidine present during the final 18 h of culture.

Optimal proliferation required that the macrophages and T lymphocytes be from the same strain. Inclusion of antibodies specific for the histocompatibility antigens of the strain under study blocked the proliferative response. Experiments in which parental strain macrophages were added to F_1 hybrid T lymphocytes showed that the interaction between the lymphocytes and macrophages could be inhibited by adding antibodies specific for histocompatibility antigens present on both the macrophages and T lymphocytes.

The role of the MHC-coded molecules in activating T lymphocytes was established in 1974; however, the mechanism for this phenomenon remained obscure. Two postdoctoral fellows in Australia designed an experiment that demonstrated the requirement for MHC compatibility in the effector phase of cytotoxic T lymphocytes.

The Zinkernagel–Doherty Experiments

Rolf Zinkernagel received his MD from the University of Basel in Switzerland before studying at the University of Lausanne for two years, where he learned immunological techniques to investigate infectious diseases, including methods for measuring the cytolytic activity of immune cells against microbially infected cells. Peter Doherty was trained as a veterinarian in Australia before traveling to the University of Edinburgh, Scotland, where he earned his PhD. He returned to Australia to assume a postdoctoral position at the University of Canberra.

Zinkernagel and Doherty demonstrated that optimal cytotoxicity of virally infected fibroblasts requires that virus-specific cytotoxic T lymphocytes and the fibroblasts share at least one set of histocompatibility (H-2) antigenic specificities. Mouse fibroblasts infected with the lymphocytic choriomeningitis virus and radiolabeled with ^{51}Cr were overlaid with spleen cells from mice previously injected with the same virus. Release of the chromium label provided a semiquantitative measure of the amount of cytotoxic activity in the mouse spleens. Zinkernagel and Doherty harvested supernatants after overnight incubation and determined the amount of radioactivity released.

As depicted in Table 20.1, optimal release of radio-isotope required that the spleen cells (containing virus-specific cytotoxic T lymphocytes) and the virally infected fibroblasts share at least one set of H-2 molecules. In the table the infected fibroblasts were all from the C3H mouse strain, which has H-2 molecules designated as H-2$^{k/k}$. Immune spleen cells from mice possessing at least one set of H-2^k molecules (CBA/H; CBA/H×C57Bl;

AKR; or C3H) lysed infected fibroblasts, resulting in the release of ^{51}Cr, while lymphocytes from strains lacking H-2$^{k/k}$ molecules failed to lyse the virally infected cells (Zinkernagel and Doherty, 1974a).

Zinkernagel and Doherty (1974b) suggested two models to explain their data: the intimacy model and the altered self model. Their original diagram distinguishing these two is reproduced in Figure 20.3.

The intimacy model (Figure 20.3) hypothesizes that T lymphocytes express a receptor that binds viral antigenic determinants displayed on the surface of the infected cell. In addition, the H-2 molecules expressed on both the T lymphocyte and the target cell interact to provide a second signal to the T lymphocyte.

The modified-self model proposed two different possibilities. In one, the virus somehow altered the H-2 molecule and this antigen–H-2 complex was recognized by the TCR. In the second model, the TCR possessed two binding sites: one for the virus and the second for the H-2 molecule of the target.

Results from further experiments performed by Zinkernagel and Doherty convinced many immunologists that the TCR interacted with both the antigen and

TABLE 20.1 Cytotoxic Activity of Lymphocytic Choriomeningitis Virus (LCM) Immune Spleen Cells from Different Mouse Strains on Monolayers of LCM Infected or Normal (Noninfected) C3H Fibroblasts

Experiment	Mouse strain	H-2 type	%^{51}Cr release[a] Infected	Normal
1	CBA/H	*k*	65.1±3.3	17.2±0.7
	Balb/C	*d*	17.9±0.9	17.2±0.6
	C57Bl	*b*	22.7±1.4	19.8±0.9
	CBA/H×C57Bl	*k/b*	56.1±0.5	16.7±0.3
	C57Bl×Balb/C	*b/d*	24.8±2.4	19.8±0.9
	nu/+ or +/+		42.8±2.0	21.9±0.7
	nu/nu		23.3±0.6	20.0±1.4
2	CBA/H	*k*	85.5±3.1	20.9±1.2
	AKR	*k*	71.2±1.6	18.6±1.2
	DBA/2	*d*	24.5±1.2	21.7±1.7
3	CBA/H	*k*	77.9±2.7	25.7±1.3
	C3TI/HeJ	*k*	77.8±0.8	24.5±1.5

[a]*%^{51}Cr release by normal spleen cells on infected targets ranged from (experiment 1) 17.1±0.3 to 20.0±0.7; (experiment 2) 20.0±1.4 to 25.3±0.7; (experiment 3) 27.2±2.0. From Zinkernagel and Doherty (1974a).*

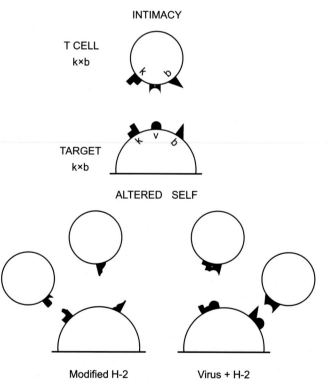

FIGURE 20.3 Diagram depicting possible ways in which T cells recognizing virally infected targets might be restricted by the H-2 antigens. The intimacy model (top) postulated that the cytotoxic T lymphocyte expressed two cell surface receptors: one specific for the viral antigens and a second that would interact with the MHC-coded molecule. The altered self models (bottom) hypothesized that T lymphocytes recognized MHC-coded molecules that had been altered by the virus. From Zinkernagel and Doherty (1974b).

the H-2 molecule (i.e., there was but a single receptor on T lymphocytes). Controversy surrounded the idea that the antigen and the histocompatibility molecule were physically linked on the APC. One argument was that an individual expresses only a few different MHC-coded molecules, thus theoretically limiting the number of different antigens to which the adaptive immune response could respond. A final verdict on the mechanism responsible for MHC restriction was not reached until the structure of the TCR was unraveled (Chapter 15).

Based on their findings and subsequent expansion of this experimental system, Zinkernagel and Doherty shared the Nobel Prize in Physiology or Medicine in 1996 "for their discoveries concerning the specificity of the cell mediated immune defence."

Three groups (Allison et al., 1982; Haskins et al., 1983; Meuer et al., 1983) unraveled the structure of the TCR in the early 1980s. Results revealed the TCR to possess a single binding site, thus favoring the idea that the receptor recognized a single entity. Previous studies demonstrated that proteins are altered prior to presentation to T lymphocytes and that the antigenic determinant recognized by a TCR involved a short (8–12 amino acid long) peptide. Emil Unanue led a collaborative effort of investigators at Washington University in St. Louis, Missouri and the Harvard Medical School in Boston, Massachusetts to prove that antigenic peptides bind directly to MHC-coded histocompatibility molecules and that antigen bound to histocompatibility molecules is recognized by the TCRs (Babbitt et al., 1985). These investigators used a 10 amino acid long peptide derived from hen egg lysozyme (HEL) known to be immunogenic yet imbedded within the native molecule rather than on its surface. A fluorescent label bound to this peptide permitted visualization of peptide binding to various isolated histocompatibility (H-2) molecules. Babbitt and his colleagues demonstrated by equilibrium dialysis that this peptide bound to class II MHC molecules from mice that responded to the peptide but not to class II MHC molecules from nonresponder mice. This binding was specific; unlabeled peptide from HEL prevented the binding while peptide from an unrelated antigen failed to impede binding.

Peptides constructed in the laboratory and containing some but not all the amino acids in the original peptide compete with binding of the HEL peptide with the class II molecules (Babbitt et al., 1986). These competitor peptides possess some structural similarities with the original peptide (i.e., lacking a tyrosine at a particular residue). In addition, a peptide corresponding to an autologous antigen was described that also inhibited the binding. These data suggest that the class II molecule fails to discriminate between foreign and self-peptides but does discriminate between unrelated foreign peptides. The authors provided additional data, indicating that immunogenic peptides contain some amino acid residues important for binding to the H-2 molecule and other residues necessary for interaction with TCRs.

Activation of CD4+ Versus CD8+ T Lymphocytes

These results support the modified-self model of antigen recognition by T lymphocytes. By the early 1970s, investigators characterized two T lymphocyte populations based on expression of surface antigens. With monoclonal antibodies all peripheral T lymphocytes could be divided into two major populations: CD4+ and CD8+ (Chapter 23). This division appeared to differentiate functionally distinct populations: CD4+ T lymphocytes are helper cells and CD8+ T lymphocytes are cytotoxic. Investigators next asked about the activation requirements of these two distinct lymphocyte populations.

Harvey Cantor and Edwin Boyse at Harvard Medical School, Boston, and the Memorial Sloan Kettering Cancer Center, New York, in 1975 demonstrated that the two T lymphocyte populations may have different requirements for activation. They determined if the generation of cytotoxic T lymphocytes to foreign H-2 antigens was augmented by the presence of helper T lymphocytes. They separated mouse T lymphocytes based on their expression of cell surface molecules into Ly1+ (CD4+) and Ly2,3+ (CD8+) populations (see Chapter 23 for nomenclature). Ly2,3+ T lymphocytes are cytotoxic while Ly1+ T lymphocytes function as helpers. Cantor and Boyse separated these two lymphocyte populations and tested them in vitro for cytotoxicity. While Ly2,3+ T lymphocytes lysed their targets, the amount of cytotoxic activity in this population could be augmented if Ly1+ cells were included in the cell cultures.

Investigators had previously shown that the target for cytotoxic T lymphocytes is an antigen coded for by class I genes in the MHC locus. When Cantor and Boyse eliminated cells expressing MHC class II coded antigens from their experiment, the amplifying activity of the Ly1+ cells was abrogated. This led them to conclude that "the amplifying Ly1+ T cells probably recognize alloantigens different from those recognized by the Ly2,3+ prekiller cells."

Using human lymphocytes stimulated by class I or class II MHC antigens, Edgar Engleman and colleagues in 1981 reached a similar conclusion. Engleman at Stanford University School of Medicine in Palo Alto, California, collaborated with colleagues at the Sloan-Kettering Institute for Cancer Research in New York to isolate lymphocytes from peripheral blood leukocytes. The investigators divided these lymphocytes into T-enriched and T-depleted populations. Engleman and colleagues further subdivided T lymphocytes based on the expression of cell surface antigens using monoclonal antibodies. Lymphocytes with a T helper phenotype (CD4+) were stimulated by class II MHC targets while lymphocytes with a T cytotoxic phenotype (CD8+) were stimulated by class I MHC antigens. Further investigation demonstrated a general rule that CD4+ T lymphocytes recognize antigen presented by MHC class II molecules while CD8+ T lymphocytes recognize antigen presented by MHC class I molecules.

ROLE OF CD3 MOLECULES IN T LYMPHOCYTE ACTIVATION

Variation in the TCR permits T lymphocytes to recognize a large array of foreign antigens. As described in Chapter 16, the intracellular tails of the α and β chains are short and most likely unable to engage the intracellular signaling mechanisms involved in transducing the environmental signal to the nucleus. This transduction function is accomplished by a series of *trans*-membrane polypeptides associated with the TCR and identified as the CD3 complex.

The CD3 complex consists of four membrane-spanning polypeptides that are noncovalently linked to α and β chains of the TCR. These four polypeptides (CD3γ, CD3δ, CD3ε, and CD3ζ) all have relatively long intracytoplasmic tails and amino acid sequences making up an immunoreceptor tyrosine-based activation motif (ITAM). Following activation ITAMs are phosphorylated and initiate the cascade of signals leading to gene transcription in the T lymphocyte.

SIGNAL 2: ROLE OF COSTIMULATORY MOLECULES

Binding of the TCR by antigen, while necessary, is insufficient for full activation of the T lymphocyte. Lafferty and Cunningham had postulated in 1975 the need for a second signal when they demonstrated that the generation of cytotoxic T lymphocytes required the stimulating cell to be viable. The second signal is supplied to the T lymphocyte by the APC; without this signal the T lymphocyte that binds its antigen will be inactivated (become anergic).

Lawrence Lum and colleagues, working at the Fred Hutchinson Cancer Research Institute at the University of Washington in 1982, identified a molecule expressed on all CD4+ T lymphocytes and a proportion of CD8+ T lymphocytes. This group used a monoclonal antibody (9.3) specific for human peripheral blood T lymphocytes to mark functionally distinct subpopulations of T lymphocytes.

Employing a protocol measuring the helper activity of T lymphocytes in an in vitro assay of immunoglobulin formation, investigators identified the function of this molecule. Peripheral blood lymphocytes secrete immunoglobulin when stimulated in vitro with pokeweed mitogen (PWM). Purified B lymphocytes fail to secrete immunoglobulin in response to PWM; however, mixing B lymphocytes with varying numbers of T lymphocytes restores immunoglobulin secretion. The helper function of the T lymphocytes is enriched by positive selection with immobilized 9.3 antibody or eliminated by treatment with antibody 9.3 plus complement, thus killing the cells.

The molecule identified by antibody 9.3 has been cloned and assigned a cluster of differentiation designation, CD28. Evidence suggesting that CD28 serves as a costimulatory molecule includes

- binding CD28 with specific antibodies failed to activate T lymphocytes unless the TCR simultaneously is binding antigen;
- the Fab portion of antibodies specific for CD28 blocked activation of T lymphocytes when APCs were used to stimulate T lymphocytes; and
- treatment of T lymphocytes with antibodies to CD28 and CD3 activated T lymphocytes even in the absence of APCs (Baroja et al., 1989).

Despite the characterization of CD28 and its function in activating T lymphocytes, the identity of the ligand for CD28 remained unknown until 1990, when Peter Linsley and colleagues at the Oncogen Division of Bristol-Myers-Squibb Pharmaceutical Research Institute and the University of Washington in Seattle transfected Chinese hamster ovary (CHO) cells with the gene coding for CD28. The transfected CHO cells expressed CD28 on their surface as detected by their reaction with a monoclonal antibody to CD28. Linsley and his coworkers labeled transfected CHO cells with ^{51}Cr and used these radiolabeled cells to detect binding to a variety of different tumor lines. The authors identified several lymphoblastoid and leukemic B lymphocyte lines that bound the CD28 expressing CHO cells. In addition, activated normal B lymphocytes also bound the CD28-positive targets. These interactions are partially blocked by adding a monoclonal antibody specific for CD28 to the assay, suggesting that these B lymphocytes contain a ligand for the CD28 molecule.

This ligand for CD28 was identified by treating one of the B lymphoblastoid cell lines (T51) with a number of monoclonal antibodies specific for B lymphocyte antigens. In all, 57 different monoclonal antibodies were tested; the antibody that most efficiently blocked binding of transfected CHO cells with T51 cells was B7/BB-1 (B7). Confirmation of the interaction between CD28 and B7 was obtained by isolating a cDNA clone for B7, transfecting CHO cells with this clone, and demonstrating specific binding of these cells with CHO cells expressing CD28. This binding was specific since it could be inhibited by treatment with monoclonal antibodies specific for CD28 or for B7.

Subsequent studies (Linsley et al., 1991a) demonstrated that interaction of T lymphocytes with either immobilized B7 or B7-positive CHO cells induced proliferation of the T lymphocytes and upregulated transcription of mRNA for the cytokine IL-2. B7 has subsequently been designated CD80 and is now known to be expressed both on B cells and on other APCs, including macrophages and dendritic cells.

Identification of the roles of CD28 and CD80 in T lymphocyte activation led to the discovery of two additional molecules, CD86 and CTLA-4 (CD154). Searching for a murine counterpart of the human CD28 molecule, Jane Gross and collaborators at the University of California, Berkley, and the Fred Hutchinson Cancer Research Center in Seattle, Washington, isolated a cDNA clone from a lymphoma library in 1990. The isolated clone had 61% homology with human CD28 and coded for a cytotoxic T lymphocyte-specific antigen (CTLA-4). The authors erroneously concluded that "these data provide strong support that we have identified the murine homologue of CD28."

Linsley et al. (1991b) showed that humans also express CTLA-4, particularly on cytotoxic T lymphocytes. They investigated the functional properties of CTLA-4 by fusing it with the constant region of an immunoglobulin gamma chain (Cγ) to produce what they termed CTLA-4-Ig. This molecule bound specifically to CD80 with high avidity. In an in vitro assay involving the interaction of T and B lymphocytes, CTLA-4-Ig dramatically inhibited T lymphocyte activation. Jeffery Bluestone and his colleagues at the University of Chicago, Illinois, adapted this observation to an in vivo model of transplant rejection in mice. In their study, they treated mice transplanted with human pancreatic islets with CTLA-4-Ig and demonstrated inhibition of graft rejection by blocking T cell recognition of CD80-positive antigen-presenting cells (Lenschow et al., 1992).

CTLA-4-Ig has been developed as an immunosuppressive agent for patients who have an autoimmune disease or who have received a kidney graft. Two drugs based on these findings are approved by the United States Food and Drug Administration. Abatacept is an inhibitor of T lymphocyte activation that binds CD80, thereby inhibiting CD80 from binding to CD28. Abatacept is approved for use in patients with rheumatoid arthritis. Belatacept, a second generation inhibitor of T lymphocyte activation, is approved for use in kidney transplant patients who are infected with the Epstein Barr virus.

Miyuki Azuma, at the Juntendo University School of Medicine in Tokyo, collaborated with colleagues in Japan and at DNAX in Palo Alto, California, to identify a second ligand for CD28 (and for CTLA-4) in 1993. This group generated a monoclonal antibody that identified a 70 kDa glycoprotein (B70) expressed by monocytes, dendritic cells, and activated (but not resting) T, B, and NK lymphocytes. This antibody inhibited the binding of CTLA-4-Ig fusion protein to human B lymphoblastoid cell lines and inhibited allogeneic mixed lymphocyte reactions. The authors conclude that "B70 is a second ligand for CD28 and CTLA-4 and may play an important role for costimulation of T cells in a primary immune response." B70 has been cloned and is now termed CD86.

CONCLUSION

Activation of T lymphocytes leads to their proliferation, differentiation, and maturation. In addition, activation results in the transcription of several genes for cytokines and chemokines. T lymphocytes recognize antigen through antigen-specific cell surface receptors, the TCR that are linked to invariant chains of the CD3 molecule. TCRs recognize short stretches of amino acids presented to the lymphocyte by other cells expressing MHC molecules. Once this recognition event occurs, a signal can be transduced to the nucleus by the CD3 complex.

The three-dimensional structure of the cell surface molecules coded by genes of the MHC provided an understanding of the mechanism by which this recognition system functions. Both class I histocompatibility molecules that present antigens to CD8+ T lymphocytes and class II histocompatibility molecules that present antigens to CD4+ T lymphocytes contain grooves or pockets in which the antigenic peptides reside. The heterogeneity of these MHC-coded molecules within the population explains differences in the spectrum of antigens any individual can recognize. This heterogeneity is most likely also responsible for the associations that are noted between the expression of certain HLA types in humans and the development of various diseases, including autoimmune disorders (Chapter 34).

Recognition of antigen through TCRs, however, is insufficient to activate a T lymphocyte, and the existence of a second signal was postulated and eventually confirmed. This second signal is mediated through molecules expressed on the T lymphocyte (CD28) and other molecules (CD80/86) expressed on the cells with which the T lymphocyte interacts (macrophages, B lymphocytes, target cells, etc.).

T lymphocyte activation is essential for initiation of the adaptive immune response, and several control mechanisms exist to inhibit overreactivity. When T lymphocytes bind antigen in the absence of a second signal, that is, if they receive signal one but not signal two, the lymphocytes are inactivated, a process termed cellular anergy. This mechanism is involved in the maintenance of immunological tolerance (Chapter 22). Additionally, the discovery of molecules involved in providing the second signal to T lymphocytes led to the development of new therapeutic approaches to regulate T lymphocyte activation, particularly in patients with autoimmune diseases and in preventing the rejection of foreign tissue grafts (Chapter 38).

References

Aisenberg, A.C., 1970. Allogeneic thymus grafts and the restoration of immune function in irradiated thymectomized mice. J. Exp. Med. 131, 275–286.

Allison, J.P., McIntyre, B.W., Bloch, D., 1982. Tumor specific antigens of murine T-lymphoma defined with monoclonal antibody. J. Immunol. 129, 2293–2300.

Azuma, M., Ito, D., Yagita, J., Okamura, K., Phillips, J.H., Lanier, L.L., Somoza, C., 1993. B70 antigen is a second ligand for CTLA-4 and CD28. Nature 366, 76–79.

Babbitt, B.P., Allen, P.M., Matsueda, G., Haber, E., Unanue, E.R., 1985. Binding of immunogenic peptides to Ia histocompatibility molecules. Nature 317, 359–361.

Babbitt, B.P., Matsueda, G., Haber, E., Unanue, E.R., Allen, P.M., 1986. Antigenic competition at the level of peptide-Ia binding. Proc. Natl. Acad. Sci. U.S.A. 83, 4509–4513.

Baroja, M.L., Lorre, K., Van Vaeck, F., Ceuppens, J.L., 1989. The anti-T cell monoclonal antibody 9.3 (anti-CD28) provides a helper signal and bypasses the need for accessory cells in T cell activation with immobilized anti-CD3 and mitogens. Cell. Immunol. 120, 205–217.

Bretscher, P.A., Cohn, M., 1968. Minimal model for the mechanism of antibody induction and paralysis by antigen. Nature 220, 444–448.

Bretscher, P.A., Cohn, M., 1970. A theory of self-nonself discrimination. Science 169, 1042–1049.

Cantor, H., Boyse, E.A., 1975. Functional subclasses of T lymphocytes bearing different LY antigens. II. Cooperation between subclasses of Ly+ cells in the generation of killer activity. J. Exp. Med. 141, 1390–1399.

Ehrlich, P., 1900. Croonian lecture: on immunity with special reference to cell life. Proc. R. Soc. London 66, 424–448.

Engleman, E.G., Benike, C.J., Grumet, F.C., Evans, R.L., 1981. Activation of human T lymphocyte subsets: helper and suppressor/cytotoxic T cells recognize and respond to distinct histocompatibility antigens. J. Immunol. 127, 2124–2129.

Gorer, P.A., 1936. The detection of antigenic differences in mouse erythrocytes by the employment of immune sera. Br. J. Exp. Pathol. 17, 42–50.

Gorer, P.A., 1937. The genetic and antigenic basis of tumor transplantation. J. Pathol. Bacteriol. 44, 691–697.

Gorer, P.A., Lyman, S., Snell, G.D., 1948. Studies on the genetic and antigenic basis of tumor transplantation. Linkage between a histocompatibility gene and "fused" in mice. Proc. R. Soc. London B Biol. Sci. 135, 499–505.

Gross, J.A., St John, T., Allison, J.P., 1990. The murine homologue of the T lymphocyte antigen CD28. Molecular cloning and cell surface expression. J. Immunol. 144, 3201–3210.

Haskins, K., Kubo, R., White, J., Pigeon, M., Kappler, J., Marrack, P., 1983. The major histocompatibility complex restricted antigen receptor on T cells. I. Isolation with a monoclonal antibody. J. Exp. Med. 157, 1149–1169.

Katz, D.H., Hamaoka, T., Benacerraf, B., 1973. Cell interactions between histoincompatible T and B lymphocytes. II. Failure of physiologic cooperative interactions between T and B lymphocytes from allogeneic donor strains in humoral response to hapten-protein conjugate. J. Exp. Med. 137, 1405–1418.

Kindred, B., Schreffler, D.C., 1972. H-2 dependence of co-operation between T and B cells in vivo. J. Immunol. 109, 940–943.

Lafferty, K.J., Cunningham, A.J., 1975. A new analysis of allogeneic interactions. Aust. J. Exp. Biol. Med. Sci. 53, 27–42.

Lafferty, K.J., Prowse, S.J., Simenovic, C.J., Warren, H.S., 1983. Immunobiology of tissue transplantation: a return to the passenger leukocyte concept. Annu. Rev. Immunol. 1, 143–173.

Lenschow, D.J., Zeng, Y., Thistlethwaite, J.R., Montag, A., Brady, W., Gibson, M.G., Linsley, P.S., Bluestone, J.A., 1992. Long-term survival of xenogeneic pancreatic islet grafts induced by CTLA4Ig. Science 257, 789–792.

Leuchars, E., Cross, A.M., Dukor, P., 1965. The restoration of immunological function by thymus grafting in thymectomized irradiated mice. Transplantation 3, 28–35.

Linsley, P.S., Brady, W., Grosmarie, L., Aruffo, A., Damle, N.K., Ledbetter, J.A., 1991a. Binding of the B cell activation B7 to CD28 costimulates T cell proliferation and interleukin 2 mRNA accumulation. J. Exp. Med. 173, 721–730.

Linsley, P.S., Brady, W., Urnes, M., Grosmarie, L.S., Damle, N., Ledbetter, J.A., 1991b. CTLA-4 is a second receptor for the B cell activation antigen B7. J. Exp. Med. 174, 561–569.

Linsley, P.S., Clark, E.A., Ledbetter, J.A., 1990. T-cell antigen CD28 mediates adhesion with B cells by interacting with activation antigen B7/BB-1. Proc. Natl. Acad. Sci. U.S.A. 87, 5031–5035.

Lum, L.G., Orcutt-Thordarson, N., Seigneuret, M.C., Hansen, J.A., 1982. In vitro regulation of immunoglobulin synthesis by T-cell subpopulations defined by a new human T-cell antigen (9.3). Cell. Immunol. 72, 122–129.

Meuer, S.C., Fitzgerald, K.A., Hussey, R.E., Hodgkin, J.C., Schlossman, S.F., Reinherz, E.L., 1983. Clonotypic structures involved in antigen-specific human T cell function: relationship to the T3 molecular complex. J. Exp. Med. 157, 705–719.

Rosenthal, A.S., Shevach, E.M., 1973. Function of macrophages in antigen recognition by guinea pig T lymphocytes. I. Requirement for histocompatible macrophages and lymphocytes. J. Exp. Med. 138, 1194–1212.

Zinkernagel, R.M., Doherty, P.C., 1974a. Restriction of in vitro T cell-mediated cytotoxicity in lymphocytic choriomeningitis within a syngeneic or semiallogeneic system. Nature 248, 701–702.

Zinkernagel, R.M., Doherty, P.C., 1974b. Immunological surveillance against altered self-components by sensitized T lymphocytes in lymphocytic choriomeningitis. Nature 251, 547–548.

TIME LINE

1900   Paul Ehrlich proposes the side-chain hypothesis to explain the interaction of antigen with antigen-reactive cells

1937   Peter Gorer demonstrates that histocompatibility antigens can induce an immune response

1968   Peter Bretscher and Melvin Cohn propose a two-signal model for activation of antigen-reactive (B) lymphocytes

1972   Berenice Kindred and Donald Shreffler demonstrate that the interaction of T and B lymphocytes requires that the lymphocytes share histocompatibility antigens

1973   Alan Rosenthal and Ethan Shevach demonstrate that the interaction between T lymphocytes and macrophages requires that the cells share histocompatibility antigens

1973   David Katz and coworkers demonstrate that interactions between T and B lymphocytes are optimal if the lymphocytes are histocompatible

1974   Rolf Zinkernagel and Peter Doherty report that interactions between cytotoxic T cells and their targets require histocompatibility

1975   Kevin Lafferty and A.J. Cunningham extend the two-signal model of activation to T lymphocytes

1975   Harvey Cantor and Edwin Boyse demonstrate that CD4+ and CD8+ T lymphocytes recognize different classes of histocompatibility antigens

1982   Jeffrey Ledbetter and colleagues provide initial evidence for the existence of CD28 on T lymphocytes

1982   James Allison isolates the β-chain of the T cell receptor (TCR)

1983   Kathryn Haskin's group and Stefan Meuer's group report the isolation and function of polypeptide chains making up the TCR

1986   Bruce Babbitt and colleagues demonstrate binding of antigen to a histocompatibility antigen

1987   Pamela Bjorkman and colleagues publish the three-dimensional structure of a class I histocompatibility molecule

1990   Peter Linsley and colleagues identify the ligand for CD28

1990   Jane Gross and collaborators identify CTLA-4, a molecule expressed on T lymphocytes that binds CD80/86

1993   Miyuki Azuma and colleagues identify CD86 as a costimulator of T lymphocyte activation

1996   Rolf Zinkernagel and Peter Doherty awarded the Nobel Prize in Physiology or Medicine

21

Development of Tolerance to Self in B Lymphocytes

INTRODUCTION

Self–non-self discrimination, one of the hallmarks of the adaptive immune response (Chapter 2), is termed tolerance, and is an acquired trait of the immune system (Chapter 8). Tolerance is a mechanism by which the individual maintains homeostasis and refrains from destroying self. Differentiation of self from non-self (foreign) is critical to protect against the development of autoimmune disease.

Tolerance differs from induced unresponsiveness. Tolerance occurs in central lymphoid organs (thymus, bone marrow, bursa of Fabricius) during differentiation of immature lymphocytes and continues throughout the life of the individual; unresponsiveness is a mechanism by which mature lymphocytes in the periphery are inhibited from reacting to antigens, including self. Unresponsiveness involves regulatory phenomena, including T_{REG} lymphocytes (Chapter 24) and cytokine interactions (Chapter 25). Today several clinical interventions manipulate the immune system, leading to inhibition of B lymphocytes (Chapter 38).

Studies in the 1950s and 1960s demonstrated that developing lymphocytes are sensitive to elimination if they express potentially autoreactive cell surface receptors. Both B and T lymphocytes differentiate from lymphoid stem cells that in turn derive from multipotent hematopoietic stem cells. Division of lymphocytes into

functionally distinct populations of T and B lymphocytes led to studies on physiologic processes by which tolerance is induced in both cell types. This chapter presents the investigations that revealed those processes responsible for inducing and maintaining self-tolerance in B lymphocytes. Experiments relevant to self-tolerance induction and maintenance in T lymphocytes are covered in Chapter 22.

The genetic rearrangements responsible for generating the B lymphocyte repertoire (Chapter 18) result in the formation of a large number of potential antibody-forming lymphocytes possessing antigen specific B cell receptors (BCRs). These BCRs are integral membrane proteins that transmit signals received from the environment to the nucleus to initiate antibody synthesis and secretion. The random rearrangement of genes in developing B lymphocytes results in the maturation of potential antibody-forming cells that may bind to and produce antibodies specific for virtually any antigen, including self. Elimination of B lymphocytes reactive to self occurs prior to export to the periphery. The surviving B lymphocytes, when activated, protect against pathogens.

Paul Ehrlich and Julius Morgenroth speculated in 1901 that a process exists ("horror autotoxicus") to protect the individual from the pathological actions of antibodies to self. Studies in the first half of the twentieth century demonstrated not only that antibodies to self are produced but that they can induce pathology in the form of autoimmune disease (Chapter 34). Several mechanisms to eliminate potentially autoreactive B lymphocytes have subsequently been described. These are divided into central tolerance and peripheral tolerance (unresponsiveness) based on the anatomical location.

In the bone marrow of mammals and the bursa of Fabricius of birds, developing B lymphocytes express surface IgM and IgD as their BCR. These receptors are tested for self-reactivity by binding to epitopes expressed in these central lymphoid organs. If the immature B lymphocyte expresses a BCR that binds self, one of three processes can occur:

- programmed cell death (apoptosis), in which case the lymphocyte is deleted;
- anergy resulting in survival of an inactive lymphocyte; or
- receptor editing, leading to expression of a new BCR that is again evaluated for binding to self.

The elimination or silencing of lymphocytes at this stage of development is referred to as central tolerance since it occurs in a central lymphoid organ (bone marrow or bursa).

If the immature B lymphocyte fails to bind self-epitopes during differentiation, it will continue to mature and eventually leave the central lymphoid organs and populate the peripheral lymphoid tissue. Even though peripheral B lymphocytes have been selected to avoid responses to self, some mature B lymphocytes may regain this reactivity and produce autoantibodies. This results from random mutations occurring in the genes coding for the variable regions of the immunoglobulins. To guard against this possibility, mechanisms exist in peripheral lymphoid organs to inhibit the activation of potentially self-reactive B lymphocytes. Inactivation that occurs once the B lymphocyte leaves the central lymphoid organs is known as peripheral tolerance.

DEVELOPMENT OF CENTRAL TOLERANCE TO SELF

Investigators designed three experimental protocols to study the development of central tolerance in B lymphocytes:

1. treatment of B lymphocytes with antibody to immunoglobulin either in vitro or in vivo followed by evaluation of antibody synthesis and secretion to foreign antigens;
2. treatment of immature B lymphocytes with antigen in vitro followed by transfer of the treated cells to irradiated mice; and

3. development of transgenic mice, in which most B lymphocytes are specific for an antigen expressed by tissues of the mouse.

These protocols demonstrated that three mechanisms exist leading to the induction of central tolerance to self in B lymphocytes: clonal deletion, clonal anergy, and receptor editing.

Clonal Deletion

Göran Möller in 1961 at the Karolinska Institute Medical School, Stockholm, Sweden, initially observed that antibody-forming lymphocytes possess immunoglobulin on their surface. By the late 1960s the presence of immunoglobulin molecules on the surface of B lymphocytes had been demonstrated by several investigators although it was not until 1971 that Ellen Vitetta and her group at the University of Texas, Dallas, provided formal proof that these immunoglobulins served as the BCR (Chapter 17).

The role of the BCR in tolerance induction was demonstrated by treating lymphocytes with antibody to gamma globulin or to IgG, IgM, or light chains. Such treatment resulted in decreased antibody secretion. In 1969, Hiroshi Fuji and Niels Jerne at the Basel Institute for Immunology, Switzerland, described the reversible suppression of an in vitro antibody response following treatment of lymphocytes with antibodies to gamma globulin. Jayne Lesley and Richard Dutton working at the University of California, San Diego in 1970 showed that treatment of mouse spleen cells with rabbit antibodies to mouse kappa chains inhibited the in vitro antibody response of these lymphocytes to sheep erythrocytes. Klaus-Ulrich Hartmann and colleagues at the Max Planck Institute in Tubingen, Germany, reported in 1971 that the primary antibody response to sheep erythrocytes in vitro is inhibited by treating mouse spleen cells with antibodies to IgG or IgM or with antibodies to the Fab portion of these molecules.

Dean Manning and John Jutila confirmed these results in 1972 using an in vivo model of antibody production. Working at Montana State University in Bozeman, these investigators injected neonatal mice with rabbit antibodies to μ-heavy chain. Four weeks later they injected these mice with sheep erythrocytes and quantitated the number of antibody-forming cells using the hemolytic plaque assay. This protocol resulted in a complete loss of both IgM and IgG antibody-forming cells. Treatment of neonatal mice with antibodies to IgG or treatment of adult mice with antibodies to μ-chain failed to completely inhibit subsequent antibody production. Paul Kincade and colleagues at the University of Alabama in Birmingham reported in 1970 that injection of newly hatched chickens with antibodies to IgM abrogated IgM production in adult chickens.

The mechanism by which treatment with antibodies to immunoglobulin led to diminished antibody secretion was investigated at the cellular level. In vitro, treatment of B lymphocytes with antibodies to immunoglobulin at 37°C induces a redistribution of the surface molecules to one pole of the cell followed by phagocytosis of the antigen–antibody complexes. This phenomenon was initially studied using mature B lymphocytes, i.e., lymphocytes isolated from the spleen that had differentiated into antibody-producing cells (Unanue et al., 1972; Katz and Unanue, 1972). Investigators studying tolerance induction in B lymphocytes eventually used this experimental design with immature lymphocytes from the bone marrow.

Two groups of investigators, Charles Sidman and Emil Unanue (1975) at Harvard Medical School and Martin Raff, working at University College, London and collaborating with colleagues at the University of Newcastle, England and the University of Alabama at Birmingham (1975), compared the effect of treating immature and mature B lymphocytes with antibodies to immunoglobulin.

Raff and coworkers isolated immature mouse lymphocytes from fetal or newborn liver or adult bone marrow or mature B lymphocytes from adult spleen or lymph nodes and treated them with antibodies specific for mouse μ-chain in vitro. Treatment of immature B lymphocytes with low concentrations of the antibody for 24h or less caused complete disappearance of the BCR; once the antibody was removed from the cultures, the effect was reversible, and the lymphocytes reexpressed their BCR. Exposure of immature lymphocytes for a longer period of time (48h) resulted in permanent loss of the BCR. Regardless of the length of time the lymphocytes were exposed, treatment of mature B lymphocytes with antibody to the μ-chain resulted in complete loss of the BCR that was reversible.

Sidman and Unanue (1975) used a similar protocol and exposed spleen lymphocytes from young or adult mice to antibodies specific for mouse IgM for 1 or 24h. Following removal of the antibody, the cells were cultured for several days, and the expression of BCR on the lymphocytes was assessed using immunofluorescence. Both immature and mature B lymphocytes treated with antibodies to IgM rapidly lost their BCRs. The reappearance of surface IgM on B lymphocytes from older animals occurred within 24h of the removal of the antibody while immature B lymphocytes treated in a similar fashion failed to reexpress their surface receptors during the duration of the experiment. Sidman and Unanue considered two explanations for the fate of the immature B lymphocytes treated with antibody to IgM: treatment either inactivated the B lymphocytes or deleted them. To determine which of these two possibilities was correct, lymphocytes from these cultures were stained with a fluorescent antibody against another protein found on B lymphocytes, the Ia antigen. Ia antigen is now known to be a class II molecule coded by the major histocompatibility complex (MHC) expressed by B lymphocytes but not T lymphocytes. Twenty-four hours after treating adult B lymphocytes with antibodies to IgM, the level of immunofluorescent staining with antibody to the Ia protein was similar to that seen before treatment. Immature B lymphocytes treated in the same manner showed Ia staining at 24h that declined by 48h. These results led the authors to speculate that "as a result of the prolonged ligand-receptor interaction, the original B lymphocytes were either dying or were changing other cellular characteristics."

Definitive evidence that immature B lymphocytes are killed as a result of treatment with antibody specific for the BCR came from studies reported by Amanda Norvell and her colleagues at the University of Pennsylvania in 1995. Using an in vitro system, immature B lymphocytes (identified as IgM+, IgD− lymphocytes) were treated with antibodies specific for IgM. Cross-linking of the BCR on immature B lymphocytes in vitro led to significant levels of apoptosis (programmed cell death) as detected by staining of the treated cells with propidium iodide. Treatment of mature B lymphocytes with the same antibody failed to induce apoptosis.

Critics questioned the relevance of the in vitro experimental model used by Raff's group, by Sidman and Unanue, and by Norvell and her colleagues to the in vivo process of tolerance induction. In the in vitro model antibody specific for IgM binds to the Fc portion of the BCR and fails to mirror the in vivo condition in which antigen binds to the Fab portion of the BCR. To answer this criticism, Gus Nossal and Beverly Pike, working at the Walter and Eliza Hall Institute of Medical Research in Melbourne, Australia, designed a second experimental protocol: treatment of immature B lymphocytes with antigen in vitro followed by transfer to irradiated mice.

In 1975, Nossal and Pike asked whether developing B lymphocytes could be silenced by interacting with antigen during maturation. Their study focused on B lymphocytes derived from adult mouse bone marrow. These immature cells possessed BCRs but could not be induced to secrete antibody. Nossal and Pike exposed lymphocytes in vitro to one of two haptens, dinitrophenol (DNP), or 4-hydroxy-3-iodo-5-nitrophenylacetate (NIP), conjugated to human gamma globulin (HGG) as a carrier. One to three days later they harvested the treated lymphocytes and injected them into irradiated mice that were subsequently injected with DNP or NIP conjugated to a different carrier protein, polymerized *Salmonella* flagellin (POL). Six to 10 days later they assayed the spleens of the reconstituted mice for the presence of antibody-forming lymphocytes as detected by a hemolytic plaque assay.

Exposure of immature B lymphocytes to haptens conjugated to HGG in culture significantly inhibited the response of those cells to the same haptens conjugated to POL when the cells were injected into irradiated recipients. An example of these results is presented in Figure 21.1. In this study exposure of bone marrow cells to DNP-HGG for 48–72 h in culture reduced the number of antibody-forming cells to DNP-POL that could be detected in the spleens of reconstituted mice.

In other experiments, Nossal and Pike characterized the unresponsiveness induced by this protocol as being

- specific for the hapten used in the original culture,
- dependent on the hapten and the cells interacting continually during B lymphocyte maturation, and
- independent of the presence of T lymphocytes in the cultures.

The authors concluded that the mechanism of B lymphocyte inhibition (which they termed clonal abortion) "may be a tolerance mechanism of great physiological significance for self-recognition."

A third experimental model designed to investigate clonal deletion in the induction of B lymphocyte tolerance involved the use of transgenic mice in which B lymphocytes develop in the presence of antigens for which they are specific. David Nemazee and Kurt Buerki (1989a), working at the Basel Institute for Immunology and the pharmaceutical company, Sandoz, in Switzerland, designed mice in which most maturing B lymphocytes express rearranged immunoglobulin genes specific for a particular histocompatibility antigen (H-2K^k). The investigators injected bone marrow cells from these transgenic mice into mice that expressed either the same or a different MHC genotype. Nemazee and Buerki assessed the presence of B lymphocytes with BCRs specific for H-2K^k. In mice expressing the H-2K^k antigen, B lymphocytes specific for H-2k^k could not be detected in the peripheral lymphoid tissue, while in mice of other H-2K genotypes, B lymphocytes specific for H-2K^k were abundant. These results suggest that the B lymphocytes reactive to self that develop in an environment expressing self are deleted as a result of interaction with antigen.

Extension of this model showed that B lymphocytes specific for H-2K^k would not develop (or were eliminated) in a mouse expressing H-2K^k antigens (Nemazee and Bürki, 1989b). Mice transgenic for B lymphocytes expressing the immunoglobulin genes coding for an antibody specific for H-2K^k were mated with mice whose MHC genes coded for H-2K^k. In the resultant F$_1$ hybrids, immature B lymphocytes were present, but no mature B lymphocytes expressing the BCR specific for H2-K^k and no antibody to H-2K^k were detected. Most of the potentially self-reactive B lymphocytes died in the bone marrow.

Clonal Anergy

A second mechanism for the development of central B lymphocyte tolerance is through a process known as clonal anergy. In immunology, anergy is defined as the lack of responsiveness to an antigen despite the presence of antigen-specific lymphocytes. Investigators hypothesized that if anergy is a credible process to explain tolerance to self, anergic cells would persist but would fail to respond to antigenic stimulation.

In 1980, Gus Nossal and Beverley Pike, working at the Walter and Elisa Hall Institute of Medical Research in Melbourne, speculated that B lymphocyte tolerance is due to the induction of anergy. Nossal and Pike injected newborn or pregnant mice with the hapten fluorescein (FLU) coupled to HGG. Spleen cells from the injected mice or from the offspring of the pregnant animals were harvested 1–6 weeks later and assayed for the number of antigen (FLU)-binding cells and the number of B lymphocytes secreting antibody to FLU. Injection of high doses of antigen resulted in a significant decrease in the number of FLU-binding cells as well as a diminished antibody response, suggesting clonal deletion. In mice treated with low doses of FLU-HGG, there was little, if any, reduction in the number of FLU-binding B lymphocytes and no difference in the avidity of binding by these cells. However, these cells failed to produce specific

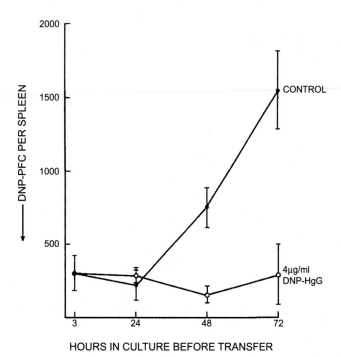

FIGURE 21.1 Effect of incubating bone marrow cells with DNP-HGG for various times on the ability of the cells to develop an anti-DNP response following immunization with DNP-POL. Cells were removed from culture and injected into irradiated, syngeneic mice that were immunized within 6 h. Spleens were assayed for antibody-forming cells 6–10 days later. *From Nossal and Pike (1975).*

antibody after stimulation with either the antigen or with a nonspecific B lymphocyte activator (mitogen). The authors concluded that the mice injected with a low dose of antigen during maturation developed tolerance to the antigens and that the B lymphocytes had been rendered anergic (i.e., the cells could bind antigen but they could not produce antibodies).

The argument could be made that the experimental design used by Nossal and Pike failed to reflect what occurs in vivo during the induction of tolerance to self in B lymphocytes. To address this criticism, Christopher Goodnow et al. (1988) at the University of Sidney, Australia, along with a number of other collaborators in Australia and at the National Institutes of Health in Bethesda, Maryland, designed a double transgenic mouse that demonstrated that anergy is operative in tolerance induction.

These investigators developed two transgenic strains of mice: one that expressed hen egg lysozyme (HEL) as a tissue antigen and a second in which most B lymphocytes expressed BCRs specific for HEL. The presence of HEL in the first transgenic strain resulted in the induction of tolerance to HEL in both T and B lymphocytes. Crosses between the two stains of mice produced hybrid animals in which B lymphocytes specific for HEL developed in an environment in which HEL is expressed as part of self. Once these hybrid mice matured, Goodnow and colleagues tested them for the presence of HEL-specific B lymphocytes and for the amount of antibody to HEL in their serum. Results showed that while the double transgenic animals possessed near normal numbers of B lymphocytes specific for HEL they failed to produce any antibody specific for HEL. The B lymphocytes that were present expressed lower numbers of IgM BCRs than did B lymphocytes from control mice; however, they expressed the usual number of IgD BCRs.

When Goodnow and coworkers transferred B lymphocytes from double transgenic mice to a nontransgenic animal and stimulated them with HEL coupled to horse erythrocytes (as a carrier), little, if any, antibody to HEL was detected, indicating that these B lymphocytes had been inactivated by maturing in the presence of HEL. The authors conclude that their "findings indicate that self-tolerance may result from mechanisms other than clonal deletion."

Receptor Editing

B lymphocytes expressing potentially self-reactive BCRs can be deleted by the induction of apoptosis or can be rendered unresponsive by induction of anergy. A third process for regulating B lymphocytes reactive to self comprises replacing the gene coding for the V region of one of the chains of the BCR of the developing B lymphocyte. This process is termed receptor editing and was

demonstrated experimentally in the early 1990s by two groups of investigators, both of which used transgenic mice.

Martin Weigert, working at the Institute for Cancer Research of the Fox Chase Cancer Center in Philadelphia, Pennsylvania, and his colleagues designed transgenic mice in which B lymphocytes possessed the genes coding for the heavy and light chains of an antibody specific for DNA, one of the autoantibodies associated with the autoimmune disease, systemic lupus erythematosus (Gay et al., 1993). Young transgenic mice had few B lymphocytes while adult transgenic animals possessed increased numbers of B lymphocytes. Analysis of the BCRs on adult B lymphocytes indicated that all of them express the heavy chain coded for by the transgene. This heavy chain was associated with light chains coded for by different genes, suggesting that the light chain gene had been altered. Examination of hybridomas derived from the spleens of the transgenic mice showed, in fact, that the B lymphocytes had rearranged the genes coding for these light chains. This resulted in the development of a messenger RNA coding for a light chain with a different amino acid sequence than the original transgene. These B lymphocytes also secreted antibody that failed to bind DNA. The authors speculate that some of these "endogenous" light chains can compete with the transgenic light chain to form a complete immunoglobulin molecule that lacks reactivity to self. They concluded that "receptor editing is a mechanism used by immature autoreactive B cells to escape tolerance."

Independently, David Nemazee at the University of Colorado Health Sciences Center in Denver led a group that discovered a similar phenomenon (Tiegs et al., 1993). These investigators employed an experimental system in which B lymphocytes specific for a particular H-2K antigen developed in an environment expressing that antigen. Peripheral blood contained only a few B lymphocytes specific for the self-antigen while the bone marrow contained significant numbers of B lymphocytes reactive to self. The B lymphocytes in the bone marrow contained high levels of the enzymes (RAG-1 and RAG-2) involved in the rearrangement of V-region genes. This implied that interaction between the BCR and its ligand (in this case a self-H-2 molecule) induces continued rearrangement of light chain genes. These results led the authors to conclude that not all lymphocytes reactive to self are deleted during selection but that some of the B lymphocytes survive by rearranging their immunoglobulin genes, resulting in the expression of a BCR of a different specificity. These results suggest a model for receptor editing presented in Figure 21.2.

While these early studies demonstrated receptor editing in light chain genes, subsequent investigations have shown that similar rearrangements also occur in the genes coding for heavy chains.

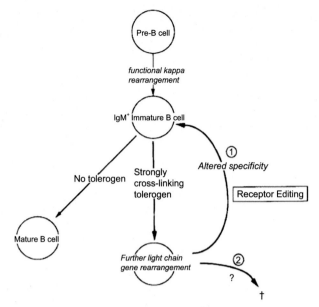

FIGURE 21.2   Model for B lymphocyte receptor editing. Immature B lymphocytes in the bone marrow express an immunoglobulin receptor molecule (BCR) that is tested against antigens in the environment. If no antigen induces strong BCR cross-linking, the B lymphocyte matures and is exported to the periphery. Strong cross-linking by an autoantigen induces rearrangement of light chain V-region genes. If the newly formed light chain competes with the original light chain for binding to the heavy chain, the B lymphocyte will acquire a new specificity. This new BCR will go through a similar process and, if self-antigens fail to cross-link this BCR, the B lymphocyte will finish differentiation and be exported to the periphery. *From Tiegs et al. (1993).*

PERIPHERAL B LYMPHOCYTE UNRESPONSIVENESS

Despite the three mechanisms described for the induction and maintenance of tolerance to self in maturing B lymphocytes, observations made during the 1970s and 1980s indicated that self-reactive B lymphocytes exist in peripheral lymphoid tissues. Several reports of B lymphocytes in normal individuals producing antibody to self were published (Primi et al., 1977a,b; Litaka et al., 1988). The systems designed to detect these lymphocytes included stimulating peripheral B lymphocytes in vitro with substances known to activate large numbers of cells (polyclonal B cell activators (PBA)) and testing the supernatants for antibody to self-antigens or injecting mice with PBA and assessing serum for antibody activity. Antibodies to a variety of self-antigens, including erythrocytes, DNA, thyroid antigens, and lymphocytes, have been detected.

In addition, genes coding for immunoglobulin in activated B lymphocytes undergo hypermutation, particularly in the variable regions of the H and L chains. This process, essential in the maturation of the antibody response, produces higher affinity antibodies. A corollary to this change in BCR is the generation of potentially self-reactive B lymphocytes (Diamond and Scharff,

1984). Since these lymphocytes are likely to produce autoantibodies if activated, mechanisms must exist in the periphery to eliminate or silence them.

Several hypotheses were formulated to explain the escape of B lymphocytes from central tolerance and subsequent migration to the periphery where they may be stimulated by infection or inflammation to synthesize and secrete antibody, resulting in pathology:

- Not all antigens are expressed in the bone marrow during development, thus precluding the maturing B lymphocytes from encountering them.
- Some self-antigens in the periphery are sequestered (i.e., brain, testes) from contact with cells of the adaptive immune system. Inflammation or infection releases these antigens to interact with immunocompetent lymphocytes.
- Self-antigens are expressed in concentrations insufficient to cross-link and activate the B lymphocytes (hormones, intracellular enzymes).
- Self-antigens bind weakly to the BCR and fail to stimulate antibody production.

It is also possible that B lymphocytes exist in a regulatory environment in which either T lymphocyte help is absent or excessive T regulation occurs.

Goodnow and colleagues in 1989 employed a double transgenic mouse model to demonstrate that mature B lymphocytes, encountering a high concentration of the antigen to which they are specific, could be rendered tolerant. These investigators designed transgenic mice expressing HEL in tissues under the control of the metallothionein promoter. As a result, the amount of HEL expressed in the tissues could be controlled by altering the amount of zinc in the water given to the mice. These mice were crossed with a second transgenic strain in which most B lymphocytes expressed BCRs specific for HEL.

F_1 hybrids maturing in the absence of zinc (and in the absence of expressed HEL) developed normal numbers of B lymphocytes that produced antibodies specific for HEL when stimulated with HEL conjugated to horse erythrocytes (HRBC). When these mice were given water-containing zinc for 1–4 days, the level of surface IgM on peripheral B lymphocytes specific for HEL decreased drastically, and these lymphocytes failed to produce antibody when transferred to nontransgenic mice and were exposed to HEL-HRBC. Such functionally silenced cells support the occurrence of peripheral anergy in B lymphocytes.

Nemazee's group in Australia designed a second experimental system involving transgenic mice to demonstrate that B lymphocytes that interact with self-antigen in the periphery are deleted (Russell et al., 1991). One of the transgenic partners had B lymphocytes, most of which expressed BCRs specific for the H-2K[b] antigen. These mice were bred with mice in which the H-2K[b] antigen was expressed only in the liver.

Analysis of the F_1 hybrids showed a decrease in the number of lymphocytes expressing IgM molecules as well as a comparable decrease in the number of B lymphocytes (measured by a second cell surface molecule—B220). These authors concluded that "B cells specific for major histocompatibility complex class I antigen can be deleted if they encounter membrane-bound antigen at a post-bone-marrow stage of development. This deletion may be necessary to prevent organ specific autoimmunity."

CONCLUSION

Research presented in this chapter describes the mechanisms that inhibit B lymphocytes from producing autoantibodies. Interaction of the BCR with antigens, including self-antigens, activates those lymphocytes to antibody production. Thus one of the goals of preventing autoantibody production is elimination or silencing of lymphocytes expressing a BCR specific for self. A plethora of studies have shown that B lymphocytes (like T lymphocytes—Chapter 22) are particularly sensitive to induction of tolerance when they are immature, and thus the mechanisms to silence potentially autoreactive B lymphocytes occur during early maturation of the cells.

A variety of mechanisms, including clonal deletion, clonal anergy, and receptor editing, exist to inhibit self-reactivity of B lymphocytes centrally (in the bone marrow) while the lymphocytes are still developing. Similar mechanisms inhibit mature B lymphocytes in the periphery from responding to autoantigens. Despite this seeming redundancy of control mechanisms, the adaptive immune response is known to produce antibodies specific for self, some of which result in autoimmune diseases. Additional mechanisms that have evolved to regulate potentially self-reactive B lymphocytes by regulatory T lymphocytes are covered in Chapter 24 while the ways in which putative tolerant B lymphocytes circumvent regulatory mechanisms to produce autoantibodies are discussed in Chapter 34.

The discovery of the phenomenon of immunological tolerance by Billingham and coworkers in the 1950s (Chapter 8) stimulated the development of potential new therapies for patients with autoimmune diseases such as systemic lupus erythematosus and rheumatoid arthritis, immune-mediated hypersensitivities such as allergy and asthma, and for recipients of organ grafts from allogeneic sources. The promise of artificially developing tolerance-based therapies for these pathologies has remained elusive for a number of reasons, including the lack of knowledge of the relevant antigens (in autoimmune diseases) and the difficulty inherent in inhibiting reactivity of already committed antibody-producing B lymphocytes.

References

Diamond, B., Scharff, M.D., 1984. Somatic mutation of the T15 heavy chain gives rise to an antibody with autoantibody specificity. Proc. Natl. Acad. Sci. U.S.A. 81, 5841–5844.

Ehrlich, P., Morgenroth, J., 1901. Ueber Hämolysine. Berl. Klin. Wochenschr. 38, 251–257.

Fuji, H., Jerne, N.K., 1969. Primary immune response in vitro: reversible suppression by anti-globulin antibodies. Ann. Inst. Pasteur (Paris) 117, 801–805.

Gay, D., Saunders, T., Camper, S., Weigert, M., 1993. Receptor editing: an approach by autoreactive B cells to escape tolerance. J. Exp. Med. 177, 999–1008.

Goodnow, C.C., Crosbie, J., Adelstein, S., Lavoie, T.B., Smith-Gill, S.J., Brink, R.A., Pritchard-Briscoe, H., Wotherspoon, J.S., Loblay, R.H., Raphael, K., Trent, R.J., Basten, A., 1988. Altered immunoglobulin expression and functional silencing of self-reactive B lymphocytes in transgenic mice. Nature 334, 676–682.

Goodnow, C.C., Crosbie, J., Jorgenson, H., Brink, R.A., Basten, A., 1989. Induction of self-tolerance in mature peripheral B lymphocytes. Nature 342, 385–391.

Hartmann, K.-U., Reeg, S., Mehner, C., 1971. The induction of haemolysin producing cells in vitro: inhibition by antiglobulin antiserum. Immunology 20, 29–36.

Katz, D.H., Unanue, E.R., 1972. The immune capacity of lymphocytes after cross-linking of surface immunoglobulin receptors by antibody. J. Immunol. 109, 1022–1030.

Kincade, P.W., Lawton, A.R., Bockman, D.E., Cooper, M.D., 1970. Suppression of immunoglobulin G synthesis as a result of antibody-mediated suppression of immunoglobulin M synthesis in chickens. Proc. Natl. Acad. Sci. U.S.A. 67, 1918–1925.

Lesley, J., Dutton, R.W., 1970. Antigen receptor molecules: inhibition by antiserum against kappa light chains. Science 169, 487–488.

Litaka, M., Aquayo, J.F., Iwatani, Y., Row, V.V., Volpe, R., 1988. In vitro induction of anti-thyroid microsomal antibody-secreting cells in peripheral blood mononuclear cells from normal subjects. J. Clin. Endocrinol. Metab. 67, 749–754.

Manning, D.D., Jutila, J.W., 1972. Immunosuppression of mice injected with heterologous anti-immunoglobulin heavy chain antisera. J. Exp. Med. 135, 1316–1333.

Möller, G., 1961. Demonstration of mouse isoantigens at the cellular level by the fluorescent antibody technique. J. Exp. Med. 114, 415–434.

Nemazee, D.A., Bürki, K., 1989a. Clonal deletion of autoreactive B lymphocytes in bone marrow chimeras. Proc. Natl. Acad. Sci. U.S.A. 86, 8039–8043.

Nemazee, D.A., Bürki, K., 1989b. Clonal deletion of B lymphocytes in a transgenic mouse bearing anti-MHC class I antibody genes. Nature 337, 562–566.

Norvell, A., Mandik, L., Monroe, J.G., 1995. Engagement of the antigen-receptor on immature murine B lymphocytes results in death by apoptosis. J. Immunol. 154, 4404–4413.

Nossal, G.J.V., Pike, B.L., 1975. Evidence for the clonal abortion theory of B-lymphocyte tolerance. J. Exp. Med. 141, 904–917.

Nossal, G.J.V., Pike, B.L., 1980. Clonal anergy: persistence in tolerant mice of antigen-binding B lymphocytes incapable of responding to antigen or mitogen. Proc. Natl. Acad. Sci. U.S.A. 77, 1602–1606.

Primi, D., Hammarström, L., Smith, C.I.E., Möller, G., 1977a. Characterization of self-reactive B cells by polyclonal B cell activators. J. Exp. Med. 145, 21–30.

Primi, D., Smith, C.I.E., Hammarström, L., Lundquist, P.G., Möller, G., 1977b. Evidence for the existence of self-reactive human B lymphocytes. Clin. Exp. Immunol. 29, 316–319.

Raff, M.C., Owen, J.J.T., Cooper, M.D., Lawton, A.R., Megson, M., Gathings, W.E., 1975. Differences in susceptibility of mature and immature mouse B lymphocytes to anti-immunoglobulin-induced immunoglobulin suppression in vitro. Possible implications for B-cell tolerance to self. J. Exp. Med. 142, 1052–1064.

Russell, D.M., Dembic, Z., Morahan, G., Miller, J.F.A.P., Bürki, K., Nemazee, D., 1991. Peripheral deletion of self-reactive B cells. Nature 354, 308–311.

Sidman, C.L., Unanue, E.R., 1975. Receptor-mediated inactivation of early B lymphocytes. Nature 257, 149–151.

Tiegs, S.L., Russell, D.M., Nemazee, D., 1993. Receptor editing in self-reactive bone marrow B cells. J. Exp. Med. 177, 1009–1020.

Unanue, E.R., Perkins, W.D., Karnofsky, M.J., 1972. Ligand-induced movement of lymphocyte membrane macromolecules I. Analysis by immunofluorescence and ultrastructural radioautography. J. Exp. Med. 136, 885–906.

Vitetta, E., Baur, S., Uhr, J.W., 1971. Cell surface immunoglobulin. II. Isolation and characterization of immunoglobulin from mouse splenic lymphocytes. J. Exp. Med. 134, 242–264.

TIME LINE

1949	F. Macfarlane Burnet and Frank Fenner hypothesize that developing antigen reactive cells are susceptible to tolerance induction
1953	Rupert Billingham, Leslie Brent, and Peter Medawar induce immunologic tolerance to foreign tissue by injecting newborn mice with alloantigens
1975	Charles Sidman and Emil Unanue and Martin Raff and colleagues independently demonstrate that prolonged treatment of immature B lymphocytes with antibody to immunoglobulin leads to cell death
1975	Gus Nossal and Beverley Pike report that treatment of immature B lymphocytes with antigen induces cell death
1980	Gus Nossal and Beverley Pike report that B cell tolerance might involve the induction of anergy
1989	David Nemazee and Kurt Bürki provide in vivo evidence that maturation of B cells in an environment in which antigen is present leads to death of B lymphocytes
1989	Christopher Goodnow and colleagues show that mature B cells can be deleted or inactivated by interaction with antigen
1993	Martin Weigert and colleagues and David Nemazee and colleagues demonstrate receptor editing in maturing B lymphocytes

22

Development of Tolerance to Self in T Lymphocytes

INTRODUCTION

Self–non-self discrimination, one of the hallmarks of the adaptive immune response (Chapter 2), is termed immunologic tolerance and is an acquired trait of the immune system (Chapter 8). Tolerance represents a mechanism by which individuals maintain homeostasis and refrain from destroying self. Differentiation of self from non-self (foreign) is critical to protect against the development of autoimmune disease.

The concept of immunologic tolerance derived from experiments performed in the 1940s and 1950s, including

- observations by Ray Owen in 1945 that some twin cattle share a common circulatory system in utero and, as a result, fail to react immunologically against their twin's red cells and skin; and
- studies by Rupert Billingham and his colleagues in 1953 in which they induced unresponsiveness to foreign alloantigens in newborn mice.

Subsequent studies focused on the lymphocyte as the central player in the development of self–non-self discrimination. F. Macfarlane Burnet and Frank Fenner in 1949 postulated that lymphocytes learn to differentiate self from non-self during maturation. Support for Burnet and Fenner's hypothesis came from studies in the 1950s

that showed that immunologic tolerance is more readily induced in immature lymphocytes than in fully differentiated cells.

The characterization of lymphocytes into functionally distinct T and B populations in the 1960s led immunologists to study the roles of T and B lymphocytes in maintaining self-tolerance. Investigators showed that potentially self-reactive B lymphocytes can be silenced by several mechanisms: deletion, anergy, or receptor editing (Chapter 21). The discovery that optimal activation of B lymphocytes requires interaction with T lymphocytes stimulated additional studies on tolerance induction in T lymphocytes.

In 1961, Jacques Miller demonstrated that the thymus is required for the maturation of a population of lymphocytes now known as T lymphocytes. Subsequent studies identified the thymus as the anatomical location in which T lymphocytes differentiate and acquire immunocompetence (Chapter 9). Thus it seemed reasonable that the thymus might be the site for the induction of immunological tolerance. Investigators showed that T lymphocytes interact with antigens through a cell-surface receptor, the T cell receptor (TCR) (Chapter 17). The TCR is synthesized by the T lymphocyte following a random rearrangement of several gene segments during differentiation in the thymus.

A Historical Perspective on Evidence-Based Immunology
http://dx.doi.org/10.1016/B978-0-12-398381-7.00022-8

The process of gene rearrangement results in the formation of large numbers of DNA sequences coding for different TCRs, each with unique antigen specificity. Expression of these TCRs on T lymphocytes provides an equally large repertoire of antigen-reactive lymphocytes. Among these lymphocytes are some that are potentially self-reactive. If self-reactive lymphocytes are released to the mature lymphocyte pool in the spleen and lymph nodes, activation of these lymphocytes might lead to the development of autoimmune diseases such as type 1 diabetes and systemic lupus erythematosus. The mechanisms that have evolved to eliminate these potentially self-reactive lymphocytes during lymphocyte development have been revealed by research performed during the past 25 years.

DIFFERENTIATION OF T LYMPHOCYTES IN THE THYMUS

Immature lymphoid precursors migrate from the hematopoietic tissue in the bone marrow to the thymus where they differentiate to competent T lymphocytes. Once these lymphocytes have matured they migrate to peripheral lymphoid tissue, including the spleen and lymph nodes. The thymus is a site of intense proliferation where many more lymphocytes are produced than are released to the peripheral lymphoid tissues. This observation led investigators to question what happened to all the newly formed thymic lymphocytes.

Don Metcalf, working at the Walter and Eliza Hall Institute of Medical Research in Melbourne, Australia, grafted 3-month-old mice with between 12 and 48 thymus glands from neonatal mice. Each graft in a multigrafted animal became populated with similar numbers of lymphocytes (as determined by the weights of the grafts). However, the presence of these additional sites of lymphopoiesis failed to significantly increase the size and weight of the peripheral lymphoid organs (Metcalf, 1963).

In subsequent investigations Metcalf and his colleagues transplanted multiple thymuses into one recipient that was injected with tritiated thymidine to label proliferating T lymphocytes in vivo. Most lymphocytes detected in the thymus grafts contained the radiolabel, indicating active proliferation in the organ. Few labeled lymphocytes were found in peripheral lymphoid tissues, suggesting that most never left the thymus but, rather, died in situ (Matsuyama et al., 1966). The authors concluded that "the majority of small lymphocytes produced in the thymus … do not migrate from these tissues but die locally at the end of their intrathymic life span of 3 to 4 days."

During these 3 to 4 days in the thymus, a sequence of events leads to the elimination of 90–95% of the newly formed lymphocytes and the release of a small population of mature, antigen-specific T lymphocytes to

peripheral lymphoid tissue. The genes responsible for coding for the TCR undergo rearrangement (Chapter 18) and the TCR is expressed on the surface of the lymphocyte. The random nature of the rearrangement process results in lymphocytes expressing a myriad of different specificities, including ones that recognize self. These lymphocytes undergo a selection process, the goal of which is to release only those T lymphocytes that bind antigens presented by cells expressing histocompatibility molecules of the individual (Chapter 20) while simultaneously failing to bind self-antigens. This process involves two steps:

- Positive selection in which the TCR is tested to determine if it can bind peptides embedded in self-histocompatibility molecules. During this stage the CD phenotype (CD4 or CD8) of the lymphocyte is set.
- Negative selection in which the developing T lymphocyte is presented with peptides representing self-antigens to eliminate potentially self-reactive clones.

Every lymphoid precursor that enters the thymus is programmed to genetically undergo cell death (apoptosis) unless it is rescued during the selection process. Developing T lymphocytes that fail to bind self-histocompatibility antigens, or bind too avidly to self-peptides, are eliminated. Only after this censoring phase of development is complete will the T lymphocyte be released to join the peripheral lymphocyte pool.

The nonlymphoid cells of the thymus comprise several unique cell types specialized to present peptides to the developing T lymphocytes. The cortex of the organ contains epithelial cells that express both class I and class II molecules coded for by the major histocompatibility complex (MHC) genes of the individual. These histocompatibility molecules contain self-peptides derived from the normal breakdown of other cells.

The thymus medulla also contains epithelial cells as well as a small number of dendritic cells. These cells express class I and/or class II histocompatibility molecules. While many of these nonlymphoid cells present self-peptides derived from tissue breakdown, some of these medullary cells express self-peptides that they synthesize under control of a transcription factor coded for by a gene termed AutoImmune REgulator (AIRE).

POSITIVE SELECTION OF T LYMPHOCYTES

Positive selection occurs in the thymus cortex and results in T lymphocytes that recognize antigenic peptides presented by histocompatibility molecules. During this process the maturing lymphocytes, which initially express both CD4 and CD8 receptors, downregulate the synthesis and expression of one of these molecules and become either a CD4+ or a CD8+ lymphocyte.

Rolf Zinkernagel and Peter Doherty (1974a, b), working at the John Curtin School of Medical Research in Canberra, Australia, demonstrated that cytotoxic T lymphocytes would only kill virally infected cells if the infected cell and the T lymphocyte shared MHC genes (Chapters 16 and 20). These investigators suggested two possible models to explain these observations (Figure 22.1):

1. the intimacy model in which cytotoxic T lymphocytes recognize two structures on the surface of the virally infected cell, one representing the viral antigen and a second coded for by the MHC; or
2. the altered self model in which the viral antigen is embedded into the structure of the histocompatibility molecule; this complex constitutes a new antigen recognized by a single receptor on the cytotoxic T lymphocyte.

Zinkernagel reasoned that these two models could be differentiated by evaluating the maturation of T lymphocyte precursors from one inbred strain of mice in an environment in which they were presented with foreign histocompatibility molecules. Working at the Scripps

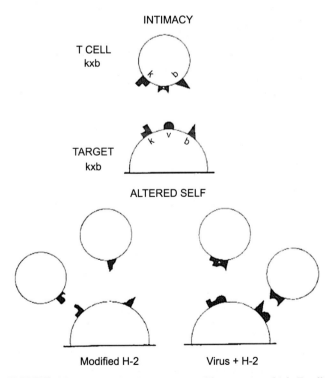

FIGURE 22.1 Diagram depicting possible ways in which T cells recognizing virally infected targets might be restricted by the H-2 antigens. The intimacy model (top) postulated that the cytotoxic T lymphocyte expressed two cell-surface receptors—one specific for the viral antigens and a second that would interact with the MHC-coded molecule. The altered self models (bottom) hypothesized that T lymphocytes recognized MHC-coded molecules that had been altered by the virus. *From Zinkernagel and Doherty (1974b)*

Clinic and Research Foundation in La Jolla, California, Zinkernagel thymectomized and irradiated F1 hybrid mice. He reconstituted these mice with bone marrow cells from one of the parent strains and determined the cytotoxic potential of the mature T lymphocytes to choriomeningitis virally infected cells (Zinkernagel, 1976).

Zinkernagel predicted that if the intimacy model were correct, parental strain lymphocytes maturing in an F1 thymus would only recognize virally infected cells of the original parental strain. Alternatively, if the altered self model were correct, the parental strain lymphocytes that matured in an F1 hybrid thymus would recognize virally infected cells expressing the histocompatibility molecules of either parent.

Cytotoxic T lymphocytes derived from precursors transferred from one strain and allowed to mature in the thymus of an F1 hybrid recognize the histocompatibility antigens of both parental strains. Similar results were reported simultaneously (1976) by two other groups of investigators: Klaus Pfizenmaier and colleagues working at the Institute of Medical Microbiology in Mainz, Germany, and Harold von Boehmer and Werner Haas at the Basel Institute for Immunology, Switzerland.

Michael Bevan at the Massachusetts Institute of Technology in Cambridge, Massachusetts, confirmed these results in 1977 using lethally irradiated parental strain mice reconstituted with hematopoietic stem cells from an F1 hybrid. In this protocol, F1 precursor cells migrate to the thymus and undergo differentiation. The epithelial cells of the thymus are resistant to the level of radiation used in these experiments, and hence the F1 precursors mature in an environment containing histocompatiblity molecules from just one of the parental strains. Bevan predicted that if the intimacy model were correct and the developing T lymphocytes expressed two receptors, one for the antigen and a second for the histocompatibility molecules, the F1 stem cells differentiating in a parental environment would recognize antigenic peptide presented by the histocompatibility molecules from either parent. Alternatively, if the altered self model were correct and the environment of the thymus participated in selecting cells, the mature peripheral T lymphocyte pool would recognize only the histocompatibility molecules of the parent in which they developed.

Results supported the second prediction (Bevan, 1977). These experiments showed that the nonlymphoid cells present in the thymus play a role in determining the specificity of the developing T lymphocytes; this phenomenon was termed "positive selection."

Selection of the CD Phenotype of T Lymphocytes

A second outcome of positive selection in the thymus is establishing the CD phenotype of the mature lymphocyte.

Precursor lymphocytes entering the thymus express neither of the CD markers (CD4 or CD8) found on mature T lymphocytes in the periphery. Shortly after arrival in the thymus, the genes coding for both CD4 and CD8 are transcribed, and the lymphocytes express both CD4 and CD8, becoming double-positive thymocytes. Following positive selection the gene coding for one or the other CD markers is silenced, and the maturing lymphocyte becomes single positive, either CD4$^+$ or CD8$^+$. The class of histocompatibility molecule involved in positive selection determines which gene is downregulated.

CD4 and CD8 molecules bind to nonpolymorphic (constant) portions of the histocompatibility molecules. CD4 binds to class II molecules expressed on antigen-presenting cells, including macrophages, dendritic cells, and B lymphocytes, while CD8 binds to class I molecules expressed on all somatic cells. Philippa Marrack, John Kappler, and their collaborators (Gay et al., 1987) at the University of Colorado Health Sciences Center, Denver, transfected a mouse T hybridoma specific for the mouse histocompatibility antigen, H-2D^b, with the gene coding for human CD4. These lymphocytes expressed a TCR that bound the histocompatibility molecule as well as the CD4 molecule. Gay and coworkers incubated these transfected mouse/human hybrids with target cells that expressed H-2D^b. These target cells were themselves transfected with genes coding for the human class II molecule HLA-DR. The level of activation of the hybridomas was measured by the amount of the cytokine IL-2 released into the culture medium.

Culture of nontransfected T hybridoma cells with transfected target cells (as control) produced a low level of IL-2 secretion. Incubation of the T hybridomas expressing human CD4 with target cells expressing a class II histocompatibility molecule, HLA-DR, resulted in synthesis and secretion of an increased amount of IL-2. Adding antibodies specific for CD4 or HLA-DR to the cultures inhibited this stimulation of the hybridoma cells. These results allowed the researchers to propose "that CD4:HLA-DR binding occurs…and that this interaction augments T-cell activation."

These results inspired additional experiments to determine the mechanism by which a T lymphocyte becomes restricted to either CD4 or CD8 in the thymus. Harold von Boehmer and his colleagues, working at the Basel Institute of Immunology in Switzerland, developed transgenic mice that contained a large proportion of T lymphocytes expressing TCRs specific for the H-Y antigen presented by a particular class I MHC molecule (H-2D^b) (Teh et al., 1988). The H-Y antigen is a minor histocompatibility antigen coded for by a gene on the Y chromosome and, hence, immunogenic only in female mice. Analysis of the phenotype of the peripheral T lymphocytes in these mice showed that mature T lymphocytes expressing the transgenic TCR were all of the CD8 phenotype despite the fact that the precursors expressed both CD molecules. The authors conclude

that "interaction of the T-cell receptor on immature thymocytes with thymic major histocompatibility complex antigens determines the differentiation of CD4$^+$8$^+$ thymocytes into either CD4$^+$8$^-$ or CD4$^-$8$^+$ mature T cells."

NEGATIVE SELECTION OF T LYMPHOCYTES

Clonal Deletion of Self-Reactive T Lymphocytes

Negative selection follows positive selection and occurs primarily in the medulla of the thymus. The end result of negative selection is elimination or silencing of those developing T lymphocytes that might react against self-antigens and induce an autoimmune response. Burnet postulated in the clonal selection theory (1959) that developing lymphocytes are susceptible to elimination if they are specific for self. Proof for this hypothesis at the level of T lymphocytes was not obtained until nearly 30 years later.

Gus Nossal and Beverley Pike at the Walter and Eliza Hall Institute of Medical Research in Melbourne, Australia, demonstrated in 1981 that induction of neonatal tolerance to antigens coded by foreign MHC genes is accompanied by a decrease in the number of cytotoxic T lymphocytes specific for those antigens. Nossal and Pike injected newborn mice of the inbred strain CBA with spleen cells from F$_1$ hybrid (CBA × BALB/c) mice to induce tolerance to the histocompatibility antigens expressed by BALB/c mice. At intervals, the investigators harvested cells from the spleens and thymuses of these tolerant mice and determined the number of cytotoxic T lymphocyte precursors specific for BALB/c antigens. Both the thymus (starting at day 5 of life) and the spleen (from day 8 of life) contained decreased numbers of T lymphocytes specific for the BALB/c antigens when compared to control mice. The authors concluded that clonal deletion of developing T lymphocytes, most likely in the thymus, is a mechanism by which tolerance is induced.

Nossal and Pike argued that the developing lymphocytes were killed; however, two additional explanations are

- the lymphocytes are silenced by clonal anergy, or
- suppressor T lymphocytes downregulate the cytotoxic activity in peripheral lymphoid tissue. (Note: In 1981, T lymphocytes that downregulated the adaptive immune response were thought to be CD8 and were known as suppressor T lymphocytes. Today immunologists agree that T regulatory lymphocytes are CD4 (Chapter 24)).

Experiments designed by John Kappler and Philippa Marrack's group at the University of Colorado in Denver addressed these possibilities.

Kappler and Marrack developed a series of hybridomas secreting monoclonal antibodies specific for TCRs. One of these antibodies, induced by immunizing BALB/c mice with T lymphocytes from SWR mice, was specific for an epitope termed Vβ17a (a variable region present on the β-chain of some TCRs). This epitope is expressed in SWR mice but not in, BALB/c or C57Bl/10 mice. T lymphocytes expressing TCRs with this determinant bind a class II histocompatibility molecule termed IE. Mice of the SWR strain (from which the original immunizing T lymphocytes were derived) are IE negative while many other strains, including BALB/c and C57Bl/10, are IE positive. The monoclonal antibody was used to identify T lymphocytes with the potential to bind this IE molecule.

Kappler and his group used this monoclonal antibody to follow the development of Vβ17a T lymphocytes in mice that express the IE molecule. In one such mouse strain, immature lymphocytes expressing TCRs possessing the Vβ17a epitope exist in the thymus while mature, peripheral lymphocytes fail to express TCRs with this epitope. Additional studies in which SWR mice were bred with strains of mice that express the IE protein showed that the number of mature Vβ17a positive T lymphocytes in peripheral lymphoid tissue decreased although the number of Vβ17a positive lymphocytes in the thymus was normal. The process resulting in the deletion of these lymphocytes appears to occur in the thymus. As the investigators summarize, "these data offer the first direct evidence for clonal elimination as a mechanism for inducing T cell tolerance to self-MHC antigens" (Kappler et al., 1987).

The mechanism of cell death caused by interaction of developing T lymphocytes with antigen was further investigated in tissue culture using the superantigen, staphylococcal enterotoxin B (SEB). Superantigens bind a large number of mature T lymphocytes based on the Vβ regions expressed on their TCRs. In 1989, Erik Jenkinson and colleagues at the University of Birmingham Medical School in England added SEB to immature T lymphocytes in cultures of thymus taken from 14-day-old mouse embryos. Treatment of immature T lymphocytes with SEB would be expected to silence any developing T lymphocytes expressing the target Vβ region. Jenkinson and coworkers observed DNA fragmentation and the initiation of a process known as apoptosis. Exposure of thymus tissue to antibodies specific for CD3 in vitro also resulted in apoptosis (Smith et al., 1989).

The main mechanism involved in the induction of central tolerance in T lymphocytes appears to involve clonal deletion. However, other studies demonstrated that maturing lymphocytes in the thymus could be rendered anergic (inactive but not killed) or could go through a process of receptor editing similar to the processes observed in B lymphocytes (Chapter 21).

Clonal Anergy in T Lymphocytes

Anergy is a state of unresponsiveness induced in a lymphocyte following interaction with an antigen in the absence of a costimulatory signal (Chapter 20). This phenomenon occurs primarily with lymphocytes in peripheral lymphoid tissue such as the spleen and lymph nodes, but some evidence exists that a similar mechanism may play a role during the development of the T lymphocyte in the thymus.

Ronald Schwartz at the National Institute of Allergy and Infectious Diseases, Bethesda, Maryland, performed much of the early work on anergy induction in T lymphocytes. He designed two experimental protocols to study induction of immunologic tolerance, both of which resulted in anergy (unresponsiveness):

1. exposure of mouse lymphocytes in vitro to pigeon cytochrome c chemically linked to spleen cells; and
2. exposure of mice in vivo to foreign histocompatibility molecules in an artificial membrane.

T lymphocyte hybridomas specific for pigeon cytochrome c proliferate when stimulated with cytochrome c. However, when these same hybridomas are exposed to pigeon cytochrome c linked to spleen cells, the proliferative response is significantly reduced. In fact, instead of a proliferative response, this treatment stimulates a long-term unresponsiveness in the hybridomas even when additional antigen-presenting cells are added to the cultures. A similar unresponsiveness is observed when spleen cells to which pigeon cytochrome c is linked are injected intravenously into control mice (Jenkins and Schwartz, 1987). As the investigators concluded, these results are "most consistent with a functional clonal deletion model of T cell tolerance induction and suggest that antigen/Ia molecule recognition under non-mitogenic conditions can result in induction of an unresponsive state."

Similar results were obtained using a model involving T lymphocyte clones that serve as inducers (helpers) of other lymphocytes. Helen Quill and Ronald Schwartz in 1987 constructed artificial membranes that expressed class II histocompatibility molecules. Pigeon cytochrome c incubated with these membranes resulted in the binding of cytochrome c to the histocompatibility molecules. Quill and Schwartz cultured T lymphocyte clones specific for cytochrome c with these membranes and assayed them for activation by measuring the increase in lymphocyte size, quantity of ^{3}H-thymidine incorporated, and the amount of the cytokines IL-2 and IL-3 secreted into the culture medium.

T lymphocyte clones treated with antigen and histocompatibility molecules in artificial membranes increased in size and secreted IL-3 but failed to proliferate or secrete IL-2. These treated lymphocytes also failed to proliferate when subsequently challenged with cytochrome *c* presented by antigen-presenting cells such as macrophages.

Interpretation of these results incorporated the idea that optimal activation of T lymphocytes required two signals: one provided by the interaction of the TCR with the antigen being presented by a histocompatibility molecule and a second by interaction between separate molecules on the T lymphocyte (CD28) and on the antigen-presenting cell (CD80/86) (Chapter 20). Quill and Schwartz conclude that their results "demonstrate that recognition by normal T cell clones of antigen and Ia" (class II histocompatibility molecules) "in the absence of other accessory cell molecules and signals results in a prolonged state of proliferative unresponsiveness possibly similar to a state of T cell tolerance in vivo."

Fiona Harding and her colleagues at the University of California, Berkeley (1992), explored the role of CD28:CD80/86 interaction in the induction of anergy. CD4+ T lymphocytes express several cell surface molecules, including CD3 and CD28. CD3 is expressed on all mature T lymphocytes where it is associated with the TCR and functions to transmit activation signals from the TCR to the nucleus. CD28 serves as the ligand for CD80/86 on antigen-presenting cells and provides a second signal in the activation of T lymphocytes. Treatment of T lymphocytes with optimal concentrations of antibodies to CD3 induces proliferation of the lymphocytes and the synthesis and secretion of the cytokine IL-2.

Harding and her colleagues added T lymphocytes to petri dishes to which a low concentration of antibody to CD3 had been bound; these lymphocytes failed to enter mitosis. Addition of a second signal in the form of antibody to CD28 to the cultures stimulated proliferation. The exposure of T lymphocytes to antibodies specific for CD3 and CD28 also increased the amount of IL-2 secreted by these cells.

The investigators extended these findings to a model of T lymphocyte anergy using T lymphocyte clones stimulated with antigen chemically linked to allogeneic spleen cells. These lymphocytes became anergic and failed to proliferate or secrete IL-2. This anergic state could be prevented if antibody specific for CD28 was present in the in vitro system while the T lymphocyte clones interacted with antigen. These results provided insights into the mechanism of T lymphocyte activation and a potential method for regulating overreactive T lymphocytes.

Receptor Editing in Developing T Lymphocytes

Developing B lymphocytes that express a cell-surface receptor specific for self may change the V genes being used to code for this receptor. This process is termed receptor editing and results in a new BCR that is subjected to selection (Chapter 21). A similar mechanism in developing T lymphocytes has been reported by several groups.

Fanping Wang and colleagues at Washington University, St. Louis, Missouri in 1998 constructed clones of T lymphocytes into which they inserted a rearranged TCR Vα and Jα gene derived from a T lymphocyte clone specific for cytochrome *c*. Most immature T lymphocytes developing in mice containing this gene expressed the introduced VαJα chain; however, once these cells progressed through maturation, the number of T lymphocytes expressing this gene declined significantly. The decrease in the number of T lymphocytes expressing this gene was due to rearrangement of the TCR α-chain and suggests that receptor editing occurs in T lymphocytes.

Using a different model, Maureen McGargill and her colleagues at the University of Minnesota provided additional evidence for receptor editing in developing thymocytes (2000). These investigators designed transgenic mice that expressed several peptides from chicken ovalbumin on thymic epithelium cells. The peptides studied differed in their affinity to bind to the TCRs. Peptides with a low binding affinity resulted in positive selection of developing T lymphocytes. McGargill and coworkers predicted that peptides with high binding affinity would induce apoptosis in the maturing T lymphocytes as an indicator of negative selection. This prediction failed confirmation and, instead, engagement of the T lymphocytes with the high affinity peptide induced internalization of the TCR and gene rearrangement in the α-chain locus. The conclusion from these observations is that immature, self-reactive T lymphocytes edit the genes coding for the TCR in a manner similar to that previously demonstrated for B lymphocytes.

CONCLUSION

Several mechanisms exist for the induction of immunological unresponsiveness in T lymphocytes. Many of these occur in the thymus, a central lymphoid organ. Maturing T lymphocytes go through positive selection during which they are selected based on binding to self-histocompatibility molecules followed by negative selection to eliminate or silence those lymphocytes capable of binding self-antigens.

Results presented in this chapter lead to additional questions that need to be addressed:

- Do the epithelial cells responsible for negative selection in the thymus express every potential self-antigen to which mature T lymphocytes might be exposed in peripheral lymphoid tissues?
- What happens to T lymphocytes that slip through the censoring function of the thymus?

Partial answers to these questions have been provided by recent investigations, including

- Investigators identified a gene expressed in the thymus medulla that codes for a transcription factor involved in synthesizing peptides representing self-antigens. This gene, known as AIRE, is under intensive study; the role of mutations in this gene in the development of autoimmune disease is covered in Chapter 34.
- Immunologists identified a population of regulatory T lymphocytes in peripheral lymphoid tissues that downregulate potentially autoreactive T lymphocytes (Chapter 24). The elimination or silencing of self-reactive T lymphocytes in the periphery occurs following activation of T lymphocytes and involves several mechanisms, including
  - activation of T regulatory lymphocytes and secretion of cytokines, including IL-10 and TGF-β (Chapter 24);
  - deletion resulting from Fas–Fas ligand interactions (Chapter 27); and
  - suppression through interaction of CD152 (CTLA4) with CD80/86 on antigen-presenting cells (Chapter 27).

Continued investigation of T lymphocyte tolerance mechanisms promises to lead to the development of ever more specific methods of regulating potentially pathogenic autoimmune responses.

References

Bevan, M.J., 1977. In a radiation chimaera, host H-2 antigens determine immune responsiveness of donor cytotoxic cells. Nature 269, 417–418.

Billingham, R.E., Brent, L., Medawar, P.B., 1953. 'Actively acquired tolerance' of foreign cells. Nature 172, 603–606.

Burnet, F.M., 1959. The Clonal Selection Theory of Acquired Immunity. Vanderbilt University Press, Nashville, TN.

Burnet, F.M., Fenner, F., 1949. Production of Antibodies, second ed. MacMillan, London.

Gay, D., Maddon, P., Sekaly, R., Talle, M.A., Godfrey, M., Long, E., Goldstein, G., Chess, L., Axel, R., Kappler, J., Marrack, P., 1987. Functional interaction between human T cell protein CD4 and the major histocompatibility complex HLA-DR antigen. Nature 328, 626–629.

Harding, F.A., McArthur, J.G., Gross, J.A., Raulet, D.H., Allison, J.P., 1992. CD-28 mediated signaling co-stimulates murine T cells and prevents induction of anergy in T-cell clones. Nature 356, 607–609.

Jenkins, M.K., Schwartz, R.H., 1987. Antigen presentation by chemically modified splenocytes induces antigen-specific T cell unresponsiveness in vitro and in vivo. J. Exp. Med. 165, 302–319.

Jenkinson, E.J., Kingston, R., Smith, C.A., Williams, G.T., Owen, J.J.T., 1989. Antigen-induced apoptosis in developing T cells: a mechanism for negative selection of the T cell repertoire. Eur. J. Immunol. 19, 2175–2177.

Kappler, J.W., Roehm, N., Marrack, P., 1987. T cell tolerance by clonal elimination in the thymus. Cell 49, 273–280.

Matsuyama, M., Wiadrowski, M.N., Metcalf, D., 1966. Autoradiographic analysis of lymphopoiesis and lymphocyte migration in mice bearing multiple thymus grafts. J. Exp. Med. 123, 559–576.

McGargill, M.A., Derbinski, J.M., Hogquist, K.A., 2000. Receptor editing in developing T cells. Nat. Immunol. 1, 336–341.

Metcalf, D., 1963. The autonomous behavior of normal thymus grafts. Aust. J. Exp. Biol. Med. Sci. 41 (Suppl.), 437–447.

Miller, J.F.A.P., 1961. Immunological function of the thymus. Lancet 278, 748–749.

Nossal, G.J.V., Pike, B.L., 1981. Functional clonal deletion in immunological tolerance to major histocompatibility complex antigens. Proc. Nat. Acad. Sci. U.S.A. 78, 3844–3847.

Owen, R.D., 1945. Immunogenetic consequences of vascular anastomoses between bovine twins. Science 102, 400–401.

Pfizenmaier, K., Starzinski-Powitz, A., Rodt, H., Rollinghoff, M., Wagner, H., 1976. Virus and trinitrophenol hapten-specific T-cell-mediated cytotoxicity against H-2 incompatible target cells. J. Exp. Med. 143, 999–1004.

Quill, H., Schwartz, R.H., 1987. Stimulation of normal inducer T cell clones with antigen presented by purified Ia molecules in planar lipid membranes: specific induction of a long-lived state of proliferative nonresponsiveness. J. Immunol. 138, 3704–3712.

Smith, C.A., Williams, G.T., Kingston, R., Jenkinson, E.J., Owen, J.J.T., 1989. Antibodies to CD3/T cell receptor complex induce death by apoptosis in immature T cells in thymic cultures. Nature 337, 181–184.

Teh, H.S., Kisielow, P., Scott, B., Kishi, H., Uematsu, Y., Blüthmann, H., von Boehmer, H., 1988. Thymic major histocompatibility complex antigens and the $\alpha\beta$ T-cell receptor determine the CD4/CD8 phenotype of T cells. Nature 335, 229–233.

von Boehmer, H., Haas, W., 1976. Cytotoxic T lymphocytes recognize allogeneic tolerated TNP-conjugated cells. Nature 261, 141–142.

Wang, F., Huang, C.-Y., Kanagawa, O., 1998. Rapid deletion of rearranged T cell antigen receptor (TCR) Vα-Jα segment by secondary rearrangement in the thymus: role of continuous rearrangement of TCR α chain gene and positive selection in the T cell repertoire formation. Proc. Nat. Acad. Sci. U.S.A. 95, 11834–11839.

Zinkernagel, R.M., 1976. Virus-specific T-cell-mediated cytotoxicity across the H-2 barrier to virus-altered alloantigen. Nature 261, 139–141.

Zinkernagel, R.M., Doherty, P.C., 1974a. Restriction of in vitro T cell-mediated cytotoxicity in lymphocytic choriomeningitis within a syngeneic or semiallogeneic system. Nature 248, 701–702.

Zinkernagel, R.M., Doherty, P.C., 1974b. Immunological surveillance against altered self-components by sensitized T lymphocytes in lymphocytic choriomeningitis. Nature 251, 547–548.

TIME LINE

1945   Ray Owen observes chimerism in twin cattle

1953   Rupert Billingham and colleagues induce unresponsiveness to foreign alloantigens in mice

1959   F. Macfarlane Burnet hypothesizes that potentially self-reactive cells are eliminated during development

1961   Jacque Miller demonstrates the role of the thymus in maturation of the cells of the immune system

1963   Donald Metcalf provides evidence that the number of lymphocytes leaving the thymus is regulated

1966   Donald Metcalf's group shows that most lymphocytes arising in the thymus never leave the organ

1974   Rolf Zinkernagel and Peter Doherty demonstrate that cytotoxic T lymphocytes (CTL) kill virally infected cells only if the cell and the CTL share MHC genes

1976   Rolf Zinkernagel demonstrates that recognition of histocompatibility antigens by T lymphocytes depends on the thymus

1977   Michael Bevan demonstrates the role of the thymus in determining the specificity of maturing T lymphocytes (positive selection)

1981   Gus Nossal and Beverley Pike reveal that induction of tolerance to a foreign MHC antigen is accompanied by a decrease in the number of cytotoxic T cells

1987   John Kappler and Philippa Marrack demonstrate that T cell tolerance to self-MHC antigens involves the elimination of reactive cells (negative selection)

1987   Marc Jenkins and Ronald Schwartz establish anergy (inactivation) as a mechanism of T cell tolerance

1988   Harold von Boehmer and colleagues demonstrate that the class of MHC molecule with which a developing T cell interacts determines the expression of CD4 or CD8

1989   Erik Jenkinson and colleagues report that cell death during tolerance induction involves the induction of apoptosis

1992   Fiona Harding and colleagues show that the interaction of T cells with antigen in the absence of a second signal results in the induction of anergy

1998   Fanping Wang and colleagues demonstrate receptor editing in T cell clones

23

T Lymphocyte Subpopulations

INTRODUCTION

Lymphocytes of the adaptive immune system are divided into B and T populations based on

- sites of maturation (Chapters 9 and 10); and
- functions (Chapters 13, 24, 26, and 27).

Bruce Glick and colleagues reported in 1956 that the cells responsible for antibody synthesis and secretion (B lymphocytes) mature in the bursa of Fabricius in birds and in the bone marrow in mammals. In 1961, Jacques Miller demonstrated that extirpation of the thymus early in the life of a mouse decreased the number of lymphocytes in the peripheral lymphoid organs in adults. The cells dependent on the thymus for maturation are called T lymphocytes and are involved in cell-mediated immune responses and immunoregulation.

When activated, T lymphocytes perform several different functions in the adaptive and innate immune systems:

- initiate inflammation,
- help B and T lymphocytes,
- reject foreign transplants,
- destroy malignantly transformed cells,
- eliminating infected cells, and
- regulating ongoing immune responses.

This multitude of functions suggested that subpopulations of T lymphocytes exist. In a search for distinct T lymphocyte populations, a variety of techniques have been employed, including

- separation by physical methods such as electrophoresis, ultracentrifugation, and gradient separation;
- evaluation of sensitivity to drugs (i.e., steroids);
- characterization of morphological differences as determined by T lymphocytes binding to and forming "rosettes" with erythrocytes from various species;
- detection of unique cell surface molecules; and
- characterization of secreted cytokines.

Studies using physical separation of cells, sensitivity to drugs, or morphological differences failed to consistently detect subpopulations of T lymphocytes. However, the antibodies induced to cell surface molecules expressed on mouse leukemias succeeded in characterizing two primary populations: CD4+ and CD8+ lymphocytes. Investigators characterized functional subpopulations of CD4+ T lymphocytes based on differential secretion of cytokines.

ANTIBODY STUDIES TO IDENTIFY T LYMPHOCYTE SUBSETS

Isoantibody Studies

Mouse lymphocytes express a number of cell-specific molecules (isoantigens) that differ antigenically between strains. Injecting one inbred strain of mice with lymphocytes from a second inbred strain induces the synthesis of isoantibodies. Edward A. Boyse and his colleagues, initially at the Sloan-Kettering Institute for Cancer Research, New York and Cornell University, Ithaca, New York, and later at Harvard Medical School, Cambridge, Massachusetts, characterized antigens present on transplantable mouse lymphoid leukemia lines. They immunized inbred strains of mice with virally induced tumors obtained from other inbred mouse strains (Boyse et al., 1968). The resulting antibodies killed the leukemic cells that induced them as well as nonmalignant lymphocytes. These antibodies detected antigens termed Ly antigens in nontumor-bearing animals that are expressed primarily by lymphocytes, including those in the thymus and in the periphery.

Boyse and Cantor described two systems of lymphocyte-specific antigens, named Ly-A and Ly-B. These are coded for by two genetic loci, *Ly-A* and *Ly-B*, each of which has two alleles. The researchers designated the allelic forms of the antigens Ly-A.1 and Ly-A.2 or Ly-B.1 and Ly-B.2. Subsequently, a third antigen with two alleles, Ly-C.1 and Ly-C.2, was discovered (Boyse et el., 1971).

The Ly-A, Ly-B, and Ly-C antigens are expressed on both naïve and activated T lymphocytes with a higher concentration of the antigens detected on lymphocytes from the thymus. Similar antibodies to these isoantigens could be induced in mouse strains immunized with thymic lymphocytes from inbred strains of mice differing at the various Ly loci (Shiku et al., 1975). By the mid-1970s, the nomenclature for these antigens had been changed to Ly-1 (Ly-A), Ly-2 (Ly-B), and Ly-3 (Ly-C).

Harvey Cantor and Edward Boyse (1975a) studied the distribution of Ly antigens in various organs. They labeled thymus, spleen, and lymph node cells from adult mice with ^{51}Cr in vitro and mixed them with antibodies to Ly antigens plus complement in a cytotoxic assay. They compared the amount of ^{51}Cr released by treatment with antibody to the total amount of ^{51}Cr released when the cells were lysed by freezing and thawing and then calculated the percentage of cells that expressed the antigen in a particular population.

Treatment with each of the antibodies to Ly antigens plus complement lysed more than 90% of lymphocytes in the thymus. These results suggest that the majority of thymic lymphocytes express all three Ly antigens. Comparatively, 35–40% of spleen lymphocytes were lysed by a mixture of antibodies to all the Ly antigens plus complement; this is similar to the number of spleen cells lysed in an identical experiment using antibodies to Thy1.2 plus complement, an antigen expressed by all T lymphocytes but not by B lymphocytes.

Treatment of spleen lymphocytes with antibodies to individual Ly antigens plus complement provided the following results:

- 30% of spleen cells express Ly-1;
- 15–20% of spleen cells express Ly-2; and
- 15–20% of spleen cells express Ly-3.

Sequential lysis of T lymphocytes from spleen and lymph node with the antibodies to Ly antigens plus complement produced the following distribution:

- 30% of peripheral T lymphocytes express predominately Ly-1 antigen;
- 7% of peripheral T lymphocytes express both Ly-2 and Ly-3 antigens but not Ly-1; and
- 50% of peripheral T lymphocytes express all three Ly antigens.

Investigators concluded that there are three unique T lymphocyte populations in peripheral lymphoid tissue based on expression of Ly antigens. Further studies focused on which of these defined populations were cytotoxic and which assisted B lymphocytes in antibody synthesis and secretion.

Cantor and Boyse (1975a) treated mouse lymphocytes with antibodies to different Ly antigens plus complement to eliminate those cells expressing the relevant antigen and subsequently tested the remaining lymphocytes in functional assays. They detected helper activity by reconstituting irradiated mice with a mixture of syngeneic B lymphocytes plus T lymphocytes depleted of one or the other Ly+ populations. The investigators injected the reconstituted mice with sheep erythrocytes and quantified the number of antibody-forming B lymphocytes detected 6 days later using a hemolytic plaque assay.

Cantor and Boyse measured T lymphocyte-mediated cytotoxicity using a similar experimental protocol. They injected irradiated mice with allogeneic T lymphocytes treated with antibodies to various Ly antigens plus complement. Five days later, they harvested spleens from these mice and cultured isolated lymphocytes with ^{51}Cr-labeled target cells expressing the same histocompatibility antigens as the irradiated mice. The amount of ^{51}Cr released during a 4-h incubation period provided a measure of the cytotoxic activity of the various Ly expressing populations.

Cantor and Boyse also generated cytotoxic T lymphocytes in vitro by culturing splenic T lymphocytes treated with antibodies to Ly antigens plus complement from one inbred strain of mice (responders) with irradiated spleen cells from a second inbred strain (stimulators). Five days later they harvested lymphocytes from these cultures and incubated them for 4 h with ^{51}Cr-labeled target cells expressing the same histocompatibility antigens as the stimulators. The amount of ^{51}Cr released after this incubation provided a measure of the activity of the various Ly$^+$ populations.

Results revealed that discrete populations of mouse T lymphocytes possess unique phenotypes. Peripheral T lymphocytes enriched for Ly-2/3$^+$ lymphocytes, following treatment with antibody against Ly-1$^+$ antigen plus complement, failed to provide help to B lymphocytes synthesizing antibodies to foreign erythrocytes but did generate cytotoxic activity. Conversely, T lymphocytes depleted of Ly-2/3$^+$ lymphocytes and hence enriched for Ly-1$^+$ lymphocytes provided help to B lymphocytes but failed to generate cytotoxicity. Cantor and Boyse concluded that helper T lymphocytes express the Ly-1 antigen while lymphocytes responsible for cell-mediated cytotoxicity express the Ly-2,3 antigen. This differential expression of the Ly antigens was seen regardless of the strains used.

At the time of these studies, T lymphocytes active in suppressing adaptive immune responses had been described (see Chapter 24); these putative T suppressor lymphocytes expressed the Ly-2,3 antigens. Finally, Ly-1$^+$ helper T lymphocytes assisted both B lymphocytes and Ly-2,3$^+$ T lymphocytes (Cantor and Boyse, 1975b).

Monoclonal Antibody Studies

In 1975, Georges Kohler and César Milstein described a method for the production of hybridomas, cloned cell lines producing monoclonal antibodies, thus providing a major technological breakthrough in the preparation of specific antibodies (Chapter 37). Several groups produced hybridomas that secreted monoclonal antibodies directed against cell surface markers on T lymphocytes.

Patrick Kung and Gideon Goldstein, working at Ortho Pharmaceutical Corporation in Raritan, New Jersey along with collaborators from the Sidney Farber Cancer Institute at Harvard in 1979 reported the development of monoclonal antibodies specific for determinants expressed on the surface of human peripheral T lymphocytes.

Kung and colleagues incubated human lymphocytes with sheep erythrocytes (SRBC). Previous researchers demonstrated that lymphocytes binding SRBCs, thus forming E-rosettes, are primarily T lymphocytes while lymphocytes that fail to form E-rosettes are mainly B lymphocytes. Kung and coworkers isolated T lymphocytes from human peripheral blood and injected mice with the isolated cells. They fused spleen cells from these mice with a mouse myeloma cell line and placed the fused cells in culture.

Culture supernatants from three hybridomas bound differentially with E-rosette positive or E-rosette negative human lymphocytes; this led to the isolation of three

monoclonal antibodies (OKT1, OKT3, and OKT4) specific for T lymphocytes. OKT1 and OKT3 antibodies bound more than 95% of peripheral T lymphocytes but fewer than 2% B lymphocytes and only 5–10% thymic lymphocytes. OKT4 antibody bound approximately 55% of peripheral T lymphocytes, less than 2% B lymphocytes, and 80% of thymic lymphocytes. (A fourth monoclonal, OKT2, possessed identical binding specificity as OKT1.)

Ellis Reinherz and colleagues determined that T lymphocytes expressing OKT4 include those that assist B lymphocytes in antibody production while OKT4-negative lymphocytes include those that become cytotoxic after stimulation of unfractionated T lymphocytes with allogeneic lymphocytes. OKT1 lymphocytes respond to T lymphocyte mitogens and soluble antigens and react in mixed lymphocyte reactions (Reinherz et al., 1979a,b).

These investigators isolated human peripheral blood lymphocytes and divided them into B lymphocytes (surface immunoglobulin positive) and T lymphocytes (surface Ig negative; E-rosette positive). T lymphocytes incubated with OKT4 antibody and a fluorescein-labeled goat antibody to mouse IgG were further separated into OKT4-positive and OKT4-negative populations by cell sorting using a fluorescence-activated cell sorter (Chapter 39).

Reinherz and coworkers cultured B lymphocytes with pokeweed mitogen, a substance that induces B lymphocyte mitosis and immunoglobulin synthesis. They supplemented these cultures with unfractionated T lymphocytes, OKT4-positive lymphocytes, or OKT4-negative lymphocytes. The addition of unfractionated T lymphocytes or OKT4-positive lymphocytes induced proliferation of the B lymphocytes and enhanced the production of immunoglobulin (Reinherz et al., 1979b). The inclusion of OKT4-negative lymphocytes failed to activate the B lymphocytes. These results demonstrate that the OKT4 monoclonal antibody defines a population of helper T lymphocytes in humans much as the antibody to the Ly-1 antigen defines helper T lymphocytes in mice.

In 1980, Reinherz and colleagues performed similar studies to define the surface markers expressed on cytotoxic T lymphocytes. By this time researchers had developed several additional monoclonal antibodies to markers on T lymphocytes, including OKT5 and OKT8. Reinherz and colleagues stimulated human peripheral blood lymphocytes in vitro with a human B lymphoblastoid cell line (Laz 156). Five days later they harvested the lymphocytes, separated them into OKT-5$^+$ and OKT-5$^-$ fractions, and tested them in a cytotoxic assay using ^{51}Cr-labeled Laz 156 cells as targets. All the cytotoxic activity segregated with the OKT-5$^+$ lymphocytes (Reinherz et al., 1980). Subsequent studies demonstrated that the antigen identified by monoclonal antibody OKT5 was also detected by a second monoclonal antibody, OKT8

(Phan-Dinh-Tuy et al., 1982). Based on the characteristics of the two antibodies, most future studies were performed using the OKT8 antibody.

The development of hybridoma technology led investigators to develop a plethora of monoclonal antibodies capable of detecting antigens expressed on populations of lymphocytes. This led to confusion since each laboratory called the resulting antibodies and the antigens they detected by different names. To reduce the confusion in comparing studies from different laboratories, the International Union of Immunology Societies (IUIS) and the World Health Organization (WHO) sponsored the First International Workshop on Human Leukocyte Differentiation Antigens in Paris in 1982. Participants at this meeting compared the specificity of 139 monoclonal antibodies submitted by 55 research groups from 14 countries. Specificity of the antibodies was determined by immunofluorescence using a panel of cultured cells. Participants in the workshop defined 15 clusters of differentiation (CD) antigens (IUIS-WHO nomenclature subcommittee, 1984). These CD antigens (CD1–11 and CDw12–w15) identified markers of various subsets of human leukocytes, including lymphocytes, granulocytes, and monocytes.

Several of the CD markers defined by this workshop are central to identifying subpopulations of T lymphocytes. Participants employed the OKT4 monoclonal antibody to characterize an antigen on some lymphocytes that is now termed CD4. CD4$^+$ T lymphocytes include those cells that provide help to B lymphocytes as well as to other T lymphocytes. Participants at the workshop also studied the monoclonal antibody detecting OKT8; the antigen detected by this antibody is called CD8 and defines a population of T lymphocytes involved in the generation of cytotoxic T lymphocyte. Most peripheral T lymphocytes express either CD4 or CD8.

Studies reviewed in Chapter 20 revealed that while the two T lymphocyte subpopulations express similar T cell receptors (TCRs), they use different mechanisms to recognize foreign antigen. TCRs expressed by CD8$^+$ lymphocytes bind antigen presented by major histocompatibility complex (MHC)-coded class I bearing antigen-presenting cells; most CD8$^+$ lymphocytes function as cytotoxic cells. TCRs expressed by CD4$^+$ T lymphocytes bind antigen presented by MHC-coded class II bearing cells, following which they perform several functions, including

- activation of B lymphocytes to efficiently synthesize antibodies,
- stimulation of CD8$^+$ T lymphocytes,
- secretion of cytokines that initiate inflammatory responses, and
- regulation of potentially pathogenic adaptive immune responses.

Measurement of CD4$^+$ and CD8$^+$ populations informs clinicians about the integrity of a patient's adaptive immune system. The human immunodeficiency virus (HIV) that causes the acquired immunodeficiency syndrome (AIDS) preferentially infects CD4$^+$ lymphocytes by binding the CD4 molecule. HIV-infected lymphocytes are destroyed, resulting in decreased numbers of these cells. The loss of CD4$^+$ lymphocytes results in a decrease in elimination of other pathogenic microorganisms, leading to recurrent and opportunistic infections, including *Pneumocystis carinii*, herpes zoster, and candida. Physicians monitor the progression of HIV infection by measuring levels of CD4$^+$ lymphocytes in the peripheral blood.

The multiple roles of CD4$^+$ lymphocytes suggested a further subdivision into functional populations; studies to assess this possibility took advantage of the finding that CD4$^+$ lymphocytes secrete a variety of different cytokines.

CYTOKINES SECRETED BY T LYMPHOCYTE SUBPOPULATIONS

T lymphocytes, unlike B lymphocytes, do not secrete antibody. T lymphocytes do, however, secrete a number of molecules, termed cytokines. Cytokines are relatively small proteins that act as intercellular messengers (Chapter 25). A variety of cells, including T and B lymphocytes and epithelial and endothelial cells, synthesize and secrete cytokines. Those secreted by T lymphocytes are critical in adaptive immune responses.

Initial studies in the 1980s separated CD4$^+$ T lymphocytes into two functional subpopulations, T helper 1(T_H1) and T helper 2 (T_H2). Both subsets of lymphocytes differentiate from a relatively immature CD4$^+$ lymphocyte called a T_H0 lymphocyte. Figure 23.1 depicts the differentiation of T_H1 and T_H2 lymphocytes as well as other populations of CD4$^+$ lymphocytes from a precursor cell that has emerged from the thymus.

In 1986, Timothy Mossman, Robert Coffman, and colleagues, working at the DNAX Research Institute of Molecular and Cellular Biology in Palo Alto, California, used long-term murine CD4$^+$ T lymphocyte clones that were specific for a variety of antigens, including chicken erythrocytes, keyhole limpet hemocyanin, or fowl gamma globulin. The investigators stimulated these clones with antigen or with the T lymphocyte mitogen, concanavalin A. Twenty-four hours later they harvested supernatants and tested them for various cytokines, including IL-2, IL-3, interferon-γ (IFN-γ), granulocyte-macrophage colony stimulating factor (GM-CSF), B-cell stimulating factor (IL-4), B-cell growth factor (IL-6), and mast cell growth factor (Chapter 25). Mossman and coworkers differentiated clones based on the cytokines each produced in response to challenge (Mossman et al., 1986). Clones designated T_H1 produce IL-2, IFN-γ, GM-CSF, and IL-3, while clones designated T_H2 produce IL-3, IL-4, IL-6, and a mast cell growth factor.

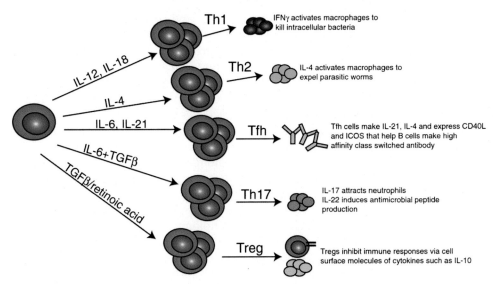

FIGURE 23.1   Diagram depicting the five functional subpopulations of CD4⁺ T lymphocytes, including the cytokines responsible for their differentiation and their unique biological functions. *From McKee et al. (2010).*

These original studies on CD4⁺ T lymphocyte subpopulations used long-term clones of lymphocytes, raising concerns about whether these results reflected the in vivo condition or if this was an in vitro artifact. Richard Locksley and his colleagues at the University of California, San Francisco, collaborated with Robert Coffman to demonstrate that, in fact, a similar phenomenon could be observed in vivo during an infection (Heinzel et al., 1989). These investigators used strains of inbred mice that responded differentially to infection with the parasite, *Leishmania major*. C57Bl mice eliminate the infection and develop lasting immunity while BALB/c mice succumb to progressive disease.

Investigators infected mice of the two strains with the parasite and then removed spleens and draining lymph nodes at weekly intervals. They extracted mRNA from isolated lymphocytes and hybridized with DNA to make probes specific for IFN-γ, IL-1, IL-2, and IL-4. Messenger RNA for IFN-γ was expressed in the lymphoid tissue of the C57Bl mice throughout the experiment while BALB/c lymphoid tissue expressed IFN-γ only transiently. The researchers reported reciprocal results when IL-4 mRNA was quantitated; lymphoid tissue from BALB/c mice expressed an IL-4 message from weeks 4–8 of the experiment, but IL-4 mRNA was not detected in the lymphoid tissues removed from C57/Bl mice. Based on these results, the authors suggest that "progression of murine leishmaniasis occurs with preferential activation of Th2...lymphocytes" while "resolution of infection occurs with preferential activation of Th1...lymphocytes."

A similar dichotomy of CD4⁺ lymphocytes is seen in the response of patients infected with *Mycobacterium leprae*, an obligate intracellular pathogen and the causative agent of leprosy. The disease is heterogeneous, ranging from patients with the lepromatous form who are unable to control the spread of the disease to tuberculoid patients who have localized granulomas without widespread dissemination of the pathogen. Investigators developed CD4⁺ T lymphocyte clones from patients with leprosy and determined the cytokine profile secreted by cells of the clones (Haanen et al., 1991; Salgame et al., 1991). In general, clones from tuberculoid patients with strong cell-mediated immunity to *M. leprae* produced primarily IFN-γ, suggesting that they are T_H1 lymphocytes, while clones from lepromatous patients who produced significant antibody secreted primarily IL-4, implying a T_H2 phenotype. mRNA extracted from skin lesions of leprosy patients and amplified in a reverse transcriptase polymerase chain reaction (PCR) using cytokine-specific primers produced similar results. The PCR product obtained from patients with the resistant form of the disease coded primarily for IL-2 and IFN-γ while mRNA from lepromatous patients coded for IL-4, IL-5, and IL-10 (Yamamura et al., 1991).

Studies over the next few years confirmed this division of CD4⁺ lymphocytes into T_H1 and T_H2 types. A Pillars of Immunology article in the *Journal of Immunology* (McGhee, 2005) summarized this division as follows:

- T_H1 lymphocytes secrete cytokines that control cell-mediated immunity.
- T_H2 lymphocytes secrete cytokines responsible for activating B lymphocytes.

Questions about these lymphocyte populations remained unanswered, including

- What is the mechanism by which CD4⁺ T lymphocytes differentiate into T_H1 or T_H2 cells?
- How do the different subpopulations of CD4⁺ T lymphocytes perform their different functions?
- What if any additional populations of CD4⁺ lymphocytes exist?

The answers to these questions emerged over the next 15 years and provide the understanding depicted in Figure 23.1.

Differentiation of CD4⁺ Subpopulations

In 1990, Graham LeGros and colleagues, working at the National Institutes of Health in Bethesda, Maryland, and Susan Swain and coworkers from the University of California, San Diego, identified the differentiation signal for T_H2 lymphocytes. Both groups of investigators used mouse lymphocytes stimulated in vitro with mitogens, antigens, or an antibody against CD3.

Naïve CD4⁺ lymphocytes synthesize low levels of IL-4 and are inefficient in activating antibody production by B lymphocytes. However, naïve T lymphocytes, stimulated in the presence of IL-2 and IL-4, develop into T_H2-cells that secrete IL-4 and IL-5 while failing to secrete IFN-γ. If IL-4 is not included in the cultures, the cells produce a cytokine profile reminiscent of T_H1 lymphocytes (IFN-γ and IL-2).

Chyi-Song Hsieh and colleagues at Washington University in St. Louis, Missouri, identified IL-12 as the differentiation signal for T_H1 lymphocytes a few years later (Hsieh et al., 1993). These investigators cultured T lymphocytes expressing a TCR specific for ovalbumin with antigen presented by macrophages. The addition of heat killed *Listeria monocytogenes* to these cultures induced maturation of T_H1 lymphocytes detected by secretion of IFN-γ. The investigators speculated that *L. monocytogenes* induced production of IL-12 that in turn stimulated differentiation of T_H1 lymphocytes. Experimental results verifying that the T_H1 phenotype is induced by IL-12 released by macrophages reacting to the added *L. monocytogenes* include the following:

- Addition of isolated IL-12 to cultures of T lymphocytes and macrophages induced the T_H1 phenotype; addition of other cytokines such as IL-1, IL-6, tumor necrosis factor-α, or transforming growth factor-β failed to induce the T_H1 phenotype.
- Separation of the *Listeria* stimulated macrophages and lymphocytes by a semipermeable membrane failed to interfere with the induction of the T_H1 phenotype, indicating that a soluble factor was involved.
- Addition of an antibody specific for IL-12 to the cultures blocked the effects of *L. monocytogenes* on the production of the T_H1 phenotype.

These results suggest separate pathways for the differentiation of T_H1 and T_H2 CD4⁺ lymphocytes. While a number of other cytokines may play supporting roles in this process (see Figure 23.1), the unique ability of IL-12 to stimulate T_H1 lymphocytes and IL-4 to stimulate T_H2 lymphocytes provides a basis for the development of potential methods to regulate the activity of these lymphocyte subpopulations.

T_H1 and T_H2 CD4⁺ lymphocytes are also differentiated based on the infectious agents they help clear (Figure 23.1). T_H1 lymphocytes secrete cytokines that activate CD8⁺ cytotoxic T lymphocytes that provide protection against intracellular pathogens such as viruses and some bacteria, including *Mycobacterium tuberculosis* and *Mycobacterium leprae*. T_H1 lymphocytes also are activated in certain pathologies, particularly autoimmune diseases, including type I diabetes and systemic lupus erythematosus. Conversely, T_H2 lymphocytes, when activated, secrete cytokines that stimulate B lymphocytes to produce antibodies (IgE) that protect against infection with protozoal parasites. The pathological counterpart of T_H2 lymphocyte activation is allergic reactions (Chapter 33).

Subsequently, researchers have described three additional subpopulations of CD4⁺ lymphocytes that are shown in Figure 23.1. These lymphocytes (T_{FH}, T_H17, and T_{REG}), like all CD4⁺ lymphocytes, mature in the thymus and perform unique functions in the adaptive immune response.

The original descriptions of T_H2 lymphocytes concluded that they help B lymphocytes switch from production of IgM to synthesis and secretion of different isotypes of antibodies. However, evidence accumulated that T_H2 lymphocytes primarily induce B lymphocytes to produce antibodies of the IgE isotype. In addition, the cytokines secreted by T_H2 lymphocytes (IL-4, IL-5, and IL-13) attract eosinophils to areas of inflammation. These observations confirmed the role of T_H2 lymphocytes in the pathology of type I (immediate) hypersensitivity reactions such as allergic asthma but left the identity of the T helper lymphocyte responsible for B lymphocyte switching to IgG and IgA antibodies unresolved.

Another molecular marker characterizing subpopulations of CD4⁺ T lymphocytes is their expression of chemokine receptors. Chemokines are small proteins that mediate cell movement in the innate and adaptive immune responses. Investigators divide chemokines into two distinct groups of molecules: CC chemokines and CXC chemokines. CC chemokines contain two adjacent cysteine residues near the amino terminus of the molecule while CXC chemokines contain a single amino acid residue between two cysteine residues.

A variety of cells secrete chemokines. They bind G-protein coupled transmembrane receptors and direct the movement and activation of cells. Like the chemokines, these receptors are named based on which group of chemokines they bind: CCR bind CC chemokines and CXCR bind CXC chemokines. Each group of receptors comprises a number of different cell surface molecules.

In 2000, two groups of investigators in Germany and Switzerland characterized a population of T lymphocytes (T_{FH}) that preferentially migrate to follicles within peripheral lymphoid tissue where they help B lymphocytes switch to IgG and IgA production. These investigators took advantage of the differential expression of chemokine receptors on populations of CD4+ lymphocytes.

T_H1 and T_H2 lymphocytes express different chemokine receptors (Mackay, 2000). For example, T_H1 lymphocytes preferentially express CCR5 and CXCR3 receptors while T_H2 lymphocytes express CCR3 and CCR4 receptors. This differential expression directs the lymphocytes to migrate to locations where certain chemokines are secreted based on the types of pathogenic microorganisms present. Expression of these receptors can be detected using monoclonal antibodies specific for each receptor.

In 2000, Dagmar Breitfeld and her colleagues, working at research institutes in Berlin and Munich, Germany, and in Bellinzona, Switzerland, identified a population of CD4+ T lymphocytes, isolated from human tonsils, that express the CXCR5 chemokine receptor. These lymphocytes localize to lymphoid follicles within peripheral lymphoid organs such as the spleen and lymph nodes. Expression of the CXCR5 chemokine receptor is also required for B lymphocyte homing to these follicles. Simultaneously, Patrick Schaerli and coworkers, working in Bern, Switzerland, and Berlin, Germany, reported similar findings. These lymphocytes expressing CXCR5 were termed "follicular B helper T cells (T_{FH})."

T_{FH} lymphocytes express costimulatory molecules, including CD40 ligand (CD154), which are required for B lymphocyte activation (Chapter 19) and for isotype switching from IgM to IgG and IgA synthesis and secretion. Thus T_{FH} lymphocytes assist antigen-stimulated B lymphocytes in switching to the production of these isotypes.

Park et al. (2005) and Harrington et al. (2005) described T_H17 lymphocytes. Several autoimmune and autoinflammatory diseases in humans and experimental animals are characterized by the presence of CD4+ T lymphocytes secreting IL-17 and IL-22. Among these diseases are experimental autoimmune encephalomyelitis and collagen induced arthritis (in mice) and rheumatoid arthritis, asthma, and systemic lupus erythematosus in humans. IL-17 is a proinflammatory cytokine inducing the synthesis and release of other inflammatory cytokines; lymphocytes that synthesize and secrete IL-17 are stimulated by other cytokines, including IL-6, TGFβ, and IL-23.

Laurie Harrington collaborated with investigators from the University of Alabama at Birmingham and Washington University in St. Louis, Missouri, to determine if T_H17 lymphocytes differentiated from T_H1 or T_H2 lymphocytes or from a precursor CD4+ T_H0 lymphocyte (Harrington et al., 2005). Harrington and her colleagues stimulated naïve mouse CD4+ lymphocytes with IFN-gamma to induce T_H1 lymphocytes or with IL-4 to induce T_H2 lymphocytes. They subsequently treated these cells with antibodies to CD3 in the presence of IL-23 and identified cytokines produced by polymerase chain reaction, ELISA for IL-17, or intracellular cytokine staining. This group found that IL-23 had little effect on T_H1 or T_H2 CD4+ lymphocytes, thus indicating that IL-23 failed to alter the cytokine synthesizing capability of already differentiated CD4+ lymphocytes. The generation of T_H17 lymphocytes was inhibited by the presence of IFN-γ or IL-4 in the cultures, indicating that T_H1, T_H2, and T_H17 lymphocytes most likely differentiate independently. The cells that secreted IL-17 in these experiments used different transcription factors during differentiation than either T_H1 or T_H2 lymphocytes.

A second group of investigators, led by Heon Park and including investigators from Seattle, Washington; Houston, Texas; and Baltimore, Maryland obtained similar results (Park et al., 2005). Park and coworkers treated T_H0 lymphocytes with IFN-γ or IL-4, both of which inhibited the development of T_H17 cells. These results confirmed that T_H1, T_H2, and T_H17 cells differentiate along separate pathways. In vivo and in vitro manipulation of the T lymphocytes secreting IL-17 provided evidence that these lymphocytes are involved in pathologic inflammation. Park and coworkers injected mice with myelin oligodendrocyte glycoprotein (MOG), an antigen capable of inducing the autoimmune disease experimental allergic encephalomyelitis. In vivo treatment of MOG-injected mice with antibodies specific for IL-17 delayed the appearance of autoimmune symptoms and inhibited the mononuclear cell infiltration of the brain as well as decreased the quantity of inflammatory cytokines secreted by spleen cells.

Transgenic mice that expressed IL-17 in the epithelial cells of the lung allowed Park's group to confirm the role of T_H17 lymphocytes in inflammatory pathology. At 3 months of age these mice were characterized by alveolar wall thickening and hypertrophic epithelium in the bronchus and bronchioles. Macrophages and CD4+ T lymphocytes infiltrated the lung parenchyma. Histologic sections of the lung tissue demonstrated the presence of a number of chemokines in greater quantity than in control, nontransgenic animals. The pathology induced in these mice is similar to that seen in patients with airway inflammation such as chronic obstructive pulmonary disease.

A fifth CD4+ subpopulation is the T-regulatory (T_{REG}) lymphocyte. In 1969, Yasuaki Nishizuka and T. Sakakura at the Aichi Cancer Center Research Institute in Nagoya, Japan, reported that thymectomy of female mice three days after birth resulted in dysgenesis of the ovaries once the animals matured. This observation led to the discovery of a population of regulatory T lymphocytes that are critical for maintaining homeostasis in the adaptive immune response. Individuals lacking these CD4+ T lymphocytes are prone to developing one or more autoimmune disorders. Chapter 24 presents the experiments that were performed to characterize these cells and their role in controlling ongoing immune responses.

CONCLUSION

Jacques Miller demonstrated the importance of the thymus in the development of lymphocytes active in the adaptive immune response in 1961. Eight years later the term T lymphocyte was added to the immunologist's lexicon, and functional studies on these lymphocytes flourished. The initial division of T lymphocytes occurred with the determination that functionally discrete populations expressed different cell surface molecules—either CD4 or CD8. While this division initially relied on the detection of cell surface molecules, immunologists now agree that these two populations also differ based on the method by which they recognize antigen.

Further characterization of the CD4 lymphocyte population depended on advances in technology, including the availability of continuously growing T cell clones, fluorescence-activated cell sorting, monoclonal antibodies, transgenic animals, and polymerase chain reactions. These techniques led to the discovery of an array of cytokines that induce T lymphocyte differentiation and function. Many of these cytokines are produced by T lymphocytes and function in regulating other cells of the adaptive immune response both positively and negatively. As a result, researchers have identified five subpopulations of the CD4 lymphocytes, each with its own signature cytokine profile. These studies led to a description of the mechanisms by which T lymphocytes regulate ongoing immune responses (Chapter 24) and to the design of unique therapeutic approaches to regulate potentially pathogenic immune responses (Chapter 38).

Additional subpopulations of CD4[+] and CD8[+] T lymphocytes may yet be described. Further investigation of lymphocytes, including their cell surface markers, the unique transcription factors they employ, and the cytokines they secrete, will provide mechanisms for regulating both beneficial and pathogenic adaptive immune responses.

References

Boyse, E.A., Itakura, K., Stockert, E., Iritani, C.A., Miura, M., 1971. Ly-C: a third locus specifying alloantigen expressed only on thymocytes and lymphocytes. Transplantation 11, 351–352.

Boyse, E.A., Miyazawa, M., Aoki, T., Old, L.J., 1968. Ly-A and Ly-B: two systems of lymphocyte isoantigens in the mouse. Proc. Roy. Soc. B 170, 175–193.

Breitfeld, D., Ohl, L., Kremmer, E., Ellwart, J., Sallusto, F., Lipp, M., Förster, R., 2000. Follicular B helper T cells express CXC chemokine receptor 5, localize to B cell follicles, and support immunoglobulin production. J. Exp. Med. 192, 1545–1551.

Cantor, H., Boyse, E.A., 1975a. Functional subclasses of T lymphocytes bearing different Ly antigens. I. The generation of functionally distinct T-cell subclasses is a differentiative process independent of antigen. J. Exp. Med. 141, 1376–1389.

Cantor, H., Boyse, E.A., 1975b. Functional subclasses of T lymphocytes bearing different Ly antigens. II. Cooperation between different subclasses of Ly[+] cells in the generation of killer activity. J. Exp. Med. 141, 1390–1399.

Glick, B., Chang, T.S., Jaap, R.G., 1956. The bursa of Fabricius and antibody production in the domestic fowl. Poult. Sci. 35, 224–225.

Haanen, J.B.A.G., Malefijt, R., Res, P.C.M., Kraakman, E.M., Ottenhoff, T.H.M., de Vries, R.R.P., Spits, H., 1991. Selection of a human T helper type 1-like T cell subset by Mycobacteria. J. Exp. Med. 174, 583–592.

Harrington, L.E., Hatton, R.D., Mangan, P.R., Turner, H., Murphy, T.L., Murphy, K.M., Weaver, C.T., 2005. Interleukin 17-producing CD4[+] effector T cells develop via a lineage distinct from the T helper type 1 and 2 lineages. Nat. Immunol. 6, 1123–1132.

Heinzel, F.P., Sadick, M.D., Holoday, B.J., Coffman, R.L., Locksley, R.M., 1989. Reciprocal expression of interferon γ or interleukin 4 during the resolution or progression of murine leishmaniasis. J. Exp. Med. 169, 59–72.

Hsieh, C.-S., Macatonia, S.E., Tripp, C.S., Wolf, S.F., O-Garra, A., Murphy, K.M., 1993. Development of T_H1 CD4[+] T cells through IL-12 produced by Listeria-induced macrophages. Science 260, 547–549.

IUIS-WHO nomenclature subcommittee, 1984. Nomenclature for clusters of differentiation (CD) of antigens defined on human leukocyte populations. Bull. WHO 62, 809–811.

Kohler, G., Milstein, C., 1975. Continuous cultures of fused cells secreting antibody of predefined specificity. Nature 256, 495–497.

Kung, P.C., Goldstein, G., Reinherz, E.L., Schlossman, S.F., 1979. Monoclonal antibodies defining distinctive human T cell surface antigens. Science 206, 347–349.

LeGros, G., Ben-Sasson, S.Z., Seder, R., Finkelman, F.D., Paul, W.E., 1990. Generation of interleukin 4 (IL-4)-producing cells in vivo and in vitro: IL-2 and IL-4 are required for in vitro generation of IL-4-producing cells. J. Exp. Med. 172, 921–929.

Mackay, C.R., 2000. Follicular homing T helper (Th) cells and the Th1/Th2 paradigm. J. Exp. Med. 192, F31–F34.

McGhee, J.R., 2005. The world of Th1/Th2 subsets: first proof. J. Immunol. 175, 3–4.

McKee, A.S., MacLeod, M.K.L., Kappler, J.W., Marrack, P., 2010. Immune mechanisms of protection: can adjuvants rise to the challenge? BMC Biol. 8, 37. http://dx.doi.org/10.1186/1741-7007-8-37.

Miller, J.F.A.P., 1961. Immunological function of the thymus. Lancet 278, 748–749.

Mossman, T.R., Cherwinski, H., Bond, M.W., Gieldin, M.A., Coffman, R.L., 1986. Two types of murine helper T cell clone. I. Definition according to profiles of lymphokine activities and secreted proteins. J. Immunol. 136, 2348–2357.

Nishizuka, Y., Sakakura, T., 1969. Thymus and reproduction: sex-linked dysgenesis of the gonad after neonatal thymectomy in mice. Science 166, 753–755.

Park, H., Li, Z., Yang, X.O., Chang, S.H., Nurieva, R., Wang, Y.H., Wang, Y., Hood, L., Zhu, Z., Tian, Q., Dong, C., 2005. A distinct lineage of CD4 T cells regulated tissue inflammation by producing interleukin 17. Nat. Immunol. 6, 1133–1141.

Phan-Dinh-Tuy, F., Niaudet, P., Bach, J.-F., 1982. Molecular identification of human T-lymphocyte antigens defined by the OKT5 and OKT8 monoclonal antibodies. Mol. Immunol. 19, 1649–1654.

Reinherz, E.L., Kung, P.C., Goldstein, G., Schlossman, S.F., 1979a. Further characterization of the human inducer T cell subset defined by monoclonal antibody. J. Immunol. 123, 2894–2896.

Reinherz, E.L., Kung, P.C., Goldstein, G., Schlossman, S.F., 1979b. Separation of functional subsets of human T cells by a monoclonal antibody. Proc. Nat. Acad. Sci. U.S.A. 76, 4061–4065.

Reinherz, E.L., Kung, P.C., Goldstein, G., Schlossman, S.F., 1980. A monoclonal antibody reactive with the human cytotoxic/suppressor T cell subset previously defined by a heteroantiserum termed T_H2. J. Immunol. 124, 1301–1307.

Salgame, P., Abrams, J.S., Clayberger, C., Goldstein, H., Convit, J., Modlin, R.L., Bloom, B.R., 1991. Differing lymphokine profiles of functional subsets of human CD4 and CD8 T cell clones. Science 254, 279–282.

Schaerli, P., Willimann, K., Lang, A.B., Lipp, M., Loetscher, P., Moser, B., 2000. CXC chemokine receptor 5 expression defines follicular homing T cells with B cell helper function. J. Exp. Med. 192, 1553–1562.

Shiku, H., Kisielow, P., Bean, M.A., Takahashi, T., Boyse, E.A., Oettgen, H.F., Old, L.J., 1975. Expression of T cell differentiation antigens on effector cells in cell-mediated cytotoxicity in vitro. Evidence for functional heterogeneity related to the surface phenotype of T cells. J. Exp. Med. 141, 227–241.

Swain, S.L., Weinberg, A.D., English, M., Huston, G., 1990. IL-4 directs the development of Th2-like helper effects. J. Immunol. 145, 3796–3806.

Yamamura, M., Uyemura, K., Deans, R.J., Weinberg, K., Rea, T.H., Bloom, B.R., Modlin, R.L., 1991. Defining protective responses to pathogens: cytokine profiles in leprosy lesions. Science 254, 277–279.

TIME LINE

1961 — Jacque Miller describes the role of the thymus in the development of lymphocytes involved in the adaptive immune response

1968 — Edward Boyse and colleagues develop antibodies against the Ly antigens of mouse T cells

1969 — Ivan Roitt introduces terms to refer to thymus-dependent T lymphocytes and bursa-dependent B lymphocytes

1969 — Yasuaki Nishizuka and T. Sakakura provide initial observations, leading to the characterization of T_{REG} lymphocytes

1975 — Harvey Cantor and Edward Boyse report the distribution of the Ly antigens on functionally different populations of T lymphocytes

1975 — Georges Köhler and César Milstein develop a method for the production of monoclonal antibodies

1979 — Patrick Kung and colleagues produce monoclonal antibodies to distinct populations of human T lymphocytes

1982 — First International Workshop on Human Leukocyte Differentiation Antigens defines cluster of differentiation (CD) markers and assigns numbers to 15 different CD antigens

1986 — Timothy Mossman and Robert Coffman divide T helper clones into T_H1 and T_H2 populations based on cytokines secreted

1990 — Graham LeGros and colleagues and Susan Swain and coworkers identify IL-4 as the cytokine responsible for differentiation of CD4 lymphocytes into T_H2 cells

1993 — Chyi-Song Hsieh and colleagues report that IL-12 stimulates maturation of T_H1 cells

2000 — Dagmar Breitfield and coworkers and Patrick Schaerli and colleagues describe a T helper population (T_{FH}) responsible for helping B lymphocytes switch to production of IgG and IgA

2005 — Heon Park and colleagues and Laurie Harrington and coworkers describe T_H17 lymphocytes

24

T Lymphocyte Control of the Immune Response: From T_S to T_{REG}

INTRODUCTION

The mammalian immune system maintains homeostasis in an environment teeming with potential pathogens. Both innate host defense mechanisms and adaptive immune responses provide a balance that requires the development of sufficiently robust responses to protect against infections while inhibiting reactions that might lead to pathologies such as autoimmune diseases and hypersensitivity.

During the first half of the twentieth century, immunologists observed that antibody levels increased following infection or vaccination and subsequently declined. They considered this pattern of antibody formation to reflect both elimination of the antigenic stimulus and the short life span of antibody-producing lymphocytes. This simplistic view became more complex during the second half of the twentieth century with the discovery of functionally different populations of lymphocytes.

In the late 1960s, groups led by Henry Claman, Anthony Davies, and Jacques Miller demonstrated that thymus-derived T lymphocytes help B lymphocytes synthesize and secrete antibody in response to antigenic challenge (Claman et al., 1966; Davies et al., 1967; Miller and Mitchell, 1968) (Chapter 13). The experimental designs that led to this conclusion involved mixing lymphocytes from various sources (bone marrow, spleen, thoracic duct, thymus) and quantitating the amount of antibody produced to antigens either in vitro or in vivo. Other investigators pursued similar experiments and

obtained contradictory results showing that mixtures of certain lymphocytes resulted in decreased antibody formation. These unanticipated findings shepherded the concept of T suppressor (T_S) lymphocytes into models of the immune system.

Between 1972 and the mid-1980s, studies on T_S lymphocytes developed into a major research focus for a cadre of cellular immunologists. In addition, the concept of T lymphocyte-mediated suppression clarified research results that were not otherwise readily explainable. Many immunologists were seduced by the notion of T_S lymphocytes, resulting in funding by the National Institutes of Health (NIH) in the United States as well as funding agencies around the world. In fact, the initial NIH grant awarded to the current author was titled Controlling Role of Thymocytes in Antibody Synthesis and dealt with T_S cells in chickens (Moticka, 1977).

By 1986, inconsistencies concerning the isolation, cloning, and genetics of T_S lymphocytes emerged, and immunologists began to question the interpretation of earlier results. This progression in concept is reflected in the number of journal articles published on the topic. A search of PubMed using the search term "suppressor T lymphocytes" yielded 15,817 papers between 1972 (1 paper) and 2014 (202 papers) with the most papers appearing in 1985 (1014). Despite the virtual absence of new research on T_S lymphocytes, the history of this concept is instructive in demonstrating that even well-established hypotheses occasionally are proven incorrect. In addition, downregulation of adaptive immune

A Historical Perspective on Evidence-Based Immunology
http://dx.doi.org/10.1016/B978-0-12-398381-7.00024-1

responses has survived with the discovery of T_{REG} lymphocytes starting in 1969 and continuing until the present.

SUPPRESSOR T LYMPHOCYTES

Several groups of investigators demonstrated suppression of the adaptive immune response by thymus-derived lymphocytes, including the following:

- In 1970, Phillip Baker and colleagues, working at the National Institutes of Health, Bethesda, Maryland, injected mice with antibodies specific for lymphocytes (an antilymphocyte serum (ALS)) at the same time they injected these mice with type III pneumococcal polysaccharide (SSS-III), an antigen that induces IgM antibodies exclusively. Mice injected with ALS produced an increased number of antibody-forming lymphocytes specific for SSS-III.
- Baker and his colleagues postulated that ALS treatment of these mice eliminated a population of regulatory lymphocytes. To test this possibility, the investigators injected mice with thymus cells prior to treatment with ALS and injection with SSS-III. This treatment restored the antibody response to the level seen in mice injected only with SSS-III. The authors conclude that "at least two functionally distinct types of presumably thymic-derived cells (a suppressor cell and an amplifier cell) act in an opposing manner to regulate the antibody response."
- In 1971, Wulf Droege, working at Harvard University, Cambridge, Massachusetts, injected mature chickens with two antigens (*Brucella abortus* and sheep erythrocytes–SRBC). He demonstrated that antibody production to both antigens was significantly decreased if the chickens had been pretreated with thymus cells from control unmanipulated donor birds; however, pretreatment with thymus cells from bursectomized animals failed to reduce the response.
- Ko Okumura and Tomio Tada, working at Chiba University, Chiba, Japan, in 1971 treated rats with a low dose (400R) of whole-body irradiation prior to injecting them with the hapten, dinitrophenol (DNP), conjugated to a carrier, *Ascaris suum* extract (DNP-As). These rats synthesized more antibody to DNP than nonirradiated control animals. In this experimental system the hapten interacts with B lymphocytes while the carrier interacts with T lymphocytes. Okumura and Tada tested whether irradiation preferentially deleted a population of T lymphocytes responsible for regulation of the antibody response by injecting irradiated rats with thymocytes from other rats hyperimmunized to *A. suum* extract prior

to immunization with DNP-As. Such treatment decreased the elevated antibody response, leading the authors to conclude "that carrier-specific, thymus-derived lymphocytes negatively regulate the (antibody) formation that is virtually hapten specific."

These studies suggest that thymus-derived lymphocytes play a suppressive role in antibody synthesis. Richard Gershon and coworkers at Yale University, New Haven, Connecticut, championed this concept and first coined the term suppressor T cells (T_S) in 1972.

Prior to these studies, investigators agreed that T lymphocytes

- help B lymphocytes synthesize antibodies;
- recognize antigen (i.e., they are specific); and
- function in cell-mediated immune responses, including delayed type hypersensitivity, graft rejection, and graft versus host reaction.

The mechanisms involved in these phenomena were yet to be explained. This was prior to the realization that thymus-derived lymphocytes comprise distinct subpopulations based on cell-surface phenotype and function (i.e., CD4:CD8; $T_H1:T_H2$, etc.). Studies performed during the following 15 years (1970–1985) provided a prodigious amount of information about T lymphocytes, including their role in both amplifying and suppressing adaptive immune responses. Despite the fact that the concept of T_S lymphocytes as originally defined is no longer accepted by scientific consensus, the dichotomy of help and suppression is valid and provides a framework for understanding homeostasis of the system.

Richard K. Gershon (1932–1983) received his medical training at Harvard and spent virtually his entire career in the pathology department at Yale University, New Haven, Connecticut. During the period from 1970 to 1983, he demonstrated that T lymphocytes both enhance and inhibit adaptive immune responses, including antibody production, induction of immunologic tolerance, and delayed type hypersensitivity. These results stimulated an enormous effort by laboratories around the world to understand the functions of suppressor T lymphocytes in virtually every conceivable immunological system.

Gershon, working with Kazumari Kondo, studied cellular interactions required for the induction of immunologic tolerance to SRBC (Gershon and Kondo, 1970). The experimental model used in these studies is shown in Figure 24.1. Gershon and Kondo thymectomized adult 7- to 8-week-old mice. Seven to 10 days later these mice received a lethal dose of irradiation, after which they were rescued by an injection of bone marrow cells. The investigators divided the mice into two groups, one of which was injected with syngeneic thymus cells while the other received no thymocytes and served as controls.

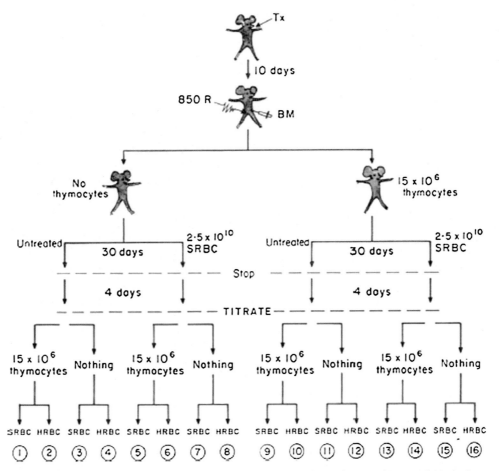

FIGURE 24.1 Experimental protocol used by Gershon and Kondo to demonstrate that induction of immunological tolerance is dependent on (suppressor) T lymphocytes. *From Gershon and Kondo (1970) Immunology, 18, 723.*

Gershon and Kondo divided these two groups into subgroups that received either a large dose of SRBC over the next month (to induce immunologic tolerance) or no SRBC. They bled the mice 4 days after the last injection of SRBC to determine serum antibody titers to SRBC; this is indicated by titrate on the figure.

None of these groups of mice produced antibodies. The investigators injected the experimental groups with syngeneic thymocytes and restimulated them with an immunizing dose of SRBC or with horse RBCs as a specificity control. Mice that received thymus cells prior to treatment with a large dose of SRBC failed to synthesize antibodies to SRBC while the control animals produced measurable antibodies. The authors conclude that "the induction of tolerance as well as the induction of immunity in thymus-dependent BMD (bone marrow-dependent) cell populations, seems to require the cooperation of TD (thymus-derived) cells."

In a subsequent study, Gershon and Kondo (1971) showed that tolerance in this system could be transferred to naïve mice. They coined the term "infectious immunological tolerance" to refer to this phenomenon. To identify the cells responsible for transferring tolerance to SRBC,

Gershon and colleagues in 1972 developed a double transfer system. They lethally irradiated a group of mice, rescued them by reconstituting them with syngeneic thymocytes, and divided them into three groups. They injected two of these groups with SRBC (either a high dose or a low dose) while the third group remained untreated. One week later they harvested splenic lymphocytes from each group of mice. These spleen cells contained T lymphocytes from the original thymus donor. Gershon and coworkers used these "educated thymocytes" to rescue a second group of irradiated syngeneic mice that were then injected with the antigen, SRBC. Some of the recipients of educated thymocytes also received 1×10^7 normal thymocytes. A control group of lethally irradiated mice received unmanipulated thymocytes.

Gershon and his group injected these recipients with SRBC and measured lymphocyte proliferation in vivo 3, 4, and 5 days later by injecting the mice with a radio-labeled precursor of DNA and determining the amount of radioactivity incorporated into the proliferating cells. The results are depicted in Figure 24.2. Group A mice received only syngeneic thymocytes while groups B, C, and D received educated thymocytes from lethally

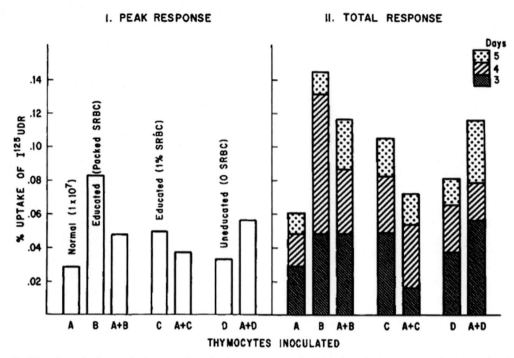

FIGURE 24.2   Proliferation of spleen cells from irradiated mice reconstituted with T lymphocytes exposed to sheep erythrocytes in donor animals. Proliferation was measured by the incorporation of ^{125}IUDR into the DNA of lymphocytes stimulated in vitro with the antigen. *From Gershon et al. (1972).*

irradiated donors. Group B mice received educated thymocytes from mice injected with a high dose of SRBC while group C recipients received educated thymocytes from mice injected with a low dose of SRBC. Donors to group D mice were not exposed to the antigen.

The primary finding from these studies is that mixing thymocytes that had not been exposed to SRBC with T lymphocytes that had been exposed to SRBC decreased the proliferative response of the recipient spleen cells. For example, mice that received thymus cells plus spleen cells from mice injected with a high dose of SRBC (A + B) responded less well than mice receiving spleen cells from SRBC-treated donors (B) alone. The authors conclude that "thymocytes are capable of suppressing the antigen-induced response of other thymocytes without the mediation of B cells or their product."

Subsequent studies on suppressor T lymphocytes focused on

- the phenotypic characterization of the lymphocytes responsible for the phenomenon, and
- the mechanisms by which such lymphocytes regulate immune responses.

John Jandinski and coworkers at Harvard Medical School, Boston, Massachusetts, demonstrated in 1976 that mouse T suppressor (T_S) lymphocytes are distinct from T helper (T_H) lymphocytes based on expression of cell-surface molecules identified by antibodies to lymphocyte antigens (Ly antigens—Chapter 23). Mathew Vadas and

colleagues in 1977 working at the Walter and Eliza Hall Institute of Medical Research in Melbourne, Australia, corroborated these results. T_S lymphocyte activity was eliminated from a population of lymphocytes by treatment with antibodies to Ly 2 but not by treatment with antibodies to Ly 1. Lymphocytes active as helpers expressed the opposite phenotype (Ly 1).

These studies characterized T lymphocyte populations and led to the division of T cells into Ly1 (CD4$^+$) and Ly2 (CD8$^+$) populations (Chapter 23). Lymphocytes that provide help express CD4, while those capable of downregulating adaptive immune responses were included, erroneously, with the population of cytotoxic lymphocytes that express CD8.

During the mid-1970s, investigators focused on the genetic control of the initiation of adaptive immune responses (Chapter 16). Proteins coded by genes in the major histocompatibility complex (MHC) regulate CD4$^+$ T_H lymphocytes. Similar studies on T_S lymphocytes concluded that different genes in the MHC regulated suppression.

A group from Harvard led by Baruj Benacerraf employed an experimental model involving the induction of antibody responses to a copolymer of glutamic acid and tyrosine (GT). Most inbred strains of mice fail to produce antibodies to GT (i.e., they are nonresponders); however, some strains (responders) produce antibodies to GT if injected with GT conjugated to methylated bovine serum albumin (GT-MBSA). Injection of mice from responder strains with GT prior to immunization with GT-MBSA inhibited subsequent antibody production to GT-MBSA. This unresponsiveness can be transferred to syngeneic mice by spleen cells or thymocytes from GT-injected animals, suggesting that the inhibition of antibody formation is due to the presence of T_S lymphocytes (Debre et al., 1975a).

Investigation of the strain distribution of this suppression as well as the inheritance of the trait in F_1 hybrids derived from mating responders with nonresponders suggested that the development of T_S lymphocytes was under control of genes in the MHC. Initially, these MHC genes were designated specific immune suppression (Is) genes (Debre et al., 1975b).

At the same time, Hugh McDevitt and coworkers at Stanford University, Palo Alto, California, provided evidence that suppressor cells could be killed by treatment with antibody directed against proteins coded for by a portion of the MHC known as the I region. The antigen detected by this antibody was expressed exclusively on T_S lymphocytes and was not detectable on either T_H or B lymphocytes. Further definition of the gene coding for this protein suggested that it was in a region of the MHC containing other genes involved in controlling the immune response; these investigators called this region I-J (Murphy et al., 1976).

The identification of a genetic region within the MHC that controlled suppression led to investigations aimed at identifying a T_S lymphocyte-secreted molecule coded for by the MHC. Tomio Tada at Chiba University in Japan, working with Chella David at Washington University in St. Louis, Missouri, identified an antigen-specific suppressive factor produced by T_S lymphocytes that functioned as a soluble inhibitor of antibody production. This factor was supposedly coded for by the I-J subregion of the MHC (Tada et al., 1976).

Through the 1970s and into the early 1980s, investigators described cell-surface markers expressed by T_S lymphocytes. Researchers isolated and characterized both antigen-specific and antigen-nonspecific suppressive factors and speculated on the mechanism of down-regulation. These speculations led to the development of elaborate proposals about the induction of suppressor cells as well as network hypotheses involving the interaction of both cell-surface and soluble mediators. Niels Jerne advanced a model consisting of idiotypes, anti-idiotypes, and anti-anti-idiotypes in a complex web of regulation (Jerne, 1985).

Idiotypes are unique antigenic determinants on immunoglobulins and on antigen-specific receptors expressed by both B and T lymphocytes. Jerne and others speculated that T lymphocyte-derived soluble factors also contained idiotypes. Idiotypes result from the unique amino acid sequence involved in forming the antigen-binding sites of these proteins. Under certain conditions, idiotypes are immunogenic, giving rise to anti-idiotypic antibodies and/or T lymphocytes (Jerne et al., 1982).

Interactions between idiotypes and anti-idiotypes were thought to be responsible for both upregulation and suppression of the adaptive immune response. Jerne was awarded the Nobel Prize in Physiology or Medicine in 1984 "for theories concerning the specificity in development and control of the immune system." This award recognized his work in the 1950s leading to the clonal selection theory as well as his contributions to the concept of an idiotype network. He shared the prize that year with Cesar Milstein and Georges Köhler for their "discovery of the principle for production of monoclonal antibodies" (Chapter 39).

Regulatory networks as well as the notion of T_S lymphocytes began to implode in the early 1980s. In 1982, Michael Steinmetz at the California Institute of Technology in Pasadena, along with colleagues at Stanford University, the University of Southern California, Los Angeles, and the University of Geneva in Switzerland, used hybrid DNA technology to produce a molecular map of the I region of the major histocompatibility region of mice. By 1982, the I region of mice had been divided into five subregions (I-A, I-B, I-J, I-E, and I-C), two of which (I-A and I-E) code for class II histocompatibility molecules. Based on their map, these investigators determined that the I-B and I-J subregions were confined to a small stretch of DNA (3.4 kb) that was insufficient to code for the proteins assigned to this area, and therefore they concluded that "the I-B and I-J subregions are not encoded in the I region between the I-A and I-E subregions."

Many of these same investigators collaborated on a study in which mRNA isolated from putative T_S hybridomas failed to hybridize with DNA that contained all of the sequences between the I-A and I-E subregions (Kronenberg et al., 1983). These authors concluded "that the genes encoding I-J serologic determinants expressed by suppressor T cells do not map between the I-A and I-E subregions." This conclusion led them to suggest three possible explanations for the discrepancy between the immunogenetic data and the molecular map of the region. These erroneous hypotheses were used for the next several years to argue that T_S lymphocytes exist.

Finally, in 1988, Goran Möller of the University of Stockholm, Sweden, published a short editorial titled "Do Suppressor T Cells Exist?" in the *Scandinavian Journal of Immunology*. While acknowledging that suppressive phenomena occur in the adaptive immune response and that T lymphocytes may mediate these phenomena, he argued against T suppressor lymphocytes being a separate population. His arguments included the following:

- "There is no marker for distinguishing suppressor from cytotoxic T cells. Thus a pure population of suppressor T cells has never been seen."
- "The suppressor I-J gene cannot be found in the place where it has been mapped."

- "Antigen-specific suppressor clones or hybridomas have nonsense rearrangements of genes for the T cell receptor or else the genes are totally deleted."

By 1990, most immunologists agreed that T_S lymphocytes do not exist and research on these lymphocytes ceased to be supported by most funding agencies, including the National Institutes of Health. Despite this shift, evidence for downregulation of the adaptive immune response continued to accumulate. This set the stage for renewed interest in a phenomenon initially described by two Japanese investigators, Yasuaki Nishizuka and Teruyo Sakakura, that led to the characterization of T regulatory lymphocytes.

RISE OF T REGULATORY LYMPHOCYTES

In 1969, Nishizuka and Sakakura, working at the Aichi Cancer Center Research Institute in Nagoya, Japan, observed that thymectomy of mice 3 days after birth resulted in dysgenesis of the ovaries in female mice once they matured but had no consistent effect on the spleen, liver, kidney, mesenteric lymph nodes, salivary or adrenal glands in females, or the testes in males. Similar results were not observed in mice thymectomized on the day of birth or at 7 days of life. Mice with malformed ovaries were infertile.

Ovarian dysgenesis was reversed if the thymectomized mice received a graft of thymus from neonatal mice on the seventh day of life. This led Nishizuka and Sakakura to postulate that the thymus functions in controlling reproduction in the female mouse. Akemi Kojima and colleagues in 1973 demonstrated that the defect in ovarian function could be overcome either by implantation with thymus or by the intraperitoneal (IP) injection of spleen cells from male mice. Kojima and coworkers hypothesized that early thymectomy in mice induces premature aging of the ovary.

During the 1970s and 1980s, other investigators extended this model of thymectomy-induced organ dysgenesis and demonstrated that removal of the thymus on the third day of life resulted in development of organ-specific autoimmune responses. For example, in 1976, Akemi Kojima and colleagues demonstrated that a proportion of mice thymectomized at 3 days of age developed spontaneous autoimmune thyroiditis characterized by the presence of antibodies reactive with thyroid extracts and infiltration of the thyroid gland with lymphocytes and plasma cells. They also observed lymphoid infiltrates in the ovary and stomach.

Osamu Taguchi and Yasuaki Nishizuka in 1980 transferred thymectomy-induced autoimmune oophoritis to newborn mice. Female mice thymectomized at 0, 3, or 7 days of life served as donors of spleen cells when they were 2–3 months old. Taguchi and Nishizuka injected newborn mice with suspensions of these cells and histologically observed their ovaries 7 days later. Twelve of fifteen recipients of spleen cells from mice thymectomized at 3 days of life developed oophoritis; none of the recipients of cells from mice thymectomized at 0 or 7 days were affected. Treatment of the spleen cells with antibody to immunoglobulin plus complement (to eliminate B lymphocytes) or with antibody to a T lymphocyte-specific antigen plus complement showed that the cells capable of transferring the autoimmune process were T lymphocytes.

In other studies, thymectomy at 3 days of life produced inflammatory damage to other organs as well as the appearance of autoantibodies to several different tissues. If thymectomized mice were maintained for a sufficient length of time, many of them developed autoimmune processes that impaired the function of the ovary, stomach, and testes as well as the thyroid and prostate glands (reviewed by Taguchi and Nishizuka, 1987).

Taguchi and Nishizuka exploited the model of thymectomy-induced autoimmune disease of the stomach and prostate to investigate the mechanisms responsible for abrogation of self-tolerance and the induction of organ-specific autoimmunity. They confirmed that an IP injection of adult spleen cells 1 day after thymectomy (day 4 of life) prevented the development of both gastritis and prostatitis. In separate experiments, they induced prostatitis (but not gastritis) in athymic (nude) mice by an IP injection of spleen cells from adult female mice into 4-day-old recipients. If the spleen cells to be injected came from mice thymectomized at 3 days of life, the recipients developed both prostatitis and gastritis.

The development of autoimmunity following early thymectomy is not restricted to mice. Similar observations have been made in rats where neonatal thymectomy of the inbred Buffalo rat increases the incidence of "spontaneous" autoimmune thyroiditis from about 20% of the animals to close to 100% (Rose et al., 1976).

Characterization of the cells responsible for regulating naturally arising autoimmune disease relied on rats with a congenital absence of thymus. Athymic rats injected with immature T lymphocytes develop wasting disease and inflammatory infiltrates in the thyroid glands, liver, lung, stomach, and pancreas. Injection of athymic rats with a mixture of immature and mature T lymphocytes inhibited the development of these autoimmune processes (Powrie and Mason, 1990).

Fiona Powrie and colleagues, working at DNAX Research Institute in Palo Alto, California and Schering-Plough Research Institute, Lafayette, New Jersey, in 1993 reported similar results when they injected severe combined immunodeficient (SCID) mice with CD4+ lymphocytes separated into immature (CD45RB^high) or memory (CD45RB^low) populations. CD45RB is a cell-surface glycoprotein expressed on thymocytes and peripheral T lymphocytes. This molecule is expressed in high levels on immature cells (CD45RB^{high}) and in low levels in mature cells (CD45RB^{low}). SCID mice injected with immature T lymphocytes developed a wasting disease, including infiltration of the colon with mononuclear cells and the secretion of large amounts of IFNγ. Injection of SCID mice with mature T lymphocytes failed to elicit the inflammatory colitis. Cotransfer of mature CD45RB^{high} T lymphocytes with CD45RB^{low} lymphocytes inhibited the wasting disease and the inflammatory colitis. These investigators concluded that "important regulatory interactions occur between the CD45RB^{high} and CD45RB^{low} CD4$^+$ T cell subsets and that disruption of this mechanism has fatal consequences."

Shimon Sakaguchi and coworkers, collaborating at several institutions in Japan, characterized the phenotype of the lymphocytes responsible for regulating potentially autoreactive T lymphocytes. In 1995, these investigators treated CD4$^+$ T lymphocytes with an antibody specific for CD25 plus complement. Antibody to CD25 binds to one of the chains of the IL-2 receptor. The IL-2 receptor binds the cytokine IL-2, a potent inducer of T lymphocyte proliferation. The gene for the IL-2 receptor is upregulated when T lymphocytes are activated and hence it is expressed on stimulated (mature) T lymphocytes. However, the IL-2 receptor is present on approximately 10% of peripheral CD4$^+$ T lymphocytes in mice prior to injection with antigen.

Sakaguchi and colleagues injected CD4$^+$ T lymphocytes depleted of CD25$^+$ lymphocytes into congenic athymic recipients. All the treated mice developed autoimmune diseases, including thyroiditis, gastritis, insulitis, sialadenitis, adrenalitis, oophoritis, glomerulonephritis, and polyarthritis. Injection of other athymic mice with CD4$^+$, CD25$^+$ lymphocytes prevented the development of these autoimmune processes. The authors conclude that T lymphocytes expressing CD4 and CD25 on their cell surface represent a naturally occurring regulatory lymphocyte involved in maintaining self-tolerance by downregulating adaptive immune responses to self-antigens; these lymphocytes are now referred to as T$_{REG}$ lymphocytes.

Clinical observations of a naturally occurring human pathology confirmed the experimental identification of T$_{REG}$ lymphocytes. Berkley Powell and collaborators at the Oregon Health Sciences Center in Portland, Oregon, in 1982 described a large family in which eight males presented with intractable diarrhea, eczema, hemolytic anemia, diabetes mellitus, or autoimmune thyroid disease, leading to death for most during the first decade of life. Eleven other males in the kindred died early in life from infections or following vaccination. Additional patients diagnosed with a similar constellation of symptoms have been described, and the disorder is designated

IPEX (immune dysregulation, polyendocrinopathy, enteropathy, X-linked syndrome) (Wildin et al., 2002). Individuals with IPEX generally succumb within the first decade of life.

A similar disease was described in males of a strain of mice with the scurfy (sf) mutation (Godfrey et al., 1991). The phenotype of these mice includes dermatological defects, anemia, cachexia (wasting), and death in the first month of life. Initially these mice were thought to serve as a model for the human disease X-linked ichthyosis (i.e., scaly skin); however, subsequent investigation revealed that defects in the hematopoietic and lymphatic system are also present. Many of the organs of affected mice are infiltrated with lymphocytes, particularly activated CD4$^+$ T lymphocytes. These activated T lymphocytes are directly responsible for the autoimmune and inflammatory processes observed in the mice.

In 2001, Mary Brunkow, working at Celltech Chiroscience in Bothell, Washington, collaborated with several colleagues to identify and map the gene responsible the pathology in scurfin mice. This gene codes for a protein (Foxp3) that is a transcriptional regulator. A frameshift mutation that results in loss of function of the protein is responsible for the disorder in scurfin mice. Investigators identified similar mutations in the human gene coding for Foxp3 in IPEX patients.

Jason Fontenot, Marc Gavin, and Alexander Rudensky, working at the Howard Hughes Medical Institute at the University of Washington, Seattle, in 2003 studied the expression of Foxp3 in CD4$^+$ lymphocytes that were either CD25 positive or CD25 negative using polymerase chain reaction analysis of mRNA isolated from the two lymphocyte populations. mRNA for Foxp3 was expressed in higher amounts in CD4$^+$ CD25 positive T lymphocytes than in CD4$^+$ CD25 negative lymphocytes. This increased expression correlated with the amount of Foxp3 protein detected by western blot analysis in the two lymphocyte populations. Several additional observations demonstrate that T$_{REG}$ lymphocytes express the Foxp3 protein, including

- targeted deletion of the gene coding for Foxp3 in male mice results in the development of an aggressive lymphoproliferative disease reminiscent of that seen in scurfin mice,
- male Foxp3-negative mice lack regulatory T lymphocytes,
- regulatory T lymphocyte development requires Foxp3, and
- transfer of regulatory T lymphocytes into newborn Foxp3-negative mice inhibits the development of the lymphoproliferation observed in these mice.

These results clarified the unregulated lymphocyte proliferation seen in patients with IPEX and in scurfin mice. More importantly, they provided a method for the detection and quantitation of T_{REG} lymphocytes in mice and humans since monoclonal antibodies to Foxp3 can be used to detect these lymphocytes.

By the first few years of the twenty-first century, immunologists accepted the concept of T lymphocyte regulation of the adaptive immune response. While T_S lymphocytes purportedly expressed CD8 on their surface and functioned through a web of interacting molecules, both cell-bound and secreted, T_{REG} lymphocytes express CD4 and regulate activation of other T lymphocytes through cell interactions and the secretion of cytokines (Chapter 25).

CONCLUSION

The concept that T lymphocytes downregulate adaptive immune responses occurred to a number of investigators once the helper function of T lymphocytes had been established (Chapter 13). Richard Gershon and his colleagues suggested that a population of suppressor T lymphocytes downregulated ongoing, adaptive immune responses such as antibody synthesis and secretion. A large number of publications identified the cell-surface phenotypes of these T lymphocytes and the genes active during suppression. At the time of the discovery of T_S lymphocytes, the mechanism by which T lymphocytes recognized foreign antigens was unknown, and an elaborate regulatory network involving idiotypes and anti-idiotypes was proposed. Once the genes coding for the mouse MHC had been mapped, and understanding of cellular immunology and immunogenetics progressed, the evidence for the existence of suppressor T lymphocytes became increasingly tenuous. By the mid-1980s, most immunologists questioned the concept of suppression as originally formulated.

The idea of downregulation of the adaptive immune responses as a mechanism of maintaining homeostasis remains appealing. Rediscovery of studies indicating that mice thymectomized early in life developed organ-specific autoimmune disease at a higher than expected incidence led to the development of the concept of T regulatory (T_{REG}) lymphocytes. These lymphocytes have a distinctive cell-surface phenotype (CD4+, CD25+) and express a unique transcription factor (Foxp3). The discovery of experimental animals and patients lacking functional T regulatory lymphocytes has reinforced the idea that these lymphocytes maintain physiological homeostasis in the adaptive immune system.

References

Baker, P.J., Stashak, P.W., Amsbaugh, D.F., Prescott, B., Barth, R.F., 1970. Evidence for the existence of two functionally distinct types of cells which regulate the antibody response to type III pneumococcal polysaccharide. J. Immunol. 105, 1581–1583.

Brunkow, M.E., Jeffery, E.W., Hjerrild, K.A., Paeper, B., Clark, L.A., Yasayko, S.-A., Wilkinson, J.E., Galas, D., Ziegler, S.F., Ramsdell, F., 2001. Disruption of a new forkhead/winged-helix protein, scurfin, results in the fatal lymphoproliferative disorder of the scurfy mouse. Nat. Gen. 27, 68–73.

Claman, H.N., Chaperon, E.A., Triplett, R.F., 1966. Immunocompetence of transferred thymus-marrow cell combinations. J. Immunol. 97, 828–832.

Davies, A.J.S., Leuchars, E., Wallis, V., Marchant, R., Elliott, E.V., 1967. The failure of thymus-derived cells to produce antibody. Transplantation 5, 222–231.

Debre, P., Kapp, J.A., Benacerraf, B., 1975a. Genetic control of specific immune suppression I. Experimental conditions for the stimulation of suppressor cells by the copolymer L-glutamic acid50-L-tyrosine50 (GT) in nonresponder BALB/c mice. J. Exp. Med. 142, 1436–1446.

Debre, P., Kapp, J.A., Dorf, M.E., Benacerraf, B., 1975b. Genetic control of specific immune suppression II. H-2 linked dominant genetic control of immune suppression by the random co-polymer L-glutamic acid50-L-tyrosine50 (GT). J Exp. Med. 142, 1447–1454.

Droege, W., 1971. Amplifying and suppressive effect of thymus cells. Nature 234, 549–551.

Fontenot, J.D., Gavin, M.A., Rudensky, A.Y., 2003. Foxp3 programs the development and function of CD4+CD25+ regulatory T cells. Nat. Immunol. 4, 330–336.

Gershon, R.K., Cohen, P., Hencin, R., Liebhaber, S.A., 1972. Suppressor T cells. J. Immunol. 108, 586–590.

Gershon, R.K., Kondo, K., 1970. Cell interactions in the induction of tolerance: the role of thymic lymphocytes. Immunology 18, 723–737.

Gershon, R.K., Kondo, K., 1971. Infectious immunological tolerance. Immunology 21, 903–914.

Godfrey, V.L., Wilkinson, J.E., Russell, L.B., 1991. X-linked lymphoreticular disease in the scurfy (sf) mutant mouse. Am. J. Pathol. 138, 1379–1387.

Jandinski, J., Cantor, H., Tadakuma, T., Peavy, D.L., Pierce, C.W., 1976. Separation of helper T cells from suppressor T cells expressing different Ly components. I. Polyclonal activation: suppressor and helper activities are inherent properties of distinct T-cell subclasses. J. Exp. Med. 143, 1382–1390.

Jerne, N.K., 1985. The generative grammar of the immune system. Science 229, 1057–1059.

Jerne, N.K., Roland, J., Cazenave, P.-A., 1982. Recurrent idiotypes and internal images. EMBO J. 1, 243–247.

Kojima, A., Sakakura, T., Tanaka, Y., Nishizuka, Y., 1973. Sterility in neonatally thymectomized female mice: its nature and prevention by the injection of spleen cells. Biol. Reprod. 8, 358–361.

Kojima, A., Tanaka-Kojima, Y., Sakakura, T., Nishizuka, Y., 1976. Spontaneous development of autoimmune thyroiditis in neonatally thymectomized mice. Lab. Invest. 34, 550–557.

Kronenberg, M., Steinmetz, M., Kobori, J., Kraig, E., Kapp, J.A., Pierce, C.W., Sorensen, C.M., Suzuki, G., Tada, T., Hood, L., 1983. RNA transcripts for I-J polypeptides are apparently not encoded between the I-A and I-E subregions of the murine major histocompatibility complex. Proc. Nat. Acad. Sci. USA 80, 5704–5708.

Miller, J.F.A.P., Mitchell, G.F., 1968. Cell to cell interaction in the immune response I. Hemolysin-forming cells in neonatally thymectomized mice reconstituted with thymus or thoracic duct lymphocytes. J. Exp. Med. 128, 801–820.

Möller, G., 1988. Do suppressor T cells exist? Scand. J. Immunol. 27, 247–250.

Moticka, E.J., 1977. The presence of immunoregulatory cells in chicken thymus: function in B and T cell responses. J. Immunol. 119, 987–992.

Murphy, D.B., Herzenberg, L.A., Okamura, K., McDevitt, H.O., 1976. A new I subregion (I-J) marked by a locus (Ia-4) controlling surface determinants on suppressor T lymphocytes. J. Exp. Med. 144, 699–712.

Nishizuka, Y., Sakakura, T., 1969. Thymus and reproduction: sex-linked dysgenesis of the gonad after neonatal thymectomy in mice. Science 166, 753–755.

Okumura, K., Tada, T., 1971. Regulation of homocytotrophic antibody formation in the rat. VI. Inhibitory effect of thymocytes on the homocytotrophic antibody response. J. Immunol. 107, 1682–1689.

Powell, B.R., Buist, N.R.M., Stenzel, P., 1982. An X-linked syndrome of diarrhea, polyendocrinopathy, and fatal infection in infancy. J. Ped. 100, 731–737.

Powrie, F., Leach, M.W., Mauze, S., Caddie, L.B., Coffman, R.L., 1993. Phenotypically distinct subsets of CD4+ T cells induce or protect from chronic intestinal inflammation in C.B-17 scid mice. Int. Immunol. 5, 1461–1471.

Powrie, F., Mason, D., 1990. OX-22high CD4+ T cells induce wasting disease with multiple organ pathology: prevention by the OX-22low subset. J. Exp. Med. 172, 1701–1708.

Rose, N.R., Bigazzi, P.E., Noble, B., 1976. Spontaneous autoimmune thyroiditis in the BUF rat. Adv. Exp. Med. Bio. 73B, 209–216.

Sakaguchi, S., Sakaguchi, N., Asano, M., Itoh, M., Toda, M., 1995. Immunologic self-tolerance maintained by activated T cells expressing IL-2 receptor α-chains (CD25). Breakdown of a single mechanism of self-tolerance causes various autoimmune diseases. J. Immunol. 155, 1151–1164.

Steinmetz, M., Minard, K., Horvath, S., McNicholas, J., Srelinger, J., Wake, C., Long, E., Mach, B., Hood, L., 1982. A molecular map of the immune response region from the major histocompatibility complex of the mouse. Nature 300, 35–42.

Tada, T., Taniguchi, M., David, C.S., 1976. Properties of the antigen-specific suppressive T-cell factor in the regulation of antibody response of the mouse. IV. Special subregion assignment of the gene(s) that codes for the suppressive T-cell factor in the H-2 histocompatibility complex. J. Exp. Med. 144, 713–725.

Taguchi, O., Nishizuka, Y., 1980. Autoimmune oophoritis in thymectomized mice: T cell requirement in adoptive cell transfer. Clin. Exp. Immunol. 42, 324–331.

Taguchi, O., Nishizuka, Y., 1987. Self tolerance and localized autoimmunity. Mouse models of autoimmune disease that suggest tissue-specific suppressor T cells are involved in self tolerance. J. Exp. Med. 165, 146–156.

Vadas, M.A., Miller, J.F.A.P., McKenzie, I.F., Chism, S.E., Shen, F.W., Boyse, E.A., Gamble, J.R., Whitelaw, A.,M., 1977. Ly and Ia antigen phenotypes of T cells involved in delayed-type hypersensitivity and in suppression. J. Exp. Med. 144, 10–19.

Wildin, R.S., Smyk-Pearson, S., Filipovich, A.H., 2002. Clinical and molecular features of the immunodysregulation, polyendocrinopathy, enteropathy, X-linked (IPEX) syndrome. J. Med. Genet. 39, 537–545.

TIME LINE

1966–1968	Henry Claman, Anthony Davies, and Jacque Miller lead groups that independently demonstrate the helper function of T lymphocytes on antibody production
1969	Yasuaki Nishizuka and Teruyo Sakakura show that thymectomy of 3-day-old but not 7-day-old mice results in ovarian dysgenesis
1970	Phillip Baker and colleagues report a thymic-derived suppressor lymphocyte sensitive to antilymphocyte serum
1971	Wulf Droege provides evidence for T suppressor lymphocytes in chickens
1971	Richard Gershon and Kazunari Kondo propose a role for T suppressor lymphocytes in tolerance induction and antigenic competition
1971	Ko Okumura and Tomio Tada demonstrate a radiation sensitive thymic-derived suppressor lymphocyte
1972	Richard Gershon coins the term suppressor T cells
1973	Akinora Kojima and colleagues report that the defect caused by thymectomy at 3 days of life can be reversed by thymic transplant, suggesting that the defect is due to a decreased number of regulatory T cells
1975	Patrice Debré and colleagues demonstrate that the genetic control of T_S lymphocytes maps to the major histocompatibility complex (MHC)
1976	Tomio Tada and Chella David identify antigen-specific suppressor factors secreted by T_S lymphocytes
1981	Akinora Kojima and Richmond Prehn observe widespread inflammation and autoimmune disease in mice thymectomized 3 days after birth
1982	Niels Jerne and coworkers provide evidence that some of the antibodies produced during a response are specific for immunoglobulin idiotypes
1982	Michael Steinmetz and colleagues develop a molecular map of the I region of the major histocompatibility complex of mice and conclude that it does not include genes for the I-J subregion
1983	Mitchell Kronenberg and coworkers fail to detect mRNA transcripts in T_S hybridomas that code for I-J polypeptides
1984	Niels Jerne awarded the Nobel Prize for Physiology or Medicine
1988	Goran Möller argues that T suppressor lymphocytes do not exist
1993	Fiona Powrie and colleagues identify T regulatory lymphocytes as a subpopulation of CD4+ T lymphocytes
1995	Shimon Sakaguchi and coworkers demonstrate that T regulatory lymphocytes express high levels of CD25
2001	Mary Brunkov and colleagues identify mutations in the gene coding for Foxp3 in scrufin mice
2002	Robert Wildin and colleagues show that IPEX, a clinical syndrome characterized by multiple autoimmune processes, occurs in individuals lacking T regulatory lymphocytes

25

Intercellular Communication in the Immune System

INTRODUCTION

Cells of the host defense mechanisms cooperate to upregulate and downregulate adaptive immune responses (Chapters 13, 14, 19, 20, and 24). While many of these interactions involve direct cell-to-cell contact, others rely on soluble factors called cytokines.

Cytokine is a general term for a class of molecules that include lymphokines, monokines, interleukins (IL), chemokines, and interferons. Cytokines have been called the hormones of the immune system (Dinarello, 2007); however, at least two characteristics differentiate cytokines from hormones:

- Hormones are produced by cells in endocrine glands (thyroid, pancreas, adrenal, ovary, testis, and others) and regulate the physiology of various other tissues and organs, while cytokines are synthesized and secreted by cells involved in host defense mechanisms.
- Hormones circulate and function systemically while cytokines function locally to regulate innate and adaptive immune responses.

Arnold Rich and Margaret Lewis described the first cytokine, macrophage migration inhibitory factor (MIF), during their studies on the response of guinea pigs to *Mycobacterium tuberculosis*. During the next 40 years, investigators defined numerous additional cytokines using both in vitro and in vivo assays and assigned names based on their functions. In addition to MIF, immunologists reported T cell growth factor (TCGF), B cell growth factor (BCGF), B cell-differentiation factor (BCDF), and many more. The application of molecular biology techniques to immunology resulted in the identification of an avalanche of additional intercellular communication molecules. Starting in 1971, the International Union of Immunological Societies organized a series of workshops during which participants compared different cytokines and agreed on a system of naming these factors based on genetic and molecular characteristics rather than their function.

Stanley Cohen and colleagues coined the term cytokine in 1974 to refer to these soluble, intercellular messengers. These molecular mediators function in both innate host defenses and in the adaptive immune response. Most cytokines have multiple functions, are produced by multiple cell types, and have multiple targets. Several cytokines possess similar if not identical functions. The expression of genes coding for cytokines can be upregulated by the entry of a foreign pathogen as well as by inflammation. Virtually every somatic cell except red blood cells produces as well as responds to cytokines.

Cytokines function by interacting through cell-surface receptors that trigger an intracellular signal, leading to altered gene regulation in the target cells. The functions ascribed to cytokines include the following (Dinarello, 2007):

- initiation of proliferation of cells, including lymphocytes and monocytes;
- enhancement of inflammation;
- abrogation of inflammation;
- activation of T and B lymphocytes;
- interference with viral infection;
- activation of apoptosis (programmed cell death); and
- directed migration of leukocytes.

Investigators in different laboratories used unique assay systems to detect cytokines—examples of these are presented in the sections of this chapter dealing with the discovery of IL-2 and IL-4. Accordingly, results obtained in different laboratories were difficult to compare. Until the mid-1980s, assay systems to quantitate cytokine concentrations did not exist, and the level of cytokine involved in any biological assay could not be determined. The publication in 1984 of the DNA sequence for IL-1 followed by similar information about other cytokines led to the synthesis of large quantities of recombinant cytokines. This, in turn, provided a source to produce monoclonal antibodies for quantitative assay systems.

EARLY STUDIES OF SOLUBLE FACTORS IN THE IMMUNE RESPONSE

Two phenomena—inhibition of macrophage migration in vitro and induction of fever in vivo—provided clues that soluble substances participate in host defenses. In both phenomena, antigen stimulates the secretion of low molecular weight proteins (cytokines) that fail to bind antigen but rather interact with other cells in the body to coordinate the innate host defenses and the adaptive immune response.

Discovery of Macrophage Migration Inhibitory Factor (MIF)

In 1932, Arnold Rich and Margaret Lewis, working at Johns Hopkins Medical School in Baltimore, Maryland, and the Carnegie Institute in Washington D.C., injected guinea pigs subcutaneously with *M. tuberculosis*. Several weeks later, they injected these animals intradermally

with an extract of *M. tuberculosis* (old tuberculin (OT)) to determine which animals had responded to the pathogen. Positive responders developed necrosis at the site of inoculation. Rich and Lewis investigated the mechanism of this reaction by isolating leukocytes from either peripheral blood or spleen from injected or control (uninjected) guinea pigs and growing them in culture.

Addition of OT to these cultures altered the migration pattern of the cells. Cells from control animals migrated randomly whether or not OT was present in the medium. Cells from *M. tuberculosis*-injected guinea pigs also migrated randomly in the absence of OT. In contrast, the addition of OT to cells from injected animals inhibited the migration of these cells. Histological evaluation of the cultures showed that the cells primarily inhibited from migrating are polymorphonuclear leukocytes and monocytes.

Twenty-five years later, in 1958, Byron Waksman and Margit Matoltsy at Harvard Medical School and Massachusetts General Hospital, Boston, exposed monolayers of peritoneal exudate (PE) cells (macrophages, polymorphonuclear leukocytes, and lymphocytes) from *M. tuberculosis*-injected guinea pigs to OT, purified protein derivative (PPD—another extract of *M. tuberculosis*), or glycerin (as a control). Exposure of PE cells from injected animals to either OT or PPD resulted in enhanced survival of the cells 72–90h later compared to exposure of these cells to glycerin or exposure of PE cells from control animals to OT, PPD, or glycerin. The authors speculated that enhanced survival may be due to the presence of lymphocytes in the mixture that "may react with antigen, releasing specific or nonspecific factors promoting the multiplication and differentiation of these other cells."

In 1962, Miriam George and John Vaughan at the University of Rochester, New York, placed PE cells from *M. tuberculosis*-injected guinea pigs into capillary tubes and incubated these tubes in tissue culture medium containing antigen. Cells from uninjected (control) animals migrated out of the capillary tube in a fan shape array, while cells from injected guinea pigs failed to migrate. The area of cell migration could be measured, providing a quantifiable assay. The amount of migration inhibition was directly related to the concentration of antigen included in the system.

John David and colleagues (1964) at New York University and Barry Bloom and Boyce Bennett (1966) at Albert Einstein College of Medicine in New York used this technique to demonstrate that, when stimulated with antigen, lymphocytes from injected animals produced a substance—macrophage MIF—that inhibited the migration of macrophages and other leukocytes.

David's group injected guinea pigs with complete Freund's adjuvant, a water-in-oil emulsion containing killed *M. tuberculosis*. They harvested peritoneal cells

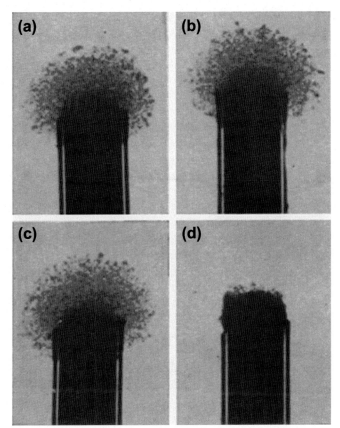

FIGURE 25.1 Antigen-induced inhibition of macrophage migration from capillary tubes. Peritoneal exudate cells obtained from normal guinea pigs are cultured with supernatants of cultures of lymphocytes from guinea pigs sensitized to *Mycobacterium tuberculosis* and treated in various ways. Chamber A contains supernatant from lymphocytes cultured with medium, chamber B is from lymphocytes incubated with an unrelated antigen (coccidioidin), and chamber C is from lymphocytes cultured with medium to which purified protein derivative (PPD)—an extract derived from the microbe—was added. Chamber D is supernatant from lymphocytes incubated with PPD. The degree of inhibition produced in these cultures could be measured and is a semiquantitative method of determining the amount of inhibitor factor being produced. *From Bloom and Bennett (1966).*

from these animals, mixed them with cells from control, uninjected guinea pigs, and placed the mixtures in capillary tubes that were incubated in tissue culture medium containing PPD. The addition of cells from injected guinea pigs inhibited migration of the control cells. In some experiments, the investigators observed inhibition of migration when cells from the injected donor made up as few as 2.5% of the total cells in the capillary tube.

Bloom and Bennett injected guinea pigs with complete Freund's adjuvant, harvested PE cells, and separated them into two populations: one that adhered to plastic containing primarily macrophages and a second that failed to adhere to plastic containing greater than 90% lymphocytes. They placed macrophages or unseparated PE cells in capillary tubes and evaluated migration with or without PPD. Unseparated cells did not migrate

from the tubes, while purified macrophages migrated even in the presence of PPD.

Bloom and Bennett prepared similar populations of cells from uninjected control guinea pigs and tested these in an identical assay. Macrophages from control animals migrated out of the tubes even in the presence of PPD. Lymphocytes from injected guinea pigs inhibited the migration of macrophages from both injected and noninjected animals when PPD was included in the mixture, while lymphocytes from noninjected animals failed to alter the migratory pattern of macrophages whether from injected or control guinea pigs (Figure 25.1).

Bloom and Bennett further demonstrated that the inhibition of cellular migration is due to secretion of a soluble factor by lymphocytes. They incubated purified lymphocytes from injected animals with PPD for 20 h and then harvested a cell-free supernatant that inhibited the migration of macrophages from capillary tubes. Bloom and Bennett offer possible explanations for these results, including that "the interaction of sensitized lymphocytes and specific antigen causes release by the cells of some pharmacologic agent which suppresses migration of macrophages without killing them."

Discovery of a Factor That Induces Fever (IL-1)

In 1785, C. Dickinson of the University of Edinburgh, Scotland, proposed that fever might be induced by breakdown products of injured tissue (referenced in Bennett and Beeson, 1953a). Throughout the next 150 years several investigators demonstrated that injection of pus or an extract of necrotic tissue induced fever in uninfected animals.

In 1944, Valy Menkin of Duke University in Durham, North Carolina, described a fever-inducing substance in inflammatory exudates. Menkin injected a sterile irritant into the peritoneal cavity of dogs to elicit a PE. Injection of this exudate intravenously into rabbits induced a fever. Menkin demonstrated that the active component of the exudate was a euglobulin that he called pyrexin. While pyrexin was originally touted as an endogenous pyrogen, other investigators raised questions as to whether the exudates from which it was isolated might have been contaminated by bacteria that are known to produce fever (Atkins, 1984).

In 1953, Ivan Bennett and Paul Beeson, working at Yale University School of Medicine, New Haven, Connecticut, injected rabbits with sterile saline to induce a PE. They cultured the cells from these exudates and harvested supernatants. When Bennett and Beeson injected these supernatants into other rabbits the recipients developed a fever (Bennett and Beeson, 1953a,b).

The investigators injected rabbits with supernatants or extracts from a variety rabbit tissues including brain, heart, lung, liver, spleen, pancreas, adrenals, skeletal muscle, bone marrow, and testis; these preparations failed to induce a fever. Bennett and Beeson determined that the substance that caused the fever was heat-labile, derived primarily from granulocytes, and was significantly different from known bacterial pyrogens.

Several investigators attempted to purify this pyrogenic factor during the following 20 years. Finally, in 1974, Patrick Murphy and coworkers at Johns Hopkins University School of Medicine in Baltimore, Maryland, purified rabbit pyrogen sufficiently to conclude that it had a molecular weight of 14,000–15,000 Da. In 1977, Charles Dinarello and colleagues, working at the National Institute of Allergy and Infectious Diseases in Bethesda, Maryland, confirmed a similar molecular weight (17,000 Da) for purified human endogenous pyrogen.

In 1971, Igal Gery, Richard Gershon, and Byron Waksman at Yale University School of Medicine, New Haven, Connecticut, described a macrophage-derived factor that potentiated the proliferative response of mouse thymocytes. Gery and his colleagues cultured mouse thymocytes with the T cell mitogen phytohemagglutinin (PHA). This treatment failed to induce proliferation although PHA was known to stimulate mitosis in peripheral T lymphocytes. The addition of human peripheral blood leukocytes to these cultures significantly enhanced proliferation. Additional studies demonstrated that the human leukocytes could be replaced by a soluble factor released by these cells.

The factor derived from macrophages (Gery and Waksman, 1972) and labeled lymphocyte-activating factor (LAF) possessed physical properties similar to those of endogenous pyrogen. In 1979, Lanny Rosenwasser and coworkers at the National Institute of Allergy and Infectious Diseases in Bethesda, Maryland, demonstrated that human endogenous pyrogen functioned in a T lymphocyte proliferation assay identically to LAF. Several other molecules described in the literature with similar properties included mitogenic peptide, helper peak-1 (HP-1), T cell-replacing factor III (TRF-III), T cell-replacing factor$_{M\varphi}$ (TRFμ), B cell-activating factor (BAF), and B cell-differentiation factor (BCDF). At a meeting held in conjunction with the Second International Lymphokine Workshop in 1979, participants reached a consensus that these were all the same molecule, and it was assigned the designation IL-1 (Aarden et al., 1979).

IDENTIFICATION OF OTHER SELECT CYTOKINES

As early as 1965, investigators described soluble factors (cytokines) that induced lymphocyte proliferation. Between 1965 and 1980, immunologists detected a large number of cytokines using a variety of in vitro and in vivo assay systems. In the following section, the studies that led to the identification of several of these factors are described. A recent review (2011) by Mübeccel Akdis

and colleagues at the University of Zurich, Switzerland, provides a comprehensive overview of the discovery, structure, receptors, signaling pathways, cellular sources and targets, and function of IL-1 to 37 plus interferon-γ.

Interleukin-2

In 1965, two groups of investigators at McGill University in Montreal, Canada, Shinpei Kasakura and Louis Lowenstein and Julius Gordon and Lloyd MacLean, added supernatants from mixed leukocyte cultures to cultures of unstimulated lymphocytes and measured proliferation by the incorporation of ^{3}H-thymidine or by counting the number of blast cells. Both groups concluded that these culture supernatants contained a blastogenic factor most likely produced by cells activated in the initial mixed leukocyte culture. They performed these studies prior to separation of lymphocytes into T and B populations; hence, neither group reported which lymphocytes proliferated.

Ten years later, in 1975, Giovanni DiSaboto, Dien-Ming Chen, and John Erickson, working at Vanderbilt University in Nashville, Tennessee, described a factor from mixed cultures of spleen cells and thymocytes that increased proliferation of the thymus cells to PHA as measured by the incorporation of ^{3}H-thymidine into DNA. This thymocyte-stimulating factor (TSF) was also found in supernatants of spleen cells cultured without thymocytes but not in cultures of bone marrow or thymus cells. TSF failed to enhance the response of spleen or lymph node cells to PHA.

In 1976, Doris Anne Morgan, Francis Ruscetti, and Robert Gallo, working at the Litton Bionetics Research Laboratory and the National Institutes of Health in Bethesda, Maryland, presented evidence for the existence of a soluble factor that stimulated T lymphocytes in humans. Morgan and her colleagues cultured human lymphocytes with PHA for 3 days. Supernatants from these cultures added to cultures of bone marrow cells activated a fraction of the cells to proliferate. The dividing cells lacked surface immunoglobulin, failed to express Epstein–Barr viral antigens, and formed rosettes with sheep erythrocytes (Ruscetti et al., 1977), all characteristics of T lymphocytes. Functionally, the cells responded to T lymphocyte mitogens (PHA, concanavalin A, and pokeweed mitogen), secreted known T lymphocyte mediators (interferon and colony-stimulating factors), and participated in mixed lymphocyte cultures as responders but not stimulators. These are all indicators that the responding cells were T lymphocytes and the factor was termed T cell growth factor (TCGF).

The physicochemical properties of TSF and TCGF proved similar. At the time of the Second International Lymphokine Workshop in 1979, several other cytokines had been described with similar functions and properties. These included thymocyte mitogenic factor, costimulator, killer cell helper factor, and secondary cytotoxic T cell-inducing factor. Participants at this workshop reached a consensus that these were all the same molecule and agreed to call it IL-2 (Aarden et al., 1979).

Cytokines That Stimulate B Lymphocytes (IL-4 and IL-6)

Macrophage-derived IL-1 induces T lymphocytes to synthesize and secrete IL-2. IL-2 in turn triggers T lymphocyte proliferation. In the 1970s and 1980s, several investigators initiated searches for cytokines that provide similar signals to B lymphocytes and described two different cytokines:

- IL-4, a factor that stimulates B lymphocyte proliferation; and
- IL-6, a factor that induces B lymphocyte differentiation to antibody production.

Richard Dutton and his group at the University of California, San Diego, initially speculated in 1971 that soluble factors existed that activated B lymphocytes to secrete immunoglobulin. In 1972, Anneliese Schimpl and Eberhard Wecker, working at the University of Würzberg, Germany, confirmed these speculations.

Schimpl and Wecker injected mice with sheep erythrocytes (SRBC), isolated B lymphocytes from the spleens of these mice, incubated these B lymphocytes in vitro with supernatants harvested from cultures of leukocytes, and quantified antibody-forming cells specific for SRBC using the hemolytic plaque assay. They tested two supernatants: one from a mixed leukocyte culture (MLC) containing cells of two different strains of mice and a second control supernatant harvested from a culture of cells of one of the two strains. Supernatants from MLCs enhanced the number of antibody-forming cells while supernatants isolated from cultures of either strain singly failed to increase the number of antibody-forming cells detected. Schimpl and Wecker called the active factor in the MLC supernatants T cell replacing factor (TRF).

Tadamitsu Kishimoto and colleagues (1975), working at the Osaka Medical School in Japan, presented the evidence that T lymphocyte-derived factors could induced immunoglobulin synthesis and secretion from naïve as well as activated B lymphocytes. Kishimoto and colleagues hypothesized that antibody production by B lymphocytes required two signals: one mediated by the binding of cell-surface immunoglobulin serving as the B lymphocyte antigen receptor and a second produced by a nonspecific soluble factor released by T lymphocytes (Chapter 19).

The investigators injected rabbits with an extract of ascaris (a parasitic worm) in complete Freund's adjuvant. They prepared a single cell suspension from the popliteal lymph nodes of these rabbits and cultured them for 24h in the presence of the ascaris extract. Supernatants from these cultures served as the source of soluble factors tested in their experimental system that involved cultured control rabbit lymphocytes treated with antibody to rabbit immunoglobulin to mimic the binding of cell-surface immunoglobulin by antigen. Twenty-four hours later, they treated these lymphocytes with the ascaris-stimulated supernatant.

Kishimoto and coworkers detected proliferation of the B lymphocytes by incorporation of ^{3}H-thymidine into DNA and measured IgG secretion in the culture fluid using a radioimmunoassay. Optimal immunoglobulin secretion required that the B lymphocytes be stimulated by both antibody to immunoglobulin and the T cell soluble factor. The factor alone, which the investigators called B cell differentiation factor (BCDF), failed to stimulate B lymphocyte proliferation. This cytokine is now called IL-6.

In the following years, other investigators reported the isolation of similar factors that caused differentiation of B lymphocytes without inducing proliferation. Researchers in different laboratories coined different names for these factors, including hybridoma growth factor, interferon β-2, B cell stimulatory factor-2, BCDF, and hepatocyte-stimulating factor. Once DNA sequences for these factors became available, investigators recognized a commonality and agreed to call the factors IL-6 (Wolvekamp and Marquet, 1990).

In 1982, Maureen Howard, working in William Paul's laboratory at the National Institutes of Health, Bethesda, Maryland, as well as Susan Swain and Richard Dutton at the University of California, San Diego, independently described a cytokine that induces proliferation of B lymphocytes. Howard and her group treated mouse B lymphocytes in vitro with antibodies to IgM and simultaneously with a supernatant harvested from a T lymphocyte hybridoma. Three days later, they added ^{3}H-thymidine and measured the incorporation of the isotope 16h later. B lymphocytes treated with both antibody to IgM and the T hybridoma-derived supernatant proliferated while treatment with either of these stimulants alone activated mitosis. Howard's group demonstrated that T lymphocytes synthesize and secrete this B cell growth factor (BCGF) that is currently called IL-4. Swain and Dutton isolated a similar B cell growth promoting factor from an alloreactive T cell line supernatant. This factor promoted B lymphocyte proliferation but failed to induce antibody production to SRBC.

Tumor Necrosis Factor (TNF)

Physicians have described spontaneous regression of tumors for several hundred years, often following an acute infection. These observations led to the development of a number of therapeutic interventions for cancer patients. William Coley described one such intervention in 1893 when he injected cancer patients with killed bacterial cultures containing *Streptococcus pyogenes* and *Serratia marcescens*. The aim of treatment with Coley's toxin, which was used until 1963, was to enhance the immune response to the tumor (Chapter 37).

The results of treating cancer patients with killed bacteria failed to consistently eliminate the tumor and advances in the areas of radiation therapy and chemotherapy supplanted this approach. Interest in the phenomenon continued, however, and focused on injection of gram negative bacteria into tumor-bearing animals to induce hemorrhagic necrosis of the tumors. In 1943, Murray Shear and coworkers at the National Cancer Institute in Bethesda, Maryland, identified the active component of gram negative bacteria as a membrane component now known as lipopolysaccharide (LPS) or endotoxin. This advance inspired studies that eventually led to the discovery of tumor necrosis factor (TNF).

Lloyd Old (1933–2011) devoted his career to tumor immunotherapy. He was trained as a physician at the University of California, San Francisco and spent his research career at the Memorial Sloan Kettering Cancer Institute in New York, where he made several major discoveries, including

- identification of cell-surface markers, leading to the differentiation of functionally different lymphocyte populations (Chapter 22);
- efficacy of Bacillus Calmette-Guérin (BCG) in cancer immunotherapy (Chapter 37);
- relationship between Epstein–Barr virus and nasopharyngeal cancer; and
- TNF.

Old and his colleagues based their investigations on the knowledge that LPS and BCG (an attenuated strain of *Mycobacterium bovis*) each inhibit tumor growth in experimental animals (Carswell et al., 1975). In vitro studies showed that neither LPS nor BCG by themselves killed or inhibited the growth of tumor cells directly. These researchers postulated that these microbial products worked through the production of an anticancer substance by the host. To test this hypothesis, Old and coworkers injected mice with BCG followed 14–21 days later with LPS. Two hours after LPS injection, they sampled blood of the mice and injected the serum intravenously into other mice that had been previously transplanted subcutaneously with a sarcoma. They measured serum activity by the amount of necrosis (on a scale of 0–3) that occurred in the tumor. During the next several days, tumors in mice injected with serum from mice treated with both BCG and LPS displayed grade 2 or 3 necrosis, while tumors in mice injected with serum from animals treated with either BCG or LPS alone exhibited minimal necrosis. They termed the active factor in these sera tumor necrosis factor (TNF).

TNF is a 150,000 Da glycoprotein that contains no residual BCG or LPS. TNF is selectively cytotoxic for malignantly transformed cells and does not inhibit the growth of several normal cell types, including mouse embryo fibroblasts and L cells (a mouse fibroblast cell line). While the cellular origin of TNF at this time remained elusive, the authors correctly speculated that TNF is produced by macrophages because both BCG and LPS activate macrophages.

Subsequent studies confirmed that TNF is produced by macrophages. In addition to killing tumor cells, TNF has several other functions, including induction of inflammation and fever, inhibition of viral replication and tumor growth, activation of apoptosis, and regulation of immunocompetent cells.

Transforming Growth Factor (TGF)

Transforming growth factors (TGF) are soluble substances secreted by virally infected cells that cause a phenotypic transformation in noninfected cells. Joseph De Larco and George Todaro, working at the National Cancer Institute, Bethesda, Maryland, described TGF in 1978. They transformed mouse fibroblasts by a sarcoma virus, grew them in culture, and harvested supernatants. De Larco and Todaro assayed these supernatants for their effect on the growth of control rat and mouse fibroblasts in soft agar. Positive results in this assay were thought to indicate that the cells had been malignantly transformed since uninfected cells fail to grow well under these conditions. The supernatant contained a factor that promoted the growth of fibroblasts in soft agar; the factor was termed sarcoma growth factor.

Subsequent characterization of this factor (now called TGF-α) confirmed that this cytokine is produced by a variety of malignantly transformed cells as well as by fetal cells and by several cells in the adult, including macrophages, brain cells, and keratinocytes. TGF-α is structurally similar to epidermal growth factor (EGF), binds to the EGF receptor, and may represent the embryonic form of EGF. In addition to its role in oncogenesis, some investigators speculate that TGF-α is important in wound healing.

In 1981, Anita Roberts and her coworkers at the National Cancer Institute in Bethesda, Maryland, described a second TGF isolated from nonneoplastic cells of various mouse organs, including skeletal muscle, heart, liver, kidney, brain, and submaxillary salivary gland. TGF-β produces effects on nontransformed cells similar to those observed with TGF-α. Unlike TGF-α, TGF-β does not compete with EGF for binding to the EGF receptors. Further study has demonstrated that the two forms of TGF do not share a common structure.

TGF-β provides both inhibitory and stimulatory signals to the adaptive immune response. Among other functions, TGF-β inhibits B lymphocyte proliferation and immunoglobulin secretion (Kehrl et al., 1986) while potentiating isotype switching of B lymphocytes from IgM to IgA (Coffman et al., 1989).

Interferon (IFN)

In 1957, Isaacs and Lindenmann discovered a substance that interferes with viral infection. Alick Isaacs (1921–1967) received his MD from the University of Glasgow in 1954. He performed his research at the National Institute for Medical Research, London. In 1956, Jean Lindenmann (1924–2015), a Swiss microbiologist/immunologist who received his MD from the University of Zurich in 1951, joined him.

Isaacs and Lindenmann studied the phenomenon of viral interference in which inactivated influenza virus inhibits the growth of live influenza virus. Heat-inactivated virus placed on the chorio-allantoic membrane (CAM) of chick embryos prevents live virus from growing on the same membrane.

Issacs and Lindenmann isolated pieces of CAM and treated them with inactivated virus for various times, ranging from 15 min to 4 h. They washed the treated membranes twice and placed them into new medium containing live virus. After an additional incubation period, they harvested the supernatants, mixed them with chicken erythrocytes (CRBC), and measured agglutination. The viability of the virus remaining in the culture medium is inversely proportional to the amount of CRBC agglutination. Isaacs and Lindenman demonstrated that incubation of the CAM with heat-inactivated virus for 15 min resulted in an 85% reduction in the amount of live virus recovered.

Several other observations in these initial studies include the following (Isaacs and Lindenmann, 1957; Issacs et al., 1957):

- Development of interference required metabolic activity; incubation of the CAM with inactivated virus at 2 °C failed to induce the interfering activity.
- Fluid recovered from cultures of CAM incubated with inactivated virus for 24 h transferred the interference to a new membrane–virus combination. Similar interfering activity was detected in the tissue culture medium derived from this second membrane.
- Culture medium derived from CAM incubated with influenza virus inhibited the growth of other viruses, indicating that the interfering activity is not virus specific.
- Antibody to influenza virus failed to neutralize the interfering activity.

Based on these results, Isaacs and Lindenmann termed the substance produced by the cells of the CAM, interferon (IFN).

Similar observations had been made 3 years previously by the Japanese virologists, Yasu-ichi Nagano and Yasuhiko Kojima (reviewed by Watanabe, 2004). Working at the University of Tokyo, they investigated the effect of injecting rabbits with inactivated vaccinia virus. They noted that a short time after injecting the rabbits intradermally with virus inactivated with ultraviolet light, the skin was resistant to an injection with live virus. They postulated that skin produced a virus inhibitory factor that they subsequently isolated and characterized (Nagano and Kojima, 1954, 1958).

Investigators have identified a large number of interferon molecules that possess similar structure and function. Each of these molecules is coded by different genes. Current convention classifies interferons based on the receptor that they bind. Type I interferons include IFN-α and IFN-β, while type II interferons include IFN-γ. All interferons function to inhibit viral infection and enhance adaptive immune responses through upregulation of the expression of genes in the major histocompatibility complex (Chapter 17). Interferons possess antitumor activity, and several of them have been approved by the US Food and Drug Administration for use in patients with malignancy (i.e., various leukemias and lymphomas), autoimmune disease (i.e., multiple sclerosis), and viral infections (i.e., hepatitis).

CHEMOKINES

Chemokines are low molecular weight proteins that induce the migration of leukocytes into areas of inflammation based on concentration gradients. Different chemokines bind to specific cell-surface receptors, and the mix of chemokines secreted during an immune response alters the types of leukocytes that enter an inflammatory locus. Researchers initially detected chemokines by stimulating cell lines in vitro with various substances such as interferon or lipopolysaccharide. Investigators isolated genes preferentially expressed by exposure to these stimuli, determined DNA sequences, deduced amino acid sequences, compared these proteins to known proteins, and speculated about their function.

The prototypical chemokine is IL-8. In 1985, Andrew Luster and his colleagues at Rockefeller University and the Memorial Sloan Kettering Cancer Center in New York used interferon-γ to stimulate a myeloid cell line that possessed monocyte characteristics. One of the genes activated in this experiment codes for a low molecular weight protein whose DNA sequence is similar to two proteins released by the degranulation of platelets. These platelet-derived proteins were chemotactic, leading the authors to speculate that the γ-interferon inducible protein "may be a member of a family of proteins involved in the inflammatory response."

Other investigators identified a similar protein during the next two years. In 1988, Kouji Matsushima and coworkers at the National Cancer Institute, Bethesda, Maryland, stimulated human monocytes with LPS, isolated a monocyte-derived neutrophil chemotactic factor (MDNCF), and cloned the DNA for this factor. The deduced amino acid sequence of MDNCF is similar to that of several other chemokines, including the γ-interferon-induced factor described by Luster, several factors released during platelet degranulation, a *v-src*-induced protein, and a growth-regulated gene product. Further study demonstrated that these molecules also shared function, and they are now designated IL-8.

NOMENCLATURE

Investigators originally named molecules involved in intercellular communication in the immune system based on the assay system used to characterize them. These functional names are confusing. In addition, following the introduction of the IL nomenclature in 1979, some investigators independently assigned IL names to new factors they characterized. This led to additional confusion since different investigators might use the same IL name to refer to different cytokines. To alleviate the chaos, the World Health Organization (WHO), in collaboration with the International Union of Immunological Societies (IUIS), established a Standing Committee on IL designation in 1991. This committee recommended procedures for the naming of secreted products of the immune systems (IUIS/WHO, 1991). These procedures require the following four criteria prior to granting of an IL designation:

1. The molecule must have been purified, the corresponding DNA cloned, and the protein expressed.
2. The nucleotide and deduced amino acid sequence must be different from any other known IL or other described molecule.
3. The molecule must be a natural product of the cells of the immune system.
4. The molecule should mediate a function (preferably multiple functions) in immune responses.

In 1991, when these criteria were initially published, the committee adopted designations for IL-1–IL-10, including IL-1α and IL-1β. Subsequent reports of this group approved designations for IL-11, 12, 13, 14, 15, and 16. While the IUIS maintains an Interleukin Subcommittee, IL designations are now listed on a Web site maintained by the Human Gene Nomenclature Committee (HGNC) available at: http://www.genenames.org/genefamilies/IL.

CONCLUSION

Cytokines refers to a group of polypeptides that allows the cells of the host defense mechanisms to communicate with one another. The term cytokine encompasses proteins that have previously been categorized as chemotactic factors (chemokines), lymphocyte-derived factors (lymphokines), monocyte-derived factors (monokines), interleukins, interferons, tumor necrosis factors, and transforming growth factors.

The initial observations that such molecules exist came from studies performed in the 1930s on the response of guinea pigs to infection with *M. tuberculosis*. These investigations formed the underpinnings for an increasing number of studies on factors secreted into cultures of various cells stimulated with a variety of antigens or microbial products. With the advent of molecular biology techniques, investigators detected many additional members of the cytokine and chemokine families based on searching DNA libraries.

The discovery of cytokines and chemokines helped explain several important phenomena in the host defense mechanisms, including

- accumulation of inflammatory cells in an area threatened by foreign material and potential pathogens,
- differentiation of various functional subpopulations of lymphocytes,
- cooperation of T and B lymphocytes in generating optimal immune responses, and
- regulation of ongoing immune responses to guard against induction of immune-mediated pathology.

Once immunologists understood the function of these small molecules they developed new and unique methods to control the innate host defense mechanisms and the adaptive immune response. Monoclonal antibodies to several of these molecules or to their receptors have been developed and are now approved for the treatment of several diseases, including rheumatoid arthritis, psoriasis, and Crohn's disease (Chapter 38).

References

Aarden, L.A., Brunner, T.K., Cerottini, J.-C., et al., 1979. Revised nomenclature for antigen-nonspecific T cell proliferation and helper factors. J. Immunol. 123, 2928–2929.

Akdis, M., Burgler, S., Crameri, R., Eiwegger, T., Fujita, H., Gomez, E., Klunker, S., Meyer, N., O'Mahony, L., Palomare, O., Rhyner, C., Quaked, N., Schaffartzik, A., Van De Veen, W., Zeller, S., Zimmermann, M., Akdis, C.A., 2011. Interleukins, from 1 to 37, and interferon-γ: receptors, functions, and roles in diseases. J. Allergy Clin. Immunol. 127, 701–721, 721e1–721e70.

Atkins, E., 1984. Fever: the old and the new. J. Inf. Dis. 149, 339–348.

Bennett, I.L., Beeson, P.B., 1953a. Studies on the pathogenesis of fever. I. The effect of injection of extracts of uninfected rabbit tissues upon the body temperature of normal rabbits. J. Exp. Med. 98, 477–492.

Bennett, I.L., Beeson, P.B., 1953b. Studies on the pathogenesis of fever. II. Characterization of fever-producing substances from polymorphonuclear leukocytes and from the fluid of sterile exudates. J. Exp. Med. 98, 493–508.

Bloom, B.R., Bennett, B., 1966. Mechanism of a reaction in vitro associated with delayed-type hypersensitivity. Science 153, 80–82.

Carswell, E.A., Old, L.J., Kassel, R.L., Green, S., Fiore, N., Williamson, B., 1975. An endotoxin-induced serum factor that causes necrosis of tumors. Proc. Nat. Acad. Sci. U.S.A. 72, 3666–3670.

Coffman, R.L., Lebman, D.A., Shrader, B., 1989. Transforming growth factor β specifically enhances IgA production by lipopolysaccharide-stimulated murine B lymphocytes. J. Exp. Med. 170, 1039–1044.

Cohen, S., Bigazzi, P.E., Yoshida, T., 1974. Similarities of T cell function in cell-mediated immunity and antibody production. Cell. Immunol. 12, 150–159.

Coley, W.B., 1893. The treatment of malignant tumors by repeated inoculations of erysipelas, with a report of ten original cases. Am. J. Med. Sci. 105, 487–511.

David, J.R., Lawrence, H.S., Thomas, L., 1964. Delayed hypersensitivity in vitro II. Effect of sensitive cells on normal cells in the presence of antigen. J. Immunol. 93, 274–278.

De Larco, J.E., Todaro, G.J., 1978. Growth factors from murine sarcoma virus-transformed cells. Proc. Nat. Acad. Sci. U.S.A. 75, 4001–4005.

Dickinson, C., 1785. An inquiry into the nature and causes of fever (with a review of the several opinions concerning its proximate cause as advanced by different authors and particularly as delivered from the practical chair in The University of Edinburgh, etc.). Abstracted in Ginger, L.C., 1952. Bacterial Pyrogens; Particularly Pyrogenic Polysaccharides of Bacterial Origin: An Annotated Bibliography. Baxter Laboratories, Morton Grove, IL.

Dinarello, C.A., 2007. Historical insights into cytokines. Eur. J. Immunol. 37, 534–545.

Dinarello, C.A., Renfer, L., Wolff, S.M., 1977. Human leukocytic pyrogen: purification and development of a radioimmunoassay. Proc. Nat. Acad. Sci. U.S.A. 74, 4624–4627.

DiSabato, G., Chen, D.-M., Erickson, J.W., 1975. Production by murine spleen cells of an activity stimulating the PHA-responsiveness of thymus lymphocytes. Cell. Immunol. 17, 495–504.

Dutton, R.W., Falkoff, R., Hirst, J.A., Hoffman, M., Kappler, J.W., Kettman, J.R., Lesley, J.F., Vann, D., 1971. Is there evidence for a non-antigen specific diffusible chemical mediator from the thymus-derived cell in the initiation of the immune response? Prog. Immunol. 1, 355–368.

George, M., Vaughan, J.H., 1962. In vitro cell migration as a model for delayed hypersensitivity. Proc. Soc. Exp. Biol. Med. 111, 514–521.

Gery, I., Gershon, R.K., Waksman, B.H., 1971. Potentiation of cultured mouse thymocyte responses by factors released by peripheral leucocytes. J. Immunol. 107, 1778–1780.

Gery, I., Waksman, B.H., 1972. Potentiation of the T-lymphocyte response to mitogens. II. The cellular source of potentiating mediator(s). J. Exp. Med. 136, 143–155.

Gordon, J., MacLean, L.D., 1965. A lymphocyte-stimulating factor produced in vitro. Nature 208, 795–796.

Howard, M., Farrar, J., Hilfiker, M., Johnson, B., Takatsu, K., Hamaoka, T., Paul, W.E., 1982. Identification of a T cell-derived B cell growth factor distinct from interleukin 2. J. Exp. Med. 155, 914–923.

Isaacs, A., Lindenmann, J., 1957. Virus interference. I. The interferon. Proc. R. Soc. Lond., B. Biol. Sci. 147, 258–267.

Isaacs, A., Lindenmann, J., Valentine, B.C., 1957. Virus interference. II. Some properties of interferon. Proc. Roy. Soc. Lond., B. Biol. Sci. 147, 268–273.

IUIS/WHO Standing Committee on Interleukin Designation, 1991. Nomenclature for secreted regulatory proteins of the immune system (Interleukins). Bull. WHO 69, 483–484.

Kasakura, S., Lowenstein, L., 1965. A factor stimulating DNA synthesis derived from the medium of leukocyte cultures. Nature 208, 794–795.

Kehrl, J.H., Roberts, A.B., Wakefield, L.M., Jakowlew, S., Sporn, M.B., Fauci, A.S., 1986. Transforming growth factor beta is an important immunomodulatory protein for human B lymphocytes. J. Immunol. 137, 3855–3860.

Kishimoto, T., Miyaka, T., Nishizawa, Y., Watanabe, T., Yamamura, Y., 1975. Triggering mechanism of B lymphocytes. I. Effect of anti-immunoglobulin and enhancing soluble factor on differentiation and proliferation of B cells. J. Immunol. 115, 1179–1184.

Luster, A.D., Unkeless, J.C., Ravetch, J.V., 1985. γ-interferon transcriptionally regulates an early-response gene containing homology to platelet proteins. Nature 315, 672–676.

Matsushima, K., Morishita, K., Yoshimura, T., Lavu, S., Kobayashi, Y., Lew, W., Appella, E., Kung, H.F., Leonard, E.J., Oppenheim, J.J., 1988. Molecular cloning of a human monocyte-derived neutrophil chemotactic factor (MDNCF) and the induction of MDNCF mRNA by interleukin 1 and tumor necrosis factor. J. Exp. Med. 167, 1883–1893.

Menkin, V., 1944. Chemical basis of fever. Science 100, 337–338.

Morgan, D.A., Ruscetti, F.W., Gallo, R., 1976. Selective in vitro growth of T lymphocytes from normal human bone marrow. Science 193, 1007–1008.

Murphy, P.A., Chesney, P.J., Wood, W.B., 1974. Further purification of rabbit leukocyte pyrogen. J. Lab. Clin. Med. 83, 310–322.

Nagano, Y., Kojima, Y., 1954. Pouvoir immunisant du virus vaccinal inactivé par des rayons ultraviolets. C. R. Seances Soc. Biol. Fil. 148, 1700–1702.

Nagano, Y., Kojima, Y., 1958. Inhibition de l'infection vaccinale par un facteur liquide dans le tissu infecté par le virus homologue. C. R. Seances Soc. Biol. Fil. 152, 1627–1629.

Rich, A.R., Lewis, M.R., 1932. The nature of allergy in tuberculosis as revealed by tissue culture studies. Bull. Johns Hopkins Hosp. 50, 115–131.

Roberts, A.B., Anzano, M.A., Lamb, L.C., Smith, J.M., Sporn, M.B., 1981. New class of transforming growth factors potentiated by epidermal growth factor: isolation from non-neoplastic tissues. Proc. Nat. Acad. Sci. U.S.A. 78, 5339–5343.

Rosenwasser, L.J., Dinarello, C.A., Rosenthal, A.S., 1979. Adherent cell function in murine T-lymphocyte antigen recognition IV. Enhancement of murine T-cell antigen recognition by human leukocytic pyrogen. J. Exp. Med. 150, 709–714.

Ruscetti, F.W., Morgan, D.A., Gallo, R.C., 1977. Functional and morphological characterization of human T cells continuously grown in vitro. J. Immnol. 119, 131–138.

Schimpl, A., Wecker, E., 1972. Replacement of T-cell function by a T-cell product. Nature New Biol. 237, 15–17.

Shear, M.J., Turner, F.C., Perrault, A., Shovelton, T., 1943. Chemical treatment of tumors. V. Isolation of the hemorrhage-producing fraction from Serratia marcescens (Bacillus prodigiosus) culture filtrate. J. Nat. Cancer Inst. 4, 81–97.

Swain, S.L., Dutton, R.W., 1982. Production of a B cell growth-promoting activity, (DL) BCGF, from a cloned T cell line and its assay on the BCL1 B cell tumor. J. Exp. Med. 156, 1821–1834.

Waksman, B.H., Matoltsy, M., 1958. The effect of tuberculin on peritoneal exudate cells of sensitized guinea pigs in surviving cell culture. J. Immunol. 81, 220–234.

Watanabe, Y., 2004. Fifty years of interference. Nature Immunol. 5, 1193.

Wolvekamp, M.C.J., Marquet, R.L., 1990. Interleukin-6: historical background, genetics and biological significance. Immunol. Lett. 24, 1–10.

TIME LINE

1785   C. Dickinson proposed that fever might be due to the action of breakdown products of necrotic tissue

1893   W.B. Coley describes a toxin (tumor necrosis factor (TNF)) induced by injecting killed bacteria

1932   Arnold Rich and Margaret Lewis describe changes in leukocyte migration in culture of immune cells produced by the addition of antigen (old tuberculin)

1944   Valy Menkin induces fever by injecting animals with a supernatant of cultured peritoneal exudate cells

1953   Ivan Bennett and Paul Beeson induce fever in a rabbit by injecting supernatants or extracts from cells derived from an inflammatory response

1954   Yasu-ichi Nagano and Yasuhiko Kojima describe a factor that inhibits the infection of cells by viruses

1957   Alick Isaacs and Jean Lindenmann describe a factor that interferes with infection cells by viruses

1958   Byron Waksman and Margit Matoltsy postulate the existence of a factor released by lymphocytes that affects the migratory behavior of macrophages

1962   Miriam George and John Vaughn devise a capillary tube method for detecting migration inhibition factor (MIF)

1964   John David and colleagues demonstrate that lymphocytes are the source of MIF

1965   Shinpei Kasakura and Louis Lowenstein and Julius Gordon and Lloyd Maclean describe a lymphocyte-stimulating factor in mixed leukocyte culture supernatants

1966   Barry Bloom and Boyce Bennett demonstrate that lymphocytes from immunized animals produce macrophage migration inhibitory factor (MIF)

1971   Richard Dutton and colleagues speculate that soluble factors exist that activate B lymphocytes to synthesize and secrete antibodies

1972   Maureen Howard and coworkers and Anneliese Schimpl and Eberhard Wecker independently describe a factor that stimulates B lymphocyte differentiation

1972   Igal Gery and Byron Waksman isolate IL-1 from macrophages

1974   Patrick Murphy and colleagues purify rabbit leukocyte pyrogen

1974   Stanley Cohen and colleagues coin the term cytokine

1975   Lloyd Old and coworkers identify TNF

1975   Giovanni DiSabato and colleagues describe thymocyte-stimulating factor (IL-2) in mice

1976   Doris Anne Morgan and coworkers describe IL-2 in humans

1977   Charles Dinarello and colleagues purify human leukocyte pyrogen

1978   Joseph DeLarco and George Todaro describe a soluble factor that transforms fibroblasts in vitro to a malignant phenotype (TGF)

1979   Participants at the Second International Lymphokine Workshop assign interleukin names to IL-1 and IL-2

1981   Anita Roberts and colleagues describe the isolation of a second transforming growth factor—TGF-β

1982   Maureen Howard and colleagues describe a B lymphocyte growth factor

1984   DNA sequence of IL-1 published

1985   Andrew Luster and collaborators describe the prototypical chemokine, IL-8

1988   Kouji Matsushima and colleagues clone the DNA for a monocyte-derived neutrophil chemotactic factor

1991   Standing committee of the World Health Organization–International Union of Immunological Societies devises criteria for designating a molecule an interleukin and approves designation of IL-1 to IL-10

CHAPTER

26

Antibody-Mediated Effector Mechanisms

INTRODUCTION

The adaptive immune response eliminates potentially pathogenic microorganisms and other foreign material by two distinct mechanisms:

- Cell-mediated responses involve activation of T lymphocytes that target and eliminate pathogens, including viruses and intracellular bacteria that exist within cells of the host (Chapter 26).
- Antibody-mediated responses involve activation of B lymphocytes that target and eliminate many microorganisms, including extracellular bacteria, fungi, and protozoal parasites, which survive outside the cells of the host.

Antibodies, synthesized and secreted by B lymphocytes, display antigenic specificity. Investigators in the late 1800s and early 1900s described antibodies based on in vitro assays used for their detection (i.e., agglutination, precipitation, toxin neutralization, complement activation). Originally, each of these assay systems was thought to detect distinct antibodies. Accordingly, investigators assigned unique names to the molecules responsible for each function: precipitins, agglutinins, amboceptors (an antibody that activated complement and caused lysis), or opsonins (an antibody that enhanced phagocytosis). Immunologists now concur that these different functions are all performed by proteins having essentially identical structures.

Hans Zinsser in 1913 working at Stanford University, Palo Alto, California, demonstrated that individual antibodies perform several different functions (the unitarian hypothesis of antibodies—Chapter 11). This hypothesis states that an antigen induces a single type of molecule capable of performing all of the in vitro functions attributed to antibody. To reach this conclusion, Zinsser showed that antibodies that precipitated an antigen in vitro also fixed (activated) complement.

Zinsser employed a two-step assay in which antibody interacted with soluble antigen to form precipitate. He harvested the supernatant from this first reaction and added it to a test tube containing erythrocytes mixed with antibody specific for these red blood cells. This assay measures the concentration of complement remaining in the supernatant determined by the degree of red blood cell lysis. Two possible results of this study were:

- the concentration of complement in the supernatant decreased with increasing precipitate, or
- the concentration of complement in the supernatant remained the same regardless of the amount of precipitate.

In fact, Zinsser showed an inverse correlation between the amount of precipitate formed in the first assay and the degree of lysis caused by the supernatant. This indicated that complement had been removed from the serum by the precipitate and that the same antibody both precipitated antigen and fixed complement.

A Historical Perspective on Evidence-Based Immunology
http://dx.doi.org/10.1016/B978-0-12-398381-7.00026-5

227

In subsequent studies, Zinsser added serum that contained complement from unimmunized animals to preformed antigen–antibody precipitates. Following incubation, he added supernatants from these mixtures to antibody-sensitized red cells and noted the presence or absence of hemolysis. As in the previous experiment, lysis of the red cells indicated that the antigen–antibody precipitates had no effect on the amount of complement in the serum, while the absence of lysis of the erythrocytes signaled that the antigen–antibody precipitate failed to remove complement. Zinsser showed that the precipitate removed complement from the serum of unimmunized animals.

From these results, Zinsser reasoned that "the fixation of alexin (complement) by precipitates is not merely a mechanical adsorption, and in that it renders more likely the supposition that the so called precipitin is actually a protein sensitizer by which a foreign protein is rendered amenable to the proteolytic action of the alexin (complement)." As Zinsser concluded, "Carried to its logical conclusion, the acceptance of this view…leads to the conception that functionally there is but one variety of specific antibodies." By 1921, Zinsser was sufficiently convinced that the unitarian view of antibodies was correct that he published a review of the topic in the *Journal of Immunology*.

When Zinsser reached this conclusion, little was known about the structure of antibodies. In 1937, Michael Heidelberger of Columbia University, New York, and Kai Pedersen of the University of Uppsala, Sweden, concluded that antibodies are modified serum proteins. In 1959, Rodney Porter at the National Institute of Medical Research, London, and Gerald Edelman working at the Rockefeller Institute, New York, independently provided experimental data leading to our contemporary understanding of the basic structure of the antibody molecule. Further study identified a division of the molecule into variable and constant regions based on the amino acid makeup (Chapter 11). This unique structure permits the molecule to bind specifically to antigen (by virtue of the amino acid sequences in the amino terminus of the molecule), and simultaneously, to interact with molecules and cells of the innate host defense systems to initiate various effector functions such as phagocytosis and inflammation (by virtue of amino acid sequences of the carboxyl terminus of the molecule).

The function of antibodies is to focus the activity of innate defense effectors on foreign material including potential pathogens. Antibody can eliminate potentially dangerous microorganisms by

- neutralization (blocking the biological activity of microorganism or their toxic products);
- activation of the classical complement pathway, leading to cell lysis and inflammation;
- opsonization (binding antigen to enhance uptake by phagocytic cells including macrophages and dendritic cells);
- participation in antibody-dependent cell-mediated cytotoxicity (ADCC), a mechanism by which nonspecific, cytotoxic lymphocytes kill foreign pathogens (Chapter 28); or
- degranulation of mast cells and eosinophils leading to release of vasoactive mediators including histamine (Chapter 33).

Investigators described the first three of these mechanisms during the initial two decades of the twentieth century. The release of vasoactive mediators from mast cells was also described in the early years of the twentieth century although the antibody responsible for this function was not determined until the mid-1960s. ADCC was described in the 1960s following a serendipitous observation during studies on optimal conditions for cell-mediated cytotoxicity (a T-lymphocyte-mediated effector mechanism).

NEUTRALIZATION

Antibody neutralization of potential pathogenic microorganisms refers to several different phenomena:

- inhibition of motility,
- interference with binding to host cells, or
- prevention of the biological effect of secreted toxins.

Neutralization was the initial function attributed to antibodies. George Nuttall (1888) working at the University of Gottingen in Germany, showed that serum taken from rabbits injected with *Bacillus anthracis* killed or neutralized the bacteria. Numerous other investigators confirmed these findings using other pathogenic microorganisms and pursued the production of antibodies that could be used to decrease the pathology induced by infections. These studies resulted in the development of a therapeutic intervention for several diseases including diphtheria and tetanus. In 1890, Emil von Behring applied the information that the disease diphtheria, resulting from infection with *Corynebacterium diphtheria,* was due not to the action of the bacteria but to the action of an exotoxin derived from the microbe. Working at the Hygiene Institute in Berlin, Germany, with Shibasaburo Kitasato, von Behring injected rabbits with diphtheria toxin and showed that transfer of the rabbit serum containing antibodies specific for diphtheria toxin protected other animals against the deleterious effects of the toxin. Extension of this result to the clinic protected patients infected with *C. diphtheria* and initiated the era of serotherapy (Chapter 3).

While physicians no longer routinely use antibodies to toxin to treat individuals with diphtheria, an FDA approved antibody is available to treat infected individuals who have not been vaccinated against the disease. A similar strategy is still used to treat individuals who may have eaten food contaminated with *Clostridium botulinum* or who have been bitten by poisonous snakes or insects (i.e., scorpions).

Other examples of antibody-mediated neutralization include antibodies induced by some vaccines developed to protect against viral infections. These vaccines are designed to induce neutralizing antibodies that inhibit the potential pathogen from binding to and invading host cells. For example, the Sabin oral polio vaccine protects against infection by a virus transmitted by the fecal–oral route. The poliovirus binds host cell surface molecules on the gastrointestinal (GI) mucosa to infect the individual. Antibodies directed against ligands expressed by the poliovirus inhibit viral entry. The Sabin vaccine proved particularly successful in inducing a local antibody response in the GI tract. While no longer used in the United States due to concerns of transmission of a live virus to immunocompromised contacts, this vaccine is still used extensively in developing countries.

Several of the vaccines that are currently under evaluation against the human immunodeficiency virus (HIV), causative agent of the acquired immunodeficiency syndrome (AIDS), are similarly directed against molecules expressed on the surface of the virus, particularly components of the gp140 complex, responsible for HIV binding to CD4+ T lymphocytes in humans. The rationale for this approach is that antibodies inhibit the binding of free virus to its target cells. Recently, researchers described patients secreting broadly neutralizing antibodies to HIV. They are investigating these antibodies to help design an improved vaccine.

The concept of neutralizing antibodies is extended to the development of several biologics that are used in treating autoinflammatory and autoimmune diseases, for example, monoclonal antibodies specific for the proinflammatory cytokine, tumor necrosis factor-alpha (TNF-α). Several different antibodies to TNF-α are approved by the FDA for use in rheumatoid arthritis, Crohn's disease, and psoriasis. Antibodies to TNF-α have decreased the pathology associated with these diseases in select patients (Chapter 38). Treatment with antibody to TNF-α is not without potential complication since chronic use renders the patient immunocompromised and increases the possibility of the development, or reemergence of, infectious diseases such as tuberculosis.

ACTIVATION OF COMPLEMENT

The complement system, a component of the innate host defense mechanism, has been commandeered by the adaptive immune response to provide protection against infections (Chapter 12). Complement consists of a group of serum proteins that are activated sequentially to eliminate potentially pathogenic microorganisms. In the absence of antibodies, activation occurs nonspecifically relying on two mechanisms termed the alternate pathway and the lectin pathway. Activation results in initiation of inflammation, induction of vasodilation, attraction of white blood cells, and lysis of both prokaryotic and eukaryotic cells. As the adaptive immune response evolved, the complement system was expropriated. IgM and IgG antibodies possess amino acid sequences in their Fc regions that bind and activate complement components thereby focusing complement activities.

Activation of complement by antigen-antibody complexes is designated the classical pathway. Jules Bordet (1870–1961) working at the Pasteur Institute in Paris investigated the protective immune response induced in guinea pigs by the injection of *Vibrio cholerae*. Other investigators had demonstrated that serum from guinea pigs injected with *V. cholerae* killed the bacteria and that this activity was abrogated by heating the serum. Bordet extended these findings and concluded that guinea pigs injected with *V. cholerae* contained a heat-stable substance that agglutinated live vibrios but failed to kill them (Bordet, 1895). Combining these observations, Bordet concluded that two substances existed: one that was heat stable termed *sensibilatrices* (antibody) and a second that was destroyed by heating named *alexine* (complement).

Bordet developed a nonmicrobial model to quantitate the interaction of antibody with complement (Bordet, 1898). He demonstrated that the addition of fresh serum to erythrocytes coated with specific antibody resulted in lysis of the red cells and release of hemoglobin. Using this model, Bordet showed that complement was not antigen specific since it lysed red cells of different species once they were coated with antibody. He also proved that red cells from different species expressed unique antigens and that complement only interacted with antibody once it bound antigen.

In 1901, Bordet assumed the directorship of a newly formed Pasteur Institute in Brussels, Belgium. Bordet developed the complement fixation assay for the detection of antibody responses to infectious microorganisms, primarily bacteria (Bordet and Gengou, 1901). In this assay, serum obtained from a patient presenting with an infection is heated at 56 °C for 30 min to inactivate complement; this treatment does not affect antibody. A standard amount of complement is added back to the heated serum, which is subsequently mixed with the bacteria. Following incubation, a standard amount of red blood cells coated with specific antibodies is added to the assay system.

If the original serum contains antibody to the bacteria, the two react and activate complement.

Antibody-coated erythrocytes added to the assay fail to lyse, and hemoglobin is not released; this represents a positive test for antibody specific to the bacteria. The presence of hemoglobin following a second incubation period indicates that the original serum lacked antibody to the bacteria.

Bordet continued his studies on the roles of antibodies and complement in providing protection against potential pathogens and made seminal contributions in other areas including phagocytosis and opsonization. Bordet was awarded the Nobel Prize in Physiology or Medicine in 1919 "for his discoveries relating to immunity."

OPSONIZATION

Almroth Wright (1861–1947) working at St. Mary's Hospital in London originally described opsonization in 1903. Opsonization is the process of enhancing phagocytosis of foreign material including bacteria. Wright received his medical degree from Dublin University in Ireland and spent his career as professor of pathology first at the Army Medical School, Netley, and then at St. Mary's Hospital, London.

Wright developed methods to immunize patients with their own bacteria in an attempt to develop therapeutic vaccines. He based these studies on the development of a vaccine by Louis Pasteur and Emile Roux in 1885 (Pasteur, 1885; reviewed by Crick, 1973) to treat individuals who had been bitten by rabid animals. Wright is best known for the development of the vaccine against typhoid fever used by the British Army during the First World War. He also pursued vaccine development against pneumonia and tuberculosis and studied serum opsonins.

Wright and his assistant S.R. Douglas studied the in vitro phagocytosis of *Staphylococcus* using white blood cells from healthy individuals (Wright and Douglas, 1903). They observed minimal phagocytosis of the bacteria in the absence of serum. Serum or plasma from healthy, noninfected individuals contained a substance that enhanced phagocytosis of the bacteria; Wright and Douglas called this substance an opsonin from the Greek word opsonein meaning to prepare for eating. They demonstrated that serum opsonin activity was destroyed by heating the serum for 10–15min to a temperature of 60°–65°C.

Wright also obtained serum from a patient who had been exposed to *Staphylococcus*; this led to the identification of a second opsonin. This opsonin resisted inactivation by heating and was subsequently identified as antibody. Immunologists have confirmed these observations and agree that two opsonins exist: one that is heat labile and a second that is heat stable.

Heat-labile opsonins exist naturally in sera from healthy, noninfected individuals. Under steady state conditions, one of the components of complement (C3) spontaneously breaks down into C3a and C3b. C3b binds microbial surfaces and other foreign particles. This complex in turn interacts with receptors on neutrophils, monocytes, macrophages, and dendritic cells and stimulates phagocytosis by these cells.

Heat-stable opsonins comprise serum antibodies that function by forming a bridge between a microbe and Fc receptors on various phagocytic cells. Both IgG and IgM antibodies bind Fc receptors on phagocytes thus providing a mechanism to eliminate pathogenic microorganisms.

ANTIBODY-DEPENDENT CELL-MEDIATED CYTOTOXICITY

In 1965, Erna Möller working at the Karolinska Institute in Stockholm, Sweden, described a fourth effector mechanism by which antibodies eliminate pathogens. Antibody dependent cell-mediated cytotoxicity (ADCC) occurs when cells (i.e., bacteria, virally infected somatic cells, or tumors) are bound by specific antibodies and then exposed to a unique population of cytotoxic lymphocytes. These lymphocytes differ from cytotoxic T lymphocytes and exist constitutively in healthy animals prior to exposure to antigen. Originally called killer (K) lymphocytes, they are now recognized as natural killer (NK) lymphocytes (Chapter 28).

Möller was investigating T-lymphocyte-mediated cytotoxicity in vitro. She injected inbred mice with allogeneic lymphocytes, harvested lymph node lymphocytes from the injected mice, and mixed these activated lymphocytes with a transplantable sarcoma expressing the same MHC-coded antigens as the allogeneic lymphocytes. She studied conditions that favored cytotoxicity of the incompatible cells and determined killing of the sarcoma cells by counting the number of cells stained by trypan blue, a vital dye excluded by living cells. This number served as a baseline for her subsequent studies.

Möller added serum from calves to the cultures as a method to enhance cell-to-cell contact. Initially, she noted that serum from 3- to 4-week-old calves increased the cytotoxic potential of harvested lymphocytes, while serum from newborn calves failed to enhance cytotoxicity. One explanation for these results is that serum from older calves contains antibodies specific for mouse cells, while newborn calf serum lacks these antibodies. Subsequent studies demonstrated that most batches of serum obtained from 3- to 4-week-old calves agglutinate mouse lymphocytes at a titer of 1:16, while newborn calf serum fails to agglutinate mouse lymphocytes. Two observations explain this dichotomy:

- calves are not exposed to mouse antigens in utero; and
- the structure of the bovine placenta (unlike the human placenta) precludes transport of serum antibodies from mother to fetus.

Möller replaced the calf serum with rabbit serum obtained either from rabbits injected with mouse cells or from uninjected controls. Addition of rabbit serum containing antibodies to mouse lymphocytes cultured with allogeneic sarcoma cells increased the killing of the sarcoma cells, while rabbit serum from uninjected controls failed to enhance lysis. Möller favored the interpretation that the role of the antibodies in this experiment was to increase contact between the effector lymphocytes and the allogeneic sarcoma cells (Möller, 1965).

Möller's initial erroneous interpretation of these results can be attributed to her original concentration on the mechanism of T-lymphocyte-mediated cytotoxicity. As a consequence, her results were not duplicated for almost 3 years.

In 1968, Ian MacLennan and G. Loewi working at the Canadian Red Cross studied immunologic nonspecific cytotoxicity of a human cell line that had been adapted to long-term growth in culture. MacLennan and Loewi labeled Chang cells with ^{51}Cr and used them as target cells in an in vitro cytotoxicity assay. They incubated labeled cells for 18h with either human peripheral blood lymphocytes or lymph node cells obtained from healthy rats or rabbits. The radioactivity released during this incubation became the baseline against which subsequent experiments were compared.

MacLennan and Loewi next injected rats or rabbits with Chang cells to prepare specific antibodies. These antibodies failed to lyse Chang cells as detected by release of an isotope from the target cells. However, when the investigators added these antibodies to parallel cultures of target cells and human lymphocytes, the amount of radioactive label released from the cells increased. Based on these results, MacLennan and Loewi conclude that "nonspecific cytotoxicity can be increased by antibody directed against the target cell."

Chang cells, used in this and numerous other investigations on lymphocyte-mediated cytotoxicity, were originally derived from normal human liver. Subsequent studies using isoenzyme analysis, DNA fingerprinting, and HeLa marker chromosomes showed that Chang cells are contaminated with HeLa cells—a cell line derived from human cervical carcinoma (Gao et al., 2011). This contamination does not decrease the validity of the conclusions derived from these experiments but cautions investigators about the purity of their reagents.

Results from early studies of ADCC suggested that antibody and effector cells be derived from different species. If true, ADCC would be a curiosity and not relate to in vivo mechanisms by which antibody eliminates pathogens. In fact, in additional studies, MacLennan and Loewi supported this possibility by reporting that they failed to observe cytotoxicity when human Rh-positive red blood cells treated with human antibodies specific for Rh antigens were cultured in the presence of human peripheral blood lymphocytes.

Subsequent studies performed with human antibodies and human effector cells demonstrated that the phenomenon worked in a homologous system (MacLennan et al., 1969). These investigators used Chang liver cells as their target. They added human serum or fluid derived from a knee aspirate to peripheral blood lymphocytes and mixed this with the target cells. Twelve out of 78 human sera enhanced Chang cell lysis. The researchers demonstrated that the factor responsible for this activity was specific for Chang cells and had the characteristics of IgG yet failed to alter Chang cell viability even in the presence of complement.MacLennan and colleagues questioned the in vivo relevancy of this observation and concluded that "there is so far no evidence showing that the mechanism described in this paper has a counterpart in vivo." Immunologists now agree, however, that ADCC is essential to protect mammals against potential pathogens and to integrate the innate and adaptive immune responses. Clinical trials based on enhancing ADCC activity in patients with various malignancies including hematologic neoplasms and solid tumors are currently underway (Chester et al., 2015).

RELEASE OF VASOACTIVE MEDIATORS

In 1902, Paul Portier and Charles Richet identified anaphylaxis as an aberrant immune response. These French scientists spent the summer of 1901 on a yacht in the Mediterranean Sea outfitted by Prince Albert of Monaco to pursue various scientific questions. Prince Albert's scientific director, Jules Richard, suggested that Portier and Richet study the reaction of fish and humans to the Portuguese man-of-war, an invertebrate found in the Mediterranean Sea. The Portuguese man-of-war captures its prey by brushing against them with its tentacles. This interaction renders the prey unable to flee. Humans who inadvertently come in contact with these same tentacles experience extreme pain sometimes accompanied with fainting.

Portier and Richet initially postulated that the tentacles gave off a poison that produced the reaction. They prepared extracts of the tentacles, injected the extracts into various experimental animals, and observed a reaction suggesting that the extract contained a powerful toxin with profound effects on the central nervous system. In an attempt to neutralize this toxin, Portier and Richet proposed producing an antibody to the toxin. This was an obvious approach in the early 1900s when treatment of diphtheria with an antibody directed to diphtheria toxin produced seemingly miraculous cures.

When the summer ended, Portier and Richet returned to their laboratory in Paris to continue this work. Since they no longer had access to Portuguese man-of-war for their studies, they switched to a related toxin from a sea anemone, *Actinia sulcata*. They injected dogs with a nonlethal dose of the sea anemone toxin and rested them for several weeks to allow the dogs to develop a protective antibody (antitoxin) response. They then reinjected the dogs with a second dose of the toxin to assess the level of protection. Instead of being protected, the dogs developed sudden onset of diarrhea and vomiting, and many of them succumbed to this second injection. This reaction was different than that observed when the dogs were injected with a lethal dose of the toxin (Chapter 33).

Portier and Richet referred to this unexpected reactivity by the term aphylaxis (shortly changed to anaphylaxis) to distinguish it from phylaxis, which was used to connote protection (Portier and Richet, 1902). Richet, to whom a Nobel Prize in Physiology or Medicine was awarded in 1913 "in recognition of his work on anaphylaxis" explained that

Anaphylaxis is the opposite of protection (phylaxis). If one injects an albuminoid substance—for example, a toxin—into the circulatory system of an animal, instead of being protected by this first injection against a further injection of the same toxin, it has become more sensitive to its action. Let us suppose that the fatal dose is 1 cg. The injection of a tenth part of that dose, that is to say 1 mg—will not make it at all ill or scarcely so. But a month later-for almost a month is required for the anaphylactic state to be produced-it has become so sensitive that a dose of 1 mg is enough to kill it by the immediate production of formidable symptoms. Therefore the first injection has caused a condition which is the opposite of protection-namely anaphylaxis (Richet, 1910).

The mechanism responsible for anaphylaxis remained elusive. Investigators showed, as early as 1910, that the reaction was transferrable by serum from a sensitized animal to a naïve one (Anderson and Frost, 1910). Passive transfer of reactivity in humans was demonstrated in 1921 by Otto Prausnitz (1876–1963) and Heinz Küstner (1897–1963) who transferred skin hypersensitivity to a normal individual (Prausnitz) using serum from an individual (Küstner) exquisitely sensitive to fish. When the recipient of the serum received an intradermal injection of fish extract, an immediate skin reaction occurred characterized by the appearance of a wheal and flare. This reaction, termed passive cutaneous anaphylaxis (PCA), resembled that seen in sensitized individuals injected with antigen.

The antibody responsible for these transfers was originally termed reagin; immunologists now agree that antibodies involved in anaphylaxis and other manifestations of similar type I hypersensitivities are of the IgE isotype. Subsequent studies showed that IgE antibodies bind to receptors on several cell types including mast cells and eosinophils. Interaction of antigen with cell-bound antibodies results in release of vasoactive chemicals including histamine, prostaglandins, and leukotrienes.

Investigators speculated about the physiological significance of IgE antibodies. Many immunologists considered that production of a class of antibodies whose function is to induce a pathological hypersensitivity made little evolutionary sense. By the early 1960s, several investigators showed that parasitic infection of several animal species including rats, monkeys, and sheep induced the production of reaginic antibody (IgE).

In 1964, Bridget M. Ogilvie working at the National Institute for Medical Research in London demonstrated that rats infected naturally with *Nippostrongylus brasiliensis* as well as rats and monkeys infected in the laboratory with *Schistosoma mansoni* and sheep infected with *Trichostrongylus colubriformis* possess serum antibodies active in PCA. PCA depends on reaginic antibodies (IgE) to bind tightly to skin cells. In these experiments, Ogilvie injected serum from infected animals into the skin of uninfected animals. Three days later she injected a mixture of antigens from the parasites and Evans blue—a dye that binds serum albumin and leaks out of capillaries in areas of increased vascular permeability. Appearance of a blue spot at the site of serum injection signals the presence of antibodies to the systemically injected antigen.

Serum from rats infected with *N. brasiliensis* produced a positive PCA reaction 19–25 days after infection that persisted for at least 7 months. Reinfection induced an enhanced antibody response within 3 days. Investigators obtained similar results using other host–parasite combinations.

During the next 10 years, several investigators demonstrated that humans infected with various parasites possessed elevated levels of serum IgE and of parasite-specific IgE antibodies. J.P. Dessaint and colleagues at the Pasteur Institute in Lille, France, reported in 1975 that patients infected with *S. mansoni* or *Schistosoma haematobium* had elevated serum IgE concentrations. Many of these patients presented with IgE antibodies specific for antigens isolated from these parasites; however, no correlation between the concentration of serum IgE and clinical course of infection was observed.

Investigators questioned the role of IgE in eliminating parasitic infections. In vitro studies showed that eosinophils and other cells to which IgE binds kill *S. mansoni* (Gounni et al., 1994). Studies using mouse and rat models of schistosomiasis produced conflicting results.

Hans Oettgen and colleagues at Case Western Reserve University in Cleveland, Ohio, designed mice lacking the genes for the constant regions of the IgE immunoglobulin (King et al., 1997). These mice failed to synthesize any IgE antibodies. King and coworkers infected these mice as well as wild-type mice with *S. mansoni* and compared the antiparasitic response of the two groups. The IgE-deficient mice proved more susceptible to infection as shown by increased worm burden and decreased granuloma formation in their livers.

Oettgen and his group also compared the response of IgE-deficient and wild-type mice to the intestinal parasite, *Trichinella spiralis* (Gurish et al., 2004). Mice lacking the gene for the constant region of IgE failed to clear *T. spiralis* from their GI track as quickly as did wild-type mice. In addition, skeletal muscle of IgE-deficient mice contained approximately twice the number of parasite larvae as did wild-type animals, and fewer of these larvae became necrotic in IgE-deficient mice as compared to larvae in skeletal muscle of wild-type animals. The authors conclude that "IgE promotes parasite expulsion from the gut following *T. spiralis* infection and participates in the response to larval stages of the parasite."

These results suggest that antibody of the IgE isotype protect mammals against parasitic infection. The most likely mechanism by which IgE functions is through the release of vasoactive mediators, particularly in the GI track. The immune response to parasitic infection includes aspects of both innate host defense mechanisms and adaptive immune responses. While many parasitic infections are accompanied by an increase in antigen specific as well as antigen nonspecific IgE synthesis, researchers continue to study the role of IgE in clearing the infecting parasites and in providing protection against reinfection.

CONCLUSION

Antibody eliminates foreign material and potentially pathogenic microorganisms using one of five methods:

- neutralization,
- complement activation,
- opsonization,
- ADCC, and
- release of vasoactive mediators from mast cells and eosinophils.

Investigators described neutralization, complement activation, and opsonization during the early decades of the twentieth century, while ADCC was serendipitously discovered in the late 1960s. The role of IgE antibodies in clearing parasitic infections remains under investigation.

Although antibodies participate in disparate mechanisms to eliminate pathogens, all antibodies are structurally similar possessing a variable Fab region that binds antigen and a relatively constant Fc region responsible for the effector functions of the molecule. Different immunoglobulin isotypes share Fab regions (and thus specificity), while each isotype has a unique Fc region.

Antibody-mediated effector mechanisms require that antibody interacts with other molecules (complement) or with cells (i.e., macrophages, NK lymphocytes, mast cells). These interactions involve the Fc portion of the immunoglobulin molecule (Chapter 11).

In humans, the classical complement pathway is activated efficiently by IgM and IgG3 antibodies and to a modest extent by IgG1 and IgG2. All of these isotypes contain amino acid sequences in the Fc region that bind the C1q protein of the complement system.

Other antibody-mediated functions involve interaction between the immunoglobulin molecule and cells. Several of the cells involved in eliminating pathogens express receptors for the Fc portion of immunoglobulin molecules. When bound, these Fc receptors transmit an intracellular signal that activates the cell. Different cell types express unique Fc receptors and hence bind different immunoglobulin isotypes. Accordingly, different isotypes perform distinct functions.

Innate host defenses eliminate many foreign substances including invading pathogens through the action of phagocytic cells particularly macrophages. Antibodies of the adaptive immune system enhance phagocytosis by serving as opsonins. All four subclasses of IgG act as opsonins although IgG1 and IgG3 are more efficient than IgG2 and IgG4. Antigen–antibody complexes bind Fc receptors on the surface of macrophages and other phagocytic cells such as dendritic cells and activate phagocytosis and intracellular destruction of potential pathogens.

Antigen coated with antibody of the IgG1 isotype preferentially binds Fc receptors expressed by NK lymphocytes activating these cells to release the contents of granules leading to lysis (ADCC; Chapter 27). NK lymphocytes destroy tumor cells as well as normal somatic cells infected with pathogenic microorganisms including viruses and intracellular bacteria.

Mast cells, basophils, and eosinophils express yet a different Fc receptor that binds the Fc portion of IgE antibodies. Cross-linking of two antibodies bound to these Fc receptors stimulates the cells to release vasoactive contents of their granules as well as to initiate enzymatic breakdown of membrane-associated arachidonic acid leading to the production of leukotrienes and prostaglandins. All of these mediators are involved in type I hypersensitivity reactions (allergy—Chapter 33) and in eliminating parasitic infections.

References

Anderson, J.F., Frost, W.H., 1910. Studies upon anaphylaxis with special reference to the antibodies concerned. J. Med. Res. 23, 31–69.

von Behring, E.A., Kitasato, S., 1890. Über das Zustandekommen der Diphtheria-immunität and der Tetanus-immunität bei Thieren. Dtsch. Med. Wochenschr. 49, 1113–1114.

Bordet, J., 1895. Les leucocytes et les proprieties actives du serum chez les vaccines. Ann. Inst. Pasteur. 9, 462–506.

Bordet, J., 1898. Sur l'agglutination et la dissolution des globules rouges par le serum d'animaux injecties de sang defibriné. Ann. Inst. Pasteur. 12, 688–695.

Bordet, J., Gengou, O., 1901. Sur l'existence de substances sensibilisatrices dans la plupart des serums anti-microbiens. Ann. Inst. Pasteur. 15, 289–302.

Chester, C., Marabelle, A., Houot, R., Kohrt, H.E., 2015. Dual antibody therapy to harness the innate anti-tumor immune response to enhance antibody targeting of tumors. Curr. Opin. Immunol. 33, 1–8.

Crick, J., 1973. The vaccination of man and other animals against rabies. Postgrad. Med. J. 49, 551–564.

Dessaint, J.P., Capron, M., Bout, D., Capron, A., 1975. Quantitative determination of specific IgE antibodies to schistosome antigens and serum IgE levels in patients with schistosomiasis (S. mansoni or S. haematobium). Clin. Exp. Immunol. 20, 427–436.

Edelman, G.M., 1959. Dissociation of γ-globulin. J. Am. Chem. Soc. 81, 3155–3156.

Gao, Q., Wang, X.-Y., Zhou, J., Fan, J., 2011. Cell line misidentification: the case of the Chang liver cell line. Hepatology 54, 1894–1895. http://dx.doi.org/10.1002/hep.24475.

Gounni, A.S., Lamkhloued, B., Ochail, K., Tanaka, Y., Delaporte, E., Capron, A., Kinet, J.-P., Capron, M., 1994. High-affinity IgE receptor on eosinophils is involved in defense against parasites. Nature 367, 183–186.

Gurish, M.F., Bryce, P.J., Tao, H., Kisselgof, A.B., Thornton, E.M., Miller, H.R., Friend, D.S., Oettgen, H.C., 2004. IgE enhances parasite clearance and regulates mast cell responses in mice infected with Trichinella spiralis. J. Immunol. 172, 1139–1145.

Heidelberger, M., Pedersen, K.O., 1937. The molecular weight of antibodies. J. Exp. Med. 65, 393–414.

King, C.L., Xianli, J., Malhotra, I., Liu, S., Mahmoud, A.A.F., Oettgen, H.C., 1997. Mice with a targeted deletion of the IgE gene have increased worm burdens and reduced granulomatous inflammation following primary infection with Schistosoma mansoni. J. Immunol. 158, 294–300.

MacLennan, I.C.M., Loewi, G., 1968. Effect of specific antibody to target cells on their specific and non-specific interactions with lymphocytes. Nature 219, 1069–1070.

MacLennan, I.C.M., Loewi, G., Howard, A., 1969. A human serum immunoglobulin with specificity for certain homologous target cells, which induces target cell damage by normal human lymphocytes. Immunology 17, 897–910.

Möller, E., 1965. Contact-induced cytotoxicity by lymphoid cells containing foreign isoantigens. Science 147, 873–874 & 879.

Nuttall, G.H.F., 1888. Experimente über die bacterien feindlichen Einflüsse des thierischen Körpers. Zeitschr. für Hygiene 4, 853–894.

Ogilvie, B.M., 1964. Reagin-like antibodies in animals immune to helminth parasites. Nature 204, 91–92.

Pasteur, L., 1885. Méthode pour prévenir la rage après morsure. Compte rendu de l'Academie des Sciences 101, 765–772.

Porter, R.R., 1959. The hydrolysis of rabbit γ-globulin and antibodies with crystalline papain. Biochem. J. 73, 119–126.

Portier, P., Richet, C., 1902. De l'action anaphylactique de certains venins. Compt. Rend. Soc de Biol. 54, 170–172.

Praustnitz, O., Küstner, H., 1921. Studien über Uberempfindlicht. Centralb. Bakterial. I Abt. Orig., 86, 160–169. Translated in Gell, P.G.H., Coombs, R.R.A., 1962. Clinical Aspects of Immunology. Blackwell, Oxford, pp. 808–816.

Richet, C., October 1, 1910. Ancient humorism and modern humorism. Brit. Med. J. 2 (2596), 921–926.

Wright, A.E., Douglas, S.R., 1903. An experimental investigation of the role of blood fluids in connection with phagocytosis. Proc. Roy. Soc. London 72, 357–370.

Zinsser, H., 1913. Further studies on the identity of precipitins and protein sensitizers (albuminolysins). J. Exp. Med. 18, 219–227.

Zinsser, H., 1921. On the essential identity of antibodies. J. Immunol. 6, 289–299.

TIME LINE

1885	Louis Pasteur and Emil Roux develop a vaccine against rabies virus
1887–1888	Jozsef von Fodor, George Nuttall, Karl Flügge, and Hans von Buchner independently describe antibacterial activity (antibody) in serum from rabbits injected with pathogenic microorganisms
1890	Emil von Behring and Shibasaburo Kitasato develop serotherapy for diphtheria and tetanus
1898	Jules Bordet discovers the complement system and the ability of complement to lyse antibody-coated sheep erythrocytes
1902	Paul Portier and Charles Richet describe anaphylaxis and conclude that it is a pathological counterpart of a protective antibody response
1903	Almroth Wright and S.R. Douglas describe opsonization and identify two serum opsonins that can be differentiated based on sensitivity to temperature
1919	Jules Bordet awarded the Nobel Prize in Physiology or Medicine
1921	Hans Zinsser publishes a review arguing that antibodies of different functions are identical in structure
1921	Otto Prausnitz and Heinz Küstner demonstrate that type I hypersensitivity can be transferred in humans by serum
1937	Michael Heidelberger and Kai Pedersen demonstrate that antibodies are serum proteins
1959	Rodney Porter and Gerald Edelman independently initiate studies leading to our contemporary understanding of antibody structure
1964	Bridget Ogilvie demonstrates that parasite infection induces production of reagin-like antibodies (IgE)
1965	Erna Möller serendipitously discovers the phenomenon of antibody-dependent cell-mediated cytotoxicity
1969	Ian MacLennan and colleagues demonstrate that ADCC functions in a homologous system (human lymphocytes, human antibody, and human target cells).
1994	Hans Oettgen and coworkers construct IgE-deficient mice that they use to investigate the role of this antibody isotype in protecting against parasite infection.

27

T-Lymphocyte-Mediated Effector Mechanisms

INTRODUCTION

Immunologists in the 1940s and 1950s discovered that some phenomena of the adaptive immune response such as graft rejection and delayed skin reactions to *Mycobacterium tuberculosis* could be transferred from sensitized animals to naïve recipients by cells (lymphocytes) but not by serum (antibodies) (Chapter 3) leading to the division of the adaptive immune system into cell-mediated and antibody-mediated responses. Further studies demonstrated that B lymphocytes synthesize and secrete antibodies, responsible for antibody-mediated responses, while cell-mediated responses are the province of T lymphocytes.

Cell-mediated responses include graft rejection, graft-versus-host reaction, delayed type hypersensitivity, induction of inflammatory responses, and lysis of virally infected and malignant cells. In addition, T lymphocytes and their products regulate, both positively and negatively, activation and suppression of other T lymphocytes as well as B lymphocytes and participate in immune-mediated pathologies including autoimmune disease and type IV hypersensitivities. This large array of functions relies on three primary mechanisms:

- target cell lysis;
- cell-to-cell interactions; and
- synthesis and secretion of cytokines leading to
  - inflammation; or
  - activation or suppression of other lymphocytes.

Antigen-specific receptors expressed on the surface of T lymphocytes, the T-cell receptor (TCR), bind short peptides derived from antigens processed by antigen-presenting cells (APC). The TCR recognizes peptides that are presented in the "context" of histocompatibility molecules of that individual (Chapter 20)—this provides the initial signal to activate the cell. Optimal activation of T lymphocytes, however, requires a second signal provided by interaction between other cell surface molecules expressed on the surfaces of T lymphocytes and APCs.

Two populations of T lymphocytes, CD4+ and CD8+, have been recognized based on expression of cell surface molecules identified by monoclonal antibodies. CD4+ T lymphocytes are helper cells, while CD8+ T lymphocytes are killers. Both CD4+ and CD8+ lymphocytes are derived from hematopoietic stem cells that originate in the bone marrow and then mature in the thymus. CD4+ T lymphocytes synthesize and secrete cytokines that induce inflammation and regulate the adaptive immune response, while CD8+ T lymphocytes lyse infected and malignant cellular targets.

Each of the populations of T lymphocytes recognizes peptides presented by different histocompatibility molecules. Antigenic peptides presented by class I histocompatibility molecules stimulate CD8+ T lymphocytes, while antigenic peptides presented by class II histocompatibility molecules stimulate CD4+ T lymphocytes. Once activated, the function of the T lymphocyte depends on the developmental history of the cell as well as the environment in which it is located.

A Historical Perspective on Evidence-Based Immunology
http://dx.doi.org/10.1016/B978-0-12-398381-7.00027-7

CELL-MEDIATED IMMUNE RESPONSES

During the first half of the twentieth century, virtually all immunologic research focused on antibody. Antibody is readily quantified, while detection of activated T lymphocytes requires sophisticated assay systems. In the clinic, the amount of antibody present in the serum of a patient with a microbial infection provides information about the course of the disease. Even in infections routinely eliminated by T lymphocytes, such as hepatitis virus, the quantity of serum antibody is used to evaluate infectivity and recovery. The concept of protective antibody led to the development of serotherapy for diphtheria and tetanus in the late 1800s and to the design of vaccines against infectious microorganisms. Unfortunately, this focus on antibodies led many clinicians to conclude erroneously that antibody could eliminate all infections.

The 1940s and 1950s ushered in studies demonstrating that certain responses of the adaptive immune system cannot be transferred to naïve animals by serum containing antibodies but rather requires activated lymphocytes. While antibody is often secreted during these responses, it is the activated lymphocytes that are critical. Merrill Chase working with Karl Landsteiner at the Rockefeller Institute in New York (Landsteiner and Chase 1942; Chase 1945) reported that delayed hypersensitivity reactions (i.e., to *M. tuberculosis*) could be transferred by cells but not by serum (Chapter 3). This observation led to studies performed independently by Avrion Mitchison at Edinburgh University, Scotland (1955), and by Peter Medawar and his group at University College, London (Brent et al., 1958).

Mitchison investigated animals reacting against allogeneic tumor grafts. Studies performed in the first half of the twentieth century demonstrated that tumors are immunogenic when transplanted to nonidentical (allogeneic) recipients (Chapter 37). In 1955, Mitchison showed that lymphocytes derived from the lymph nodes draining a tumor allograft transferred the immune response to the tumor to naïve, syngeneic animals. Serum from the tumor-bearing animal failed to transfer immunologic rejection of transplanted tumors. Mitchison concluded that tumors are immunogenic and that this immune response involves the activation of lymphocytes.

Medawar's group similarly demonstrated that lymphocytes, but not serum, transferred immunologic memory from animals that had rejected skin grafts. These results suggest that antibody is not involved in the rejection of normal skin grafts or tumors.

Antibodies failed to transfer other immunological reactions from a sensitized animal to a naïve one including graft-versus-host reactivity and positive tuberculin skin tests; however, lymphocytes did transfer these responses (Chapter 3). Investigators asked how the passive transfer of lymphocytes in the absence of antibody could elicit adaptive immune reactions. The discovery of functional subpopulations of T and B lymphocytes (Chapters 9 and 10) aided in answering this question. Subsequently, investigators demonstrated several functions they attributed to T lymphocytes including lymphocyte-mediated cytotoxicity.

Lymphocyte-Mediated Cytotoxicity

In 1960, Andre Govaerts working at the Pasteur Institute in Brussels, Belgium, transplanted kidney grafts from outbred dogs to unrelated recipients. Six to 16 days later, the transplanted kidneys ceased to function, signaling graft rejection. At autopsy, Govaerts noted that the transplanted kidneys were necrotic.

At the time of transplantation, Govaerts established cultures of kidney cells from the donor dogs. He harvested serum and lymphocytes from the recipients before, during, and after rejection. He mixed the recipient's serum with donor kidney cells both in the presence and absence of complement to test for antibody activity. He detected antibody-mediated lysis by observing the kidney cells for the signs of cytotoxicity (swelling, agglutination, cytoplasmic vesiculation, rupture of cell membrane, failure to exclude vital dyes including trypan blue and eosin). Serum from dogs bearing or having rejected a foreign kidney failed to lyse donor kidney cells. As a control, Govaerts treated similar cultures with antibodies to dog kidneys induced in rabbits; these antibodies damaged the cultured cells.

In parallel studies, Govaerts added lymphocytes from the thoracic duct of the graft recipients to cultures of donor kidney cells and assessed damage. Lymphocytes harvested during and after rejection induced destruction of the cultured kidney cells. Based on these results, the author concluded that "living lymphocytes from the recipient animal showed a clear-cut cytopathogenic effect on the renal culture from the donor."

Addition of serum plus lymphocytes to kidney cell cultures increased the percentage of cells injured compared to cultures treated with only serum or lymphocytes. These results led Govaerts to postulate that the damage may be due to the presence of "cell-bound antibodies" on recipient lymphocytes. As such this represents an early description of antibody-dependent cell-mediated cytotoxicity (ADCC) although Govaerts failed to recognize the significance of this finding. ADCC, discovered initially by Erna Möller in 1965, is one of the mechanisms by which antibody functions in eliminating foreign material and pathogens (Chapter 26).

Govaerts performed his studies before investigators described separate populations of T and B lymphocytes. Thus, he did not realize that functional subpopulations existed. Two lines of investigation in the early 1970s identified T lymphocytes as cytotoxic cells:

- Jean-Charles Cerottini and coworkers at the Swiss Institute for Experimental Cancer Research in Lausanne, injected mice with allogeneic cells to induce a cytotoxic response that they detected in vitro. They reported in 1970 that treatment of spleen cells from the injected mice with an antibody specific for T lymphocytes (anti-theta) inhibited cytotoxicity against the foreign cells.
- Pierre Golstein and colleagues working at the Karolinska Institute in Stockholm, Sweden, in 1972, immunized mice with an allogeneic tumor. Spleen cells from these mice proved cytotoxic to the tumor cells in vitro. Golstein and coworkers removed B lymphocytes from these spleen cells and demonstrated that B-lymphocyte-depleted populations were as cytotoxic to the tumor as were untreated spleen lymphocytes.

Pavel Kisielow and colleagues working with Edward Boyse at the Memorial Sloan-Kettering Cancer Center in New York questioned if cytotoxic T lymphocytes (CTLs) could be differentiated from T lymphocytes responsible for other immunological functions. Boyse and colleagues had previously developed a series of antibodies specific for mouse T lymphocytes (Boyse et al., 1968, 1971). Each antibody recognized unique antigens termed Ly. Initially, three Ly antigens were identified: Ly-1, Ly-2, and Ly-3 (Chapter 23). Treatment of mouse lymphocytes with antibodies to one of the Ly antigens plus complement eliminated the lymphocytes expressing that Ly antigen. Using this experimental protocol, Kisielow and coworkers determined the Ly phenotype of mouse cytotoxic lymphocytes.

In 1975, these investigators injected inbred mice either once or multiple times with spleen cells expressing foreign histocompatibility antigens. Lymphocytes, isolated from the peritoneal exudates of these mice 3 to 5 days after a final stimulation, lysed target cells possessing the same foreign histocompatibility antigens as the immunizing cells. Kisielow and coworkers treated aliquots of these cytotoxic lymphocytes with antibodies to either the Ly-1 antigen plus complement or to the Ly-2 antigen plus complement. The investigators reported that lymphocytes treated with antibody to the Ly-2 antigen plus complement failed to lyse the allogeneic targets, while lymphocytes treated with antibodies to Ly-1 plus complement lysed the allogeneic cells as effectively as untreated cells.

These studies defined a population of T lymphocytes that are cytotoxic to various targets including allogeneic cells and cells expressing tumor or virally coded cell surface antigens. Such lymphocytes are now classified as CD8+ lymphocytes based on studies performed with monoclonal antibodies (Chapter 23). TCRs expressed by CD8+ T lymphocytes specifically recognize target cell antigens presented by class I histocompatibility molecules. This interaction activates CD8+ T lymphocytes to lyse target cells expressing the same antigen. Activated CD8+ T lymphocytes possess two independent mechanisms to produce cell lysis:

- release of cytotoxic mediators perforin and granzyme; or
- interaction of a recently synthesized cell surface molecule (Fas ligand (FasL)) with a complementary molecule, Fas, expressed on target cells.

Both of these interactions activate genes in the target cell that result in apoptosis (programmed cell death).

Perforin is preformed in cytoplasmic granules of CTLs (and in natural killer (NK) and NKT lymphocytes—Chapter 28). These granules also contain serine proteases (granzymes). When CTLs bind to their target, granules fuse with the cell membrane, and the contents are released into the intracellular space. Perforin polymerizes and forms a transmembrane pore in the target cell through which granzymes enter and activate apoptotic death pathways (reviewed by Voskoboinik et al., 2010).

Eckhard Podack and colleagues working at New York Medical College and the Rockefeller University in New York in 1985 identified perforin in the granules of CTLs by disrupting these cells and determining which components were responsible for cell lysis. Red blood cells (RBC), incubated with antibody plus complement, develop membrane lesions leading to lysis. Podack and coworkers observed similar lesions in RBCs incubated with a 72–75 kDa protein isolated from granules of CTLs in the presence of Ca^{++}. Treated RBCs hemolyzed. The investigators named the protein perforin and speculated that perforin produced pores in the RBC leading to an osmotic alteration and consequent lysis.

Additional studies, however, demonstrated that the simple punching of holes in the cell membrane was not the mechanism of lysis in nucleated cells. In addition to perforin, granules in CTLs contain a series of enzymes known collectively as granzymes. CTLs release these enzymes that then enter the targeted cell and activate the caspase genetic pathway leading to programmed cell death (apoptosis).

A second mechanism by which CTLs induce cell death in their targets is through interaction between complementary receptors on the two cells. Virtually every cell expresses a molecule called Fas (APO-1; CD95). Fas is a death receptor that, when bound, activates the caspase pathway leading to DNA damage and apoptosis. Activated CTLs express a cell surface molecule called FasL (CD178). The binding of Fas by FasL initiates apoptosis of the Fas expressing cell.

In 1989, Bernhard Trauth and collaborators at the German Cancer Research Center in Heidelberg, Germany, and Shin Yonehara and colleagues at the Tokyo Metropolitan Institute of Medical Science in Japan, independently developed monoclonal antibodies that identified Fas. Trauth and his group developed monoclonal antibodies to a human B lymphoblast cell line to identify cell surface antigens that might be useful in controlling the growth of human malignant lymphocytes. One of the antibodies they developed recognized a lymphocyte expressed 52 kDa antigen (APO-1). Interaction of the antibody with APO-1-induced programmed cell death.

Yonehara and coworkers developed monoclonal antibodies to characterize cell surface receptors (Yonehara et al., 1989). These investigators injected mice with the human fibroblast line FS-7, harvested spleen cells from these mice, and prepared monoclonal antibodies. One of these monoclonal antibodies lysed the FS-7 fibroblasts. This group named the antigen recognized by this antibody "FS-7-associated surface antigen" or Fas.

Shige Nagata led a group of investigators at the Osaka Bioscience Institute in Japan to determine the mechanism responsible for lysis of the FS-7 expressing fibroblasts by the monoclonal antibody (reviewed by Nagata, 2004). He reasoned that Fas was a receptor involved in cell survival and considered two explanations:

• Fas bound a growth or survival factor, or
• Fas bound a death-inducing factor.

Nagata reasoned that if the first possibility is correct, then the monoclonal antibody developed by Yonehara blocked the uptake or activity of some important nutrient or growth factor. If the second postulate is correct, the monoclonal antibody acted as an agonist mimicking the action of the death factor. Subsequent investigations showed that Fas is, in fact, a receptor for a death-inducing factor.

Nagata's group demonstrated that binding of the Fas protein by a monoclonal antibody induced cell death by apoptosis (Itoh et al., 1991). Itoh and coworkers transfected mouse cell lines with the gene for human Fas and treated these cells with a monoclonal antibody against human Fas. The antibody failed to bind mouse Fas, which these transformed cell lines also expressed; however, the binding of the monoclonal antibody to human Fas was sufficient to kill the mouse cells. This result argues against Fas serving as a receptor for a growth or survival factor and rather demonstrates that human Fas transmitted a signal to upregulate the apoptotic pathway.

Pierre Golstein and his group at the Karolinska Institute in Stockholm, Sweden, identified a CTL line in 1993 that expressed a ligand that bound Fas and induced apoptosis (Rouvier et al., 1993). They used this lymphocyte line to isolate the receptor for Fas, a molecule initially called FasL. It is now renamed CD178. Takashi Suda and colleagues in 1993 working at the Osaka Bioscience Institute in Osaka, Japan, used a soluble form of Fas to probe CTLs that bound Fas and isolated DNA

from these lymphocytes. They transfected a gene coding for a transmembrane protein into COS cells (a fibroblast-like immortalized cell line from green monkey kidney). When transfected COS cells interacted with target cells expressing Fas, the target cells underwent apoptosis.

Subsequent studies have demonstrated the importance of apoptosis induced by interaction of Fas with FasL in several biological phenomena including embryogenesis, maintenance of homeostasis, development of the lymphocyte repertoire, and protection against virally infected and malignantly transformed cells. Defects in these interactions play a role in an array of pathologies including autoimmune disease, malignant transformation, and neurodegenerative diseases.

Induction of Inflammation

Inflammation, a key component of innate host defenses, serves as a major mechanism by which organisms protect themselves from pathogens. The adaptive immune system has evolved methods to target inflammation to areas of pathogen invasion. The primary mechanism by which the adaptive immune response induces inflammation is through secretion of proinflammatory cytokines including IL-1, IL-6, IL-17, and TNF-α by antigen-specific CD4+ T lymphocytes.

Investigators described the first cytokines using an in vitro model of a delayed hypersensitivity reaction (Chapter 25). Guinea pigs injected systemically with antigens from M. tuberculosis generate a T-lymphocyte-mediated response. Ten or more days following this initial injection, investigators injected these animals intradermally with M. tuberculosis antigen to evaluate reactivity to the pathogen. If the animal had responded immunologically to the original injection, a lesion characterized by induration (hardening) of the skin accompanied by cellular infiltration and redness appeared at the test site in 24–72 h. An identical reaction occurs in humans previously exposed to M. tuberculosis. This reaction monitors clinical exposure to the pathogen.

Cells that infiltrate the skin lesions are predominately mononuclear (lymphocytes and macrophages). Originally, investigators postulated that most of the cells present in the lesion were antigen specific. However, in 1967, Stanley Cohen, Robert McCluskey, and Baruj Benacerraf at the New York University School of Medicine demonstrated that this postulate was erroneous. Cohen and colleagues injected guinea pigs with two different antigens both known to elicit a delayed hypersensitivity reaction. They spaced the two injections 6 days apart and injected the guinea pigs with tritiated thymidine on days 1–4 following the initial injection to label cells reacting specifically to the first antigen. Cohen and colleagues skin tested these animals with both antigens and demonstrated that the numbers of radiolabeled cells in the two skin lesions were identical. These results led the authors to conclude that "specifically sensitized cells which are believed to initiate the inflammation of delayed hypersensitivity reactions are too few to be detected." This, and other studies, led the researchers to conclude that most of the cells in the lesion were present nonspecifically.

If the cells appearing in a delayed hypersensitivity reaction are not antigen specific, what types of cells migrate into the lesion, and how do those cells get there? Today, immunologists agree that soluble factors (cytokines) released by antigen-specific sensitized lymphocytes are responsible for these reactions. However, initial descriptions of soluble factors released by sensitized lymphocytes were met with skepticism.

Detection of soluble factors depended on the development of an in vitro model system to study delayed hypersensitivity. Arnold Rich and Margaret Lewis developed such a model in 1932. Working at Johns Hopkins University in Baltimore, Maryland, Rich and Lewis injected guinea pigs with *M. tuberculosis*. They cultured peripheral blood leukocytes and fragments of the spleens from injected animals and from uninjected controls. Rich and Lewis noted that over time mononuclear cells migrated from the peripheral blood and spleen fragments. Addition of tuberculin antigens to cultures of cells from tuberculin-injected animals inhibited the migration of the cells; addition of these same antigens to cultures of cells derived from control animals failed to inhibit this migration.

Thirty years later in 1962, Miriam George and John Vaughn, working at the University of Rochester in New York revisited this finding and developed a method for detailed study of the reaction. George and Vaughn injected guinea pigs with antigens to induce a delayed hypersensitivity reaction. They loaded cells derived from the peritoneal exudates of these animals into capillary tubes and placed them in petri dishes. Over time, the cells migrated out of the capillary tubes onto cover slips in the petri dishes to produce a fan-like zone of migration, the extent of which could be quantified. Addition of the antigen with which the animal had been injected inhibited the migration of cells from the tube. Measurement of the degree of inhibition provided a semiquantitative indication of the strength of the immune response.

George and Vaughn demonstrated that this in vitro system was immunologically specific by adding different antigens to the cells. The inhibition of migration only occurred when they incubated the cells with the antigen to which the cells had been sensitized.

Barry Bloom and Boyce Bennett (1966; 1968) at the Albert Einstein College of Medicine in New York used this technique to investigate the mechanism of inhibition. They injected guinea pigs with tuberculin to induce a delayed hypersensitivity reaction, harvested peritoneal exudate cells from the injected animals, and placed them

in culture with tuberculin. Bloom and Bennett prepared a supernatant from these cells that they added to peritoneal exudate cells from control animals that had not been injected with tuberculin. The supernatant inhibited migration of cells from uninjected guinea pigs. These results suggested that cells in the peritoneal exudate from injected animals secreted a factor that inhibited migration of cells from control guinea pigs.

Bloom and Bennett determined the cellular source of the inhibitory factor. They separated peritoneal exudate cells from tuberculin-injected animals into lymphocyte-rich and lymphocyte-depleted populations based on adherence to plastic or glass petri dishes. They added tuberculin to both populations, harvested supernatants, and added these supernatants to peritoneal exudate cells from uninjected animals. Figure 27.1

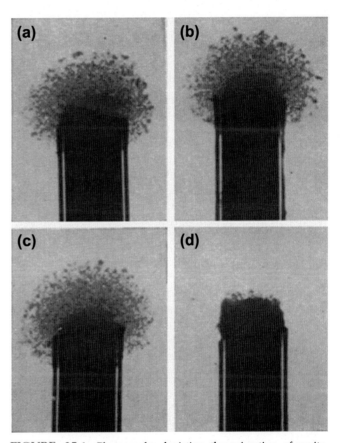

FIGURE 27.1 Photographs depicting the migration of peritoneal exudate cells from capillary tubes demonstrating that inhibition of migration is due to a substance elaborated by lymphocytes from injected animals. All tubes contain peritoneal exudate cells from a normal, noninjected guinea pig. Peritoneal exudate (PE) cells obtained from tuberculin-injected guinea pigs were incubated under various conditions, and the supernatants from these mixtures were added to the capillary tube cultures. (a) Supernatant from PE cells incubated with tissue culture medium only. (b) Supernatant from PE cells incubated with an unrelated antigen, coccidioidin. (c) Supernatant from PE cells from which lymphocytes had been removed prior to incubation with tuberculin antigen. (d) Supernatant from PE cells incubated with tuberculin antigen. *From Bloom and Bennett (1966).*

presents photographs of a representative experiment. Supernatants from lymphocyte-depleted populations failed to inhibit migration of the cells from the capillary tubes (panel C), while supernatants from tuberculin-sensitized peritoneal exudate cells inhibited migration (panel D). The investigators concluded that sensitized (immune) lymphocytes secrete a soluble substance into the tissue culture medium that they called migration inhibitory factor (MIF).

Investigators have sequenced and crystallized MIF and identified its receptor. While not antigen specific, MIF is a cytokine produced by T lymphocytes in response to activation by antigen. The late 1960s, researchers have described an array of additional cytokines involved in the initiation of inflammation including IL-1, IFN-γ, IL-6, IL-17, IL-19, IL-22, IL-23, IL-26, IL-31, IL-36, and TNF-α. These are synthesized and secreted by a variety of cell types including lymphocytes, monocytes/macrophages, dendritic cells, fibroblasts, and epithelial and endothelial cells.

Cytokines produced by different cell types function by interacting with cell surface receptors and initiate distinct activities such as induction of fever, stimulation of the acute phase response, regulation of hematopoiesis, and promotion of apoptosis. The resulting redundancy afforded by cytokines that induce similar functions provides several pathways for the adaptive immune system to activate inflammation. In addition, the overlapping functions provide several pathways to induce inflammation in the event a gene for one of these cytokines is mutated.

Immune Regulation

The adaptive immune response maintains a balance between responding adequately to eliminate potential pathogens and other foreign material and responding too aggressively leading to autoimmune diseases such as type 1 diabetes and systemic lupus erythematosus or hypersensitivities including allergy. Several regulatory mechanisms including T helper and T regulatory lymphocytes (Chapters 13 and 24) and feedback systems that rely on cytokines maintain this homeostatic balance.

Three independent groups of investigators described T helper cells in the late 1960s (Claman et al., 1966; Davies et al., 1967; Miller and Mitchell, 1968). These investigators demonstrated that while thymus-derived (T) lymphocytes do not themselves produce antibody, they are essential to help bone marrow-derived (B) lymphocytes synthesize optimal amounts of antibody. The mechanism of collaboration between T helper and B lymphocytes involves both cell-to-cell contact and the release of cytokines. Details of the experimental design used by these three groups are presented in Chapter 13.

T helper lymphocytes express CD4 on their cell surfaces. In the absence of CD4$^+$ T lymphocytes (Chapter 32), B lymphocytes synthesize and secrete some antibody but only of the IgM isotype. This suggests that T-lymphocyte-mediated help is most likely a late evolutionary addition to adaptive immune responses. Activation of B lymphocytes in the presence of T lymphocytes alters the isotype of antibody produced, thus increasing the number of protective mechanisms (complement activation and ADCC by IgG, survival of IgA in the gastrointestinal and respiratory tracts, degranulation of mast cells by IgE) that can be recruited in response to potential pathogens. In addition, B lymphocytes assisted by T lymphocytes develop into memory cells that respond rapidly and with greater vigor upon subsequent challenge with the sensitizing antigen.

CD4$^+$ T lymphocytes assist other T lymphocytes activated by foreign antigens (Chapter 20). Activated CD4$^+$ T lymphocytes produce cytokines including IL-2 that induce proliferation in both CD4$^+$ and CD8$^+$ T lymphocytes. In addition, T lymphocytes synthesize and secrete several cytokines that are involved in the differentiation of the subpopulations of CD4$^+$ T lymphocytes (Chapter 23). Differentiation of these subpopulations is crucial in determining which of the many protective mechanisms are activated to rid the individual of potential pathogens. Currently, investigators describe five populations of CD4$^+$ T lymphocytes each with a different function (Chapter 23). These include

- T_H1 lymphocytes that provide help to CD8$^+$ CTLs.
- T_H2 lymphocytes that help B lymphocytes switch to the synthesis and secretion of IgE antibodies.
- T_{FH} (follicular helper) lymphocytes that help B lymphocytes switch to the synthesis and secretion of IgA and IgG.
- T_H17 lymphocytes that secrete cytokines involved in inflammatory responses.
- T_{REG} lymphocytes that downregulate ongoing immune responses.

The concept of suppression or regulation (Chapter 24) of ongoing immune responses provides an attractive model for developing therapeutic interventions for diseases in which the immune system is hyperactive such as allergies and autoimmunity or in clinical situations such as allogeneic tissue or organ grafts where inhibition of the adaptive immune response would be therapeutic.

CONCLUSION

T lymphocytes eliminate nascent tumors and intracellular microorganisms such as viruses and some bacteria, and regulate the strength of adaptive immune responses. Functionally, T lymphocytes lyse malignant or infected cells, induce inflammatory responses, and synthesize and secrete soluble intercellular messengers called cytokines. Immunologists have characterized two main categories of T lymphocytes based on expression of lymphocyte-specific cell surface markers—CD4+ and CD8+. CD4+ lymphocytes comprise at least five functionally separate populations (T_H1, T_H2, T_{FH}, T_H17, T_{REG}) that

- induce inflammation through the release of low-molecular weight soluble factors; and
- regulate, both positively and negatively, activation and suppression of other T lymphocytes as well as B lymphocytes.

CD8+ T lymphocytes release contents of intracellular granules that contain perforin and granzymes. These mediators form pores in the cell membrane of target cells resulting in the induction of the caspase system leading to programmed cell death (apoptosis). CD8+ T lymphocytes also mediate apoptosis through the expression of a cell surface molecule (FasL) that binds Fas on target cells.

The effector functions of T lymphocytes require an array of populations each of which have matured through unique developmental paths. This chapter reviewed the studies that led to the description of cell-mediated cytotoxicity and the induction of inflammation. Previous chapters reviewed studies pertaining to the role of T lymphocytes in activating B lymphocytes (Chapter 13) and the role of T regulatory lymphocytes (Chapter 24). T lymphocyte effector mechanisms provide protection against infectious microorganisms and tumors and are responsible for the pathology displayed in some autoimmune and autoinflammatory diseases (Chapters 31 and 34) and certain hypersensitivity diseases (Chapter 33).

References

Bloom, B.R., Bennett, B., 1966. Mechanism of a reaction in vitro associated with delayed-type hypersensitivity. Science 153, 80–82.

Bloom, B.R., Bennett, B., 1968. Migration inhibitory factor associated with delayed-type hypersensitivity. Fed. Proc. 27, 13.

Boyse, E.A., Itakura, K., Stockert, E., Iritani, C.A., Miura, M., 1971. Ly-C: a third locus specifying alloantigen expressed only on thymocytes and lymphocytes. Transplantation 11, 351–352.

Boyse, E.A., Miyazawa, M., Aoki, T., Old, L.J., 1968. Ly-A and Ly-B: two systems of lymphocyte isoantigens in the mouse. Proc. Roy. Soc. B 170, 175–193.

Brent, L., Brown, J., Medawar, P.B., 1958. Skin transplantation immunity in relation to hypersensitivity. Lancet 272, 561–564.

Cerottini, J.C., Nordin, A.A., Brunner, K.T., 1970. Specific in vitro cytotoxicity of thymus-derived lymphocytes sensitized to alloantigens. Nature 228, 1308–1309.

Chase, M.W., 1945. The cellular transfer of cutaneous hypersensitivity to tuberculin. Proc. Soc. Exp. Biol. Med. 59, 134–135.

Claman, H.N., Chaperon, E.A., Triplett, R.F., 1966. Immunocompetence of transferred thymus-marrow cell combinations. J. Immunol. 97, 828–832.

Cohen, S., McCluskey, R.T., Benacerraf, B., 1967. Studies on the specificity of the cellular infiltrate of delayed hypersensitivity reactions. J. Immunol. 98, 269–273.

Davies, A.J.S., Leuchars, E., Wallis, V., Marchant, R., Elliott, E.V., 1967. The failure of thymus-derived cells to produce antibody. Transplantation 5, 222–231.

George, M., Vaughan, J.H., 1962. In vitro cell migration as a model for delayed hypersensitivity. Proc. Soc. Exp. Biol. Med. 111, 514–521.

Golstein, P., Wigzell, H., Blomgren, H., Svedmyr, D.A.J., 1972. Cells mediating specific in vitro cytotoxicity II. Probable autonomy of thymus-processed lymphocytes (T cells) for the killing of allogeneic target cells. J. Exp. Med. 135, 890–906.

Govaerts, A., 1960. Cellular antibodies in kidney homotransplantations. J. Immunol. 85, 516–522.

Itoh, N., Yonehara, S., Ishil, A., Yonehara, M., Mizushima, S.-I., Sameshima, M., Hase, A., Seto, Y., Nagata, S., 1991. The polypeptide encoded by the cDNA for human cell surface antigen Fas can mediate apoptosis. Cell 66, 233–243.

Kisielow, P., Hirst, A., Shiku, H., Beverley, P.C.L., Hoffmann, M.K., Boyse, E.A., Oettgen, H.F., 1975. Ly antigens as markers for functionally distinct subpopulations of thymus-derived lymphocytes of the mouse. Nature 253, 219–220.

Landsteiner, K., Chase, M.W., 1942. Experiments on transfer of cutaneous sensitivity to simple compounds. Proc. Soc. Exp. Biol. Med. 49, 688–690.

Miller, J.F.A.P., Mitchell, G.F., 1968. Cell to cell interaction in the immune response I. Hemolysin-forming cells in neonatally thymectomized mice reconstituted with thymus or thoracic duct lymphocytes. J. Exp. Med. 128, 801–820.

Mitchison, N.A., 1955. Studies on the immunological response to foreign tumor transplants in the mouse. J. Exp. Med. 102, 157–177.

Möller, E., 1965. Contact-induced cytotoxicity by lymphoid cells containing foreign isoantigens. Science 147, 873–874 & 879.

Nagata, S., 2004. Early work on the function of CD95, an interview with Shige Nagata. Cell Death Differ. 11, S23–S27.

Podack, E.R., Young, J.D.-E., Cohn, Z.A., 1985. Isolation and biochemical and functional characterization of perforin 1 from cytolytic T-cell granules. Proc. Nat. Acad. Sci. U.S.A. 82, 8629–8633.

Rich, A.R., 1932. The nature of allergy in tuberculosis as revealed by tissue culture studies. Bull. Johns Hopkins Hosp. 50, 115–131.

Rouvier, E., Luciani, M.-F., Golstein, P., 1993. Fas involvement in Ca2+ -independent T cell mediated cytotoxicity. J. Exp. Med. 177, 195–200.

Suda, T., Takahashi, T., Golstein, P., Nagata, S., 1993. Molecular cloning and expression of the Fas ligand, a novel member of the tumor necrosis factor family. Cell 75, 1169–1178.

Trauth, B.C., Klas, C., Peters, A.M.J., Matzku, S., Möller, P., Falk, W., Debatin, K.-M., Krammer, P.H., 1989. Monoclonal antibody-mediated tumor regression by induction of apoptosis. Science 245, 301–305.

Voskoboinik, I., Dunstone, M.A., Baran, K., Whisstock, J.C., Trapani, J.A., 2010. Perforin: structure, function and role in human immunopathology. Immunol. Rev. 235, 35–54.

Yonehara, S., Ishii, A., Yonehara, M., 1989. A cell-killing monoclonal antibody (anti-Fas) to a cell surface antigen co-downregulated with the receptor of tumor necrosis factor. J. Exp. Med. 169, 1747–1756.

TIME LINE

| 1932 | Arnold Rich and Margaret Lewis describe an in vitro method to study immunity to *Mycobacterium tuberculosis* |

1945 Merrill Chase demonstrates that skin sensitivity to simple chemical can be transferred by cells

1955 Avrion Mitchison transfers tumor rejection to naïve animals by lymphocytes

1958 Peter Medawar and colleagues transfer skin graft rejection by lymphocytes

1960 Andre Govaerts describes cytotoxic effects of lymphocytes on target cells

1962 Miriam George and John Vaughan devise a capillary method to study migration of tuberculin-sensitive cells in vitro

1966 Stanley Cohen, Robert McCluskey, and Baruj Benacerraf describe the lymphocyte as the antigen-specific cell responsible for delayed type hypersensitivity reaction

1968 Barry Bloom and Boyce Bennett define macrophage migration inhibitory factor (MIF)

1966–1968 Henry Claman, Anthony Davies, and Jacque Miller independently demonstrate that thymus-derived lymphocytes help bone marrow-derived lymphocytes to produce an optimal antibody response

1970 J.C. Cerottini and colleagues demonstrate that antitheta antiserum eliminates cells responsible for cell-mediated cytotoxicity

1971 Pierre Golstein and coworkers show that B cells are not cytotoxic to allogeneic tumor cells

1975 Pavel Kisielow and colleagues identify cytotoxic T cells as Ly-2$^+$, Ly-1$^-$

1985 Eckhard Podack and colleagues isolate and characterize perforin from the granules of cytotoxic T lymphocytes

1989 Shin Yonehara and coworkers identify a cell surface antigen, Fas, the binding of which induces the apoptotic pathway.

28

Lymphocytes that Kill: Natural Killer (NK) and Natural Killer T (NKT) Lymphocytes

INTRODUCTION

Hematopoietic stem cells generate all the cells of the peripheral blood. Located in the bone marrow, these stem cells give rise to myeloid and lymphoid progenitors. The myeloid progenitor is the source for erythrocytes, neutrophils, basophils, eosinophils, monocytes, and platelets. The lymphoid progenitor differentiates into functionally distinct populations of T, B, and NK lymphocytes. T lymphocytes mature in the thymus where they express antigen-specific receptors (T cell receptors, TCRs). Interaction of T lymphocytes with foreign antigens activates the cell leading to gene transcription and synthesis and secretion of soluble mediators. During the 1970s, investigators identified two populations of T lymphocytes that are distinguished by expression of cell-surface molecules (CD4 or CD8) as well as by function (helper vs cytotoxic).

B lymphocytes mature in the bone marrow (or in the bursa of Fabricius in birds). During maturation B lymphocytes express antigen-specific receptors. Interaction of B lymphocytes with foreign antigens activates the cell leading to the synthesis and secretion of specific antibody. Both T and B lymphocytes are constituents of the adaptive immune response.

Natural killer (NK) lymphocytes constitute a third lineage of lymphocytes derived from lymphoid progenitors.

NK lymphocytes, a component of the innate host defenses, are large cells that contain cytoplasmic granules, mature from lymphoid precursors, and express a unique set of surface receptors. Once activated, NK lymphocytes release the contents of their granules and kill both malignantly transformed and pathogen-infected cells.

DISCOVERY OF NK LYMPHOCYTES

Neuroblastoma is a childhood malignancy that has a relatively high rate of spontaneous regression. In 1968, Ingegerd Hellström and her colleagues at the University of Washington in Seattle investigated immune responses against neuroblastoma using a colony inhibition assay. Hellström and her coworkers isolated tumor cells from patients and established them in tissue culture. They added patient serum or lymphocytes to the cultures and observed growth of the neuroblastoma cells. The investigators surmised that inhibition of tumor growth in vitro was an indication of an induced immune response, either antibody-mediated or cell-mediated to tumor-associated antigens.

Hellström and colleagues observed growth inhibition when they added peripheral blood lymphocytes from patients with neuroblastoma to autochthonous tumors

A Historical Perspective on Evidence-Based Immunology
http://dx.doi.org/10.1016/B978-0-12-398381-7.00028-9

or to tumors from other patients with neuroblastoma. The investigators interpreted this as an indication that neuroblastoma cells from different patients express cross-reactive antigens. They then added lymphocytes from the peripheral blood of mothers whose infants presented with neuroblastoma to the cultures of tumor cells and observed that these lymphocytes also inhibited the growth of their child's tumor as well as the growth of similar tumors from other children. To explain this phenomenon the authors suggested, erroneously, that neuroblastoma cells express a virally induced antigen that crossed the placenta and sensitized the mothers during pregnancy.

Other reports of naturally occurring, lymphocyte-mediated cytotoxicity against tumors appeared in the early 1970s. For example, Eugene Rosenberg and colleagues at the National Cancer Institute, Bethesda, Maryland, in 1972 studied families with identical twins, one of whom presented with lymphocytic leukemia. They isolated peripheral blood lymphocytes from family members and tested them, in vitro, for cytotoxic activity against the leukemic cells and against healthy lymphocytes from the unaffected twin. These investigators showed that lymphocytes from family members killed the leukemic cells but not the healthy lymphocytes. They also reported that some individuals unrelated to the twins possessed lymphocytes that lysed the leukemic cells. Rosenberg and coworkers proposed, incorrectly, that a leukemia-associated virus activated the cytotoxic cells in both leukemic and nonleukemic individuals.

By the early 1970s, additional investigators reported natural cytotoxicity by lymphocytes from individuals who had not previously been exposed to the target antigen. Some investigators suggested viral infections as the source of antigenic stimulation of these lymphocytes. The National Cancer Institute sponsored a conference in 1972 to evaluate results obtained by investigators in different laboratories (Herberman and Gaylord, 1973). Since some investigators considered differences in technology as an explanation for these observations, attendees evaluated the techniques used by different groups. By the end of the conference most participants agreed that some healthy, nontumor-bearing individuals possess lymphocytes that kill radiolabeled tumor cells in vitro (Oldham, 1983). The phenomenon is called natural cytotoxicity, and the responsible lymphocytes are today referred to as NK lymphocytes.

NK LYMPHOCYTES

NK lymphocytes kill various cellular targets, particularly tumor cells and cells infected with a variety of intracellular microbes. Morphologically, these cells

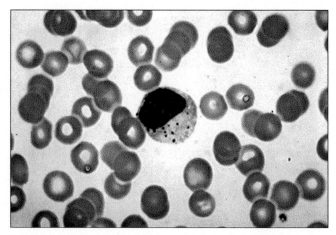

FIGURE 28.1 Large granular lymphocyte in a blood smear. This lymphocyte is significantly larger than small lymphocytes usually found in the peripheral blood. http://www.pathnet.medsch.ucla.edu/educ/lecture/pathrev/casestudy/case9/case9q.htm.

are large granular lymphocytes (Figure 28.1). NK lymphocytes are present constitutively and are activated by malignant or infected cells within hours. NK lymphocytes lack antigen-specific receptors such as those found on T and B lymphocytes and are considered part of the innate host defense system. As with other components of the innate immune system, NK lymphocytes fail to develop a memory response.

Most of the early investigations of NK lymphocytes focused on the cytotoxic killing of tumor cells. Ronald Herberman's group (1973) at the National Cancer Institute of the National Institutes of Health in Bethesda, Maryland, suggested that lymphocytes capable of killing tumor cells exist in healthy mice. These investigators injected mice with murine sarcoma virus (MSV) and identified the lymphocytes responsible for tumor-specific immunity. MSV induces localized sarcomas that, in some strains of mice (i.e., C57Bl/6N), regress within 3 weeks implying the development of an adaptive immune response. Herberman and colleagues removed lymphocytes from MSV-injected mice and incubated these lymphocytes with ⁵¹Cr-labeled sarcoma cells. The amount of radiolabel released into the tissue culture medium correlated with the amount of antitumor cytotoxicity present.

As anticipated, mice in which the tumor regressed developed significant levels of cytotoxic activity. Herberman's group characterized the lymphocytes responsible for this killing activity. They harvested lymphocytes from MSV-injected mice and treated them with antibodies specific for an antigen expressed on T lymphocytes (theta) or with antibodies against immunoglobulin (a B lymphocyte-specific marker). Treatment with antibodies to theta antigen in the presence of complement eliminated most of the cytotoxic activity while treatment with antibodies to immunoglobulin in the presence of complement failed to decrease killing of the sarcoma cells. These results showed that T lymphocytes were primarily responsible for the lytic activity.

Unexpectedly, Herberman and his colleagues discovered that lymphocytes from control, noninjected mice also possessed cytotoxic activity to the sarcoma cells. The amount of isotope released by tumor cells exposed to lymphocytes from control animals was significantly greater than that released spontaneously by the tumor cells. The cytotoxic lymphocytes from control mice proved insensitive to treatment with antitheta antibody indicating they were not T lymphocytes.

In 1975, Herberman's group tested lymphoid cells from several strains of nontumor-bearing mice for natural cytotoxicity against syngeneic and allogeneic tumor cells in a similar ^{51}Cr release assay (Herberman et al., 1975a,b). Control mice of all ages possessed lymphocytes that killed tumor cells; however, lymphocytes from mice between 5 and 8 weeks of age possessed the greatest level of natural cytotoxicity. Lymphocytes from all lymphoid organs as well as those from peripheral blood and peritoneal exudates served as killers in the assay. Even lymphocytes from athymic (nude) mice killed tumor cells reinforcing the previous observation that the cytotoxic cells were most likely not cytotoxic T lymphocytes.

Herberman and his coworkers further characterized cytotoxic lymphocytes from nude mice and concluded that they were not macrophages or T lymphocytes—they failed to express immunoglobulin on their surface, and they did not kill target cells coated with antibody. They proposed that this "natural cytotoxicity against mouse tumor cells is mediated by a unique subpopulation of lymphoid cells" that they termed N cells (Herberman et al., 1975b). These lymphocytes were subsequently renamed NK lymphocytes by Rolf Kiessling and colleagues.

Kiessling working in the Department of Tumor Biology of the Karolinska Institute in Stockholm, Sweden, with Hans Wigzell and Eva Klein injected mice with the Molony leukemia virus to induce tumors. These investigators radiolabeled tumor lines established from these mice and incubated them in vitro with lymphocytes from various lymphoid organs of nontumor-bearing mice (Kiessling et al., 1975a,b). One to 4 h later the investigators quantified the amount of radioisotope released into the culture medium and demonstrated the presence of natural cytotoxicity.

Utilizing protocols commonly used in the 1970s, Kiessling and colleagues characterized the cytotoxic cells. They treated the cells with antibody to the theta antigen plus complement to remove T lymphocytes, incubated them on plastic petri dishes to remove adherent cells (macrophages and dendritic cells), and filtered them through a column to which antibody to

immunoglobulin was bound to remove B lymphocytes. The lymphocytes recovered from these procedures killed the leukemic cells to the same extent as did the original population of lymphocytes. The authors concluded that these lymphocytes constituted a population of lymphocytes possessing natural cytotoxicity that they termed NK cells.

Erna Möller in 1965 identified a related type of cytotoxic activity in which lymphocytes kill target cells coated with antibodies (Chapter 26). The lymphocytes responsible for this activity develop in the absence of an intact thymus (Van Boxel et al., 1972) and were termed Killer (or K) cells to reflect their unique function. K lymphocytes lack most T and B lymphocyte markers but do express Fc receptors allowing them to bind antibody molecules. For several years debates persisted concerning the differences (or similarities) of NK and K cells. Most immunologists now agree that both natural cytotoxicity by NK lymphocytes and antibody-dependent cell-mediated cytotoxicity (ADCC) by K lymphocytes reflect the functioning of a single cell type. (Möller, 1965)

SELF–NON-SELF RECOGNITION BY NK LYMPHOCYTES

Cells of the host defense systems recognize foreignness using several different mechanisms. B lymphocytes express cell-surface immunoglobulin that possesses the same antigenic specificity as the antibody that B lymphocyte will eventually synthesize and secrete. T lymphocytes express TCRs that bind short peptides processed and presented by antigen-presenting cells. The receptors on both B and T lymphocytes derive from rearrangement and recombination of several genes during maturation of the cells (Chapter 18).

Macrophages and other phagocytic cells express a series of pattern recognition receptors (PRRs—Chapter 29) that are genetically coded. PRRs bind molecular patterns common to pathogens. This binding initiates phagocytosis and activates the cell leading to transcription of a variety of genes involved in inflammation.

NK lymphocytes fail to express TCRs, cell-surface immunoglobulin, or PRRs. The cells that serve as targets for NK activity express a variety of cell-surface molecules, none of which appear to be obvious targets for NK lymphocyte binding and activation. Between the early 1970s and late 1980s several different groups of scientists performed studies to determine the mechanism of recognition used by NK lymphocytes. Investigators designed experiments based on the model of cytotoxic T lymphocytes. These lymphocytes express antigen-specific TCR that recognize foreign antigen presented to them by cells expressing cell-surface molecules coded for by major histocompatibility complex (MHC) genes. However, since NK lymphocytes fail to express a TCR, other recognition mechanisms were sought.

In the late 1970s several groups of investigators reported that some lymphocytes treated with interferon (a cytokine secreted in response to stimuli including viral infection) become more efficient killers of tumor cells (Einhorn et al., 1978; Herberman et al., 1979; Trinchieri et al., 1978). Other immunologists xploited this information to determine how NK lymphocytes kill both allogeneic and syngeneic tumor cells (Carlson et al., 1980; Vanky et al., 1980).

Farkas Vanky and colleagues working in Eva Klein's laboratory at the Karolinska Institute in Stockholm, Sweden, harvested peripheral blood lymphocytes from tumor patients and tested them in an in vitro assay against autologous or allogeneic tumor biopsy cells. Patient lymphocytes killed their own tumor cells in 28% of the assays while these same lymphocytes killed allogeneic tumors in 5% of the assays. Patient lymphocytes treated with interferon maintained the level of killing of their own tumors; however, these lymphocytes killed allogeneic tumors in approximately 50% of the assays. These results suggest that interferon-induced lymphocytes preferentially lyse allogeneic targets rather than syngeneic targets. The authors concluded, inaccurately, that interferon treatment resulted in the polyclonal activation of those lymphocytes committed to recognizing foreign transplantation antigens.

In 1980, George Carlson and coworkers working at the University of Alberta in Edmonton, Canada, injected different strains of inbred mice with leukemia cells labeled with ^{3}H-thymidine. They used whole body gamma counting to detect tumor cell survival. Leukemia cells survived better in a syngeneic rather than an allogeneic environment. Carlson and colleagues initially postulated that tumors fail to survive in allogeneic mice due to the induction of an adaptive immune response to foreign histocompatibility antigens. However, they observed a decreased survival of tumors in allogeneic mice within 24h of cell injection arguing against the likelihood of an induced response. Allogeneic tumor cells also failed to survive in mice with congenital or induced deficiency of T lymphocytes. Neither circulating antibody nor macrophages could be implicated in the elimination of the leukemic cells in allogeneic mice. The authors therefore suggested this might be an example of NK lymphocyte activity.

Hans Wigzell and colleagues (Stern et al., 1980) working at the Karolinska Institute in Stockholm, Sweden, demonstrated that certain tumor cells could be killed by lymphocytes in an experimental model designed to preclude activation of cytotoxic T lymphocytes. Teratocarcinomas are germ cell cancers that fail to express antigens coded by genes in the MHC on their cell surfaces and therefore are not susceptible to killing by cytotoxic T lymphocytes. Wigzell and coworkers reported that mouse teratocarcinomas are highly susceptible to killing by NK lymphocytes. These cytotoxic lymphocytes are insensitive to an antibody to T lymphocytes and are not B lymphocytes or macrophages. Teratocarcinoma cells treated with retinoic acid differentiate to more mature cell types that express MHC molecules and become less sensitive to lysis by NK lymphocytes.

The Missing-Self Hypothesis

Stern's results prompted Klas Kärre of the Karolinska Institute, Stockholm, Sweden, to develop the missing-self hypothesis in 1985. This hypothesis states that NK lymphocytes are most efficient in killing targets that have reduced or absent expression of self-MHC-coded gene products on their cell surface (Kärre, 1985; Kärre et al., 1986; Ljunggren and Kärre, 1990).

Studies using a B lymphocyte cell line (Daudi) derived from a patient with Burkitt lymphoma supported the missing-self hypothesis. Daudi cells are used as a common target for studies on NK lymphocyte activity. Due to a mutation in the gene coding for the β2-microglobulin polypeptide, these lymphoma cells fail to express cell-surface HLA class I molecules (HLA refers to the human histocompatibility molecules coded by the MHC). While β2-microglobulin is not coded for by genes in the MHC, the polypeptide is required for the expression of all class I MHC molecules.

Anne Quillet and her colleagues at research institutes in France and the Netherlands (1988) induced Daudi cells to express class I HLA molecules by transfecting these cells with the gene coding for the β2-microglobulin polypeptide. These transfected cells resisted killing by NK lymphocytes thus suggesting that the expression of class I MHC-coded molecules by a cell protects it against NK lymphocyte-mediated lysis. While supporting the missing-self hypothesis, these results failed to identify the target molecule responsible for NK lymphocyte activation.

Malignant transformation as well as viral infection often downregulate the genes coding for class I MHC molecules. Investigators have cited this observation as a mechanism by which virally infected and malignant cells escape elimination by cytotoxic T lymphocytes since MHC class I molecules present antigens to CD8^{+} cytotoxic T lymphocytes. As a part of the innate host defenses, NK lymphocytes therefore must play a crucial role in the initial response to viral infections and to developing malignancies. NK lymphocytes express a variety of cell-surface receptors that bind to ligands on malignant or virally infected cells. The binding of these receptors to their ligands transmits either positive (stimulatory) or negative (inhibitory) signals to the NK lymphocyte. The balance of these signals determines whether or not the lymphocyte kills the target cell (Yonehara et al., 1989).

Stimulatory Receptors on NK Lymphocytes

NK lymphocytes are activated by cells that are damaged as a result of infection, malignant transformation, or stress. While the absence of HLA class I molecules on potential NK lymphocyte targets may be sufficient to unleash the lytic activity of these cells, NK lymphocytes express additional cell-surface receptors that bind ligands on damaged cells that activate the lytic response. These stimulatory receptors are not as specific as the receptors expressed by B and T lymphocytes.

The search for stimulatory receptors involved two different strategies:

- identification of genes that are preferentially expressed in NK lymphocytes using differential hybridization and cDNA subtraction methodology, and
- identification of NK lymphocyte-specific cell-surface molecules by monoclonal antibodies.

Jeffrey Houchins and colleagues, working with Fritz Bach at the University of Minnesota in Minneapolis, employed the first strategy and focused on genes that encode membrane-bound proteins. In 1990, they isolated a cDNA clone from NK lymphocytes. This group used this cDNA (NKG2) to probe a DNA library prepared from an NK lymphocyte clone (Houchins et al., 1991). This process identified four transcripts (NKG2-A, NKG2-B, NKG2-C, and NKG2-D) each of which was sequenced. The investigators inferred the amino acid sequence for each transcript. While the peptides coded by NKG-2A and NKG-2B appear to be alternatively spliced products of the same gene, peptides coded by NKG-2C and NKG-2D represent products of two distinct genes. The authors conclude "that the NKG2 peptides are members of a supergene family characterized by the presence of a C-type animal lectin domain" with "transmembrane signaling capability."

Subsequent investigation demonstrated that NKG2-D is an NK lymphocyte-activating receptor. NKG2-D binds to stress-induced glycoproteins termed MIC-A (MHC class I chain-related gene A) and MIC-B. MIC-A and MIC-B are coded by genes in the MHC and are related to the alpha chains of class I histocompatibility molecules, but they do not bind peptides or β2-microglobulin. In 1999, Stefan Bauer collaborated with scientists at the Fred Hutchinson Cancer Research Institute in Seattle, Washington, and DNAX Research Institute in Palo Alto, California, to identify NKG2-D as the receptor for MIC-A. They further demonstrated that cells expressing NKG2-D, including NK lymphocytes and CD8+ cytotoxic T lymphocytes, could be stimulated by ligation of the NKG2-D receptor thus

concluding that their "results define an activating immunoreceptor-MHC ligand interaction that may promote antitumor NK and T cell responses."

Simona Sivori and colleagues at the University of Genoa in Italy used the second strategy to identify several additional NK lymphocyte-activating receptors. They immunized mice with human NK lymphocytes (CD3-, CD16+, CD56+), harvested their spleens, and constructed hybridomas secreting monoclonal antibodies specific for the NK lymphocytes (Pessino et al., 1998; Sivori et al., 1997). Sivori and her colleagues selected antibodies that enhanced the natural killing activity of NK lymphocyte clones. In this manner they identified an NK lymphocyte-specific surface protein with a molecular weight of 46 kDa. These researchers detected NKp46 on all NK lymphocytes, both activated and resting, but not on other cell types. They cross-linked NKp46 by treatment with the monoclonal antibody and observed NK lymphocyte activation as measured by Ca++ uptake, cytokine production, and induction of cytotoxicity.

Investigators identified two additional activating receptors, NKp30 and NKp44, using monoclonal antibodies to molecules expressed on NK lymphocytes (Pende et al., 1999; Vitale et al., 1998). All three of these receptors bind forms of heparin sulfate, a polysaccharide expressed on many cell types including tumor cells.

Inhibitory Receptors on NK Lymphocytes

Based on the missing-self hypothesis, researchers postulated that inhibitory receptors expressed by NK lymphocytes bind to MHC-coded class I molecules. Studies proved the validity of this postulate, however the receptors on NK lymphocytes from humans and mice are different; human NK lymphocytes express a series of killer-cell immunoglobulin-like receptors while mouse receptors are lectin-like and are termed Ly-49. When these receptors bind class I MHC molecules, they inhibit the activation of the NK lymphocytes rather than down-regulating an already activated killer.

Franz Karlhofer, Randall Ribaudo, and Wayne Yokoyama working at the University of California, San Francisco and the National Institutes of Health, Bethesda, Maryland, identified a class I binding molecule on the surface of mouse NK lymphocytes in 1992. Karlhofer and colleagues separated NK lymphocytes from C57Bl/6 mice (H-2b) into two populations based on expression of the Ly-49 cell-surface molecule. They activated these two populations with IL-2 and used them in an in vitro cytotoxicity assay with a series of 51Cr-labeled allogeneic mouse cell lines. NK lymphocytes that express Ly-49 fail to lyse allogeneic target cells expressing H-2d or H-2k while NK lymphocytes that are Ly-49-negative kill targets expressing these histocompatibility antigens. Transfection of a susceptible tumor target with the gene for H-2D^d rendered the cell line resistant to lysis by Ly-49$^+$ lymphocytes. Monoclonal antibodies against either Ly-49 or against the α-chain of the H-2D^d molecule inhibited the interaction between NK lymphocytes and transfected tumor cells. Based on these data, the authors speculated that "NK cells may possess inhibitory receptors that specifically recognize MHC class I antigens."

In 1993, Alessandro Moretta and collaborators at the Universities of Genoa and Turin in Italy identified inhibitory receptors on human NK lymphocytes. These investigators developed monoclonal antibodies specific for a 58 kDa molecule (p58) expressed on subsets of NK lymphocytes. Clones of NK lymphocytes that express p58 recognize an MHC class I-coded molecule called Cw3. These NK lymphocytes kill P815 target cells (a mouse mastocytoma tumor line that does not express the Cw3 molecule). Moretta and colleagues transfected P815 target cells with the gene coding for Cw3; these transfected cells proved resistant to NK-mediated killing. Addition of F(ab')$_2$ fragments of monoclonal antibodies specific for p58 to cultures of NK lymphocytes and P815 targets expressing Cw3 resulted in target cell death (Moretta et al., 2001).

These results suggest that HLA class I molecules like Cw3 bind the p58 molecule on NK lymphocytes and inhibit activation of the NK lymphocytes. Additional studies demonstrated that soluble p58 binds HLA class I molecules. Studies using monoclonal antibodies to a second NK-specific molecule, p70, produced similar results (Litwin et al., 1994).

Molecular identification of the receptors responsible for inhibiting NK lymphocyte activity revealed the existence of several gene families coding inhibitory receptors. These receptors all bind various HLA class I molecules, the expression of which on nonmalignant cells guards against the killing of healthy, somatic cells.

Functions of NK Lymphocytes

NK lymphocytes protect the mammalian host from destruction by intracellular pathogens, particularly viruses, and from the establishment of tumors. NK lymphocytes possess the same killing mechanisms as do CD8$^+$ cytotoxic T lymphocytes. As described in Chapter 27, perforin as well as serine proteases (granzymes) are present in the cytoplasmic granules of both cytotoxic T lymphocytes and NK lymphocytes. When NK lymphocytes bind to their target, granules fuse with the cell surface, and the contents are released into the intracellular space. Perforin polymerizes and forms a transmembrane pore through which granzymes enter and induce apoptotic death pathways (reviewed by Voskoboinik et al., 2010).

A second mechanism by which both NK cells and cytotoxic T lymphocytes induce death in susceptible cells is through interaction between Fas (CD95) on target cells and Fas ligand (CD178) on NK lymphocytes. Virtually every somatic cell expresses Fas, a death receptor that, when bound, activates the caspase pathway leading to DNA damage and cell death. Fas ligand is not normally expressed on NK lymphocytes but is induced during activation by IFNγ and TNF-α, two cytokines secreted by several cells during the early phases of the inflammatory response.

NKT LYMPHOCYTES

In 1987, Ralph Budd and collaborators in Lausanne, Switzerland, described a population of phenotypically immature T lymphocytes in mice that express low levels of surface TCR. These lymphocytes are CD4-negative and CD8-negative. Simultaneously B.J. Fowlkes and her colleagues at the National Institutes of Health in Bethesda, Maryland, defined a similar lymphocyte population that shares characteristics of both NK lymphocytes and cytotoxic T lymphocytes and are today called NKT lymphocytes.

NKT lymphocytes mature in the thymus where the genes coding for the TCR normally undergo rearrangement. The TCRs expressed by NKT lymphocytes represent a small fraction of the total repertoire available to T lymphocytes. Fowlkes and coworkers in 1987 reported that NKT lymphocytes predominately express the products of a single V$_β$ gene family—V$_β$8. In 1992, Hisashi Arase and colleagues at the Hokkaido University in Sapporo, Japan, collaborating with Robert Good at the University of South Florida St. Petersburg, described a population of NKT lymphocytes that express an NK-specific cell-surface molecule (NK1.1) as well as a TCR. When the TCR β-chain variable region was analyzed, most of these lymphocytes expressed V regions coded for by the V$_β$7 or V$_β$8.2 genes.

Researchers evaluated the α-chain of the TCR on NKT lymphocytes and reached a similar conclusion. Olivier Lantz and Albert Bendelac working at the National Institutes of Health in Bethesda, Maryland, demonstrated in 1994 that mouse NKT lymphocytes express TCRs that have amino acid sequences coded for by the V$_α$14 gene while human NKT lymphocytes express TCRs with amino acid sequences coded for by the V$_α$24 gene, a homolog of the mouse V$_α$14.

The alpha chain of the TCR of NKT lymphocytes in both mice and humans also uses a single J region: J$_α$281 in mice and J$_α$Q in humans. These alpha chains are paired with V$_β$8, V$_β$7, or V$_β$2 chains in mice and with V$_β$11 chains in humans. Relying on the knowledge that CD4$^+$ T lymphocytes bind peptides presented by molecules coded for by MHC class II genes and that CD8$^+$ T lymphocytes recognize peptides presented by molecules coded for by MHC class I genes, investigators searched for similar NKT ligands.

Several investigators demonstrated that NKT lymphocytes develop in mice devoid of class I or class II molecules suggesting that binding of MHC-coded molecules by NKT lymphocytes is not necessary for cell maturation. In 1995, Albert Bendelac and colleagues working at Princeton University in New Jersey and the National Institute of Allergy and Infectious Diseases showed that mouse NKT lymphocytes recognize CD1 molecules. CD1 has been assigned by the Human Leukocyte Differentiation Antigens Workshops to a series of glycoproteins (CD1a, b, c, d, e) expressed on antigen-presenting cells (dendritic cells, B lymphocytes, monocytes) as well as on Langerhans cells, cortical thymocytes, and intestinal epithelia cells. Although not coded directly by MHC genes, CD1 molecules are structurally related to molecules coded for by MHC class I genes.

During the following 2 years several investigators searched for peptides that might associate with CD1 molecules. These studies were based on the assumption that CD1 on antigen-presenting cells functioned to present antigens to NKT lymphocytes similar to the way class I or class II molecules present antigens to T lymphocytes. In 1997 a group of investigators led by Masuru Taniguchi at Chiba University in Japan identified the ligand for the NKT TCR as a glycosylceramide (Kawano et al., 1997). Taniguchi and colleagues demonstrated that NKT lymphocytes treated with glycosylceramide proliferated and that this proliferative response could be abrogated by treating the lymphocytes with monoclonal antibodies specific for either $V_\beta 8$ or CD1d.

NKT lymphocytes provide an evolutionary bridge between the innate host defense mechanisms and the adaptive immune response. NKT lymphocytes recognize glycolipids on cellular targets, lyse these targets, and react rapidly by the synthesis and secretion of cytokines including IL-4, a critical cytokine in the activation of CD4+, T_H2 lymphocytes that induce B lymphocytes to switch to IgE antibody synthesis. IgE antibody is essential in protecting mammals against infection by parasites (MacDonald, 2007).

CONCLUSION

Several different populations of lymphocytes function in the innate host defense mechanisms and the adaptive immune responses. In the adaptive immune system, B lymphocytes synthesize and secrete antibodies that bind to extracellular pathogens while CD8+ cytotoxic T lymphocytes bind to and eliminate cells infected with intracellular pathogens. The innate host defenses also possess lymphocytes with cytotoxic

potential—these include NK lymphocytes and NKT lymphocytes that express a conserved TCR.

NK lymphocytes kill malignantly transformed somatic cells and protect the host from the establishment of tumors. They also participate in some effector functions that involve products of the adaptive immune system. NK lymphocytes expressing Fc receptors bind antibody-coated targets and focus their cytotoxic mechanisms. This helps the host defenses eliminate pathogens through a process termed ADCC. NK lymphocytes also recognize potential targets in the absence of antibody—recognition requires that the targets fail to express self-histocompatibility molecules. NK lymphocytes express both stimulatory and inhibitory receptors and function using the same cytotoxic effectors as cytotoxic T lymphocytes.

NKT lymphocytes, identified in the 1980s, protect the individual against potential pathogens by mechanisms that remain under investigation. Among the possibilities that have been proposed, NKT lymphocytes

- provide protection against bacteria including *Sphingomonas* and *Ehrlichia* that express glycolipids on their surface: mice congenitally devoid of NKT lymphocytes fail to develop a response to these microbes;
- regulate the differential maturation of the T_H2 subpopulation of CD4+ T lymphocytes through rapid secretion of cytokines, especially IL-4, resulting in synthesis and secretion of IgE antibodies;
- eliminate malignantly transformed cells that express glycolipids on their surface; and
- contribute to microbial-induced pathology (septic shock) due to release of inflammatory cytokines including TNF-α.

References

Arase, H., Arase, N., Ogasawara, K., Good, R.A., Onoé, K., 1992. An NK1.1+ CD4+8- single-positive thymocyte subpopulation that expresses a highly skewed T-cell antigen receptor V_β family. Proc. Nat. Acad. Sci. U.S.A 89, 6506–6510.

Bauer, S., Groh, V., Wu, J., Steinle, A., Phillips, J.H., Lanier, L.L., Spies, T., 1999. Activation of NK cells and T cells by NKG2D, a receptor for stress-inducible MICA. Science 285, 727–729.

Bendelac, A., Lantz, O., Quimby, M.E., Yewdell, J.W., Bennink, J.R., Brutkiewicz, R.R., 1995. CD1 recognition by mouse NK1+ T lymphocytes. Science 268, 863–865.

Budd, R.C., Miescher, G.C., Howe, R.C., Lees, R.K., Bron, C., MacDonald, H.R., 1987. Developmentally regulated expression of T cell receptor beta chain variable domains in immature thymocytes. J. Exp. Med. 166, 577–582.

Carlson, G.A., Melnychuk, D., Meeker, M.J., 1980. H-2 associated resistance to leukaemia transplantation: natural killing in vivo. Int. J. Cancer 25, 111–122.

Einhorn, S., Blomgren, H., Strander, H., 1978. Interferon and spontaneous cytotoxicity in man. I. Enhancement of the spontaneous cytotoxicity of peripheral lymphocytes by human leukocyte interferon. Int. J. Cancer 22, 405–412.

Fowlkes, B.J., Kruisbeek, A.M., Ton-That, H., Weston, M.A., Coligan, J.E., Schwartz, R.H., Pardoll, D.M., 1987. A novel population of T-cell receptor alpha beta-bearing thymocytes which predominately express a single V beta gene family. Nature 329, 251–254.

Hellström, I., Hellström, K.E., Pierce, G.E., Bill, A.H., 1968. Demonstration of cell-bound and humoral immunity against neuroblastoma cells. Proc. Nat. Acad. Sci. U.S.A 60, 1231–1238.

Herberman, R.B., Gaylord, C.E., 1973. Conference and workshop of cellular immune reactions to human tumor-associated antigens. Nat. Cancer Inst. Monogr. 37, 221.

Herberman, R.B., Nunn, M.E., Lavrin, D.H., 1975a. Natural cytotoxic reactivity of mouse lymphoid cells against syngeneic and allogeneic tumors. I. Distribution of reactivity and specificity. Int. J. Cancer 16, 216–229.

Herberman, R.B., Nunn, M.E., Holden, H.T., Lavrin, D.H., 1975b. Natural cytotoxic reactivity of mouse lymphoid cells against syngeneic and allogeneic tumors. II. Characterization of effector cells. Int. J. Cancer 16, 230–239.

Herberman, R.B., Nunn, M.E., Lavrin, D.H., Asofsky, R., 1973. Effect of antibody to θ antigen on cell-mediated immunity induced in syngeneic mice by murine sarcoma virus. J. Nat. Cancer Inst. 51, 1509–1512.

Herberman, R.B., Ortaldo, J.R., Bonnard, G.D., 1979. Augmentation by interferon of human natural and antibody-dependent cell-mediated cytotoxicity. Nature 277, 221–223.

Houchins, J.P., Yabe, T., McSherry, C., Bach, F., 1991. DNA sequence analysis of NKG2, a family of related cDNA clones encoding type II integral membrane proteins on human natural killer cells. J. Exp. Med. 173, 1017–1020.

Houchins, J.P., Yabe, T., McSherry, C., Miyokawa, N., Bach, F.H., 1990. Isolation and characterization of NK cell and NK/T cell-specific cDNA clones. J. Mol. Cell. Immunol. 4, 295–304.

Karlhofer, F.M., Ribaudo, R.K., Yokoyama, W.M., 1992. MHC class I alloantigen specificity of Ly-49+ IL-2 activated natural killer cells. Nature 358, 66–70.

Kärre, K., 1985. Role of target histocompatibility antigens in regulation of natural killer activity: a reevaluation and a hypothesis. In: Herberman, R. (Ed.), Mechanisms of Cytotoxicity by Natural Killer Cells, Academic Press, New York, pp. 81–92.

Kärre, K., Ljunggren, H.G., Piontek, G., Kiessling, R., 1986. Selective rejection of H-2-deficient lymphoma variants suggest alternative immune defence strategy. Nature 319, 675–678.

Kawano, T., Cui, J., Koezuka, Y., Toura, I., Kaneko, Y., Motoki, K., Ueno, H., Nakagawa, R., Sato, H., Kondo, E., Koseki, H., Taniguchi, M., 1997. CD1d-restricted and TCR-mediated activation of Vα14 NKT cells by glycosylceramides. Science 278, 1626–1629.

Kiessling, R., Klein, E., Wigzell, H., 1975a. "Natural" killer cells in the mouse. I. Cytotoxic cells with specificity for mouse Moloney leukemia cells. Specificity and distribution according to genotype. Eur. J. Immunol. 5, 112–117.

Kiessling, R., Klein, E., Pross, H., Wigzell, H., 1975b. "Natural" killer cells in the mouse. II. Cytotoxic cells with specificity for mouse Moloney leukemia cells. Characteristics of the killer cell. Eur. J. Immunol. 5, 117–121.

Lantz, O., Bendelac, A., 1994. An invariant T cell receptor α chain is used by a unique subset of major histocompatibility class I-specific CD4+ and CD4-8- T cells in mice and humans. J. Exp. Med. 180, 1097–1106.

Litwin, V., Gumperz, J., Parham, P., Phillips, J.H., Lanier, L.L., 1994. NKB1: a natural killer cell receptor involved in the recognition of polymorphic HLA-B molecules. J. Exp. Med. 180, 537–543.

Ljunggren, H.-G., Kärre, K., 1990. In search of the "missing-self": MHC molecules and NK cell recognition. Immunol. Today 11, 237–244.

MacDonald, H.R., 2007. NKT cells: in the beginning. Eur. J. Immunol. 37, S111–S115.

Möller, E., 1965. Contact-induced cytotoxicity by lymphoid cells containing foreign iso-antigens. Science 147, 873–874 & 879.

Moretta, A., Bottino, C., Vitale, M., Pende, D., Cantoni, C., Mingari, M.C., Biassoni, R., Moretta, L., 2001. Activating receptors and coreceptors involved in human natural killer cell-mediated cytolysis. Annu. Rev. Immunol. 19, 197–223.

Moretta, A., Vitale, M., Bottino, C., Orengo, A.M., Morelli, L., Augugliaro, R., Barbaresi, M., Ciccone, E., Moretta, L., 1993. P58 molecules as putative receptors for major histocompatibility complex (MHC) class I molecules in human natural killer (NK) cells. Anti-p58 antibodies reconstitute lysis of MHC class I-protected cells in NK clones displaying different specificities. J. Exp. Med. 178, 597–604.

Oldham, R.K., 1983. Natural killer cells: artifact to reality: an odyssey in biology. Cancer Metast. 2, 323–336.

Pende, D., Parolina, S., Pessino, A., Sivori, S., Augugliaro, R., Morelli, L., Marcenaro, E., Accame, L., Malaspina, A., Biassoni, R., Bottino, C., Moretta, L., Moretta, A., 1999. Identification and molecular characterization of NKp30, a novel triggering receptor involved in natural cytotoxicity mediated by human natural killer cells. J. Exp. Med. 190, 1505–1516.

Pessino, A., Sivori, S., Bottino, C., Malaspina, A., Morelli, L., Moretta, L., Biassoni, R., Moretta, A., 1998. Molecular cloning of NKp46: a novel member of the immunoglobulin superfamily involved in triggering of natural cytotoxicity. J. Exp. Med. 188, 953–960.

Quillet, A., Presse, F., Marchiol-Fournigault, C., Harel-Bellan, A., Benbunan, M., Ploegn, H., Fradelizi, D., 1988. Increased resistance to non-MHC-restricted cytotoxicity related to HLA A, B expression. Direct demonstration using β2-microglobulin transfected Daudi cells. J. Immunol. 141, 17–20.

Rosenberg, E.B., Herberman, R.B., Levine, P.H., Halterman, R.H., McCoy, J.L., Wunderlich, J.R., 1972. Lymphocyte cytotoxicity reactions to leukemia-associated antigens in identical twins. Int. J. Cancer 9, 648–658.

Sivori, S., Vitale, M., Morelli, L., Sanseverino, L., Auguliaro, R., Bottino, C., Moretta, L., Moretta, A., 1997. p46, a novel natural killer cell-specific surface molecule which mediated cell activation. J. Exp. Med. 186, 1129–1136.

Stern, P., Gidlund, M., Örn, A., Wigzell, H., 1980. Natural killer cells mediate lysis of embryonal carcinoma cells lacking MHC. Nature 285, 341–342.

Trinchieri, G., Santoli, D., Koprowski, H., 1978. Spontaneous cell-mediated cytotoxicity in humans: role of interferon and immunoglobulin. J. Immunol. 120, 1849–1855.

Van Boxel, J.A., Stobo, J.D., Paul, W.E., Green, I., 1972. Antibody-dependent lymphoid cell-mediated cytotoxicity: no requirement for thymus-derived lymphocytes. Science 175, 194–196.

Vanky, F.T., Argov, S.A., Einhorn, S.A., Klein, E., 1980. Role of alloantigens in natural killing. Allogeneic but not autologous tumor biopsy cells are sensitive for interferon-induced cytotoxicity of human blood lymphocytes. J. Exp. Med. 151, 1151–1165.

Vitale, M., Bottino, C., Sivori, S., Sanseverino, L., Casticoni, R., Marcenaro, E., Augugliaro, R., Moretta, L., Moretta, A., 1998. NKp44, a novel triggering surface molecule specifically expressed by activated natural killer cells, is involved in non-major histocompatibility complex-restricted tumor cell lysis. J. Exp. Med. 187, 2065–2072.

Voskoboinik, I., Dunstone, M.A., Baran, K., Whisstock, J.C., Trapani, J.A., 2010. Perforin: structure, function and role in human immunopathology. Immunol. Rev. 235, 35–54.

Yonehara, S., Ishii, A., Yonehara, M., 1989. A cell-killing monoclonal antibody (anti-Fas) to a cell surface antigen co-downregulated with the receptor of tumor necrosis factor. J. Exp. Med. 169, 1747–1756.

TIME LINE

1965	Erna Möller serendipitously discovers the phenomenon of antibody-dependent cell-mediated cytotoxicity
1968	Ingegerd Hellström and colleagues describe cytotoxic lymphocytes in the peripheral blood of mothers whose children present with neuroblastoma
1972	Conference held at the National Cancer Institute to evaluate the research identifying natural killer (NK) lymphocytes
1973	Ronald Herberman and colleagues describe NK lymphocytes in mice
1975	Rolf Kiessing and colleagues coin the term natural killer cells
1980	Hans Wigzell's group demonstrates that NK lymphocytes preferentially lyse tumor cells that fail to express MHC-coded class I molecules
1985	Klas Kärre postulates the missing-self hypothesis to explain how NK lymphocytes recognize targets
1987	Ralph Budd and colleagues and B.J. Fowlkes and coworkers independently identify a population of CD4-, CD8- lymphocytes that express characteristics of both NK and T lymphocytes (NKT lymphocytes)
1987	B.J. Fowlkes and coworkers report that double negative lymphocytes express a TCR using a single Vβ region
1988	Anne Quillet and collaborators provide evidence for the missing-self hypothesis
1990	Jeffrey Houchins and collaborators identify NKG2, a gene coding for transmembrane molecules expressed in NK cells involved in transmitting a stimulatory signal
1992	Franz Karlhofer and colleagues identify Ly-49 as an inhibitory receptor on NK lymphocytes
1992	Wayne Yokoyama and coworkers identify an inhibitor molecule expressed by mouse NK lymphocytes that binds a class I molecule
1993	Alessandro Moretta and collaborators identify inhibitory receptors on human NK lymphocytes
1994	Olivier Lantz and Albert Bendelac show that mouse and human NKT lymphocytes express relatively invariant TCRs
1995	Albert Bendelac and collaborators demonstrate that mouse NKT lymphocytes recognize CD1 molecules on antigen-presenting cells
1997	Simona Sivora and colleagues develop monoclonal antibodies specific for NK lymphocytes and describe NK-activating receptors
1997	Masuru Taniguchi and coworkers identify glycosylceramide as the ligand for CD1 molecules

Role of Dendritic Cells in the Adaptive Immune Response

INTRODUCTION

Dendritic cells (DCs) are one of the antigen-presenting cells (APCs) that capture antigen, engulf and process it, and present it to lymphocytes to induce an adaptive immune response. All APCs (macrophages, B lymphocytes, and DCs) express both major histocompatibility complex (MHC)-coded class I and class II molecules as well as costimulatory molecules such as CD80/86. Of the three APCs, DCs are unique since they alone activate resting, naïve T lymphocytes.

DCs derive from hematopoietic stem cells in the bone marrow. Investigators have identified DCs that differentiate from both lymphoid and myeloid precursors. Lymphoid precursors generate plasmacytoid DCs, while myeloid precursors give rise to myeloid DCs. In this chapter, the focus will be on myeloid DCs.

DCs are found in all lymphoid and many nonlymphoid organs of the body including the skin (where they are called Langerhans cells, LCs) and the gastrointestinal and respiratory tracks. Immature DCs are present in the peripheral blood. In nonlymphoid organs, DCs interact with antigen and transport it to local lymph nodes or spleen, where the processed antigen activates the adaptive immune response.

The history of the discovery and characterization of DCs covers almost 150 years. As a medical student at the Universities of Jena and Berlin, Paul Langerhans (1847–1888) first described DCs in human skin in 1868. Langerhans relied on newly developed histological stains to study the innervation of the skin. He stained sections of skin with gold chloride and visualized "stellate corpuscles" that appeared similar to cells of the central nervous system. Langerhans erroneously assumed the cells to be part of the nervous system. These skin DCs were subsequently named LCs. During the ensuing 100 years, the function of LCs was unknown; in fact in the 1974 edition of Ham's *Histology*, the author concludes "Their function and why they should have an association with stratified squamous epithelium, present problems. They are probably macrophages." Immunologists now recognize LCs as one of the APCs that perform a critical function in protecting skin from potential pathogens.

Langerhans made other important discoveries during his career. He described the groups of cells in the pancreas that also bear his name, the islets of Langerhans. The function of the cells in these islets was not known during Langerhans' life however the cells are now recognized as the source of insulin in the body and the target of the autoimmune response in type 1 diabetes.

A Historical Perspective on Evidence-Based Immunology
http://dx.doi.org/10.1016/B978-0-12-398381-7.00029-0

253

DENDRITIC CELLS IN THE ADAPTIVE IMMUNE SYSTEM

The discovery of DCs and their role in the adaptive immune system stemmed from a collaboration between Ralph Steinman and Zanvil Cohn that started in the late 1960s and continued for over 20 years. In 1969, Steinman (1943–2011) joined the Cohn laboratory at the Rockefeller University in New York as a postdoctoral fellow. Steinman, who received his MD degree from Harvard, noted in a 2012 autobiographical sketch that the following question stimulated his research: "How does the body decide to make an immune response, especially a cell-mediated one, when antigen enters the body. Or…how is Burnet's selection of T cell clones initiated?"

In 1969, immunologists knew that optimal antibody production required collaboration between B and T lymphocytes (Chapter 13). They also knew that a third cell type, characterized as a plastic adherent cell, was necessary to initiate an antibody response in vitro (Mosier, 1967; Chapter 14). Information about the mechanisms responsible for these cell interactions including MHC restriction of antigen presentation, costimulatory molecules, and the identity of cytokines involved in cell-to-cell communication remained undiscovered.

In 1973, Steinman and Cohn cultured single-cell suspensions of mouse lymphoid organs including spleen, lymph nodes, and Peyer's patches on plastic petri dishes or glass cover slips. They observed several different cell types that adhered to these surfaces after 60 min including macrophages, granulocytes, and lymphocytes. They also noted a large stellate cell present in small numbers for which they proposed the term dendritic cells (DCs). DCs possess a large nucleus and one or two nucleoli and comprise between 0.1% and 1.6% of the total nucleated cells in mouse lymphoid organs. The cytoplasm contains numerous mitochondria and is arranged in dendrite-like processes that move as if sampling the environment. Steinman and Cohn conclude that DCs are unlike macrophages since DCs "do not appear to engage in active endocytosis." Figure 29.1 depicts DCs viewed by phase contrast microscopy.

During the next 6 years, Steinman and Cohn along with other collaborators published a series of papers describing the function of DCs in vitro and in vivo, methods for identification and purification of DCs, and methods for maintaining the cells in tissue culture (Steinman and Cohn, 1974; Steinman et al., 1974; Steinman et al., 1975; Steinman et al., 1979). Steinman, who spent his entire career at Rockefeller University, continued to study DCs until his death, which occurred 3 days prior to the announcement that he had received one-half of the 2011 Nobel Prize in Physiology or Medicine for "his discovery of the dendritic cell and its role in adaptive immunity."

CHARACTERIZATION OF DENDRITIC CELLS

In 1974, Steinman and Cohn studied DCs in vitro and showed that they differ significantly from other cells in peripheral lymphoid tissue, particularly macrophages. They centrifuged single-cell suspensions of lymphoid organs in bovine serum albumin, a method that separates cells based on cell density. Most DCs remained suspended at the surface of the centrifuge tube, where they were enriched 7–20-fold. By contrast macrophages occurred at the surface and in the pellet.

Steinman and Cohn performed assays for endocytic activity on adherent cell populations. The investigators exposed the cells to a variety of substances including horse radish peroxidase (HRP), immune complexes containing HRP and antibody to HRP, sheep erythrocytes (SRBC) bound with antibodies to SRBC, polystyrene particles, and heat-killed *Staphylococcus albus*. Macrophages in these preparations served as a positive control since they are known to actively endocytose various substances. Greater than 90% of macrophages contained the test markers while fewer than 5% of DCs internalized any of them. These studies confirmed and extended previous observations that DCs failed to actively endocytose foreign particles even when specific antibodies are bound to the particles.

Steinman and Cohn investigated the expression of several DC cell surface molecules using antibodies known to bind to lymphocytes and macrophages. DCs express molecules coded by genes in the MHC (both class I and class II) but failed to react with antibodies to a T lymphocyte antigen or to antibodies to immunoglobulin heavy or light chains. DCs stained weakly with an antibody that detected more than 95% of macrophages in the same preparations.

Spleen cells injected into lethally irradiated, syngeneic mice rescue these mice and repopulate the peripheral blood and lymphoid tissue with mature erythroid, lymphoid, and myeloid cell lines. Based on morphology, Steinman and Cohn speculated that DCs might be these primitive stem cells. They injected spleen cells devoid of DCs by adherence on glass into lethally irradiated mice. These preparations of DC-depleted spleen cells reconstituted the treated mice as efficiently as did control spleens indicating that in fact, DCs are not stem cells.

Other investigators proposed that DCs bind antigen or antigen–antibody complexes during an immune response. Steinman and Cohn removed spleens from unimmunized mice or at various times following one or two injections of SRBC. DCs from these spleens failed to bind SRBC or SRBC coated with specific antibody although macrophages from these same animals both bound and internalized antigen or antibody–antigen complexes.

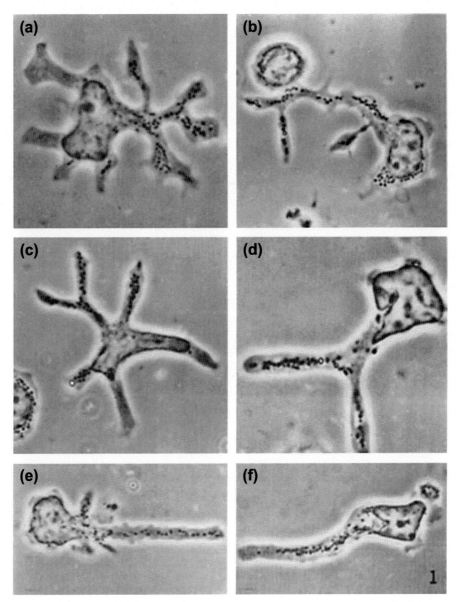

FIGURE 29.1   Phase contrast photographs of stellate-shaped (dendritic) cells from mouse spleen (a–d), lymph node (e), and Peyer's patches (f). *From Steinman and Cohn (1973).*

In summarizing these results, Steinman and Cohn argue that DCs are morphologically and functionally distinct from other cell types present in the mouse spleen. Steinman and colleagues subsequently described the characteristics of DCs in vivo that differentiate them from lymphocytes and from monocytes/macrophages including their ontogeny, their sensitivity to steroids and irradiation, their kinetics and turnover, and their response to antigen stimulation (Steinman et al., 1974).

Mice treated with whole-body irradiation showed a dramatic decrease in the number of DCs but not macrophages that could be recovered from their spleens. Steinman and colleagues reconstituted lethally irradiated mice with bone marrow or spleen cells from syngeneic mice or from F_1 donors. Cells from both sources reconstituted the lymphoid organs of the recipients including DCs. The DCs in the reconstituted animals expressed the histocompatibility molecules of the donor animal.

Thymus cells failed to reconstitute DCs in irradiated mice although spleen cells devoid of DCs (by adherence to glass) did reconstitute the DC population. The investigators concluded that DCs derived from a precursor found in glass nonadherent spleen and bone marrow but absent in thymus. This precursor is morphologically different from the DC itself.

Steinman and his coworkers measured the proliferation of DCs both in vivo and in vitro. They treated cultures of DCs with 3H-thymidine. Simultaneously they injected mice with a dose of ^{3}H-thymidine followed by an infusion of nonlabeled thymidine. Both intravenous and intraperitoneal injection labeled a small proportion (1.5–2.5%) of DCs in the first hour. This confirmed their in vitro findings. When ^{3}H-thymidine was continuously present in vivo, approximately 10% of splenic DCs turned over every 24 h. This does not reflect an increase in the total number of DCs but a replacement of unlabeled DCs with newly formed cells. Companion studies in mice immunized with SRBC as an antigen revealed only a modest increase in the total number of DCs. The investigators concluded that these data "further distinguish dendritic cells as a novel cell type, distinct from mononuclear phagocytes and lymphocytes."

Steinman and coworkers presented additional studies that demonstrated that DCs are a unique cell type present in small numbers in splenic white pulp (Steinman et al., 1975). They maintain their morphology during purification and in short-term tissue culture, and they express both cell surface molecules coded by both class I and class II MHC genes (Steinman et al., 1979).

FUNCTIONAL CHARACTERIZATION OF DENDRITIC CELLS

Steinman and Witmer (1978) next investigated the role of DCs as stimulator cells in a mixed leukocyte reaction. They harvested spleen cells from C57Bl mice and cultured them with various cell populations derived either from allogeneic DBA/2 mice or semiallogeneic (C57Bl × DBA/2) F$_1$ mice. One to 5 days later they added ^{3}H-thymidine to the cultures and quantitated the amount of radioactivity incorporated into DNA. They treated the cultured cells with antibodies specific for the H-2 antigens of either the responding or stimulating strains of mice to identify the source of the cells that incorporated the radiolabeled thymidine.

Steinman and Witmer reported that C57Bl spleen cells cultured with DCs from either semiallogeneic or allogeneic mice proliferated optimally. C57Bl spleen cells incorporated significantly more ^{3}H-thymidine when cultured with DCs than when cultured with purified lymphocytes. The investigators compared DCs as stimulators with other cells expressing class II antigens such as B cells and macrophages and reported that DCs induced a greater response in a mixed leukocyte reaction than did the other cells. This led the authors to predict that "DCs and not macrophages will prove to be a critical accessory cell required in the generation of many immune responses."

Robert Lechler and J. Richard Batchelor in 1982 working at the Hammersmith Hospital in London provided additional information about the role of DCs in stimulating an immune response. These researchers studied the role of DCs in kidney graft rejection. They injected the potential graft recipients (AS rats) with donor (AS × AUG)

F$_1$ spleen cells 11 days before transplant. One day later they injected these AS rats with antibodies specific for AUG rats. Rats of the AS strain received kidneys from (AS × AUG)F$_1$ mice and a second dose of anti-AUG antibodies. This protocol results in the long-term survival of kidneys in the recipients. Four weeks later, the investigators removed successful grafts and retransplanted them to new AS strain rats along with an intravenous injection of various populations of cells from F$_1$ donors.

Injection of small numbers (1–5 × 10^4) of DCs in this protocol resulted in acute rejection of the graft while injection of larger doses of peripheral blood or 5 × 10^6 B or T lymphocytes failed to trigger graft rejection. Lechler and Batchelor proposed that donor-strain DCs provide the major immunogenic stimulus in graft rejection.

In 1984, Denise Faustman and colleagues working at Washington University in St. Louis, Missouri, collaborated with Ralph Steinman and confirmed this conclusion in a model of allogeneic pancreatic islet cell transplantation. Faustman and coworkers injected C57Bl/6 mice with streptozotocin, a drug known to induce diabetes. They monitored onset of the disease by measuring serum glucose levels; once the level of glucose exceeded 400 mg/dL, the mice received a transplant of isolated islets from an allogeneic strain of mice, B10BR. The investigators treated some of the islets to be transplanted with a monoclonal antibody specific for a DC antigen and complement. Other islets were untreated or were treated only with complement.

Faustman and colleagues monitored the transplanted mice by measuring serum glucose levels. Levels greater than 250 mg/dL signaled graft rejection. All five of the mice transplanted with untreated islets as well as five of six of the mice receiving complement-treated islets rejected the transplants within 20 days. By contrast, transplants treated with antibodies to DC antigens survived for more than 65 days and some rats maintained normal glucose levels for up to 200 days.

These researchers subsequently injected some of the mice bearing successful grafts with allogeneic cells enriched for DCs. This treatment led to rapid graft rejection. The investigators conclude that their results "indicate that dendritic cells are a potentially important component of transplantation rejection reactions."

Subsequent experiments demonstrated that DCs present antigens in an MHC-restricted manner to both CD8$^+$ and CD4$^+$ T lymphocytes. In 1980, Michel Nussenzweig and colleagues generated CD8$^+$ cytotoxic T lymphocytes (CTL) specific for trinitrophenyl (TNP) by incubating lymphocytes with TNP-coated T lymphocytes. They measured cytotoxicity against TNP-coated targets by the release of ^{51}Cr. When Nussenzweig and coworkers attempted to generate anti-TNP-specific CTLs using purified T lymphocytes rather than unseparated lymphoid populations, they discovered that the stimulation step required an accessory cell, a function most efficiently performed by DCs.

In 1983 Kayo Inaba, working in Steinman's laboratory partially purified lymphocytes from mouse spleen cells either by passage through a column of Sephadex G-10, a procedure that removed adherent cells including DCs, or by treatment with a monoclonal antibody specific for DCs plus complement. He cultured these lymphocytes under conditions designed to stimulate a primary immune response to SRBC in vitro. Isolated lymphocytes failed to mount an antibody response to red blood cells. Addition of small numbers of DCs to the cultures enhanced the antibody response to the level observed with unseparated spleen cells. Isolated macrophages failed to restore the antibody response to the same extent as did DCs. These results demonstrate that DCs are essential accessory cells for the activation of helper T cells (CD4[+]) in antibody production.

The conclusion of these studies demonstrated that DCs serve as the primary APC for activation of

- mixed leukocyte reactions,
- allogeneic kidney and pancreatic islets cell graft rejection,
- cytotoxic T lymphocytes, and
- helper cells in an antibody response.

RELATIONSHIP BETWEEN LANGERHANS CELLS AND DENDRITIC CELLS

The morphological similarities between DCs in lymphoid organs and LCs in the skin posed a natural question about the relationship between the two cells types. Several groups of scientists working with LCs demonstrated that they express both class I and II MHC-coded antigens on their surface (Rowen et al., 1977), are derived from hematopoietic stem cells in the bone marrow (Katz et al., 1979), express several cell surface molecules (i.e., Fc and C3 receptors) similar to those expressed by macrophages (Stingl et al., 1977), and present antigen to T lymphocytes (Stingl et al., 1978).

Gerold Schuler and Steinman (1985) isolated LCs from mouse skin and cultured them for various periods of time. This model allowed Schuler and Steinman to characterize LCs and compare them to macrophages. These investigators confirmed that isolated LCs express class II MHC-coded molecules. When initially isolated from skin, LCs bind monoclonal antibodies specific for macrophage antigens but not those specific for T and B lymphocytes. Freshly isolated LCs also fail to bind antibodies specific for DCs. However during 3 days of culture, staining with antibodies to macrophages decreased while staining with antibodies to DCs increased.

Freshly isolated LCs failed to act as accessory cells in a mixed leukocyte assay; following 2–3 days in vitro LCs acquired this stimulatory function. Based on these findings, Schuler and Steinman concluded "LC seem to be immunologically immature, but acquire many of the features of spleen DC during culture. We suggest that functioning lymphoid DC may, in general, be derived from less mature precursors located in nonlymphoid tissues."

DENDRITIC CELL VACCINES

Clinical investigators treating patients presenting with malignant tumors proposed that DCs could be modified to be used as vaccines. This led to the development of DC vaccines to malignancies including metastatic melanoma, non-Hodgkin's lymphoma, metastatic colorectal cancer, and cancers of the breast, ovaries, pancreas, and prostate. Several of these vaccines are currently in clinical trials.

Investigators performed proof of concept experiments originally in experimental animals. In 1990, Kayo Inaba and colleagues along with Ralph Steinman isolated adherent cells (containing both macrophages and DCs) from mouse spleens and incubated them with one of several protein antigens (sperm whale myoglobin, conalbumin, human gamma globulin, or ovalbumin). They then purified DCs, macrophages, and B lymphocytes and injected these cells individually into the foot pads of naïve mice. Five days later, they removed draining lymph nodes from these mice, prepared single-cell suspensions, and cultured the lymphocytes for 3 days with antigen. Twelve to 16 hours prior to termination of the cultures, they added ^{3}H-thymidine; uptake of this DNA precursor signaled activation of lymphocytes by the antigen.

The researchers detected proliferation of antigen-specific T lymphocytes when the mice received antigen-pulsed DCs but not when they received antigen-pulsed macrophages or B lymphocytes. The interaction between DCs and T lymphocytes is MHC-restricted suggesting that the DCs present antigen in the context of histocompatibility molecules. These results stimulated efforts to develop vaccines with syngeneic DCs.

Clinical investigators develop DC-based vaccines for tumors as a means of either enhancing tumor immunogenicity or for prevention of malignant transformation. The protocols involve modifying a patient's DCs in vitro with tumor-specific antigens that are then returned to the patient, where they theoretically activate T lymphocytes to become cytotoxic. Requirements for this therapy include identification of tumor-specific antigens and isolation of sufficient DCs from a patient to create an individualized vaccine. Development of DC vaccines required new methods to separate, purify, and grow

DCs. A major breakthrough came with the discovery that granulocyte–macrophage colony-stimulating factor (GM-CSF) stimulates the growth of DCs from hematopoietic stem cells.

Kayo Inaba and colleagues in Ralph Steinman's laboratory at the Rockefeller University and Christopher Caux and coworkers at the Schering Plough Laboratory for Immunological Research and INSERM in France simultaneously described this breakthrough in 1992 that allowed the development of vaccines for a number of different tumor antigens. The first DC-based vaccine was licensed by the Food and Drug Administration, USA, in 2010 for metastatic, asymptomatic, hormone refractory prostate cancer (Chapter 38).

CONCLUSION

Paul Langerhans observed in the 1860s a unique cell type that he thought was a component of the nervous system of the skin. Over 100 years later, Ralph Steinman and Zanvil Cohn described a similar cell, the DC, in spleens of mice. Immunologists now agree that the skin LC and the lymphoid DC constitute two Maturational stages of the same cell lineage.

Studies performed over the last 40 years resulted in the characterization of DCs as the primary APC for the induction of adaptive immune responses. Ralph Steinman persisted in these investigations and finally convinced other immunologists of the existence and function of DCs. For this work, Steinman was awarded the Nobel Prize in Physiology or Medicine in 2011.

Much remains to be discovered about DCs and how to manipulate them to enhance adaptive immune responses. Researchers recently demonstrated that there are several different subpopulations of DCs that derive from different hematopoietic precursor cells. While most investigators demonstrated that DCs function as stimulators of an adaptive immune response, some studies have shown that these cells might also downregulate ongoing responses. Little is known about the APCs required to activate various subpopulations of CD4$^+$ T lymphocytes (Chapter 22), and further studies are required.

DC vaccines represent a major potential addition to the oncologist's armamentarium in the fight against cancer, but even in this area several questions persist. These include

- What is the best method to generate DC vaccines that cause tumor regression? Can DC vaccines provide protection prior to development of a tumor?
- What are the requirements for activating various subpopulations of CD4$^+$ T lymphocytes? How can DC vaccines that induce T$_{REG}$ cells be avoided while

vaccines that activate CD4$^+$ T$_H$1 lymphocytes be preferentially constructed?
- What are the design options for DC vaccines that will activate NK lymphocytes?

As a recent review of DC-based cancer immunotherapy concludes, "Even though the approach of using tumour antigen-presenting DCs in therapeutic vaccination strategies has been shown to work effectively in mice and looks promising in *in vitro* studies, the actual clinical benefit for patients with cancer has been marginal. There clearly is still room for improvement" (Yi and Appel, 2013).

References

Caux, C., Dezutter, C., Schmitt, D., Banchereau, J., 1992. GM-CSF and TNF-α cooperate in the generation of dendritic langerhans cells. Nature 360, 258–261.

Faustman, D.L., Steinman, R.M., Gebel, H.M., Hauptfeld, B., Davie, J.M., Lacy, P.E., 1984. Prevention of rejection of murine islet allografts by treatment with anti-dendritic cell antibody. Proc. Nat. Acad. Sci. U.S.A. 81, 3864–3868.

Ham, A.W., 1974. Histology, seventh ed. J.B. Lippincott Co., Philadelphia, PA, p. 616.

Inaba, K., Inaba, M., Romani, N., Aya, H., Deguchi, M., Ikehara, S., Muramatsu, S., Steinman, R.M., 1992. Generation of large numbers of dendritic cells from mouse bone marrow cultures supplemented with granulocyte/macrophage colony-stimulating factor. J. Exp. Med. 176, 1693–1702.

Inaba, K., Metlay, J.P., Crowley, M.T., Steinman, R.M., 1990. Dendritic cells pulsed with protein antigens in vitro can prime antigen-specific, MHC-restricted T cells in situ. J. Exp. Med. 172, 631–640.

Inaba, K., Steinman, R.M., Van Voorhis, W.C., Maramatsu, S., 1983. Dendritic cells are critical accessory cells for thymus-dependent antibody responses in mouse and in man. Proc. Nat. Acad. Sci. U.S.A. 80, 6041–6045.

Katz, S.L., Tamaki, K., Sachs, D.H., 1979. Epidermal langerhans cells are derived from cells originating in the bone marrow. Nature 282, 324–326.

Langerhans, P., 1868. Über die nerven der menschlichen haut. Virchows Arch. (B) 44, 325–337.

Lechler, R.I., Batchelor, J.R., 1982. Restoration of immunogenicity to passenger cell-depleted kidney allografts by the addition of donor strain dendritic cells. J. Exp. Med. 155, 31–41.

Mosier, D.E., 1967. A requirement for two cell types for antibody formation in vitro. Science 158, 1573–1575.

Nussenzweig, M.C., Steinman, R.M., Gutchinov, B., Cohn, A.A., 1980. Dendritic cells are accessory cells for the development of anti-trinitrophenyl cytotoxic T lymphocytes. J. Exp. Med. 152, 1070–1084.

Rowen, G., Lewis, M.G., Sullivan, A.K., 1977. Ia antigen expression on human epidermal langerhans cells. Nature 268, 247–248.

Schuler, G., Steinman, R.M., 1985. Murine epidermal langerhans cells mature into potent immunostimulatory dendritic cells in vitro. J. Exp. Med. 161, 526–546.

Steinman, R.M., 2012. Decisions about dendritic cells: past, present and future. Annu. Rev. Immunol. 30, 1–22.

Steinman, R.M., Adams, J.C., Cohn, Z.A., 1975. Identification of a novel cell type in peripheral lymphoid organs of mice. IV. Identification and distribution in mouse spleen. J. Exp. Med. 141, 804–820.

Steinman, R.M., Cohn, Z.A., 1973. Identification of a novel cell type in peripheral lymphoid organs of mice. I. Morphology, quantitation, tissue distribution. J. Exp. Med. 137, 1142–1162.

Steinman, R.M., Cohn, A.A., 1974. Identification of a novel cell type in peripheral lymphoid organs of mice. II. Functional properties in vitro. J. Exp. Med. 139, 380–397.

Steinman, R.M., Kaplan, G., Witmer, M.D., Cohn, Z.A., 1979. Identification of a novel cell type in peripheral lymphoid organs of mice. V. Purification of spleen dendritic cells, new surface markers and maintenance in vitro. J. Exp. Med. 149, 1–16.

Steinman, R.M., Lustig, D.S., Cohn, Z.A., 1974. Identification of a novel cell type in peripheral lymphoid organs of mice. III. Functional properties in vivo. J. Exp. Med. 139, 1431–1445.

Steinman, R.M., Witmer, M.D., 1978. Lymphoid dendritic cells are potent stimulators in the primary mixed leukocyte reaction in mice. Proc. Nat. Acad, Sci. U.S.A. 75, 5132–5136.

Stingl, G., Katz, S.I., Clement, L., Green, I., Shevach, E.M., 1978. Immunologic functions of Ia-bearing epidermal langerhans cells. J. Immunol. 121, 2005–2013.

Stingl, G., Wolff-Schreiner, E., Pichler, W.J., Gschnait, F., Knapp, W., Wolff, K., 1977. Epidermal langerhans cells bear Fc and C3 receptors. Nature 268, 245–246.

Yi, D.H., Appel, S., 2013. Current status and future perspectives of dendritic cell-based cancer immunotherapy. Scand. J. Immunol. 78, 167–171.

TIME LINE

1868	Paul Langerhans describes dendritic cells in the skin; concludes they are part of the nervous system of the skin
1967	Donald Mosier demonstrates that initiation of an in vitro antibody response requires adherent cells
1973	Ralph Steinman and Zanvil Cohn publish their initial description of dendritic cells in mouse lymphoid organs
1974	Ralph Steinman and coworkers present evidence that dendritic cells function by presenting antigens to T lymphocytes
1980	Michel Nussenzweig working with Ralph Steinman demonstrates that dendritic cells are required to stimulate CD8$^+$ cytotoxic T lymphocytes
1982	Robert Lechler and J. Richard Batchelor transfer dendritic cells to induce graft rejection in rats rendered nonresponsive to allogeneic antigens
1983	Kayo Inaba and colleagues demonstrate that dendritic cells serve as accessory cells for the activation of helper T cells (CD4$^+$) in antibody production
1984	Denise Faustman and colleagues in Steinman's laboratory inhibit rejection of transplanted allogeneic pancreatic islets by depleting the grafts of dendritic cells
1985	Gerold Schuler and Ralph Steinman report that Langerhans cells are immature dendritic cells
1990	Kayo Inaba in Steinman's laboratory induces an adaptive immune response in vivo using dendritic cells that phagocytize protein antigen in vitro
1992	Kayo Inaba and colleagues and Christophe Caux and coworkers identify GM-CSF as an important cytokine in the maturation of dendritic cells
2010	FDA approves the first dendritic cell-based vaccine for prostate cancer
2011	Ralph Steinman awarded the Nobel Prize in Physiology or Medicine for his discovery of dendritic cells

The Mucosal Immune System and Secretory IgA

INTRODUCTION

Humans and other mammals exist within a complex ecosystem teeming with microorganisms, some of which are normal microbiota while others are potential pathogens. Mammalian hosts maintain homeostasis with this microbiota by a variety of mechanisms. Interactions with normal microbiota are minimized while protection against potential pathogens requires intact defense mechanisms at the interface between host and environment.

The primary boundaries between the body and the environment occur at the skin and the mucous membranes lining many of the internal organs including the gastrointestinal, respiratory, and genital–urinary systems. Both innate host defenses and adaptive immune response provide effector mechanisms at these sites. Responses to the normal microbiome include induction of an unresponsive state in lamina propria dendritic cells and upregulation of $CD4^+$ T_{REG} lymphocytes. In addition some bacterial products such as capsular polysaccharide from *Bacteroides fragilis* stimulate the synthesis of the anti-inflammatory cytokine IL-10. These effects balance the induction of inflammatory responses in submucosal locations to decrease potentially pathogenic reactions to normal flora.

Protection against potential pathogens also involves both nonspecific innate host defense mechanisms and specific adaptive immune responses. The innate host defenses include mechanical barriers, secreted antimicrobial substances, and nonspecific mechanisms such as low pH and inflammation that inhibit microbial attachment, penetration, and growth. Once these defenses are breeched, components of the adaptive immune system are activated. While some of the mechanisms of the adaptive immune system described elsewhere in this book play a role in protecting the gastrointestinal, respiratory, and genital–urinary tracts, a unique, secretory immune system has evolved to provide effective defenses at these internal sites. This system differentiates innocuous material (i.e., food and digestive products in the gastrointestinal tract) from matter that is potentially pathogenic.

Immunologists divide the adaptive immune system into systemic and mucosal components. The systemic component includes peripheral lymphoid tissues such as the spleen and lymph nodes as well as cells present in various organs and in peripheral blood and lymphatics. The mucosal or secretory immune system includes a collection of lymphoid organs such as the tonsils, adenoids, Peyer's patches, and appendix as well as aggregates of

A Historical Perspective on Evidence-Based Immunology
http://dx.doi.org/10.1016/B978-0-12-398381-7.00030-7

lymphocytes associated with mucous membranes. These lymphoid tissues are called the mucosal-associated lymphoid tissue (MALT). Researchers described the mucosal immune system as a separate system in the 1960s.

Both B and T lymphocytes reside in the MALT. The predominate effector mechanism active in the secretory immune system involves a unique isotype of antibody, secretory IgA (sIgA). Although IgA is also present in the systemic immune response, sIgA functions primarily to provide immunity along mucosal surfaces. The studies presented in this chapter describe the research that identified and characterized this mucosal immune system.

IDENTIFICATION OF MUCOSAL-ASSOCIATED LYMPHOID TISSUE (MALT)

The gastrointestinal, respiratory, and genital–urinary systems are mucosal-lined structures continually exposed to environmental antigens. These antigens include potential pathogens against which the body must be protected by either innate or adaptive immune responses. However, many of these antigens such as food are innocuous and typically do not induce a pathogenic response. Others including dust, pollen, and sperm can induce potentially deleterious responses. To counter these threats and maintain homeostasis at the interface between body and environment, a unique immune system has evolved along mucosal surfaces. This unique system includes aggregates of lymphoid tissue, the MALT, that function analogous to the peripheral lymphoid tissues of lymph nodes and spleen.

Johann Conrad Peyer, a Swiss physician and professor of medicine, originally described the presence of lymphoid aggregates along the intestinal tract in 1677. Peyer originally thought that these structures represented glands of the intestine. Subsequent observations revealed that these structures are lymphoepithelial organs although their function was only described in the twentieth century. In fact during the search for the bursa equivalent in mammals, some immunologists speculated erroneously that these structures served as a site of differentiation of B lymphocytes (Chapter 10). These aggregates of lymphocytes are now called Peyer's patches (Brandtzaeg, 1996).

Histologic studies of mucosal-lined organs identified other components of the MALT including scattered lymphoid follicles and organized lymphoid tissues such as the tonsils and adenoids, the appendix, and draining (mesenteric) lymph nodes. Macrophages and dendritic cells in these structures sample the environment and identify potential pathogens. Pathogens deemed potentially dangerous induce an immune response that effectively eliminates the threat. As a result, cells within these lymphoid structures constitute a local

immune system responsible for maintaining the integrity of the gastrointestinal, respiratory, and genital–urinary systems.

EVIDENCE FOR A SEPARATE MUCOSAL IMMUNE SYSTEM

In the 1920s, investigators in Russia and in France noted that individuals infected with *Shigella* and other pathogens possessed antibodies to these bacteria in their gastrointestinal tract in the absence of serum antibodies to the same microorganisms. Researchers in the 1960s and 1970s identified a unique immunoglobulin isotype in gastrointestinal and other secretions and confirmed the existence of a secretory immune system that provides protection to anatomical sites contiguous with the environment.

In 1919, Alexandre Besredka working at the Pasteur Institute in Paris fed rabbits *Shigella dysenteriae* and demonstrated that they were protected against fatal dysentery even in the absence of serum antibodies (Brandtzaeg, 1996). Arthur Davies, a physician serving with the British army in Jerusalem, in 1922 confirmed this observation. He detected antibodies to dysentery *bacillus* in stools from infected soldiers earlier in the infection than he detected serum antibodies. He concluded that early in the infection, "agglutinins for the *B. dysenteriae* group were absent in the blood but were present in the intestinal exudate."

The discordance in antibody levels reported in these and similar studies suggested the presence of separate immune systems, one protecting the mucosal organs and a second involved in systemic defense. Researchers confirmed the existence of these two systems that are relatively exclusive based on

- identification and preferential location of IgA antibody in secretions, and
- migration of cells involved in the mucosal immune system.

DISCOVERY OF SECRETORY IgA

Joseph Heremans and colleagues described IgA as a separate class of serum antibody in 1959 (Chapter 16). Four years later W.B. Chodirker and Thomas Tomasi (1963) at the University of Vermont reported that IgA is the predominant immunoglobulin in a number of secretory fluids. Tomasi, trained as a physician at the University of Vermont, earned his PhD from The Rockefeller University in 1965. During his PhD studies he interacted with investigators including Halstead Holman evaluating patients with protein-losing enteropathies;

in such individuals the albumin:globulin ratio in intestinal fluids is reversed compared to serum, with the intestinal fluids containing a large amount of gamma globulin. This result could not be explained by normal transudation of plasma from the circulation, leading Tomasi to pursue identification of the immunoglobulins present in body fluids (Tomasi, 1992).

Once Tomasi arrived at the University of Vermont as a faculty member he focused on identifying the proteins present in human secretions. As Tomasi recollected in 1992, "a junior medical student and former dentist, Sheldon Zigglebaum asked to do a summer project in my laboratory. He was familiar with obtaining fluid directly from the parotid duct with a simple device called a Curby cap. This secretion lacked mucus and could be obtained in a sterile and painless manner from myself and all 'volunteers' from my own lab and other surrounding labs. We were often seen with plastic tubes coming out of our mouths leading to test tubes in the upper pocket of our lab jackets when we were walking in the halls or even when we were in meetings."

Tomasi and his coworkers demonstrated that saliva from the parotid gland contained excess gamma globulin compared to serum. They evaluated saliva using an antibody specific for IgA and showed that most of this gamma globulin was, in fact, IgA. Subsequently they demonstrated that secretions from other sources (tears, bile, colostrum, and small intestine) also contained predominately IgA. As Tomasi recalled in 1992 they "recruited volunteers: collected sweat by wrapping plastic around arms; tears by gently persuading the lab members to peel onions or to look at the sun glaring off the Vermont snow, and nasal secretions by washing the nares with saline. For this last secretion I was the first 'volunteer'—we mistakenly used distilled water…this brought tears to my eyes (no sympathy, but another lacrimal collection)."

They demonstrated that IgA is the predominate immunoglobulin in secretions bathing mucous surfaces. This led to studies designed to determine

- the structure of serum and sIgA, and
- the source of sIgA.

The Structure of Serum and sIgA

Tomasi and his colleagues (1965) investigated the IgA present in parotid gland saliva and colostrum from healthy individuals and in ascites fluid from patients with advanced cirrhosis. They initially showed that the IgA in ascites fluids and in serum are immunochemically similar. Ultracentrifugation studies on IgA isolated from ascites, serum, and secretions demonstrated that IgA exists in two molecular forms: serum and ascites IgA sediments predominately as a 7S molecule like IgG while

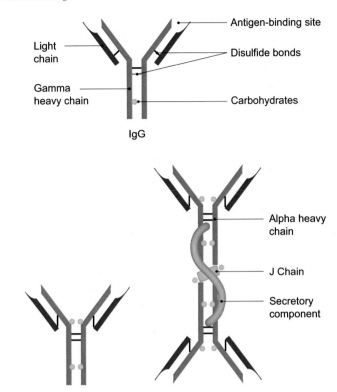

FIGURE 30.1   Diagram comparing the structure of IgG, monomeric IgA, and secretory IgA. The dimeric form of sIgA includes J chain and secretory component. *From http://spot.pcc.edu/~jvolpe/b/bi234/lec/8_9defe nses/9_outline.htm.*

IgA in secretions is mainly 11S. Thus IgA in secretions is larger than serum IgA leading Tomasi to suggest that serum IgA is monomeric and consists of the basic four-chain structure of most other immunoglobulin isotypes (Chapter 11) while IgA found in secretions is polymeric, most likely consisting of two monomers (Figure 30.1).

Immunological analysis of sIgA and serum IgA with an antibody specific for serum IgA showed no differences between the two molecules. However analysis of these samples with an antibody specific for sIgA revealed an antigenic determinant in sIgA missing in serum IgA. Absorption of the antibody against sIgA with normal human serum removed immunological activity against serum IgA while retaining activity against sIgA. The authors conclude from their immunodiffusion data that sIgA contains not only heavy and light chains but an additional unique polypeptide chain called secretory component.

Identification of Secretory Component

Mary Ann South and her colleagues at the University of Minnesota presented additional information about the unique polypeptide associated with sIgA in 1966. She collected saliva from patients with congenital agammaglobulinemia or with isolated deficiency of IgA. These secretions possessed a polypeptide chain that contained the unique immunological determinants seen in Tomasi's studies even in the absence of sIgA. Transfusion of these patients with 1 or 2 L of plasma from healthy donors resulted in the appearance of IgA in saliva of some of the patients. This IgA contained the unique polypeptide chain leading to the hypothesis that the chain transports the IgA across the epithelial barrier.

In 1969, Donald Tourville working with Tomasi at the State University of New York in Buffalo, demonstrated by immunofluorescence that this secretory component, absent from plasma cells, is found in and on epithelial cells lining mucous membranes. The researchers concluded

1. IgA and secretory component are synthesized by separate cell types, and
2. secretory component is actively involved in the transport of sIgA across the epithelial barrier into the glandular lumen.

Figure 30.2 presents Tourville and colleagues' model to explain this transport mechanism. This model fails to indicate where secretory component is synthesized; subsequent investigations showed that it is synthesized by the epithelial cells of the mucous membrane.

In 1978, Silvia Crago and colleagues working in Jiri Mestecky's laboratory at the University of Alabama, Birmingham (Crago et al., 1978) demonstrated that epithelial cells from human fetuses bind polymeric, but not monomeric, IgA both on their surface and within the cell. They further demonstrated that secretory component, produced by these epithelial cells, serves as a receptor for IgA.

Keith Mostov and his colleagues at the Rockefeller University in New York in 1980 isolated messenger RNA

specific for secretory component from rabbit mammary gland. They characterized the translation products of this mRNA and deduced the structure of four polypeptide chains. These chains, which are larger than the secretory component associated with sIgA, exist in epithelial cells as transmembrane proteins. Mostow and coworkers developed a hypothesis to explain the transport of sIgA across the epithelial cell:

> …secretory component is synthesized as a 120 kDa glycoprotein complex by epithelial cells and integrated into the basal and lateral membranes of these cells where it serves as a receptor for sIgA. Binding of sIgA to this receptor induces the formation of a vesicle that transports the complex across the cell. During the process of transport, proteolytic cleavage removes the polypeptides associated with transmembrane binding so that the complex that is deposited into the glandular lumen contains a single molecule of secretory component (80 kDa) attached to a dimer of IgA.

In addition to secretory component, polymeric IgA as well as other polymeric forms of immunoglobulin (i.e., IgM) contains an additional polypeptide termed a joining (J) chain. Plasma cells synthesize J chains as well as the heavy and light chains of the IgA molecule. Polymers consisting of four heavy chains, four light chains, and one J chain are assembled prior to secretion thus assuring that the molecules possess only a single specificity.

Identification of J Chain

In 1970, Michael Halpern and Marian Koshland working at the University of California, Berkeley described the existence of a novel polypeptide associated with sIgA. Halpern and Koshland isolated rabbit sIgA from colostrum, purified it by treatment with detergent, and fractionated it on a molecular weight sieve to remove the secretory component. Reduction and alkylation of the remaining sIgA resulted in two fractions that had molecular weights consistent with heavy and light chains. Electrophoresis of the isolated fractions revealed a band that migrated more rapidly than the light chain. This polypeptide chain had a molecular weight of approximately 23 kDa and an amino acid composition different from light chains. The authors termed this component J chain and demonstrated a similar chain in sIgA isolated from human colostrum.

Halpern and Koshland evaluated human IgA myeloma proteins to address the possibility that this J chain was a light chain unique to IgA molecules. They studied both monomeric and dimeric forms of myeloma proteins and demonstrated that J chain was associated with dimeric forms but not with monomeric forms. They concluded that J chain is "synthesized in the same plasma cell as the heavy and light chains" and functions to link monomeric units into a dimer.

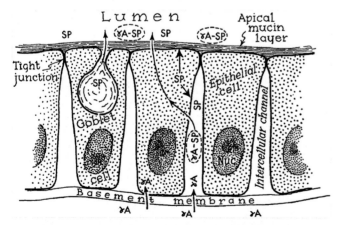

FIGURE 30.2 Hypothetical model for the transport of sIgA across the epithelial barrier along mucosal membranes. This model was generated as a result of information obtained concerning the separate cellular origins of sIgA and secretory component. *From Tourville et al., 1969.*

Jiri Mestecky and his group (1971) reported the presence of a similar J chain in human colostrum and associated with human serum IgM. They reduced the disulfide bonds of these immunoglobulins and separated heavy and light chains by electrophoresis. The light chain fractions of both colostral IgA and IgM contained unique polypeptide chains that shared electrophoretic mobilities, molecular weights, peptide composition, and antigenic determinants that differed from immunoglobulin light chains. The investigators concluded that J chain is produced by plasma cells synthesizing polymeric forms of immunoglobulin including IgA and IgM. J chain is bound covalently to heavy chains and functions by linking the monomeric units together prior to secretion.

The Cellular Source of sIgA

Immunologists considered two options to explain the source of sIgA. Either it is synthesized

- locally in the lymphoid tissues of the gastrointestinal, respiratory, and genital–urinary systems; or
- systemically in peripheral lymphoid tissue and then transudated from serum.

During the late 1960s, several investigators used fluorescent antibody specific for IgA to determine the location of the immunoglobulin in cells of specimens resected from the gastrointestinal tract including parotid glands, tonsils, stomach, and rectum (Crabbé and Heremans, 1966, 1967; Gelzayd et al., 1967). These investigators observed staining in the lamina propria and the interstitial tissue in cells resembling plasma cells and in some of the epithelial cells. Use of antibody specific for sIgA absorbed with serum from healthy donors (to remove antibodies to the immunoglobulin while leaving antibodies to secretory component) demonstrated staining almost exclusively in epithelial cells.

Based on these results, the authors proposed the existence of a distinct host defense mechanism in the external secretions. This system is characterized by a unique type of antibody (sIgA) that is produced locally and that contains a polypeptide chain not found associated with serum IgA. This polypeptide chain is produced by the epithelial cells of the gland in which the sIgA is synthesized and is involved in transport of the immunoglobulin into the secretions.

MIGRATORY PATH OF LYMPHOCYTES IN THE MUCOSAL IMMUNE SYSTEM

The mucosal immune system responds to a large number of different antigens. In 1971, Susan Craig and John Cebra working at Johns Hopkins University, Baltimore, Maryland, transferred lymphocytes from rabbit Peyer's patches, peripheral blood, or popliteal lymph node to irradiated, allogeneic recipients. They harvested various organs from the recipients and identified the origin of cells by immunofluorescence. They showed that lymphocytes from Peyer's patches reconstituted both Peyer's patches and spleens with lymphocytes that preferentially synthesized IgA. Additionally, Peyer's patch lymphocytes reconstituted gut-associated lymphoid tissue in the irradiated animals better than did lymphocytes from peripheral blood or popliteal lymph node. They concluded that Peyer's patches are an enriched source for IgA precursors.

Craig and Cebra discussed the mechanism leading to the preferential reconstitution of intestinal lymphoid tissues with lymphocytes from Peyer's patches and concluded, erroneously, that the distribution of the injected cells is random rather than dependent on a homing mechanism.

In 1979, Mark McDermott and John Bienenstock at McMaster University, Ontario, Canada, designed studies to support the concept of a common mucosal immune system in which lymphocytes from one mucosal site preferentially migrate to other mucosal sites. McDermott and Bienenstock labeled mouse mesenteric lymph node lymphocytes with ^{3}H-thymidine and transferred them intravenously into syngeneic female recipients. Within 24h of transfer, they detected labeled lymphocytes in several mucosa-associated organs including the gastrointestinal tract, cervix, vagina, uterus, mammary glands, and mesenteric lymph nodes. They stained the labeled lymphocytes from these mucosal associated organs by immunofluorescence and observed that 60% of the cells produced IgA while 25% synthesized IgG. By contrast, labeled lymphocytes from peripheral lymph nodes of these reconstituted mice stained predominately with IgG (44%); only a minority of the lymphocytes stained with IgA (8%). The authors concluded "these results support the concept of a mucosal immunologic system in which different mucosal surfaces are linked by migrating IgA plasmacyte precursors."

These results led to further studies to determine the mechanism by which lymphocytes involved in the mucosal immune system selectively return to mucosal sites. The lamina propria underlying mucous membranes contains dendritic cells and other antigen-presenting cells (APCs). These cells engulf materials present in the lumen of the organ and transport potential antigens to local (i.e., mesenteric) lymph nodes. Naïve lymphocytes continually migrate from peripheral blood into mesenteric lymph nodes, where they sample the antigens transported there by APCs. If B or T lymphocytes are activated, they proliferate, develop effector capabilities, and migrate back to the MALT.

Investigators sought the mechanism responsible for selective migration of lymphocytes to mucosal sites and determined that lymphocytes express a number of molecules (integrins) on their surfaces that interact with ligands on vascular endothelial cells.

The intergrin responsible for mucosal homing of lymphocytes is designated as α4β7. The α4β7 integrin preferentially binds a ligand—mucosal addressin cell adhesion molecule-1 (MAdCAM-1)—expressed on high endothelial venules in Peyer's patches, the lamina propria, and the lactating mammary gland. Cornelia Berlin and her colleagues at Stanford University, Palo Alto, California, demonstrated in 1993 that antibodies to α4 and β7 integrin chains but not to other integrins inhibit lymphocyte binding to purified MAdCAM-1 or to MAdCAM-1 transfectants. Researchers in the late 1990s demonstrated that the gene coding for α4β7 is selectively upregulated in lymphocytes stimulated to proliferate in a mucosal site (reviewed by Salmi and Jalkanen, 2005).

DISCOVERY OF MICROFOLD (M) CELLS AND THEIR FUNCTION

Epithelial cells separate lymphoid follicles in the gastrointestinal tract from the gastrointestinal lumen. Antigens to which the secretory immune system responds are in the lumen and must traverse this epithelial layer. Researchers observed potential antigens, particularly pathogenic microorganisms, crossing the mucosal epithelium; however, experimental proof for a unique transport system first appeared in 1973. Dale Bockman working with Max Cooper at the University of Alabama, Birmingham, demonstrated a selective uptake and transport of inert particles such as India ink, and a potential antigen (ferritin), by epithelial cells overlying the lymphoid follicles in the gastrointestinal tracts of chickens, rabbits, and mice.

In 1974, Robert Owen and Albert Jones, working at the Veterans Administration Hospital and the University of California, San Francisco, performed a histological study of human intestinal mucosal cell types. They obtained tissue from the small intestine from patients undergoing intestinal bypass surgery for treatment of obesity and dissected Peyer's patches from the mucosa. Owen and Jones prepared these tissues for light, scanning, and transmission electron microscopy. They examined these sections and observed a unique cell type present in the mucosa directly overlying the lymphoid follicles of Peyer's patches. Instead of microvilli characteristic of most mucosal epithelium, M cells displayed numerous microfolds on their luminal surface and were thus called microfold (M) cells. M cells are thinner than the columnar epithelium cells typical of the intestinal tract and contain vesicles in their cytoplasm. The authors postulated that M cells have "a transport function, possibly for luminal antigenic material or for secretory immunoglobulin."

M cells in the follicle-associated epithelium endocytose a variety of substances including inert particles (latex spheres and India ink), antigens (ferritin and horseradish peroxidase), and microorganisms (viruses and bacteria) (reviewed by Bockman et al., 1983). M cells transport these substances to an environment rich in macrophages and B and T lymphocytes, where antigen phagocytosis and processing occurs.

CONCLUSION

The history of the secretory immune system spans several centuries starting with the initial description of Peyer's patches by J.C. Peyer in 1677. In the 1920s, investigators in Russia and in France noted that individuals infected with *Shigella* and other pathogens possessed antibodies to these bacteria in their gastrointestinal tract in the absence of serum antibodies to the same microorganisms. These observations hinted at the presence of an immune system associated with external secretions that differed from the systemic adaptive immune response. Researchers identified mucosal-associated lymphoid tissue including tonsils, adenoids, and appendix in the mid-1900s. Finally, in 1963, a unique immunoglobulin molecule was described in secretions and called secretory (s) IgA.

The description of a secretory immune system impacted medical practice. sIgA present in colostrum and milk provides protection for the neonate against potential pathogens that might infect through the gastrointestinal tract. As a result breastfeeding of infants has assumed added importance, particularly in third world countries and in areas of poor sanitation.

Albert Sabin developed an effective polio vaccine designed to be taken orally thus inducing a local immune response in the gastrointestinal tract. Poliovirus is transmitted by the fecal–oral route. The Sabin vaccine induces a local response consisting of IgA antibodies that inhibit the binding of virus to epithelial cells of the gastrointestinal tract.

Certain immunopathologies of the gastrointestinal tract are known to involve aberrant responses to self-antigens or to environmental antigens. For example, patients presenting with celiac disease possess antibodies to antigens derived from gluten, a constituent of many grains. In addition, the immune response in inflammatory bowel disease is an abnormal response to some of the normal microbiome of the gut. The description of host defense mechanisms in these clinical situations suggests a scientific rationale for development of effective therapies (Chapter 38).

References

Berlin, C., Berg, E.L., Briskin, M.J., Andrew, D.P., Kilshaw, P.J., Holzmann, B., Weissman, I.L., Hamann, A., Butcher, E.C., 1993. Alpha 4 beta 7 integrin mediates lymphocyte binding to the mucosal vascular addressin MAdCAM-1. Cell 74, 185–195.

Besredka, A., 1919. De la vaccination contre les états typhoides par la voie buccale. Ann. Inxt. Pasteur. 33, 882–903.

Bockman, D.E., Boydston, W.R., Beezhold, D.H., 1983. The role of epithelial cells in gut associated immune reactivity. Ann. NY Acad. Sci. 409, 129–144.

Bockman, D.E., Cooper, M.D., 1973. Pinocytosis by epithelium associated with lymphoid follicles in the bursa of Fabricius, appendix and Peyer's patches. An electron microscopic study. Am. J. Anat. 136, 455–477.

Brandtzaeg, P., 1996. History of oral tolerance and mucosal immunity. Ann. NY Acad. Sci. 778, 1–27.

Chodirker, W.B., Tomasi, T.B., 1963. Gamma-globulin quantitative relationships in human serum and nonvascular fluids. Science 142, 1080–1081.

Crabbé, P.A., Heremans, J.F., 1966. The distribution of immunoglobulin-containing cells along the human gastrointestinal tract. Gastroenterology 51, 305–316.

Crabbé, P.A., Heremans, J.F., 1967. Distribution in human nasopharyngeal tonsils of plasma cells containing different types of immunoglobulin polypeptide chains. Lab. Invest. 16, 112–123.

Crago, S.S., Kulhavy, R., Prince, S.J., Mestecky, J., 1978. Secretory component on epithelial cells is a surface receptor for polymeric immunoglobulins. J. Exp. Med. 147, 1832–1837.

Craig, S.W., Cebra, J.J., 1971. Peyer's patches: an enriched source of precursors for IgA-producing immunocytes in the rabbit. J. Exp. Med. 134, 188–200.

Davies, A., 1922. An investigation into the serological properties of dysentery stools. Lancet 200, 1009–1012.

Gelzayd, E.A., Kraft, S.C., Fitch, F.W., 1967. Immunoglobulin A: localization in rectal mucosal epithelial cells. Science 157, 930–931.

Halpern, M.S., Koshland, M.E., 1970. Novel subunit in secretory IgA. Nature 228, 1276–1278.

Heremans, J.F., Heremans, M-Th, Schultze, H.E., 1959. Isolation and description of a few properties of the β2A–globulin of human serum. Clin. Chim. Acta 4, 96–102.

McDermott, M.R., Bienenstock, J., 1979. Evidence for a common mucosal immunologic system I. Migration of B immunoblasts into intestinal, respiratory, and genital tissues. J. Immunol. 122, 1892–1898.

Mestecky, J., Zikan, J., Butler, W.T., 1971. Immunoglobulin M and secretory immunoglobulin A: presence of a common polypeptide chain different from light chains. Science 171, 1163–1165.

Mostov, K.E., Kraehenbuhl, J.P., Blobel, G., 1980. Receptor mediated transcellular transport of immunoglobulin: synthesis of secretory component as multiple and larger transmembrane forms. Proc. Nat. Acad. Sci. U.S.A. 77, 7257–7261.

Owen, R.L., Jones, A.L., 1974. Epithelial cell specialization within human Peyer's patches: an ultrastructural study of intestinal lymphoid follicles. Gastroenterology 66, 189–203.

Salmi, M., Jalkanen, S., 2005. Lymphocyte homing to the gut: attraction, adhesion, and commitment. Immunol. Rev. 206, 100–113.

South, M.A., Cooper, M.D., Wolheim, F.A., Hong, R., Good, R.A., 1966. The IgA system I. Studies of the transport and immunochemistry of IgA in saliva. J. Exp. Med. 123, 615–627.

Tomasi, T., 1992. The discovery of secretory IgA and the mucosal immune system. Immunol. Today 13, 416–418.

Tomasi, T.B., Tan, E.M., Solomon, A., Pendergast, R.A., 1965. Characteristics of an immune system common to certain external secretions. J. Exp. Med. 121, 101–124.

Tourville, D.R., Adler, R.H., Bienenstock, J., Tomasi, T.B., 1969. The human secretory immunoglobulin system: immunohistological localization of γA, secretory "piece" and lactoferrin in normal human tissues. J. Exp. Med. 129, 411–429.

TIME LINE

1677	Johann Conrad Peyer describes aggregates on lymphoid tissue in the small intestine
1920s	Alexandre Besredka and Arthur Davies independently demonstrate that antibody to a pathogen may exist in secretions yet be absent in blood
1959	Joseph Heremans and colleagues describe serum IgA
1963	W.B. Chodirker and Thomas Tomasi report that IgA is the predominant immunoglobulin in saliva
1965	Thomas Tomasi and colleagues demonstrate that IgA in secretions (colostrum and saliva) is 11S
1966	Mary Ann South and coworkers identify secretory component associated with sIgA
1969	Donald Tourville and colleagues demonstrate that secretory component is produced by epithelial cells
1970	Michael Halpern and Marian Koshland describe a novel polypeptide, the J chain, associated with secretory IgA in the rabbit
1971	Jiri Mestecky and colleagues isolate J chain associated with human secretory IgA as well as with serum IgM
1971	Susan Craig and John Cebra report that Peyer's patches are an enriched source for IgA-secreting B lymphocytes
1973	Dale Bockman and Max Cooper observe selective antigen transport across the epithelium by cells overlying lymphoid follicles in the gastrointestinal tract
1974	Robert Owen and Albert Jones describe a unique epithelial cell type in human gastrointestinal mucosa called a microfold (M) cell
1978	Silvia Crago and colleagues report that secretory component on epithelial cells binds polymeric immunoglobulin
1979	Mark McDermott and John Bienenstock demonstrate a common mucosal immune system
1980	Keith Mostov and coworkers provide evidence that secretory component functions by transporting sIgA across the epithelium to the intestinal lumen
1993	Cornelia Berlin and colleagues identify the cell surface molecules involved in the selective migration of lymphocytes in the secretory immune system

31

Disorders of the Innate Host Defenses

INTRODUCTION

Host defenses to potential pathogens involve two separate but interacting systems. Innate host defenses include physical barriers such as the skin and mucous membranes, immunologically nonspecific cells including granulocytes, monocytes/macrophages, dendritic cells, and natural killer (NK) lymphocytes, and soluble mediators such as defensins, lysozyme, the complement system, and inflammatory cytokines. Adaptive host defenses include T and B lymphocytes and the effector mechanisms of these immunologically specific cells.

The International Union of Immunological Societies sponsors an expert committee on primary immunodeficiencies that meets periodically to update the classification of primary (congenital) immunodeficiencies (Al-Herz et al., 2014). This group divided these disorders into eight groups, several of which involve the innate host defenses:

- defects in innate immunity,
- congenital defects of phagocyte number function or both,
- defects of NK lymphocytes,
- complement deficiencies, and
- autoinflammatory disorders.

Patients with defects in any of the components of the innate host defenses often present with infections. Such deficiencies may be either congenital or acquired. Congenital deficiencies include several discrete diseases resulting from diminished number and/or function of cells (e.g., monocytes, granulocytes, NK lymphocytes) or from decreased synthesis of proteins (e.g., complement). These defects result from mutations in the genes responsible for the proper maturation or function of these nonspecific cells and proteins.

Acquired deficiencies of the innate host defenses develop as a consequence of trauma (burns), surgery, exposure to irradiation and chemotherapeutic agents, or secondary to other disease processes (e.g., autoimmune neutropenia).

Recently clinicians have described a group of pathologies characterized by inflammatory responses in the absence of any obvious stimulus. Patients with these autoinflammatory disorders present with recurrent episodes of unexplained fever. While rare, they occur in families and result from mutations in genes regulating the synthesis of inflammatory cytokines, particularly IL-1.

This chapter, the first of four dealing with pathologies of host defense systems, encompasses clinical situations developing from defects in the innate host defenses. Subsequent chapters focus on other immunopathologies resulting from

- deficiencies of the adaptive immune responses (Chapter 32);
- aberrant responses of adaptive immunity to foreign antigens (hypersensitivities) (Chapter 33); and
- adaptive immune responses to self (autoimmunity) (Chapter 34).

DEFICIENCIES OF THE CELLS OF INNATE HOST DEFENSE MECHANISMS

Innate host defenses respond rapidly to potential pathogens. While trauma causes defects of the physical barriers of skin and mucous membranes, other deficiencies involve genetic mutations that result in decreased cell numbers, abnormalities in cell functions, or defects in the molecules responsible for providing protection. Due to the genetic nature of these deficiencies, many appear in newborns and infants.

Defects of White Blood Cells—Quantitative

Cells of the innate host defenses include monocytes/macrophages, neutrophils, dendritic cells, and NK lymphocytes. Individuals with inadequate cell numbers or function present as distinct clinical entities characterized by an inability to confront infectious microorganisms and destroy them. Cells involved in the innate defenses differentiate from either myeloid precursors (neutrophils and monocytes) or lymphoid precursors (NK lymphocytes).

In 1922, Werner Schultz in Munich, Germany, described several female patients who presented with sore throat, prostration (exhaustion), and neutropenia; he termed this disorder agranulocytosis (referenced in Stiehm and Johnston, 2005). Subsequent investigators described patients with Schultz disease characterized by recurrent infections, particularly involving the oral cavity, pharynx, skin, perirectal and anal areas, and the respiratory tract. These patients also demonstrate poor wound healing (Jacobson and Berliner, 2014).

Although associated with infections, chemotherapy, radiation, exposure to chemicals, or the use of any of several drugs including clozapine and penicillin, the underlying cause of agranulocytosis in adults currently remains unknown. In 1956, Rolf Kostmann, a physician working in Northern Sweden, described an extended family, several members of which presented with neutropenia. Individuals with Kostmann syndrome present early in life with recurrent bacterial infection. Kostmann syndrome is a congenital disease due to a mutation in a nuclear gene (HAX-1) coding for a mitochondrial protein that protects developing myeloid cells from apoptosis. Researchers have identified several other mutations leading to maturational arrest of granulocyte differentiation in the bone marrow. Patients with these mutations also present with recurrent bacterial infections early in life.

Beginning in the 1960s, clinicians described at least 10 additional congenital defects in neutrophil differentiation. In 1964, Wolf Zuelzer of Wayne State University College of Medicine in Detroit, Michigan, described a 10-year-old female who presented with recurrent bacterial infections of the respiratory tract associated with chronic granulocytopenia in her peripheral blood. Evaluation of this patient's bone marrow revealed an increased number of myeloid cells including "an abundance of granulocytes at all levels of differentiation, and an actual increase in the percentage of segmented mature forms." Many of the nuclei in these mature granulocytes appeared to be degenerating—hematologists now recognize that these cells are undergoing apoptosis prior to release from the bone marrow. Zuelzer concluded that these granulocytes are unable to leave the bone marrow and proposed the term myelokathexis to describe this condition.

Neutrophils released to the peripheral blood migrate to areas of infection in tissue. This process, requiring interaction of integrins on neutrophils with selectins on endothelial cells of blood vessels, results in diapedesis of neutrophils. Patients with leukocyte adhesion deficiency lack integrins. Thus, despite sufficient neutrophils in the peripheral blood, these cells fail to reach the infectious loci, where they are needed.

In 1982 Amin Arnaout and colleagues from the Children's Hospital Medical Center in Boston, Massachusetts, described increased susceptibility to infection with pyogenic bacteria in an 8-year-old boy. Arnaout and coworkers demonstrated that leukocytes from this patient were defective in several receptor-coupled functions including uptake of particles coated with antibody, superoxide generation, and degranulation stimulated by phagocytosis. These defects correlated with the absence of a typically expressed cell surface glycoprotein of approximately 150,000 Da.

One year previously in 1981, Robert Todd and colleagues at Harvard Medical School in Boston developed two monoclonal antibodies specific for human monocytes. The antigen identified by one of these monoclonal antibodies is a heterodimer expressed by granulocytes as well as by monocytes. One of the chains of this antigen has a molecular weight of approximately 155,000 Da. Collaborative studies between Todd and his colleagues and Arnaout's group demonstrated that this monoclonal antibody was specific for the cell surface glycoprotein absent from the 8-year-old boy's white blood cells (Dana et al., 1984). Further study revealed that patients with one form of leukocyte adhesion deficiency have a mutation in the gene coding for this glycoprotein—the common β2 chain (CD18) of the β2 integrin family.

Decreased numbers of monocytes are also associated with impaired phagocytosis of microorganisms, particularly intracellular bacteria including *Mycobacterium tuberculosis* and *Salmonella*, viruses (varicella zoster), and fungi (*Histoplasma capsulatum*, *Coccidioides* spp.). Monocytes and their progeny including macrophages and dendritic cells present engulfed antigen to CD4+ T lymphocytes of the adaptive immune response.

Investigators have described several mutations in the genes coding for receptors or signaling molecules in macrophages. Melanie Newport and colleagues working at the Imperial College School of Medicine at St. Mary's, London and Erasmus University, Rotterdam, Netherlands, in 1996 analyzed the genomes of four related children who were unusually susceptible to mycobacterial infections. Newport's group identified mutations in a segment of chromosome 6 that contains the gene coding for the interferon (IFN)-γ receptor. The leukocytes of these children fail to express the IFN-γ receptor, and as a result their macrophages cannot respond to IFN-γ by producing the inflammatory cytokine, TNF-α. Patients with these mutations fail to mount an effective inflammatory response necessary to clear mycobacterial infections—the disease has been referred to as Mendelian susceptibility to mycobacterial diseases.

Defects of White Blood Cells—Qualitative

In 1957, Robert Good and his colleagues working at the University of Minnesota defined chronic granulomatous disease (CGD) as an X-linked syndrome (Berendes et al., 1957). They described four boys presenting with recurring infections due to *Staphylococci* and other catalase-positive bacteria. In 1966, Beulah Holmes working with Good and colleagues at the University of Minnesota demonstrated that granulocytes, from patients with this X-linked recessive condition, phagocytize but fail to kill bacteria. Holmes and her colleagues isolated polymorphonuclear leukocytes from three patients diagnosed with CGD and from unaffected individuals as controls. They incubated these cells with *Staphylococcus aureus* for 1 to 2h. At the end of the incubation period, they divided the cultures in half preparing stained smears with one portion and plating a second aliquot on nutrient agar.

In the stained smears, granulocytes from both sources contained bacteria indicating that phagocytosis was intact. Quantitation of the number of viable bacteria following incubation revealed a larger concentration of bacteria in preparations from CGD patients than in cells from healthy individuals. They saw similar results when they incubated patient granulocytes with a second, catalase-positive bacteria, *Aerobacter aerogenes*, leading Holmes and her coworkers to conclude "leukocytes of patients with granulomatosis seem to be capable of phagocytosis but defective in ability to kill or digest microorganisms."

Holmes and her group speculated that the defect in CGD may be due to a deficiency in an enzyme involved in the functioning of the lysosomes in white blood cells. Robert Baehner and David Nathan working at Harvard Medical School in Boston, Massachusetts, demonstrated in 1967 that phagocytes from patients with CGD failed to activate the hexose monophosphate shunt (respiratory burst) during phagocytosis of inert styrene particles thus inhibiting the production of hydrogen peroxide. This group further showed that phagocytes from CGD patients failed to reduce the dye nitroblue tetrazolium (NBT). Phagocytes from unaffected individuals reduce this dye from yellow to blue. These observations provided a laboratory test (the NBT test) that readily detects individuals with this defect.

Researchers have described mutations in genes coding for at least four different proteins involved in the generation of reactive oxygen species in CGD patients. While CGD is the most common congenital defect of the phagocytes of the innate host defenses, affecting approximately 4–5 of every 1,000,000 live births, additional phagocytic disorders have subsequently been described. These include mutations resulting in defects in chemotaxis, adhesion, and bacterial destruction.

Paul J. Edelson and collaborators at the University of California, San Francisco, in 1973 described three patients with recurrent bacterial infections including 2 females (6 months and 24 years of age) and a 9-year-old boy. Edelson isolated neutrophils from these patients and assessed their random migration from capillary tubes, their adhesion to a nylon wool column, and their mobility across a polycarbonate filter in response to a filtrate of an *Escherichia coli* culture.

The results of the random migration test and the adherence assay varied between the three patients, but in each instance at least one of the patients showed a defect in activity. Neutrophils from all three patients failed to migrate in response to the *E. coli* chemotactic signal. Based on these results, the authors conclude that an array of defects including those that involve cell membrane associated events can lead to deficiencies in neutrophil function.

Bernard Babior from the New England Medical Center Hospital in Boston, Massachusetts, collaborated with investigators from Tufts New England Medical Center, the National Institute of Allergy and Infectious Diseases, Duke University, and Harvard Medical School in a study of a 5-year-old boy with recurrent pyogenic infections (Crowley et al., 1980). Neutrophils isolated from this boy failed to respond to a chemotactic signal and showed decreased phagocytic activity. These researchers isolated proteins from neutrophils of the patient and of healthy individuals as controls. They compared the electrophoretic mobility of these proteins and reported that neutrophils from healthy individuals possess a glycoprotein with a molecular weight of 110 kDa (gp110) that was absent in the patient's neutrophils. Moreover, neutrophils from the patient's mother revealed a slight decrease in the amount of gp110 while neutrophils from his father and a brother contained the expected concentration of the protein. These results suggest that gp110 is a membrane protein involved in the response to chemotactic signals.

Defects of Natural Killer (NK) Lymphocytes

NK lymphocytes, a component of the innate host defenses, mediate cytotoxicity and produce cytokines (Chapter 28). They primarily protect the host against viral infections and malignantly transformed cells and differentiate from lymphoid stem cells. Human NK lymphocytes express several unique cell surface molecules including CD56; however, they fail to express the T lymphocyte marker, CD3, or a T cell receptor.

While physicians observe defects of NK lymphocytes in some patients with congenital immunodeficiencies of the adaptive immune response (Peter et al., 1983; Chapter 32), individuals with isolated defects of NK lymphocytes are rare. NK lymphocyte deficiencies are either quantitative or qualitative.

In 1989, Christine Biron working with John Sullivan at the University of Massachusetts Medical School in Worcester and Kevin Byron from Brown University in Providence, Rhode Island, described a 17-year-old female who presented with a herpes simplex virus infection of the skin. The patient's past medical history included recurrent bouts of otitis media and leukopenia. At age 13, she was hospitalized with a life-threatening varicella infection during which she developed varicella pneumonia.

Evaluation of this patient's immune system revealed decreased numbers of lymphocytes. During her hospitalization, her serum immunoglobulin levels decreased but returned to levels within acceptable reference range following recovery from the infection. T lymphocyte activity, measured by delayed hypersensitivity to tetanus toxoid, and in vitro proliferation to allogeneic lymphocytes and T lymphocyte mitogens was unaffected when compared to healthy individuals. Flow cytometric determination of lymphocytes from the patient's peripheral blood revealed numbers of T lymphocytes within the established reference range. Biron and her colleagues analyzed the phenotype of these T lymphocytes and demonstrated the presence of both CD4+ and CD8+ lymphocytes.

The patient's peripheral blood lacked lymphocytes that stained with NK lymphocyte markers including CD16 and NKH-1 (CD56). Functionally her peripheral blood lymphocytes failed to lyse several NK-sensitive target cell lines including K562 and Daudi, a B lymphocyte cell line derived from a patient with Burkitt lymphoma. Lysis of these targets was not increased when Biron and colleagues incubated the patient's lymphocytes with interferon-γ, a cytokine known to enhance NK lymphocyte activity, or with antibody, a treatment that leads to antibody-dependent cell-mediated cytotoxicity, another function of NK lymphocytes.

Investigators have described several mutations that lead to a reduced number of NK lymphocytes in peripheral blood and lymphoid tissue (Orange, 2013).

Mutations in the GATA2 gene, coding for a transcription factor involved in early events in hematopoiesis, result in deficiencies of several different lymphocyte populations including B, T, and NK. The MCM4 gene is responsible for NK lymphocyte maturation. Mutations in this gene, originally identified in a family with a history of recurrent viral infections as well as lymphoproliferative disease stimulated by Epstein–Barr virus, result in severely reduced numbers of NK lymphocytes. The peripheral blood of three members of this family had fewer than 1% of the expected numbers of NK lymphocytes.

Patients have also presented with qualitative defects due to loss-of-function mutations in genes coding for proteins involved in NK lymphocyte functions. These rare mutations usually affect more than just NK lymphocytes. For example, mutations in genes involved in the biosynthesis of perforin and granzyme affect both NK lymphocyte and cytotoxic T lymphocyte function. Similarly investigators have described patients with increased susceptibility to infections that have mutations in genes involved in other aspects of NK lymphocyte biology including (Wood et al., 2011)

- recognition of target cells,
- intracellular signaling and cell activation,
- granule biogenesis, and
- exocytosis of granules.

DEFICIENCIES OF THE COMPLEMENT SYSTEM

The complement system is a component of the innate host defenses that is co-opted by the adaptive immune response as an effector mechanism to eliminate potential pathogens (chapter12). Complement consists of approximately 30 different serum and cell membrane bound proteins that are sequentially activated. The complement cascade is triggered by the classical, the alternate, or the lectin pathway. All three pathways converge on activated C3 and result in initiation of inflammation and lysis of pathogens. The classical pathway requires interaction of the first component of complement (C1) with antibody bound to antigen. The alternate and lectin pathways are activated independent of antibody.

Researchers have described individuals that lack one or more of the complement components. Some of these individuals exhibit no signs or symptoms; others present either with difficulty eliminating infectious microorganisms or with manifestations of various autoimmune diseases, particularly immune complex disorders. Malnourished individuals often present with complement deficiencies resulting in defective responses to infectious microorganisms. Other individuals present with congenital complement deficiencies caused by mutations in genes coding for individual proteins of the complement cascade. Autosomal recessive (C2, C3, and others) as well as autosomal dominant (C1 inhibitor) and X-linked recessive (properdin) inheritance patterns have been reported.

Arthur Silverstein working at the Armed Forces Institute of Pathology in Washington, D.C., in 1960 first described a case of an individual lacking serum complement. The individual, David Pressman, was one of Silverstein's colleagues in the laboratory and originally donated some of his own blood for use as a source of complement (Rosen, 2000). Between 1952 and 1960, investigators tested hemolytic activity of Pressman's serum six times and compared it to the hemolytic activity of serum from individuals with intact complement systems. They used an assay in which the serum was added to antibody-coated sheep erythrocytes, and the amount of hemoglobin released was measured. In each assay, researchers measured the hemolytic activity of Pressman's serum and found it to be between 5% and 10% of the expected activity of healthy individuals.

Analysis of the individual complement components known at that time demonstrated a deficiency of C2 (in the early 1960s four components of complement were recognized—subsequent investigations revealed that the classical path of complement activation involves nine individual proteins). Despite this defect in C2, Pressman remained healthy.

In 1966, Martin Klemperer and colleagues working at Children's Hospital Medical Center in Boston, Massachusetts, described a second individual with a complement deficiency due to a mutation in the gene coding for complement component C2. These investigators demonstrated that this defect had an autosomal recessive mode of inheritance.

Congenital C2 deficiency is a relatively common defect in humans. During the 1970s, investigators described individuals lacking other complement components. While some individuals with complement deficiencies present with no adverse medical consequences, other patients have increased susceptibility to infections and develop immune complex-mediated pathologies including systemic lupus erythematosus.

In addition to deficiencies of the complement components involved in the cascade, clinicians have described patients with mutations in the genes coding for several of the regulatory proteins of the complement system. Patients with hereditary angioedema (HAE) present with periodic episodes of edema due to an inherited defect in production of an inhibitor of C1 esterase. The edema occurs at various anatomical locations but is most severe when it affects the respiratory tract leading to obstruction of the airway. In 1888, William Osler at the University of Pennsylvania provided an initial description of HAE in members of three families. During the ensuing 75 years

several additional reports of HAE appeared in the medical literature with little information about possible etiology.

In 1963, Virginia Donaldson and Richard Evan working at the Cleveland Clinic and Western Reserve School of Medicine in Cleveland, Ohio, discovered that patients with the disease lacked serum C1 esterase inhibitor, and they postulated erroneously that some serum factor destroyed or inactivated C1 esterase inhibitor. To test this hypothesis, they mixed serum from these patients with serum from unaffected individuals and measured the function of C1 esterase inhibitor in the mixture. Surprisingly, they demonstrated that the level of C1 esterase inhibitor in the mixture remained within the established reference range. Subsequently investigation showed that patients presenting with HAE have a mutation in the gene coding for C1 esterase inhibitor leading to either total absence or malfunction of the molecule. Current treatment involves periodic infusion of C1 esterase inhibitor.

Properdin, a serum protein originally described by Louis Pillemer and colleagues in 1954, stabilizes C3b and initiates the alternate complement pathway. In 1982, Anders Sjöholm and colleagues in Lund, Sweden, described three males in an extended family whose sera were deficient in properdin. One of these individuals died of fulminant infection with *Neisseria meningitidis* group C. Three other individuals in the same family died from *Neisseria* infections. Surprisingly, patients deficient in serum properdin are not unusually susceptible to infection with other bacteria.

Investigators have identified other families with a similar properdin deficiency. Members of these families are characterized by unusual sensitivity to infection with *Neisseria* but not to other bacteria. This disorder is transmitted as an X-linked recessive trait.

AUTOINFLAMMATORY DISEASES

Autoinflammatory disorders, a group of diseases characterized by periodic episodes of exaggerated inflammation and fever in the absence of microbial infection, are associated with mutations in genes regulating the production of inflammatory cytokines including IL-1. Clinicians have described both congenital and acquired forms of these diseases.

Familial Mediterranean fever (FMF), a prototype of the autoinflammatory disorders, and one of the most common, has been observed by physicians for thousands of years. Investigators estimate that in specific ethnic groups (Turks, Armenians, Arabs, Sepharidic Jews, and Italians) as many as 20% of the population carry the mutated gene. In 1945, Sheppard Siegal at Mt. Sinai Hospital in New York described a case of paroxysmal peritonitis. The patient presented with recurrent bouts of abdominal pain accompanied with fever as high as

105 °F. Subsequently other clinicians described patients with similar symptoms. These individuals all had a Middle Eastern ancestry and the disease segregated into families suggesting an underlying genetic cause.

In 1997, two groups identified the gene mutation responsible for this disease. The International FMF Consortium cloned a gene on chromosome 16. Individuals with FMF have one of three missense mutations not found in unaffected individuals. The mutated gene codes for pyrin, a protein expressed in the nuclei of granulocytes.

The French FMF Consortium likewise identified a candidate gene for FMF on chromosome 16. They called the protein coded by this gene marenostrim. Immunologists and geneticists now agree that the two proteins are identical and most investigators have adopted the pyrin name.

The function of the pyrin protein remains unknown at this time although it most likely interacts with other proteins in the cell to regulate the level of the inflammatory response. Absence of the protein results in unregulated inflammation resulting in the fever associated with FMF.

CONCLUSION

Innate host defense mechanisms provide the initial defense against invading pathogens thereby maintaining immunological homeostasis of the mammalian host in a potentially hostile, microbial environment. Defects in these defenses lead to a variety of pathologies. In addition to recurrent infections with pathogenic and opportunistic microorganisms, some patients with defective innate defenses present with immune complex-mediated autoimmune diseases.

Both acquired and congenital immunodeficiencies occur. Acquired defects result from malnutrition, trauma, surgery, exposure to radiation or chemotherapeutic drugs, or secondary to other disease processes including cancer or autoimmunity. These acquired deficiencies are likely to affect several of the individual components of the response and may reverse when the causative stimulus is removed or overcome.

Congenital defects are usually characterized by reduced numbers or function of white blood cells as well as decreased synthesis of defense-related mediators such as cytokines and chemokines or secretion of immunologically nonspecific reactants including components of the complement system. Investigations of these patients with these deficits reveal mutations in one or more genes crucial to the normal functioning of the innate host defense system. As a result, these deficiencies usually present early in life. Most of the diseases resulting from these mutations are rare; however, studies performed on affected patients provide valuable information about the mechanisms involved in protecting against potential pathogenic microorganisms.

A second type of pathology associated with abnormal innate host defense mechanisms results from overreactive responses leading to the spontaneous induction of fever and inflammation in the absence of any underlying cause. These autoinflammatory diseases are similar to autoimmune diseases involving the adaptive immune response (Chapter 34).

References

Al-Herz, W., Bousfiha, A., Casanova, J.-L., et al., 2014. Primary immunodeficiency diseases: an update on the classification from the International Union of Immunological Societies expert committee for primary immunodeficiency. Front. Immunol. 5, 1–33.

Arnaout, M.A., Pitt, J., Cohen, H.J., Melamed, J., Rosen, F.S., Colten, H.R., 1982. Deficiency of a granulocyte-membrane glycoprotein (gp150) in a boy with recurrent bacterial infections. N. Engl. J. Med. 306, 693–699.

Baehner, R.L., Nathan, D.G., 1967. Leukocyte oxidase: defective activity in chronic granulomatous disease. Science 155, 835–836.

Berendes, H., Bridges, R.A., Good, R.A., 1957. A fatal granulomatosus of childhood: the clinical study of a new syndrome. Minn. Med. 40, 309–312.

Biron, C.A., Byron, K.S., Sullivan, J.L., 1989. Severe herpesvirus infections in an adolescent without natural killer cells. N. Engl. J. Med. 320, 1731–1735.

Crowley, C.A., Curnutte, J.T., Rosin, R.E., André-Schwartz, J., Gallin, J.I., Klempner, M., Synderman, R., Southwick, F.S., Stossel, T.P., Babior, B.M., 1980. An inherited abnormality of neutrophil adhesion – its genetic transmission and its association with a missing protein. N. Engl. J. Med. 302, 1163–1168.

Dana, N., Todd, R.F., Pitt, J., Springer, T.A., Arnaout, M.A., 1984. Deficiency of a surface membrane glycoprotein (Mo1) in man. J. Clin. Invest. 73, 153–159.

Donaldson, V.H., Evan, R.R., 1963. A biochemical abnormality in hereditary angioneurotic edema: absence of serum inhibitor of C'1-esterase. Am. J. Med. 35, 37–44.

Edelson, P.J., Stites, D.P., Gold, S., Fudenberg, H.H., 1973. Disorders of neutrophil function. Defects in the early stages of the phagocytic process. Clin. Exp. Immunol. 13, 21–28.

Holmes, B., Quie, P.G., Windhorst, D.B., Good, R.A., 1966. Fatal granulomatous disease of childhood. An inborn abnormality of phagocytic function. Lancet 287, 1225–1228.

Jacobson, C.S., Berliner, N., 2014. Neutropenia. In: Greer, J.P. (Ed.), Wintrobe's Clinical Hematology. Lippincott, Williams and Wilkins, Philadelphia, PA. pp. 1279-1288.

Klemperer, M.R., Woodworth, H.C., Rosen, F.S., Austen, K.F., 1966. Hereditary deficiency of the second component of complement (C'2) in man. J. Clin. Invest. 45, 880–890.

Kostmann, R., 1956. Infantile genetic agranulocytosis; agranulocytosis infantilis hereditaria. Acta Paediatr. 45 (Suppl. 105), 1–78.

Newport, M.J., Huxley, C.M., Huston, S., Hawrylowicz, C.M., Oostra, B., Williamson, R., Levin, M., 1996. A mutation in the interferon-γ-receptor gene and susceptibility to mycobacterial infection. N. Engl. J. Med. 335, 1941–1946.

Orange, J.S., 2013. Natural killer cell deficiency. J. Allergy Clin. Immunol. 132, 515–525.

Osler, W., 1888. Hereditary angioneurotic edema. Am. J. Med. Sci. 95, 362–367.

Peter, H.H., Friedrich, W., Dopfer, R., Müller, W., Kortmann, C.C., Pichler, W.J., Heinz, F., Rieger, C.H., 1983. NK cell function in severe combined immunodeficiency (SCID): evidence of a common T and NK cell defect in some but not all SCID patients. J. Immunol. 131, 2332–2339.

Rosen, F.S., 2000. A brief history of immunodeficiency disease. Immunol. Rev. 178, 8–12.

Schultz, W., 1922. Über eigenartige Halserkrankungen. Dtsch. Med. Wochenschr. 48, 1495–1497.

Siegal, S., 1945. Benign paroxysmal peritonitis. Ann. Intern. Med. 23, 1–21.

Silverstein, A.M., 1960. Essential hypocomplementemia: report of a case. Blood 16, 1338–1341.

Sjöholm, A.G., Braconier, J.-H., Söderström, C., 1982. Properdin deficiency in a family with fulminant meningococcal infections. Clin. Exp. Immunol. 50, 291–297.

Stiehm, E.R., Johnston, R.B., 2005. A history of pediatric immunology. Ped. Res. 57, 458–467.

The French FMF Consortium, 1997. A candidate gene for familial Mediterranean fever. Nat. Genet. 17, 25–31.

The International FMF Consortium, 1997. Ancient missense mutations in a new member of the RoRet gene family are likely to cause familial Mediterranean fever. Cell 90, 797–807.

Todd, R.F., Nadler, L.M., Schlossman, S.F., 1981. Antigens on human monocytes identified by monoclonal antibodies. J. Immunol. 126, 1435–1442.

Wood, S.M., Ljunggren, H.-G., Bryceson, Y.T., 2011. Insights into NK cell biology from human genetics and disease associations. Cell. Mol. Life Sci. 68, 3479–3493.

Zuelzer, W.W., 1964. "Myelokathexis" – a new form of chronic granulocytopenia. Report of a case. N. Engl. J. Med. 270, 699–704.

TIME LINE

1888	William Osler describes three families with hereditary angioedema
1922	Werner Schultz describes clinical picture of patients with neutropenia
1956	Rolf Kostmann defines a congenital form of neutropenia resulting in severe recurrent infections in childhood
1957	Robert Good and colleagues describe four boys with "fatal granulomatosus"
1960	Arthur M. Silverstein reports a case of hypocomplementemia
1963	Virginia Donaldson and Richard Evan discover that patients with hereditary angioedema lack serum C1 esterase inhibitor
1964	Wolf Zuelzer describes an individual in which granulocytes fail to be released from the bone marrow (myelokathexis)
1966	Beulah Holmes and coworkers describe the underlying defect in granulocytes from patients with chronic granulomatous disease
1973	Paul Edelson and collaborators identify patients with recurrent bacterial infections in whom peripheral blood leukocytes failed to respond to chemotactic stimuli
1982	Andres Sjöholm and colleagues describe three males in an extended family with deficient serum properdin
1982	Amin Arnaout and colleagues describe an 8-year-old male lacking cell surface adhesion molecules (integrins) that make him susceptible to pyogenic infections
1989	Christine Biron and colleagues report a 13-year-old girl with severe and recurrent herpesvirus infections resulting from a lack of NK lymphocytes
1996	Melanie Newport and coworkers identify a mutation in the gene coding for the IFN-γ receptor leading to decreased inflammation and increased susceptibility to mycobacterial diseases

Defects in the Adaptive Immune Response Leading to Recurrent Infections

INTRODUCTION

The adaptive immune system is activated by pathogens that escape innate host defense mechanisms. Individuals with deficiencies in the adaptive immune system often present with a history of repeated infections. Defects of the adaptive immune response (immunodeficiencies) may be either congenital (primary) or acquired. Congenital immunodeficiencies are rare but serious disorders characterized by an unusual susceptibility to recurrent infections with the same microorganism or by infections with microbes that are rarely pathogenic. The etiology of these immunodeficiencies involves mutations in a variety of genes coding for proteins required for the proper development or functioning of the adaptive immune system. Investigation of these mutations and the diseases they cause has provided insights into the differentiation and operation of the adaptive immune system.

Prior to the development of antibiotics, most patients with congenital immunodeficiencies developed recurrent infections within the first year of life that failed to readily resolve; many died prematurely. The advent of antibiotics in the 1940s permitted some of these infants to survive for various periods of time although the threat of infection was ever present. Over 100 different congenital immunodeficiency disorders have been

categorized leading to a deeper understanding of the function of the healthy human adaptive immune system. Robert Good, one of the leaders in the study of these congenital defects, termed these diseases "experiments of nature."

Acquired immunodeficiencies have existed for centuries and, until fairly recently, were caused either by other underlying diseases (e.g., cancer, malnutrition) or as a complication from some medical treatment (e.g., bleeding and purging, drugs that kill lymphocytes). Since the early 1980s clinicians recognized another example of acquired immunodeficiency caused by infection of CD4$^+$ T lymphocytes with the human immunodeficiency virus (HIV).

The International Union of Immunological Societies established an expert committee for primary immunodeficiencies that meets periodically to update the classification of these diseases and to develop guidelines for diagnosis and management. This committee works with the World Health Organization and Orpha.net, a Web portal for rare diseases and orphan drugs (http://www.orpha.net/consor/cgi-bin/index.php) to update and revise the International Classification of Disease codes for primary immunodeficiencies. A recent publication by this committee (Al-Herz et al., 2014) divides these disorders into eight groups and provides key clinical and laboratory features for each disease as well as presumed etiology. The historical background of some of these disorders involving the adaptive immune system is covered in this chapter.

PRIMARY (CONGENITAL) IMMUNODEFICIENCIES

Early Examples of Immunodeficiency in Children

Between 1920 and 1950, clinicians identified several patients with immunodeficiencies including ataxia–telangiectasia, chronic mucocutaneous candidiasis, and Wiskott–Aldrich syndrome (Stiehm and Johnston, 2005). While the mechanisms responsible for these immunodeficiencies remained obscure at the time, subsequent research demonstrated that these diseases result from mutations in one or more genes.

Ataxia–telangiectasia (A–T): Ladislav Syllaba and Kamil Hemmer in 1926 described three Czech siblings with progressive cerebellar ataxia and ocular telangiectasia. In 1941, Denise Louis-Bar reported a 9-year-old girl with similar presenting symptoms. In addition to neurological problems, these patients present with recurrent sinopulmonary infections, dilated blood vessels in the eye and on the skin, immune system abnormalities including defective immunoglobulin synthesis of one or more of the immunoglobulin classes, and decreased circulating T lymphocytes. This constellation of symptoms is called A-T and is considered a primary immunodeficiency.

A-T patients are susceptible to increased numbers of respiratory infections with opportunistic microorganisms. The gene responsible for this syndrome is transmitted as an autosomal recessive trait. Investigators discovered a mutation in a gene (ATM) coding for a protein involved in regulating the cell cycle and repairing double stranded DNA breaks. This protein also regulates expression of the tumor suppressor gene, p53. As a result, approximately 20–25% of patients with A-T develop cancer (usually lymphoma or leukemia) during the second or third decade of life.

Chronic mucocutaneous candidiasis: In 1929, Edward S. Thorpe and Harry E. Handley at the University of Pennsylvania described a young girl who presented with tetany associated with chronic mycelial infection of the mouth, a syndrome now termed chronic mucocutaneous candidiasis. Patients present with recurrent or persistent infection of their mucous membranes, skin, and nails with *Candida albicans* or with another *Candida* species. These patients lack mature, functioning T lymphocytes; several different gene mutations have been implicated.

Wiskott-Aldrich syndrome: Alfred Wiskott in 1937 and Robert Aldrich in 1954 independently described patients with the Wiskott–Aldrich syndrome. Patients presenting with this syndrome are characterized by a history of recurrent infections, eczema, and thrombocytopenia. This X-linked disease is caused by mutations in the Wiskott–Aldrich syndrome (*WAS*) gene that codes for a protein expressed in all blood cells. This protein is involved in the development and function of the actin cytoskeleton of cells. In lymphocytes, mutations of the *WAS* gene inhibit interactions between lymphocytes, macrophages, and pathogens thereby interfering with transmission of activation signals. Mutations in the *WAS* gene are associated with other congenital immunodeficiencies including X-linked thrombocytopenia and severe congenital neutropenia (http://ghr.nlm.nih.gov/gene/WAS).

Deficiencies of Antibody Production— Agammaglobulinemia

In 1952, Colonel Ogden C. Bruton (1908–2003), a pediatrician at Walter Reed Army Hospital in Washington D.C., described an 8-year-old male patient with a 4-year history of recurrent infections. The patient originally presented at 4.5 years of age with a 2-day history of fever and bone pain. His physician diagnosed him with osteomyelitis and treated him with penicillin. During the next 3.5 years, he developed numerous episodes of fever and apparent infection that were treated with sulfa drugs and/or antibiotics. When Bruton saw the patient he reviewed this history and summarized the frequency of infections, the type of the pneumococcus isolated, other diseases documented, and attempted therapies; this summary is reproduced in Figure 32.1.

Bruton thoroughly evaluated the patient at 8 years of age and hypothesized that he failed to make antibodies based on the observation that the same microorganism was isolated on numerous occasions. Bruton developed a pneumococcal vaccine containing the strains isolated from the patient and administered it over a period of 5 months. No evidence of antibody production was obtained. Administration of a commercially prepared polysaccharide vaccine incorporating a number of different pneumococcal strains likewise failed to induce antibody production.

Tests for the presence of antibody to other microorganisms also were negative. The patient had a positive Schick test despite having received the normal pediatric immunizations with diphtheria toxoid. (A Schick test involves injecting a small amount of dilute diphtheria toxin intradermally to test for susceptibility to infection with diphtheria. A positive reaction is manifested by a cutaneous reaction. Individuals with antitoxin antibodies will fail to react to the toxin and have a negative reaction.) Antibodies to a typhoid vaccine could not be elicited, and the patient's serum was negative for antibody to mumps despite having had this disease three

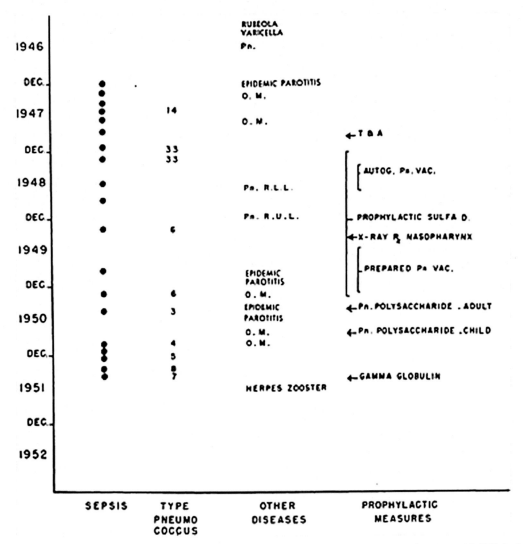

FIGURE 32.1   Time course of symptoms recorded and prophylactic measures attempted in the initial patient with X-linked agammaglobulinemia. OM = otitis media; Pn = pneumococcal infection; T + A = tonsillectomy and adenoidectomy; Pn Vac = pneumococcal vaccine. *From Bruton, O.C., 1952. Pediatrics 9, 722.*

times. Bruton proposed that there might be a defect in the patient's gamma globulin and ordered a serum electrophoresis.

Arne Tiselius developed serum electrophoresis in the 1930s (Chapter 11). In 1939, Tiselius and Kabat demonstrated that virtually all serum antibody activity migrated electrophoretically with the gamma globulin fraction. In 1952, when Bruton sent the serum of his patient to the laboratory for analysis, serum electrophoresis was a relatively new diagnostic tool. The initial laboratory report showed a complete absence of gamma globulin. Thinking there had been an error, Bruton sent a second sample. The laboratory once again reported no detectable gamma globulin. Based on this result, Bruton concluded that the patient lacked antibodies and initiated a series of subcutaneous injections with normal human serum globulin containing gamma globulin. This treatment resulted in elevated levels of serum gamma

globulin that declined over a 6-week period. Continued monthly treatment with gamma globulin provided protection for this patient for nearly 60 years against most bacterial infections.

Researchers subsequently demonstrated that the genetic basis for Bruton agammaglobulinemia is a mutated gene on the X chromosome. Boys with X-linked agammaglobulinemia (XLA) usually present with recurrent bacterial infections although they occasionally have difficulty with persistent viral and parasitic infections as well. They are unable to produce antibodies of any isotype.

Mechanistically, there is a block in the development of B lymphocytes. XLA patients have normal numbers of pre-B lymphocytes in their bone marrow but lack circulating, mature B lymphocytes and plasma cells. Two groups of investigators cloned the responsible gene using positional cloning (Tsukada et al., 1993; Vetrie et al., 1993). These researchers demonstrated that the mutated gene normally codes for a protein–tyrosine kinase. This tyrosine kinase, expressed in all hematopoietic cells, is particularly important for development of B lymphocytes. This enzyme, known as Bruton tyrosine kinase (Btk), is required for the differentiation of pre-B cells into mature, functioning B lymphocytes. Mutations in this gene inhibit transmission of signals from the pre-B cell receptor to the nucleus.

Investigators subsequently reported several other congenital defects affecting antibody production. These defects result from mutations in genes coding for several different proteins including

- the μ-heavy chain,
- proteins that transmit the signal from the B cell receptor to the nucleus, and
- structural components of the B cell receptor and cell-surface molecules that receive second signals for activation and/or isotype switching.

Deficiencies of T Lymphocytes—Thymic Dysplasia

Beginning in the 1960s investigators described several disorders affecting T lymphocytes. Deficiencies of T lymphocytes lead to a more severe set of clinical findings than is seen with B lymphocyte defects due to the numerous roles of T lymphocytes in many of the protective functions of the adaptive immune response. Patients with deficiencies of T lymphocytes present earlier in life with infections caused by a variety of microorganisms including viruses, fungi, and intracellular bacteria. This section presents two examples of T lymphocyte deficiencies both due to failure of thymic development, Nezelof syndrome and DiGeorge syndrome.

Christian Nezelof (1922–2015), a pediatrician and pathologist at Necker Hospital, Paris, initially reported a case of thymic hypoplasia in 1964 just 3 years after Jacques Miller's seminal work at the Walter and Eliza Hall Institute in Melbourne, Australia, demonstrating the role of the thymus in the development of lymphocytes (Miller, 1961). Nezelof syndrome, a rare, congenital, autosomal recessive immunodeficiency that affects both males and females, is characterized by a lack of T lymphocyte-mediated immune responses in patients with levels of serum immunoglobulin near or within established reference ranges. Individuals affected with Nezelof syndrome lack a thymic shadow on radiological examination and present with severe, recurrent infections within the first 6 months of life. These infections are primarily due to pathogens that parasitize living cells, including viruses, fungi, and intracellular bacteria. Individuals with Nezelof syndrome often die before the age of two unless they receive a graft of fetal thymus.

Three years later Angelo DiGeorge and his colleagues working at the University of São Paulo, Brazil, reported a group of patients lacking a functional thymus (Lischner et al., 1967). DiGeorge, a pediatric endocrinologist, attended a lecture by Max Cooper at the 1965 meeting of the Society for Pediatric Research (Cooper et al., 1965). Cooper's data, obtained from thymectomized and bursectomized chickens, supported the division of the immune system into distinct functional components (Chapter 10). At this presentation, DiGeorge realized that Cooper's results helped make sense of patients he had been treating.

DiGeorge's patients initially presented with tetany due to a congenital absence of the parathyroid glands responsible for calcium homeostasis. Despite adequate control of serum calcium levels, all four initial patients succumbed, most likely to infections. On autopsy pathologists failed to find any trace of the thymus gland. Patients with this syndrome present with a history of recurrent infections, absence of delayed hypersensitivity reactions, retention of skin allografts, and a failure to produce antibodies following immunization with several antigens. Additional findings, obvious at birth, include cardiac malformations and structural defects in the palatal region. Researchers confirmed that these findings are related and can be traced to abnormal development of the third and fourth pharyngeal pouches during embryogenesis. This defect results from a deletion in chromosome 22; the severity of the disease is related to the size of the deletion. What was formerly termed DiGeorge syndrome is now called 22q11.2 deletion syndrome (Fomin et al., 2010).

Severe Combined Immunodeficiency (SCID)

In the late 1950s and early 1960s, investigators in Switzerland described several patients who presented with immunodeficiencies that affected both antibody production (B lymphocytes) and cell-mediated responses including delayed hypersensitivity and allograft rejections (T lymphocytes) (Hitzig et al., 1958; Tobler and Cottier, 1958; Hitzig and Willi, 1961; Freycon et al., 1961). Infants from consanguineous marriages constituted an unusual share of the initial cohort of these patients, and some pediatricians felt this was a unique form of immunodeficiency due to inbreeding. Initially termed Swiss type agammaglobulinemia, it is now included in a group of diseases known as severe combined immunodeficiency (SCID).

In 1962, Fred Rosen, David Gitlin, and Charles Janeway at The Children's Hospital Medical Center at

Harvard reported a case of a 15-month-old infant who presented with similar signs and symptoms. This boy demonstrated both agammaglobulinemia and defects in delayed type hypersensitivity and allograft rejection. The patient presented with a history of recurrent respiratory infections and failure to gain weight. Laboratory evaluation revealed decreased serum gamma globulin as well as neutropenia. The researchers reported an absence of isohemagglutinins to the B blood group antigen despite typing the boy's red cells as type A. He also failed to generate a delayed hypersensitivity skin reaction to an antigen from *C. albicans* despite having been infected with the fungus.

Rosen and his colleagues reported decreased numbers of peripheral blood lymphocytes and lymphoid tissues that lacked germinal centers, small lymphocytes, or plasma cells. They transplanted thymus from a 5-month-old donor in an attempt to correct these deficiencies, but this failed to reverse the immunodeficiency. At autopsy, the patient's thymus weighed less than 1 g and no lymphocytes or Hassall's corpuscles were noted.

While the underlying mechanism of the defect in these patients was not known, subsequent studies have defined several mutations that can lead to similar clinical pictures. Geneticists have identified both X-linked and autosomal recessive modes of inheritance among the numerous forms of SCID. X-linked forms of SCID result from mutations in genes coding for either a polypeptide chain common to the receptors for several interleukins including IL-2, IL-4, IL-7, IL-9, IL-15, and IL-21 or for cell-surface molecules involved in T and B lymphocyte activation. Autosomal recessive forms of SCID result from mutations in genes coding for several important regulatory mechanisms in the adaptive immune response including proteins involved in the expression of major histocompatibility complex-coded molecules on the cell surface.

Clinicians use the information garnered from genetic studies of SCID patients to confirm the mechanisms responsible for the functioning of the healthy adaptive immune response and to provide novel therapeutic interventions to try to correct the defect. Many children with congenital immunodeficiency disease are treated with bone marrow transplantation while others respond better to transfusions of their own cells that have been genetically manipulated with an unmutated gene (Chapter 38).

Bare Lymphocyte Syndrome

In 1978, Jean-Louis Touraine and colleagues in Lyon, France, described an individual whose cells failed to express class I histocompatibility (HLA) molecules on their surface. A 4-month-old male with refractory oral candidiasis was referred to Touraine and colleagues. One month later he was hospitalized with pneumonia caused by *Pneumocystis carinii (jiroveci)*. Despite aggressive treatment, he succumbed to respiratory failure at 8 months of age.

The patient presented with lymphopenia, virtually absent T lymphocytes, and a B lymphocyte count that was at the lower limit of the established reference range. Delayed hypersensitivity skin tests to *Candida* and to dinitrofluorobenzene (a skin sensitizer) proved equivocal. Antibody levels were virtually undetectable including isohemagglutinins to the A and B blood group antigens (patient had O type blood). Complement levels were within reference range.

Touraine and her colleagues incubated peripheral blood leukocytes from the patient, his parents, and a sibling with antibodies to several HLA-A and HLA-B cell-surface molecules. The patient's leukocytes failed to stain with any of the antibodies while leukocytes from his parents and sibling stained positively. The authors conclude that the patient cells failed to express class I HLA molecules. The patient's peripheral blood leukocytes stimulated allogeneic lymphocytes in a mixed leukocyte reaction (MLR). A positive MLR indicates that the stimulator cells express class II HLA molecules.

At the time that Touraine and colleagues reported this case the immunologic role of the HLA molecules in presenting antigenic epitopes to T lymphocytes was still controversial (Chapter 20). Immunologists now appreciate that class I HLA molecules are required to present peptides from antigens to CD8+ cytotoxic T lymphocytes. Based on this knowledge, the fact that this patient suffered recurrent fungal infections (*Candida* and *Pneumocystis*) is expected.

Patients who fail to express both HLA class I and class II molecules on the surface of their cells are characterized by severe immunodeficiency that affects both antibody production and cell-mediated immunity. In 1980, Claude Griscelli and colleagues working at the Hôpital Neckar Enfants-Malades in Paris, France, described five children who presented with diarrhea, failure to thrive, and recurrent respiratory infections starting at 3 months of age. The numbers of B and T lymphocytes in these patients were variable but not drastically reduced from the numbers in unaffected, age-matched controls. The expression of class I and class II HLA molecules on peripheral blood leukocytes was reduced—the authors concluded that "since ... HLA antigens (are) necessary for a full expression of immune responses ... immunocompetent cells may not cooperate, especially in responses to T dependent antigens, in patients with defective HLA expression."

ACQUIRED IMMUNODEFICIENCY SYNDROME (AIDS)

In June 1981, Michael Gottleib and colleagues working in Los Angeles, California, published a description in *Morbidity and Mortality Weekly Report* of five cases of *Pneumocystis* pneumonia in young, homosexual males. Two of the patients died prior to publication of the report while the three survivors had severely depressed numbers of T lymphocytes. Within a month a second report appeared in *Morbidity and Mortality Weekly Report* describing 26 homosexual men aged 26–51 years who presented with Kaposi sarcoma, a rarely diagnosed malignancy. Several of these men, who lived in California or New York, presented with pneumonia, the causative agent of which, *P. carinii* (now *Pneumocystis jiroveci*), is pathogenic only in immunocompromised individuals (Friedman-Kein et al., 1981). These two brief publications as well as several others prompted the U.S. Centers for Disease Control and Prevention (CDC) to establish a task force to investigate the relationship between Kaposi sarcoma and opportunistic infections; the task force concluded that these cases represented a new infectious disease, acquired immunodeficiency syndrome (AIDS) (CDC, 1982).

This finding prompted several research groups to search for the causative agent of this immunosuppressive disease. Two groups, one led by Luc Montagnier at the Pasteur Institute in Paris and a second led by Robert Gallo at the National Cancer Institute of the National Institutes of Health, Bethesda, Maryland, isolated HIV and demonstrated that HIV causes AIDS.

HIV is a retrovirus in which the genetic material is coded in RNA rather than DNA. During the 1970s, virologists achieved significant advances in characterizing RNA tumor viruses culminating in 1980 when Gallo and his group isolated the first human retrovirus from a patient with a T cell leukemia (Poiesz et al., 1980). They called this virus human T cell leukemia virus type I (HTLV-I). Researchers isolated a second retrovirus, HTLV-II, from a cell line derived from a patient with hairy cell leukemia. During a workshop on AIDS held at the Cold Spring Harbor Laboratory, Long Island, New York, in 1982, Gallo speculated that AIDS is most likely caused by a retrovirus that is a variant of HTLV-I or II.

In 1983, Francoise Barré-Sinoussi working with Luc Montagnier and coworkers in Paris isolated a retrovirus from cultures of T lymphocytes derived from a patient with lymphadenopathy, a syndrome known to increase a patient's risk of developing AIDS. This virus, different from either HTLV-I or II, was named lymphadenopathy associated virus (LAV). The authors speculated that "this virus … belongs to a general family of T-lymphotropic retroviruses that are horizontally transmitted in humans and may be involved in several pathological syndromes, including AIDS."

The issue of *Science* in which this report appeared included four other papers suggesting a link between human T cell leukemia virus and AIDS (summarized by Marx, 1983). The evidence contained in these papers includes the isolation of HTLV from some AIDS patients, detection of HTLV DNA from the T cells of some AIDS patients, and the presence of antibody to HTLV in AIDS patients at a level greater than that found in unaffected individuals.

During the next 2 years, there was a flurry of activity including sharing of cultures and reagents between Montagnier's laboratory at the Pasteur Institute and Gallo's laboratory at the National Institutes of Health. Gallo and his colleagues isolated a virus similar to LAV from T lymphocytes obtained from AIDS patients; they named this virus HTLV-III (Popovic et al., 1984). Gallo's group in 1984 demonstrated that HTLV-III could be isolated from the majority of AIDS and pre-AIDS patients but not from healthy individuals. AIDS patients also consistently presented with antibodies in their serum against HTLV-III. These papers are now generally accepted as strengthening an association between infection with HTLV-III/LAV (HIV) and eventual development of AIDS. Additional background and references on the early history of the search for the AIDS virus is reported in a joint paper by Gallo and Montagnier (1987).

The search for the AIDS virus engendered intense rivalry for priority both between the scientists and at the level of the national leadership of France and the United States. In 1987, Prime Minister Jacques Chirac of France and President Ronald Regan of the United States met and agreed that the groups led by Montagnier and Gallo should jointly share credit for the discovery of the AIDS virus. This dispute was about more than national pride since the United States had filed a patent for a diagnostic test for HIV, and the potential monetary return on this patent was significant. The history of this search has been recounted numerous times including in a series of historical statements published in *Science* in 2002 (Gallo, 2002; Gallo and Montagnier, 2002; Montagnier, 2002).

Cells that express surface CD4 markers along with the chemokine receptor type 5 (CCR5) serve as the target for HIV infection. Evidence for the role of CD4 in HIV infectivity came from two observations:

- vesicular stomatitis virus expressing retroviral envelope antigens infected CD4+ lymphocytes but not lymphocytes expressing other cell-surface markers (Dalgleish et al., 1984); and

- antibodies to CD4 but not to other cell-surface markers interfered with HIV infectivity (Dalgleish et al., 1984; Klatzman et al., 1984).

By the mid to late 1980s, most scientists accepted the proposition that HIV causes AIDS although at least one prominent biologist disputed this fact (i.e., Duesberg, 1988, 1996). The early evidence was primarily epidemiological, and it was only during the decade between 1985 and 1996 that immunologists obtained evidence to demonstrate fulfillment of Koch's postulates. In 1996, Stephen O'Brien and James Goedert published a review in which they argued that HIV fulfills Koch's postulates. In addition to the epidemiological evidence, they make the following points:

- HIV has been isolated from many AIDS patients. In some patients in which HIV itself cannot be isolated, the genetic material coding for the virus is detectable using polymerase chain reaction.
- Accidental infection of laboratory workers while working with HIV resulted in a marked decrease in $CD4^+$ T lymphocytes and the occurrence of opportunistic infections, both indicators of AIDS. Recent data (CDC, 2011) report that there have been 57 healthcare workers who seroconverted to HIV due to occupational exposure.
- Several patients treated by an HIV-positive dentist tested positive for HIV antibodies even though they had no risk factors except invasive dental procedures performed by the dentist. The dentist and at least two of the infected patients have subsequently died of AIDS-related complications.
- A strain of HIV (HIV-2) causes an AIDS-like disease when injected into baboons.
- Transfer of HIV to SCID mice that have been reconstituted with human lymphoid stem cells results in an infection characterized by decreased $CD4^+$ T lymphocytes.

$CD4^+$ T lymphocytes serve as helpers for B lymphocytes and $CD8^+$ T lymphocytes. They also activate the inflammatory response. As a result they are instrumental in providing protection against many potentially pathogenic microorganisms. Once infected with HIV a $CD4^+$ T lymphocyte has a shortened half-life especially if it is activated by the antigen for which it is specific. As a result, HIV-infected individuals gradually lose $CD4^+$ T lymphocytes and are subject to a myriad of life-threatening infections and malignancies. HIV infection and the resulting AIDS epidemic attracted the interest of many immunologists, both clinicians and basic scientists, and stimulated significant funding from the National Institutes of Health in the United States and from similar national and private research funding organizations around the world. This funding in turn stimulated several novel approaches to control the progression of the disease. A future goal of ongoing investigations is the development of a vaccine that inhibits viral transmission and destroys virally infected lymphocytes.

The discovery of HIV and its role in AIDS are two of the most significant advances in medicine made during the second half of the twentieth century. The Nobel Prize in Physiology or Medicine for 2008 was awarded to Luc Montagnier and François Barré-Sinoussi "for their discovery of HIV." They shared the prize with Harald zur Hausen who discovered the role of human papilloma virus in cervical cancer. Several commentators (e.g., Vahine, 2009) suggested that Robert Gallo should have shared in this prize—the Nobel Prize Committee makes no comment on the rationale for including or excluding any scientist.

CONCLUSION

The adaptive immune system functions efficiently to eliminate potential pathogens that escape innate host defenses. Defects of the adaptive system result in overwhelming infections with a variety of microorganisms. These immunodeficiencies may be either congenital or acquired. Prior to the availability of antibiotics, clinicians in several countries sporadically reported children with histories of recurrent infections. The first description of a congenital immunodeficiency disease is attributed to Col. Ogden Bruton in 1952 with his publication of a case report of an 8-year-old boy with XLA. Since 1952, investigators have described patients with more than 100 different congenital immunodeficiencies affecting T lymphocytes, B lymphocytes, and antigen-presenting cells.

The study of immunodeficiency disorders confirmed and broadened our understanding of the adaptive immune responses. Although rare, congenital immunodeficiencies demonstrate the intricate interactions of the cells and molecules of the system. For many of the congenital immunodeficiencies the underlying genetic defects have been described. Therapy for some of these patients is now available, and new interventions are under development.

The HIV epidemic leading to AIDS has fostered an explosion of basic science and clinical research in the field of immunology. Before the causative agent for AIDS was identified, the virus spread relatively unimpeded through unprotected sex, childbirth, needle sharing, and a contaminated blood supply. Once a test for HIV was developed, transmission by blood transfusion was drastically curtailed especially in the developed countries; however, AIDS transmission remains a major epidemic around the world.

References

Al-Herz, W., Bousfiha, A., Casanova, J.-L., et al., 2014. Primary immunodeficiency diseases: an update on the classification from the International Union of Immunological Societies expert committee for primary immunodeficiency. Front. Immunol. 5, 1–33.

Aldrich, R., Sternberg, A.G., Campbell, D.C., 1954. Pedigree demonstrating a sex-linked recessive condition characterized by draining ears, eczematoid dermatitis and bloody diarrhea. Pediatrics 13, 133–139.

Barré-Sinoussi, F., Chermann, J.C., Rey, F., Nugeyre, M.T., Chamaret, S., Gruest, J., Dauget, C., Axel-Blin, C., Vézinet-Brun, R., Rouzioux, C., Rozenbaum, W., Montagnier, L., 1983. Isolation of a T-lymphotropic retrovirus from a patient at risk for acquired immune deficiency syndrome (AIDS). Science 220, 868–871.

Bruton, O.C., 1952. Agammaglobulinemia. Pediatrics 9, 722–728.

CDC, 1982. Epidemiological aspects of the current outbreak of Kaposi's sarcoma and opportunistic infections. N. Eng. J. Med. 306, 248–252.

CDC, 2011. Surveillance of occupationally acquired HIV/AIDS in healthcare personnel, as of December 2010. http://www.cdc.gov/HAI/organisms/hiv/Surveillance-Occupationally-Acquired-HIV-AIDS.html.

Cooper, M.D., Peterson, R.D.A., Good, R.A., 1965. A new concept of the cellular basis of immunity. J. Ped. 67, 907–908.

Dalgleish, A.G., Beverley, P.C.L., Clapham, P.R., Crawford, D.H., Greaves, M.F., Weiss, R.A., 1984. The CD4 (T4) antigen is an essential component of the receptor for the AIDS retrovirus. Nature 312, 763–767.

Duesberg, P.H., 1988. HIV is not the cause of AIDS. Science 241, 514.

Duesberg, P., 1996. Inventing the AIDS Virus. Regenery Pub., Washington, D.C.

Fomin, A.B.F., Pastorino, A.C., Kim, C.A., Pereira, A.C., Carneiro-Sampaio, M., Jacob, M.A., 2010. DiGeorge syndrome: a not so rare disease. Clinics 65, 865–869.

Freycon, F., Jeune, M., Larbre, F., Germain, D., 1961. Lymphoplasmocytic aplasia in infants with alymphocytosis and hypogammaglobulinemia. J. Med. Lyon 42, 147–192.

Friedman-Kien, A., Lauberstein, L., Marmor, M., et al., 1981. Kaposi's sarcoma and *Pneumocystis* pneumonia among homosexual men—New York City and California. MMWR. 30, 305–308. http://www.jstor.org.ezproxy1.lib.asu.edu/stable/pdf/23300179.pdf.

Gallo, R.C., 2002. Historical essay. The early years of HIV/AIDS. Science 298, 1728–1730.

Gallo, R.C., Montagnier, L., 1987. The chronology of AIDS research. Nature 326, 435–436.

Gallo, R.C., Montagnier, L., 2002. Historical essay. Prospects for the future. Science 298, 1730–1731.

Gottlieb, M.S., Schanker, H.M., Fan, P.T., Saxon, A., Weisman, J.D., Pozalski, I., 1981. *Pneumocystis* pneumonia-Los Angeles. MMWR. 30, 250–252. http://www.jstor.org.ezproxy1.lib.asu.edu/stable/pdf/23295554.pdf?&acceptTC=true&jpdConfirm=true.

Griscelli, C., Durandy, A., Virelizier, J.L., Hors, J., Lepage, V., Colombani, J., 1980. Impaired cell-to-cell interaction in partial combined immunodeficiency with variable expression of HLA antigens. In: Seligmann, M., Hitzig, W.H. (Eds.), Primary Immunodeficiencies, INSERM Symposium No. 16. Elsevier/North Holland, Amsterdam, pp. 499–503.

Hitzig, W.H., Biro, Z., Bosch, H., Huser, H.J., 1958. Agammaglobulinemia and alymphocytosis with atrophy of lymphatic tissue. Helv. Paediatr. Acta 13, 551–585.

Hitzig, W.H., Willi, H., 1961. Hereditary lymphoplasmacytic dysgenesis ("alymphocytosis with agammaglobulinemia"). Schweiz. Med. Wochenschr. 91, 1625–1633.

Klatzman, D., Champagne, E., Chamaret, S., Gruest, J., Guetard, D., Hercend, T., Gluckman, J.-G., Montagnier, L., 1984. T-lymphocyte T4 molecule behaves as the receptor for human retrovirus LAV. Nature 312, 767–768.

Lischner, H.W., Punnett, H.H., DiGeorge, A.M., 1967. Lymphocytes in the absence of the thymus. Nature 214, 580–582.

Louis-Bar, D., 1941. Sur un syndrome progressif comprenant des télangietasies capillaires cutanées et conjonctivales symétriques, ä disposition naevoide et des troubles cérébelleux. Confin. Neurol. (Basel) 4, 32.

Marx, J.L., 1983. Human T-cell leukemia virus linked to AIDS. Science 220, 806–809.

Miller, J.F.A.P., 1961. Immunological function of the thymus. Lancet 278, 748–749.

Montagnier, L., 2002. Historical essay. A history of HIV discovery. Science 298, 1727–1728.

Nezelof, C., Jammet, M.L., Lortholary, P., Labrune, B., Lamy, M., 1964. Hereditary thymic aplasia: its place and responsibility in a case of lymphocytic, normoplasmocytic and normoglobulinemia aplasia in an infant. Arch. Fr. Pediatr. 21, 897–920.

Poiesz, B.J., Ruscetti, F.W., Gazdar, A.F., Bunn, P.A., Minna, J.D., Gallo, R.C., 1980. Detection and isolation of type C retrovirus from fresh and cultured lymphocytes of a patient with cutaneous T cell lymphoma. Proc. Nat. Acad. Sci. U.S.A. 77, 7415–7419.

Popovic, M., Samgadharan, M.G., Read, E., Gallo, R.C., 1984. Detection, isolation, and continuous production of cytopathic retroviruses (HTLV-III) from patients with AIDS and pre-AIDS. Science 224, 497–500.

Rosen, F.S., Gitlin, D., Janeway, C.A., 1962. Alymphocytosis, agammaglobulinemia, homografts, and delayed hypersensitivity: study of a case. Lancet 280, 380–381.

Stiehm, E.R., Johnston, R.B., 2005. A history of pediatric immunology. Ped. Res. 57, 458–467.

Syllaba, L., Hemmer, K., 1926. Contribution a L'independence de l'athetose double idiopathique et congenitale: atteinte familiae, syndrome dystrophique, signe du reseauvasculaire conjonctival, integrite psychique. Rev. Neurol. (Paris) 1, 541–562.

Thorpe, E.S., Handley, H.E., 1929. Chronic tetany and chronic mycelia stomatitis in a child aged four and one-half years. Am. J. Dis. Child. 38, 328–338.

Tiselius, A., Kabat, E.A., 1939. An electrophoretic study of immune serum and purified antibody preparations. J. Exp. Med. 69, 119–131.

Tobler, R., Cottier, H., 1958. Familial lymphopenia with agammaglobulinemia and severe moniliasis: the essential lymphocytophthisis as a special form of early childhood agammaglobulinemia. Helv. Paediatr. Acta 12, 215–240.

Touraine, J.-L., Betuel, H., Souillet, G., Jeune, M., 1978. Combined immunodeficiency disease associated with absence of cell-surface HLA-A and -B antigens. J. Pediatr. 93, 47–51.

Tsukada, S., Saffran, D.C., Rawlings, D.J., Parolini, O., Allen, R.C., Kllsak, I., Sparkes, R.S., Kubagawa, H., Mohandas, T., Quan, S., Belmont, J.W., Cooper, M.D., Conley, M.E., Witte, O.H., 1993. Deficient expression of a B cell cytoplasmic tyrosine kinase in human X-linked agammaglobulinemia. Cell 72, 279–290.

Vahine, A., 2009. A historical reflection on the discovery of human retroviruses. Retrovirology. 6, 40. http://www.retrovirology.com/content/6/1/40.

Vetrie, D., Vorechovsky, I., Sideras, P., Holland, J., Davies, A., Flinter, F., Hammarstrom, L., Kinnon, C., Levinsky, R., Bobrow, M., Smith, C.I.E., Bentley, D.R., 1993. The gene involved in X-linked agammaglobulinemia is a member of the *src* family of protein-tyrosine kinases. Nature 361, 226–233.

Wiskott, A., 1937. Familiarer angeborener Morbus Werihofii. Montschr. Kinderheilk 68, 212–216.

TIME LINE

1926   Ladislav Syllaba and Kamil Henner describe three Czech siblings with cerebellar ataxia and dilated blood vessels in the eye and skin (ataxia-telangiectasia)

1929   Edward Thorpe and Harry Handley report a patient presenting with tetany and chronic mucocutaneous candidiasis

1931   Alfred Wiskott describes three brothers with recurrent infections, eczema, and thrombocytopenia

1941   Denise Louis-Bar reports on children with ataxia-telengiectasia and characterizes the disease

1952   Ogden Bruton describes the initial case of X-linked agammaglobulinemia

1954   Robert Aldrich reports a family in which several members have Wiskott–Aldrich syndrome

1958   Walter Hitzig and colleagues and R. Tobler and H. Cottier publish cases of individuals with defects of both antibody and cell-mediated immunity (Swiss type agammaglobulinemia; severe combined immunodeficiency)

1964   Christian Nezelof reports on a case of thymic hypoplasia

1967   Angelo DiGeorge and colleagues present patients with thymic dysplasia, cardiac malformations, absent parathyroids, and facial structural defects

1978   Jean-Louise Touraine and colleagues report the initial case of bare lymphocyte syndrome

1980   Claude Griscelli and coworkers report patients who fail to express class II HLA molecules

1980   Robert Gallo and colleagues identify the first human retrovirus, HTLV-I

1981   Initial description of acquired immunodeficiency syndrome (AIDS) among homosexual males

1982   CDC task force concludes that AIDS is an infectious disease

1983   Francoise Barré-Sinoussi, Luc Montagnier, and colleagues isolate a retrovirus (LAV) from a patient with lymphadenopathy

1984   Robert Gallo's group isolates a retrovirus (HTLV-III) from most AIDS patients

1987   French and American governments agree to share credit for the discovery of the AIDS virus

2008   Luc Montagnier and Francoise Barré-Sinoussi share the Nobel Prize for Physiology or Medicine

33

Pathologies Resulting from Aberrant Immune Responses

INTRODUCTION

The adaptive immune system responds to potential pathogens by the production of antibodies and specifically sensitized T lymphocytes. Antibodies eliminate infections caused by extracellular bacteria, fungi, and some parasites while T lymphocytes eliminate viruses and intracellular bacteria. These two systems (along with innate host defenses) protect against most infectious agents; however, occasionally the adaptive immune response reacts to antigens not associated with infectious microorganisms. Such aberrant immune responses often lead to pathology.

Early in the twentieth century, clinicians linked several diseases including serum sickness and anaphylaxis to aberrant immune responses. These disorders involve antibodies of various classes (isotypes) as well as activated T lymphocytes. In the 1890s, several investigators described experiments in which animals injected repeatedly with small doses of substances (serum, egg albumin, antibodies) from other species reacted with systemic manifestations often leading to death (Cohen and Mazzullo, 2009). In all situations, the initial injection of the foreign substance failed to elicit any clinical

signs or symptoms. Emil von Behring observed in 1894 that animals injected multiple times with horse antibodies to diphtheria toxin developed cardiovascular and/or pulmonary distress. Since he proposed that the animals had developed increased sensitivity to some toxic property of the substance, he named such reactions hypersensitivity.

Following the descriptions of anaphylaxis by Portier and Richet in 1902 and of serum sickness by von Pirquet and Schick in 1905, other investigators attributed a variety of pathologies to hypersensitivity, and this number increased dramatically during the next 50 years. Clinicians developed methods to detect these hypersensitivities that involved subcutaneous or intradermal injections of the antigens considered responsible for the clinical symptoms. Classification of the hypersensitivities relied on the time course required to detect skin reactivity following these injections. Immediate skin reactions occur within minutes to hours of injection and are mediated by antibody while delayed skin reactions manifest in 24–72 h and are mediated by T lymphocytes.

In 1963, Robin Coombs and Phillip Gell established a classification system of four types of hypersensitivity based on the underlying immunologic phenomena causing the damage which, with minor alterations, remains useful:

- Type I—IgE-mediated hypersensitivity such as allergies, anaphylaxis, and some forms of asthma;
- Type II—antibody-mediated hypersensitivity in which nonsoluble antigens, such as cells or tissues, interact with antibody thus resulting in lysis of, or damage to, the cell or tissue;
- Type III—immune complex hypersensitivity in which soluble antigen, such as protein, binds antibody, activates complement, and induces inflammation in small blood vessels located in the kidney, joints, skin, and elsewhere; and
- Type IV—cell-mediated hypersensitivity in which activated T lymphocytes bind soluble or cell-associated antigens causing lysis of the cells and inducing inflammation.

The studies reviewed in this chapter include both clinical observations and laboratory investigations that provided insight into the underlying pathophysiology.

TYPE I HYPERSENSITIVITIES

Type I hypersensitivities occur in individuals who synthesize IgE antibodies to foreign antigens. IgE binds to specialized Fc receptors on mast cells and eosinophils. Subsequent exposure to the same antigen cross-links cell-bound IgE resulting in mast cell degranulation and rapid release of several pharmacologically active mediators including histamine, prostaglandins, and leukotrienes as well as cytokines, chemokines, and enzymes. These mediators induce vasodilation and smooth muscle contraction leading to increased vascular permeability, bronchial constriction, increased mucus production, vomiting and diarrhea, and, sometimes, death.

Initial documented descriptions of type I hypersensitivities appeared during the 1890s (Cohen and Mazzullo, 2009). Emil von Behring in 1894 observed that the initial exposure of an animal to antibody specific for diphtheria toxin produced in horses induced no clinical symptoms. Animals repeatedly injected with antibody, however, developed cardiovascular and/or pulmonary distress; he termed this reaction hypersensitivity. Contemporaneously several other investigators reported similar findings in experimental animals repeatedly injected with other foreign substances. The reaction, induced by extremely small doses of the foreign substance, occasionally resulted in death of the animal. Originally investigators attributed these reactions, erroneously, to an increased susceptibility to an intrinsic toxic property of the injected substance. At that time, investigators failed to recognize the possible connection with the immune

system. Two French scientists identified the immunologic mechanism responsible for this phenomenon in 1902.

Prince Albert I of Monaco had an interest in science, particularly oceanography. He outfitted a number of yachts for scientific study and staffed them with scientists, scientific equipment, and experimental animals. These yachts sailed the Mediterranean Sea every summer with scientists working on questions of interest to the Prince. In 1901, Prince Albert invited Paul Portier (1866–1962) and Charles Richet (1850–1935) to sail on one of these yachts. Prince Albert's scientific director, Jules Richard, suggested that Portier and Richet study the reaction of fish and humans to the Portuguese man-of-war, an invertebrate found in the Mediterranean Sea (May, 1984; Cohen and Mazzullo, 2009; Boden and Burks, 2011).

The Portuguese man-of-war (*Physilia*) captures its prey by brushing against them with its tentacles and immobilizes them. The effect on humans who inadvertently come in contact with these same tentacles includes stinging, burning, redness, extreme pain, and lymphadenopathy. In previously exposed individuals who develop hypersensitivities, a subsequent exposure may result in difficulty breathing and cardiac arrest.

Portier and Richet initially postulated that the tentacles released a poison that produced the reaction. They prepared extracts of the tentacles, which they injected into various experimental animals, and observed respiratory distress and other reactions suggestive of a powerful toxin with profound effects on the central nervous system. Portier and Richet proposed producing an antibody to the toxin to neutralize it. Theirs was a reasonable approach in the early 1900s and was based on the model of treatment of diphtheria with an antibody directed to diphtheria toxin that produced seemingly miraculous cures (Chapter 3). The summer ended and Portier and Richet returned to their laboratory in Paris to continue this work. Since they no longer had access to Portuguese man-of-war for these studies, they switched to a related toxin from a sea anemone, *Actinia sulcata*.

Portier and Richet injected dogs with a dose of the sea anemone toxin and rested them for several weeks to allow the dogs to develop an expected protective antibody (antitoxin) response. None of the injected dogs demonstrated any adverse reaction. They then reinjected the dogs with a second dose of the toxin to assess the level of protection. Instead of being protected, the dogs developed sudden onset of diarrhea and vomiting, and many of them succumbed to this second injection.

Portier and Richet referred to this unexpected result by the term aphylaxis (shortly changed to anaphylaxis) to distinguish it from phylaxis, a term defined as protection against infection (Portier and Richet, 1902). Richet, awarded the Nobel Prize in Physiology or Medicine in 1913 "in recognition of his work on anaphylaxis," recounted in an address delivered to the International Congress of Physiology in 1910:

> Anaphylaxis is the opposite of protection (phylaxis). If one injects an albuminoid substance—for example, a toxin—into the circulatory system of an animal, instead of being protected by this first injection against a further injection of the same toxin, it has become more sensitive to its action. Let us suppose that the fatal dose is 1 cg. The injection of a tenth part of that dose, that is to say 1 mg—will not make it at all ill or scarcely so. But a month later-for almost a month is required for the anaphylactic state to be produced-it has become so sensitive that a dose of 1 mg is enough to kill it by the immediate production of formidable symptoms. Therefore the first injection has caused a condition which is the opposite of protection-namely anaphylaxis.

The Immune System in Anaphylaxis

Because the mechanism of anaphylaxis was not immediately obvious researchers suggested two possibilities (reviewed by Cohen and Mazzullo, 2009):

- a humoral theory that hypothesized the formation of an enzymatic cleavage product released from the toxin more rapidly on second injection of the toxin (Vaughan and Wheeler, 1907); or
- a cellular theory that proposed that antibody was synthesized in response to the original sensitization and that this antibody was taken up by cells within the target organs (e.g., in the cardiovascular and respiratory systems) prior to the second challenge (Besredka, 1907).

Attempts to detect specific antibody in serum from injected animals met with failure although some investigators demonstrated that the reaction could be transferred to naïve animals using serum. John Anderson and W.H. Frost working in the Hygiene Laboratory of the U.S. Public Health and Marine Hospital Service, Washington, D.C., demonstrated in 1910 that serum from a hypersensitive animal could transfer anaphylaxis to naive animals. Anderson and Frost injected guinea pigs with horse serum to induce hypersensitivity. They then injected naïve guinea pigs with serum from these hypersensitive guinea pigs. Subsequent injection of the recipient guinea pigs with horse serum induced an anaphylactic reaction. The time required between injection of the serum and demonstration of a hypersensitivity reaction was less than 24 h. Anderson and Ford incubated the original guinea pig serum with horse serum to absorb out any antibody. The treated guinea pig serum failed to transfer the hypersensitivity thus suggesting that antibody was involved in this transfer.

In 1910, Werner Schultz (1878–1947) also working at the Hygiene Laboratory of the U.S. Public Health and Marine Hospital Service in Washington, D.C., developed an in vitro technique that led to an explanation to the mechanism by which anaphylaxis caused tissue damage. Schultz injected guinea pigs with horse serum. He dissected muscle strips from the ileum of these animals and suspended them in isotonic saline. He then added either horse serum or serum from other species as control to the preparations. Horse serum induced muscle contraction in preparations from hypersensitive animals while addition of serum from other species failed to produce contraction.

In 1911, Henry Hallett Dale (1875–1968) and Patrick Laidlaw (1881–1940) working at the Wellcome Physiological Research Laboratories in London demonstrated the role of histamine in this reaction. They suspended uterine muscle from nonsensitized guinea pigs in saline, added histamine (β-iminapolyethylamine), and observed muscle contraction identical to that seen when antigen was added to muscle from a sensitized animal. Despite the fact that Werner Schultz and Henry Dale never collaborated, the phenomenon they studied is called the Schultz–Dale reaction, and investigators used this model for almost 50 years to dissect, diagnose, and explain antibody-mediated type I hypersensitivity.

Dale received his MD from Cambridge and pursued physiological and pharmacological investigations while at University College and the National Institute of Medical Research, both in London. Dale pursued other studies including ones on the transmission of nerve impulses and shared the Nobel Prize for Physiology or Medicine in 1936 with Otto Loewi "for their discoveries relating to chemical transmission of nerve impulses."

Type I hypersensitivity reactions in humans were not immediately recognized despite anecdotal evidence that humans developed anaphylaxis. In 1896, Gottstein reported human fatalities following administration of horse antibodies specific for diphtheria toxin (Cohen and Mazzullo, 2009). Other investigators observed fatal consequences of bee stings.

In 1921, Otto Prausnitz (1876–1963) and Heinz Küstner (1897–1963) working at the Hygiene Institute of the University of Breslau in Germany, reported the transfer of skin hypersensitivity from an allergic to a healthy individual. They collected serum from Küstner, who was exquisitely sensitive to fish, and injected it subcutaneously into Prausnitz. Twenty-four hours later they applied a fish extract locally to Prausnitz' skin and observed an immediate skin reaction characterized by the appearance of a wheal and flare. This Prausnitz–Küstner (P-K) reaction proved useful to demonstrate the pathophysiology of hypersensitivity in humans. In fact Ishizaka and his coworkers employed the P-K reaction in the mid-1960s to identify the antibody isotype responsible for allergy to ragweed pollen (Ishizaka et al., 1967).

While these early studies showed that antibody transferred one of the models of type I hypersensitivity, the identity of the specific antibody isotype responsible was described 45 years later. Kimishige Ishizaka working with his wife Teruka and colleagues at the University of Colorado Medical School (1966) and S. Gunnar O. Johansson and Hans Bennich (1967) working at University Hospital, Uppsala, Sweden, described a novel isotype of antibody, IgE, involved in type I hypersensitivities (Chapter 11).

Humans synthesize IgE antibodies to provide protective immunity against protozoal parasites. However, a group of genetically susceptible individuals produce IgE to foreign antigens that subsequently activate an immediate hypersensitivity upon reexposure to the antigen. The most common antigens to which IgE is synthesized are foods (e.g., peanuts, seafood), drugs (e.g., penicillin, codeine), and insect venom (e.g., wasps, bees). IgE antibodies induced by these antigens bind to effector cells (mast cells) throughout the body. Reintroduction of the sensitizing antigen cross-links two IgE molecules causing release of vasoactive mediators (e.g., histamine) leading to the signs and symptoms associated with hypersensitivity including shortness of breath, asthma, allergic rhinitis, hypotension, irregular heartbeat, eczema, urticaria, and gastrointestinal disorders.

TYPE II HYPERSENSITIVITY

Karl Landsteiner (1868–1943) working at the University of Vienna, Austria, discovered the ABO blood groups in 1900. He mixed blood from two individuals and observed agglutination of the erythrocytes in some of the mixtures. This agglutination is due to the presence of naturally occurring antibodies (isohemagglutinins) in one individual's serum that bind antigens on red cells from the second individual. Through testing a large number of blood specimens, Landsteiner initially described three groups of individuals based on their blood type—A, B, and O. Blood group AB was discovered 1 year later. Landsteiner also showed that transfusion of blood between two individuals succeeded if they shared blood type. This finding led to successful clinical blood transfusions, the first of which was performed by Ruben Ottenberg in 1907 at Mount Sinai Hospital in New York (Ottenberg, 1908).

Investigators described additional blood group antigens (e.g., MN, P) in the 1920s and 1930s. None of these induced naturally occurring antibodies as did the A and B blood groups, and hence incompatibility at these markers posed little problem during initial transfusions. However, patients transfused repeatedly with blood incompatible at these and other red blood cell antigens may develop antibodies.

In 1939, Phillip Levine (1900–1987) and Rufus E. Stetson (1886–1967) working at Newark Beth Israel Hospital in New Jersey described a 25-year-old woman who delivered a stillborn infant during the thirty-third week of gestation. Following delivery, the woman bled profusely requiring a blood transfusion. Both she and her husband were blood group O thus allowing him to serve as the donor of the initial transfusion. Almost immediately the patient suffered a transfusion reaction characterized as chills and pain in her legs and head. The following day she received a transfusion of O blood from a different donor without adverse reaction. Subsequent testing showed that the patient's serum agglutinated her husband's erythrocytes as well as the red cells of 42 out of 50 group O blood donors from the Blood Transfusion Betterment Association.

Clinicians had previously detected similar agglutinating antibody in individuals following multiple, ABO-matched blood transfusions. However, this woman had no history of previous transfusions, and Levine and Stetson guessed that the stimulus for antibody production came from antigens in the fetus inherited from the father. Such an antibody explained both the demise of the fetus and the transfusion reaction elicited by the husband's blood.

In 1941, Karl Landsteiner and Alexander Wiener at the Rockefeller Institute for Medical Research injected rabbits with blood from rhesus monkeys. These rabbits produced an antibody that reacted with a human red blood cell antigen different from A, B, M, or N. They called this blood group Rh and showed that Rh antigen occasionally induced an antibody response following blood transfusions.

Levine and Stetson thought that the antibody produced by their patient against her husband's red cells was identical to the rabbit antibody used by Landsteiner and Wiener and thus called the blood group antigen Rhesus factor. Investigators subsequently demonstrated that the two antibodies detected different antigens; however, the terminology currently in use assigns Rh factor to the antigen described by Levine and Stetson while the antigen detected by the antibodies to rhesus blood is called the LW (Landsteiner–Weiner) antigen.

The Rh blood group system refers to antigens expressed on red blood cells. Several of these antigens including D, C, c, E, and e induce antibodies in transfusion reactions. In blood typing an individual is either Rh positive or Rh negative; Rh positive connotes the presence of the D antigen on red cells. Incompatibility at the Rh (D) antigen is the major stimulator of antibodies during pregnancy resulting in erythroblastosis fetalis and hemolytic disease of the newborn.

Hemolytic disease of the newborn is a type II hypersensitivity reaction. Approximately 85% of humans express the Rh (D) antigen on their red blood cells.

When a woman who is Rh negative is pregnant with an Rh positive fetus, fetal Rh positive erythrocytes enter the maternal circulation, late in gestation or at delivery, and stimulate an antibody response in the mother. The first antibody synthesized, IgM, is excluded from crossing the placenta and entering the fetus. Second and subsequent pregnancies with Rh positive fetuses provide a stimulus that induces isotype switching to IgG. IgG antibodies are actively transported across the placenta during pregnancy where they bind the fetal Rh-positive erythrocytes and destroy them. Destruction of red blood cells releases hemoglobin that is catabolized to bilirubin, which in turn is excreted in bile and urine. While bilirubin is a usual product of red blood cell turnover, excess bilirubin leads to symptoms ranging from mild (jaundice—yellowing of the skin and eyes and fatigue) to severe (kernicterus—brain damage, hydrops fetalis—edema, seizures, mental retardation, difficulties in hearing and speaking, and death). The underlying mechanism of this disease led to an intervention to prevent the formation of such antibodies in Rh-negative women thus protecting Rh-positive fetuses in subsequent pregnancies (Chapter 38).

Investigators identified other type II hypersensitivities. More than 100 years ago Julius Donath and Karl Landsteiner detected antibodies specific for red blood cell antigens in patients with paroxysmal cold hemoglobinuria (Chapter 8). These antibodies bind a patient's erythrocytes in the extremities, where the temperature is less than 37 °C, and are destroyed by complement activation when the red cells return to the core of the body (Donath and Landsteiner, 1904).

During the ensuing 100 years, investigators reported other examples of type II hypersensitivity reactions leading to autoimmune diseases (Chapter 34). In addition to red cells these pathologies affect other cells of the blood (e.g., neutrophils, platelets) as well as various tissues and organs (neuromuscular junctions in myasthenia gravis, thyroid cells in Grave disease, myelin-producing cells of the peripheral nervous system in multiple sclerosis). Once formed, these autoantibodies bind their targets and initiate the same effector mechanisms (complement activation, opsonization, antibody-dependent cell-mediated cytotoxicity, neutralization) that the adaptive immune system employs to eliminate potential pathogens (Chapter 26).

TYPE III HYPERSENSITIVITY

In 1905, Clemens von Pirquet and Bela Schick described a clinical complication observed in some patients injected with horse antibodies to diphtheria toxin. Some patients developed fever, skin rash, joint pain, cardiac abnormalities, and kidney malfunction

within 10–14 days of the initial dose of horse antibodies. Patients who received a second injection of the horse antibodies presented with similar symptoms more rapidly. von Pirquet and Schick (1905) proposed that this was an example of a pathologic immune response and named this constellation of presenting signs and symptoms serum sickness.

von Pirquet (1874–1929) received his medical training at the University of Graz in Austria. He specialized in pediatrics and worked at the Children's Clinic in Vienna at the time of the discovery of serum sickness. Bela Schick (1877–1967) was also trained as a physician at the University of Graz and was a faculty member at the University of Vienna in the early 1900s.

In 1911, von Pirquet realized that the symptoms of serum sickness occurred simultaneously with the appearance of antibodies against the foreign serum and reasoned that the antibody combined with the foreign antigen to form a "toxic compound" that caused the disease. The identity of this "toxic compound" required 50 years of investigation.

In 1922, Alexander Glenny and Barbara Hopkins at the Wellcome Physiological Research Laboratories in London investigated the elimination of antibodies injected into a foreign animal. They injected rabbits with horse antibodies induced against diphtheria toxin and harvested serum from these rabbits periodically during the next several days. Glenny and Hopkins assayed the rabbit serum to determine how much activity against diphtheria toxin remained. When activity was plotted against time (Figure 33.1) they observed that the foreign antibody disappeared in three phases. Within the first 24 h approximately 50% of the antibody disappeared;

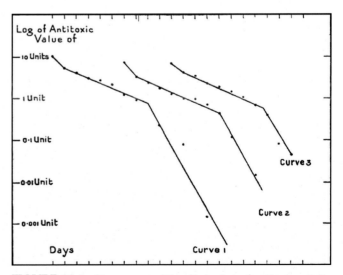

FIGURE 33.1 Time course of the elimination of antitoxic activity measured in three rabbits injected with horse antibody to diphtheria toxin. Rabbits were injected with 0.5 ml of horse serum containing 750 units of antitoxin activity. *From Glenny and Hopkins (1922).*

this is due to serum protein equilibrating between the vascular and extravascular compartments of the rabbit's body. A second phase of constant percentage loss occurred over the next 6–7 days. Approximately 25% of the remaining antibody vanished each day, this is attributed to catabolism of horse proteins. Finally, Glenny and Hopkins observed a phase of accelerated loss of antibody that they hypothesized was the result of immune clearance due to formation of antibodies to the horse serum proteins (Glenny and Hopkins, 1922).

Glenny and Hopkins pursued these studies to determine the duration of protection that might be expected following treatment of a patient with antitoxin serotherapy. Within a year, in 1923, Glenny, Hopkins, and Gaston Ramon developed a vaccine against *Corynebacterium diphtheria* toxin (toxoid) that eventually superseded the use of horse antitoxin in the clinic.

David Talmage and his colleagues at Washington University, St. Louis, Missouri, in 1951 observed a similar time course of antigen elimination. They injected rabbits with radiolabeled bovine gamma globulin (BGG) and followed the elimination of the radioisotope over time. Simultaneously they measured the appearance of antibodies to BGG in the serum of the injected rabbits and correlated the rate of antigen elimination with the appearance of antibody. From their results they concluded that the rapid phase of antigen elimination is an "early and sensitive manifestation of the immune response."

These studies confirmed that serum proteins from one species (e.g., horse, cattle) are immunogenic in animals of a second species (i.e., humans and rabbits). Antibodies induced by foreign serum proteins might explain the occurrence of serum sickness in some patients treated with antibodies to diphtheria toxin raised in horses (serotherapy).

Further investigation identified other situations in which type III hypersensitivity reactions induce pathology including autoimmune diseases (i.e., systemic lupus erythematosus), drug hypersensitivities (i.e., allopurinol, cephalosporin), and allergens (inhaled hay dust). Some type III hypersensitivities result from antibody responses induced to infectious microorganisms. Examples include reactive arthritis (associated with various bacteria including *Chlamydia trachomatis*), polyarteritis nodosa (associated in some patients with hepatitis B infection), and poststreptococcal glomerulonephritis (GN).

Infection with group A *Streptococcus* results in several diseases including pharyngitis, impetigo, and scarlet fever. Sequelae of infection with group A *Streptococcus* include rheumatic fever and rheumatic heart disease, toxic shock syndrome, and poststreptococcal GN.

Bela Schick and Clemens von Pirquet in the first decade of the twentieth century independently suggested that immune complexes play a role in pathology of acute poststreptococcal GN. Schick in 1907 (referenced in Michael et al., 1966) compared the time course of serum sickness seen in patients injected with horse antibody to diphtheria toxin with the interval between the appearance of scarlet fever (a streptococcal-mediated infection) and the development of acute nephritis. In 1906, von Pirquet (referenced in Huber, 2006) postulated that a reaction similar to that involved in serum sickness was responsible for the kidney damage observed after a bout of scarlet fever. These early observations stimulated investigators to develop animal models of immune complex-mediated disease.

In 1958, Kimishige Ishizaka and Dan Campbell working at the California Institute of Technology developed an experimental model of immune complex disease that they visualized in skin. First, they injected guinea pigs intravenously with Evans blue, a dye that leaks from the vascular system only in areas with increased permeability. They then injected the guinea pigs intracutaneously with either preformed antigen–antibody complexes or with physiological saline. Ishizaka and Campbell observed the injection site for the appearance of blue dye and reported that injection of antigen–antibody complexes led to release of the dye into the skin while injection of physiological saline failed to produce a reaction. Ishizaka and Campbell concluded that immune complexes increased vascular permeability locally and led to the leakage of the dye. Today immunologists agree that the increased vascular permeability is caused by activation of the complement system by the immune complexes.

In 1961, Frank Dixon and coworkers at the University of Pittsburgh, Pennsylvania, developed a second animal model to study immune complex-mediated disease. They injected rabbits daily with one of several protein antigens including bovine serum albumin, human serum albumin, BGG, or human gamma globulin to induce an antibody response. Dixon and colleagues bled the rabbits weekly and tested their sera for the presence of antigen (detected by precipitation using a predetermined amount of antibody) and antibody (measured by a quantitative precipitin assay). Dixon and coworkers also collected 24 h urine samples that they analyzed for the presence of urinary protein. They biopsied the kidney weekly and prepared the tissue for histologic evaluation.

Individual rabbits developed clinical signs (proteinuria) and morphological changes (proliferation of glomerular capillary endothelium and infiltration of polymorphonuclear leukocytes) similar to those seen in humans with acute, subacute, or chronic GN. Rabbits that developed acute GN possessed greater amounts of antibody to the injected antigen in their peripheral blood than did those developing chronic GN.

Immunohistochemical staining of sections of kidney biopsies demonstrated the presence of antigen deposited along the basement membrane in a granular pattern along with rabbit gamma globulin. This histological picture is similar to that seen in sections from humans with serum sickness.

Based on these observations, Dixon and his colleagues concluded that

- "the renal injury is precipitated by antigens with no known affinity for, or immunologic relationship to kidney"; and
- "antigen–antibody complexes localize in the kidney, apparently on the basis of nonimmunologic factors, and may be the etiologic agent of renal injury."

By the 1960s, investigators proposed an immunological mechanism for poststreptococcal GN in humans based on the following clinical findings (Michael et al., 1966):

- serum complement levels are decreased in the early stages of GN;
- gamma globulin is deposited in the kidneys of patients with GN; and
- IgG and streptococcal antigen (immune complexes) are detectable in glomeruli of most patients with GN.

Alfred Michael and his collaborators at the University of Minnesota confirmed these clinical findings when they studied kidney biopsies from 16 children with acute poststreptococcal GN. They stained biopsies with fluorescent antibody to immunoglobulin or to complement and demonstrated the presence of IgG and complement components on the epithelial surface of the glomerular basement membranes. Biopsies from some of the patients also stained with antibody to streptococcal antigens.

Michael and collaborators speculated that the mechanism of production of acute GN "may be similar to that occurring in experimental antigen–antibody complex disease. The presence of streptococcal antigen in the glomeruli of some patients with this disease tends to support but does not prove the antigen–antibody complex hypothesis."

TYPE IV HYPERSENSITIVITY

Skin reactions to antigen injection are divided into two types based on the time course: immediate reactions appearing within minutes to a few hours of injection and resolving after a relatively short period of time, and delayed reactions, appearing only after an interval of several hours and reaching a peak in intensity 48–72h after injection. Hans Zinsser working at Columbia University in New York reported the temporal differences in these reactions in 1921. Zinsser compared the skin reactivity of groups of guinea pigs injected intraperitoneally with horse serum or with an extract of *Mycobacterium tuberculosis*.

Zinsser injected guinea pigs with horse serum and tested them 2–3 weeks later by an intradermal injection of horse serum. This procedure induced a wheal (a round elevation of the skin white in the center with a pale periphery) within 5–10 min, and Zinsser concluded that these guinea pigs had developed an antibody-mediated hypersensitivity. He also demonstrated a similar reaction in naïve guinea pigs injected with serum from a sensitized guinea pig.

Zinsser injected additional groups of guinea pigs with antigens from *M. tuberculosis*. Skin tests of these animals with *M. tuberculosis* antigen (tuberculin) resulted in a delayed skin reaction (48–72h). Zinsser postulated that this reaction was due to antibodies and tested this hypothesis by exposing uteri from positive guinea pigs to tuberculin antigen in a tissue bath. Contraction of uterine muscle in the presence of antigen is a measure of antibody-mediated anaphylaxis as described by Schultz and Dale (section on type I hypersensitivity in this chapter). Antigen failed, in most cases, to induce uterine muscle contraction.

Based on these studies, Zinsser concluded that "in guinea pigs two fundamentally different types of intradermal reactions may be observed. One of these is the immediate, transitory reaction which develops in animals sensitized against proteins (horse serum, etc.)...the other is the tuberculin type of skin reaction which develops more slowly, leads to a more profound injury of the tissues and is independent of anaphylaxis."

In 1921, the identity of the cell or cells responsible for antibody production and the functional differentiation of T and B lymphocytes was yet to be discovered. Several other investigators studied the skin reactivity to various antigens derived from *M. tuberculosis* during the 1920s and 1930s. These studies culminated in the discovery in 1942 by Merrill Chase and Karl Landsteiner working at the Rockefeller Institute in New York that tuberculin skin reactivity could be transferred by cells isolated from a sensitized animal but not by serum.

Chapter 3 presents other experimental models in which cells rather than antibodies are responsible for immunological reactions. Avrion Mitchison in 1955 working at Edinburgh University, Scotland, reported that cells, but not serum, transferred protection against transplanted tumors from immune animals to naïve animals. In 1958, Leslie Brent and colleagues at University College in London showed that graft rejection is dependent on cells and not antibodies. Subsequently investigators identified adaptive immune responses as well as several pathologies that involve type IV hypersensitivity reactions. These include the normal adaptive immune response to viral infections, allergic contact dermatitis to plants (poison oak, sumac, or ivy) and metals (nickel, gold), and several autoimmune diseases such as rheumatoid arthritis, psoriasis, and Hashimoto thyroiditis (Chapter 34).

IMMUNE-MEDIATED PATHOLOGIES SECONDARY TO INFECTIONS

Several pathological processes including granuloma formation in response to infection by *M. tuberculosis*, lysis of red cells in malaria, destruction of liver cells during hepatitis C infection, and deposition of antigen–antibody complexes in kidney glomeruli in poststreptococcal GN develop as sequelae of immune responses to potential pathogens. The mechanisms responsible for these pathologies can be grouped according to the hypersensitivity classification system developed by Coombs and Gell. Other immune-mediated pathologies include damage caused by the massive release of inflammatory mediators (cytokine storm) induced by superantigens released during bacterial infections, especially staphylococci.

Poststreptococcal Rheumatic Fever and Rheumatic Heart Disease

Sequelae from infection with group A *Streptococcus* include GN and rheumatic fever. Poststreptococcal GN results from deposition of antigen–antibody complexes in kidney glomeruli and is an example of a type III hypersensitivity.

Patients with rheumatic fever present with one or more of the following symptoms: skin rash, subcutaneous nodules, joint pain, Sydenham chorea, and carditis. These manifestations are likely due to the activity of antibodies to streptococcal bacteria that cross-react with antigens on various organs including heart, cerebellum, synovium, and skin. Cardiac involvement can develop into rheumatic heart disease characterized by destruction of the mitral valve.

In 1962, Melvin Kaplan and Mary Meyeserian from Western Reserve University, Cleveland, Ohio, described an 11-year-old boy hospitalized with sore throat, fever, and joint pain. Laboratory evaluation demonstrated the presence of antibodies specific for *Streptococcus* although throat cultures proved negative for β-hemolytic *Streptococcus*. The patient's hospital course included recurrent fevers and episodes of congestive heart failure and peripheral edema that led to his demise 5.5 months after the onset of his illness. On autopsy Kaplan and Meyeserian noted infiltration of the heart muscle with lymphocytes and plasma cells and, by immunofluorescence, the presence of gamma globulin throughout the myocardium.

The association of infection with β-hemolytic *Streptococcus* and the presence of gamma globulin in the heart led Kaplan and Meyeserian to hypothesize that an antibody to an antigen of *Streptococcus* might cross-react with an antigen on myocardium. They injected rabbits with group A β-hemolytic *Streptococcus* and evaluated the antibodies formed for their specificity for human heart tissue. By immunofluorescence and complement fixation they detected antibody binding to myofibers and to smooth muscle in arteries. The antibody specific for heart muscle could be adsorbed from the rabbit serum by streptococcal cells.

Additional studies performed by Kaplan's group demonstrated that

- a goat antibody to rabbit or human heart precipitated extracts of streptococcal cell walls (Kaplan and Suchy, 1964); and
- some patients with streptococcal infection produced an antibody that reacted with both streptococcal cell walls and human heart tissue (Kaplan and Svec, 1964).

Since this cross-reactive antibody was present in many patients with poststreptococcal rheumatic heart disease, but not in patients with other bacterial infections, the authors concluded that the streptococcal infection induced antibody that bound human heart tissue.

Toxic Shock Syndrome

Toxic shock syndrome, a systemic disease induced by the immune system's response to toxins secreted by staphylococcal and other Gram-positive microorganisms, is characterized by sudden onset of a high fever (greater than 102 °F), accompanied with vomiting and/or diarrhea, a skin rash, mental confusion, and hypotension. Franklin Stevens of Columbia University College of Physicians and Surgeons in New York initially described this constellation of symptoms in 1927 when he reported three patients with a skin rash similar to scarlet fever but from whom *Staphylococcus aureus* rather than *Streptococcus* was isolated. James Todd and colleagues working at the Children's Hospital of Denver, University of Colorado, Ohio State University, and Herkimer Memorial Hospital in New York, in 1978 described seven children who developed these symptoms following infection with *Staphylococcus*. They named the disease toxic shock syndrome. The causative microorganism produces a toxin that is responsible for the symptoms; however, the pathophysiological mechanism was unknown at that time.

Investigators subsequently isolated and identified several staphylococcal toxins responsible for toxic shock syndrome. In 1981, Patrick Schlivert working with collaborators at the University of California, Los Angeles, and the Centers for Disease Control and Prevention in Atlanta, Georgia, isolated an enterotoxin from strains of *S. aureus* obtained from patients with toxic shock syndrome. In 1981, Merlin Bergdoll and his group at the University of Wisconsin, Madison, isolated a similar enterotoxin. This toxin, now called toxic shock syndrome toxin 1 (TSST1), when injected into rabbits produced fever and caused T lymphocyte proliferation. In 1985, Roland Carlsson and Hans Olov Sjögren working at the University of Lund, Sweden, demonstrated that activation of T lymphocytes by TSST1 induced the synthesis and secretion of cytokines including IL-2 and IFN-γ.

Researchers proposed that TSST1 activated T lymphocytes by binding a cell surface receptor. While stimulating cytokine secretion from unpurified lymphocytes, the toxin failed to activate purified T lymphocytes. Roland Carlsson and colleagues in 1988 compared TSST1 with other known T lymphocyte mitogens including phytohemagglutinin and concanavalin A (Con A). They demonstrated that activation of T lymphocytes by toxin required the presence of an accessory cell such as monocytes, B lymphocytes, or B lymphomas. Carlsson and coworkers further demonstrated that the interaction between accessory cells and T lymphocytes requires that the two cells share genes in the major histocompatibility complex (MHC).

The identification of accessory cells as well as the MHC restriction of their interaction provided a clue to the binding specificity of the toxin. Cells that serve as accessory cells for TSST1 stimulation also serve as classical antigen-presenting cells (APCs) to activate CD4+ T lymphocytes in the adaptive immune response. APCs express histocompatibility molecules coded for by class II MIIC genes. Within a year of Carlsson's identification of the requirement for accessory cells in the stimulation of T lymphocytes, two groups showed that *S. aureus* toxin preferentially bound a human class II MHC coded molecule called HLA-DR (Fischer et al., 1989; Fraser, 1989).

John Fraser working at the University of Auckland, New Zealand, used toxin radiolabeled with ^{125}I to detect this binding. He incubated cells expressing class II HLA molecules with the radioactive toxin. Following lysis of these cells, he precipitated the extract with a monoclonal antibody specific for the HLA molecule. Analysis of the precipitate demonstrated that the toxin bound specifically to HLA-DR molecules.

Contemporaneously, Hans Fischer working in the laboratory of Roland Carlsson at the University of Lund, Sweden, used flow cytometry and electrophoresis to characterize the molecules recovered from accessory cells that bound staphylococcal enterotoxin A (SEA). Fischer incubated SEA with Raji cells, a cell line derived from a Burkitt lymphoma and maintained in culture since 1963. He stained these cells with antibodies specific to either SEA or to one of the class II molecules expressed by Raji cells, HLA-DR. Fischer analyzed these stained cells by flow cytometry and demonstrated that SEA and class II molecules were both expressed on the surface of the cells. He solubilized Raji cells that bound SEA by treatment with detergent and electrophoresed the extract resulting in the appearance of a single protein band containing both SEA and HLA class II molecules. Finally he demonstrated that a monoclonal antibody that blocked the binding of SEA to Raji cells also bound HLA-DR molecules. These results led Fischer and his group to conclude that "the HLA-DR molecule is the main functional molecule for binding of SEA to accessory cells and that this binding of SEA to HLA-DR is a necessary requirement for SEA-induced T cell activation."

Toxins presented by class II MHC molecules stimulate many but not all T lymphocytes. In 1989, Janice White and her colleagues working in the laboratories of John Kappler and Philippa Marrack at the University of Colorado, Denver, employed two approaches to identify the portion of the T cell receptor (TCR) on mouse T lymphocytes to which these toxins bind:

- Staining T lymphocytes stimulated by staphylococcal toxin with monoclonal antibodies specific for various Vβ segments of TCRs. Nearly every dividing T lymphocyte contained Vβ3, Vβ8.1, Vβ8.2, or Vβ8.3 as part of their TCRs.
- Developing T lymphocyte clones from lymphocytes that responded to staphylococcal toxin and determining the expression of the V region on the beta chain of the TCR expressed by these clones. Twenty-five of twenty-seven responding clones expressed one of the four Vβ regions (Vβ3, Vβ8.1, Vβ8.2, or Vβ8.3) identified by monoclonal antibodies.

Investigators performed similar studies in humans and concluded that staphylococcal toxins produce their pathology by binding to MHC-coded class II molecules on APCs. These cells then present this toxin to a large number (10% or more) of T lymphocytes expressing TCRs using a limited repertoire of Vβ regions. Presentation by APCs induces systemic inflammation created by the synthesis and secretion of large amounts of cytokines (cytokine storm) resulting in the symptoms associated with toxic shock syndrome.

CONCLUSION

The immune response, originally thought to protect the individual against potentially pathogenic microorganisms, is now concomitantly implicated in an array of clinical pathologies. Several observations made at the turn of the twentieth century focused attention on aberrations induced by immune responses, particularly those to nonmicrobial antigens. Investigators described anaphylaxis, serum sickness, hemolytic disease of the newborn, and tuberculin sensitization prior to 1950. In 1962, Coombs and Gell classified the seemingly large numbers of different mechanisms responsible for these pathologies to four distinct types of hypersensitivity. This classification remains useful today although other schemes have been presented (Sell, 1978). Recent advances to unravel the cellular, molecular, and genetic underpinnings of these mechanisms inspired the development of novel therapeutic interventions including monoclonal antibodies to IgE and CD3 and biologics to TNF-α and other inflammatory mediators.

Diseases classified as immune mediated encompass an ever increasing number of clinical syndromes. Clinicians have described more than 80 autoimmune diseases (Chapter 34). Many of these including immune-mediated thrombocytopenia and autoimmune polyglandular syndrome are rare; however, some, such as rheumatoid arthritis, systemic lupus erythematosus, type I diabetes, and multiple sclerosis affect 0.5% or more of the population. Many nonautoimmune syndromes are also included in the panoply of immune-mediated disorders including allergies to foods, insect venoms, and drugs, certain forms of asthma, poststreptococcal GN, and toxic shock syndrome.

The immunological mechanisms responsible for the pathology in these clinical entities include the formation of antibodies and specifically sensitized T lymphocytes as well as inflammatory cytokines. More and more of these diseases are targeted by novel therapies as described in Chapter 38.

References

Anderson, J.F., Frost, W.H., 1910. Studies upon anaphylaxis with special reference to the antibodies concerned. J. Med. Res. 23, 31–69.

Behring, E., 1894. Infektion and Desinfektion. Thomas, Leipzig.

Bergdoll, M.S., Cross, R.A., Reise, R.F., Robbins, R.N., Davis, J.P., 1981. A new staphylococcal enterotoxin F, associated with toxic-shock-syndrome Staphylococcus aureus isolates. Lancet 317, 1017–1021.

Besredka, A., 1907. Du mecanisme de l'anaphylaxie vis-à-vis du derum de cheval. Comp. Rend. Soc. De. Biol. 59, 294–296.

Boden, S.R., Burks, A.W., 2011. Anaphylaxis: a history with emphasis on food allergy. Immunol. Rev. 242, 247–256.

Brent, L., Brown, J., Medawar, P.B., 1958. Skin transplantation immunity in relation to hypersensitivity. Lancet 272, 561–564.

Carlsson, R., Fischer, H., Sjögren, H.O., 1988. Binding of staphylococcal enterotoxin A to accessory cells is a requirement for its ability to activate human T cells. J. Immunol. 140, 2484–2488.

Carlsson, R., Sjögren, H.O., 1985. Kinetics of IL-2 and interferon-γ production, expression of IL-2 receptors, and cell proliferation in human mononuclear cells exposed to staphylococcal enterotoxin A. Cell. Immunol. 96, 175–183.

Cohen, S.G., Mazzullo, J.C., 2009. Discovering anaphylaxis: elucidation of a shocking phenomenon. J. Allergy Clin. Immunol. 124, 866–869.

Coombs, R.R.A., Gell, P.G.H., 1963. In: Gell, P.G.H., Coombs, R.R.A. (Eds.), Clinical Aspects of Immunology. Blackwell, Oxford, p. 317.

Dale, H.H., Laidlaw, P.P., 1911. Further observations on the physiological action of β-iminapolylethylamine. J. Physiol. 43, 182–195.

Dixon, F.J., Feldman, J.D., Vazquez, J.J., 1961. Experimental glomerulonephritis. The pathogenesis of a laboratory model resembling the spectrum of human glomerulonephritis. J. Exp. Med. 113, 899–920.

Donath, J., Lansteiner, K., 1904. Uber paroxysmale Hamoglobinurie. Munchener Med. Wochenschr. 51, 1590–1593.

Fischer, H., Dohlstein, M., Lindvall, M., Sjogren, H.-O., Carlsson, R., 1989. Binding of staphylococcal enterotoxin A to HLA-DR on B cell lines. J. Immunol. 142, 3151–3157.

Fraser, J.D., 1989. High-affinity binding of staphylococcal enterotoxins A and B to HLA-DR. Nature 339, 221–223.

Glenny, A.T., Hopkins, B.E., 1922. Duration of passive immunity. J. Hyg. 21, 142–148.

Huber, B., 2006. 100 Jahre Allergie: Clemens von Pirquet-sein Allergiebegriff und das ihn zugrunde liegende Krankheitsverständnis. Wien. Klin. Wochen 118, 573–579.

Ishizaka, K., Campbell, D.H., 1958. Biological activity of soluble antigen-antibody complexes. I. Skin reactive properties. Proc. Soc. Exp. Biol. Med. 97, 635–638.

Ishizaka, K., Ishizaka, T., Hornbrook, M., 1966. Physiochemical properties of reaginic antibody. IV. Presence of a unique immunoglobulin as a carrier of reaginic activity. J. Immunol. 97, 75–85.

Ishizaka, K., Ishizaka, T., Menzel, A.E.O., 1967. Physicochemical properties of reaginic antibody. VI. Effect of heat on γE-, γG- and γA-antibodies in the sera of ragweed sensitive patients. J. Immunol. 99, 610–618.

Johansson, S.G.O., Bennich, H., 1967. Immunological studies of an atypical (myeloma) immunoglobulin. Immunology 13, 381–394.

Kaplan, M.H., Meyeserian, M., 1962. An immunological cross-reaction between group-A streptococcal cells and human heart tissue. Lancet 279, 706–710.

Kaplan, M.H., Suchy, M.L., 1964. Immunologic relation of streptococcal and tissue antigens. II. Cross-reaction of antisera to mammalian heart tissue with a cell wall constituent of certain strains of group A streptococci. J. Exp. Med. 119, 643–649.

Kaplan, M.H., Svec, K.H., 1964. Immunologic relation of streptococcal and tissue antigens. III. Presence in human sera of streptococcal antibody cross-reactive with heart tissue. Association with streptococcal infection, rheumatic fever and glomerulonephritis. J. Exp. Med. 119, 651–665.

Landsteiner, K., 1900. Zur Kenntnis der antifermentativen, lytischen und agglutinierenden Wirkungen des Blutserums und der Lymphe. Centralblatt f. Bakteriol. Parasitenkd. U. Infekt. 27, 357–362.

Landsteiner, K., Chase, M.W., 1942. Experiments on transfer of cutaneous sensitivity to simple compounds. Proc. Soc. Exp. Biol. Med. 49, 688–690.

Levine, P., Stetson, P.E., 1939. An unusual case of intra-group agglutination. J. Amer. Med. Assoc. 113, 126–127.

May, C.D., 1984. The ancestry of allergy: being an account of the original experimental induction of hypersensitivity recognizing the contribution of Paul Portier. J. Allergy Clin. Immunol. 75, 485–495.

Michael, A.F., Drummond, K.N., Good, R.A., Vernier, R.L., 1966. Acute poststreptococcal glomerulonephritis: immune deposit disease. J. Clin. Invest. 45, 237–248.

Mitchison, N.A., 1955. Studies on the immunological response to foreign tumor transplants in the mouse. J. Exp. Med. 102, 157–177.

Ottenberg, R., 1908. Transfusion and arterial anastomosis. Some experiments in arterial anastomosis and a study of transfusion with presentation of two clinical cases. Ann. Surg. 47, 486–505.

Portier, P., Richet, C., 1902. De l'action anaphylactique de certains venins. Compt. Rend. Soc. Biol. 54, 170–172.

Praustnitz, C., Küstner, H., 1921. Studien über Uberempfindlicht. Cent. Bakt. Abt. Orig. 86, 160–169. Translated to English in Gell, P.G.H., Coombs, R.R.A. (Eds.), 1962. Clinical Aspects of Immunology. Blackwell, Oxford, pp. 808–816.

Richet, C., 1910. Ancient humorism and modern humorism. Brit. Med. J. 2 (2596), 921–926.

Schick, B., 1907. Die Nachkrankheiten des Scharlach. Jb. Kinderheilk 65, 132.

Schlivert, P.M., Shands, K.N., Dan, B.B., Schmid, G.P., Nishimura, R.D., 1981. Identification and characterization of an exotoxin from *Staphylococcus aureus* associated with toxic-shock syndrome. J. Inf. Dis. 143, 509–516.

Schultz, W.H., 1910. Physiological studies in anaphylaxis: I the reaction of smooth muscle of the guinea pig sensitized with horse serum. J. Pharmacol. Exp. Ther. 1, 549–567.

Sell, S., 1978. Immunopathology. Amer. J. Pathol. 90, 211–279.

Stevens, F.A., 1927. The occurrence of *Staphylococcus aureus* infection with a scarlatiniform rash. JAMA 88, 1957–1958.

Talmage, D.W., Dixon, F.J., Bukantz, S.C., Dammin, G.J., 1951. Antigen elimination from blood as an early manifestation of the immune response. J. Immunol. 67, 243–255.

Todd, J., Fishaut, M., Kapral, F., Welch, T., 1978. Toxic-shock syndrome associated with phage-group-I staphylococci. Lancet 312, 1116–1118.

Vaughan, V.C., Wheeler, S.M., 1907. The effects of egg white and its split products on animals: a study of susceptibility and immunity. J. Infect. Dis. 4, 476–508.

von Pirquet, C.E., 1911. Allergy. Arch. Intern. Med. 7, 259–288.

von Pirquet, C.E., Schick, B., 1905. Die Serumkrankheit. Franz Deuticke, Leipzig/Wien.

White, J., Herman, A., Pullen, A.M., Kubo, R., Kappler, J.W., Marrack, P., 1989. The Vβ-specific superantigen staphylococcal enterotoxin B: stimulation in mature T cells and clonal deletion in neonatal mice. Cell 56, 27–35.

Zinsser, H., 1921. Studies on the tuberculin reaction and on specific hypersensitivities in bacterial infection. J. Exp. Med. 34, 495–524.

TIME LINE

1902	Paul Portier and Charles Richet discover anaphylaxis
1904	Jules Donath and Karl Landsteiner describe the presence of anti-red cell antibodies in paroxysmal cold hemoglobinuria
1905	Clemens von Pirquet and Bela Schick describe serum sickness
1909	Werner Schultz develops an in vitro method to measure anaphylaxis using muscle from guinea pig ileum
1910	John Anderson and W.H. Frost transfer anaphylaxis sensitivity to unsensitized animals by serum
1911	Clemens von Pirquet identifies antibodies to foreign serum as the etiological agent in serum sickness
1911	Henry Hallett Dale demonstrates the role of histamine in anaphylaxis
1913	Paul Portier awarded the Nobel Prize for Physiology or Medicine
1921	Hans Zinsser describes the tuberculin skin reaction
1921	Otto Prausnitz and Heinz Küstner demonstrate the transfer of anaphylactic sensitivity in humans
1939	Phillip Levine and Rufus Stetson report the initial case of erythroblastosis fetalis
1942	Merrill Chase and Karl Landsteiner transfer delayed type hypersensitivity with cells
1958	Kimishige Ishizaka and Dan Campbell demonstrate the mechanism of immune complex-mediated pathology
1962	Frank Dixon and colleagues develop an animal model of immune complex-mediated hypersensitivity
1962	Phillip Gell and Robin Coombs define four types in immune-mediated hypersensitivity reactions
1962	Melvin Kaplan and Mary Meyeserian describe cross-reaction between group A *Streptococcus* and heart tissue
1966	Alfred Michael and collaborators report the presence of antigen–antibody complexes in the kidneys of children with poststreptococcal glomerulonephritis
1967	Kimishige Ishizaka and colleagues and Gunnar Johansson and Hans Bennich discover IgE
1978	James Todd and colleagues describe toxic shock syndrome and its association with infections with *staphylococcus*
1981	Merlin Bergdoll and coworkers and Patrick Schlivert and collaborators isolate toxic shock syndrome toxin 1 (TSST1)
1989	Hans Fischer and coworkers and John Fraser report that TSST1 preferentially binds HLA-DR molecules
1989	Janice White and colleagues determine that staphylococcal enterotoxin binds specific Vβ regions expressed by T cells on their T cell receptor

34

Immune Responses Directed Against Self

INTRODUCTION

Two adaptive immune mechanisms have evolved to provide protection against potentially pathogenic microorganisms, malignantly transformed cells, and other dangerous invaders: antibodies synthesized by B lymphocytes that react primarily against extracellular bacteria, fungi, and protozoa parasites and specifically sensitized T lymphocytes that react against intracellular pathogens as well as against nascent tumors. The genetic mechanisms that permit the adaptive immune response to recognize and react to this wide variety of pathogenic microorganisms and other dangerous intruders result in an incredibly large array of unique specificities. These specificities are represented by the binding capability of cell surface receptors on individual B and T lymphocytes (Chapter 18). Due to the random nature of the generation of these receptors, some of the resultant cells inevitably express cell surface receptors directed toward self. Adaptive immune responses targeted to self-antigens disrupt homeostasis of the defense mechanisms of the body and induce pathology. To guard against the possibility of self-reactivity, the developing immune system has evolved several mechanisms to eliminate potentially autoreactive lymphocytes and assure immunologic tolerance thus maintaining homeostasis (Chapters 8, 21, and 22).

Tolerance-inducing mechanisms protect the integrity of the adaptive immune system; aberrations of tolerance lead to a large number of diseases characterized by activation of autoreactive B and/or T lymphocytes. Some of these disorders including Hashimoto thyroiditis, myasthenia gravis, and type 1 diabetes affect a single organ although the effects may impinge on homeostasis throughout the body. Others such as systemic lupus erythematosus (SLE) and rheumatoid arthritis (RA) affect tissues throughout the body producing systemic symptoms. Pathological damage is due to the direct action of antibodies, the deposition of antigen–antibody complexes, or the action of T lymphocytes. The mechanisms responsible for pathology are presented in the chapter on hypersensitivities (Chapter 33).

Before the adaptive immune system was identified, clinicians described many of the diseases now characterized as autoimmune. During the 1950s and 1960s, investigators reported associations between the presence of autoantibodies and certain pathologies such as SLE, Hashimoto thyroiditis, and immune-mediated anemia. In 1957, Ernest Witebsky and coworkers at the State University of New York, Buffalo, published a series of criteria required to prove that a disease is, in fact, autoimmune in nature. These criteria, based on Koch's postulates, have become known as Witebsky's postulates and include:

- "the direct demonstration of free, circulating antibodies that are active at body temperature or of cell-bound antibodies by indirect means;
- the recognition of the specific antigen against which this antibody is directed;
- the production of antibodies against the same antigen in experimental animals;
- the appearance of pathological changes in the corresponding tissues of an actively sensitized experimental animal that are basically similar to those in the human disease."

When Witebsky published these postulates, the division of immunocompetent cells into T and B lymphocytes as well as the basis of cell-mediated immunity had yet to be described. Immunological research focused on antibodies and investigators sought evidence for the presence of autoantibodies for those diseases thought to have an autoimmune etiology. More recently immunologists identified cell-mediated responses in many of these disorders. Now clinicians and immunologists agree that the clinical symptoms seen in many of the autoimmune processes primarily depend on activated T lymphocytes and that the presence of serum antibodies constitutes an epiphenomenon. A contemporary listing of Witebsky's postulates would, therefore, include the requirement for the demonstration of autoantibodies or specifically sensitized T lymphocytes.

The following sections review the historical background for several autoimmune diseases and the studies that led to identification of the underlying pathologic mechanisms.

EARLY STUDIES ON AUTOIMMUNE REACTIVITY AND DISEASE

In 1901, Paul Ehrlich and Julius Morgenroth, working at the Institute for Sera Research and Serum Testing (now renamed the Paul Ehrlich Institute) in Frankfurt, Germany, coined the term "horror autotoxicus" to refer to the concept that the adaptive immune system could not produce a pathological response against self. This idea derived from their studies of goats injected with their own red blood cells, with red blood cells from other goats, or with red blood cells from other species. Ehrlich and Morgenroth assayed sera from these animals for the presence of antibodies against red blood cells. While they detected antibody directed against erythrocytes of other species and of other members of their own species, they detected no antibody against self-red blood cells (Chapter 8).

However, a few years later other investigators demonstrated that animals, including humans, could in fact produce antibodies to a variety of self-antigens. Julius

Donath and Karl Landsteiner, working at the University of Vienna, Austria, documented the first autoimmune disease when they described antibodies in patients with paroxysmal cold hemoglobinuria (PCH) in 1904.

Patients with PCH, a rare disease characterized by the spontaneous lysis of red cells during exposure to cold temperatures, present with anemia and hemoglobinuria. Donath and Landsteiner described the presence of a hemolysin in the serum of three patients with PCH. This antibody binds red blood cells at temperatures below 37 °C (i.e., in the extremities). The red cells lyse as a result of complement activation when they return to the body core.

In the mid-1880s, Louis Pasteur and Emile Roux working at the Pasteur Institute in Paris described a second autoimmune process, postvaccine encephalomyelitis. They had developed a rabies vaccine derived from the dried spinal cord of rabbits infected with rabies virus. Clinicians administered this vaccine, which contained some rabbit nervous tissue, to patients exposed to a rabid animal using a protocol that involved a series of injections over several days. The vaccine protected most individuals who had been infected by the rabies virus; however, patients in whom the vaccine "failed" often received a second round of vaccine injections. Some of these patients developed ascending paralysis (loss of muscle activity starting in the lower limbs and ascending throughout the body) with a mortality rate of approximately 30%.

Investigators postulated that the vaccine activated the patient's immune response to synthesize and secrete antibodies to rabbit nervous tissue that cross-reacted with human nervous tissue thereby inducing inflammation in both the peripheral and central nervous systems leading to demyelination and the resulting paralysis.

Francis Schwentker and Thomas Rivers working at the Rockefeller Institute of Medical Research in New York in 1934 tested this postulate by injecting rabbits multiple times with brain extracts or emulsions. They quantitated antibodies to brain and showed that injection of fresh emulsions failed to induce antibody while emulsions of brain that had been allowed to sit for five or more days and then injected, or brain tissue that had been mixed with an immunological stimulant such as vaccinia virus, induced significant amounts of antibodies specific for myelin. Schwentker and Rivers reported that several of the injected rabbits producing these antibodies became partially paralyzed. Histological observations of the brains of these animals revealed foci of perivascular infiltration and necrosis surrounded by inflammation.

Despite these initial descriptions of diseases in humans and experimental animals associated with the presence of antibodies to self, another 20 years passed before investigators accepted the concept of clinically relevant autoimmune diseases.

AUTOIMMUNE DISEASES—NEW PATHOLOGIC MECHANISMS FOR OLD DISEASES

While ancient writings attributed to Egyptian, Greek, Roman, and Indian physicians contain descriptions of many of the autoimmune diseases, investigators only recently unraveled the pathophysiology of many of these disorders. The following sections highlight the historical evidence supporting an autoimmune etiology for a few of the more than 80 diseases that have been described.

Type 1 Diabetes

Egyptian and Indian physicians described diabetes almost 3500 years ago when they observed that patients produced copious amounts of urine that was sweet to taste. Apollonius of Memphis, a Greek physician, coined the term diabetes (siphon, to pass through) 1500 years ago. Indian physicians divided the disease into type 1 and type 2 based on the age of onset with type 1 occurring in young individuals while type 2 was seen in older patients. This division continued until well into the twentieth century when researchers determined that the two diseases had different pathologic mechanisms. Type 1 diabetes involves an autoimmune response against the insulin-secreting cells of the pancreas, while type 2 diabetes is (usually) characterized by a nonautoimmune etiology.

Unraveling the pathophysiology of type 1 diabetes depended on the development of an animal model of the disease. Joseph von Mering (1849–1908) and Oskar Minkowski (1858–1931) working at the University of Strasbourg, France, reported in 1890 that a dog from which the pancreas had been surgically removed developed all the signs and symptoms of diabetes including the presence of glucose in urine.

Eugene Opie (1873–1971), a medical student at Johns Hopkins University in Baltimore, Maryland, provided evidence of a connection between the pancreatic islets of Langerhans and diabetes (Opie, 1901a,b). Further study led Edward Albert Sharpy-Schafer working at the University of Edinburgh, Scotland, to hypothesize that individuals with type 1 diabetes were missing a chemical normally produced by the islets. He termed this chemical insulin from insula, the Latin word for islet (Garrison, 1925).

In 1922, Frederick Banting (1891–1941) and his colleagues at the University of Toronto repeated the studies of von Mering and Minkowski and demonstrated they could reverse diabetes by providing the dogs with an extract made from the islets of Langerhans of intact, healthy dogs. Isolation and purification of insulin used in the treatment of patients with type 1 diabetes soon followed. For this work, Frederick Banting and John McLeod were awarded the Nobel Prize

in Physiology or Medicine in 1923 "for their discovery of insulin."

The role of an adaptive immune response in the pathophysiology of type 1 diabetes remained unrecognized for another 50 years. In 1974, Gian Franco Bottazzo and colleagues working at the Middlesex Hospital Medical School in London reported the presence of antibodies specific for cells of the islets of Langerhans in patients with type 1 diabetes. Autopsy observations of the pancreas from these patients revealed the presence of an ongoing inflammatory response and infiltration of the organ by lymphocytes and plasma cells. Bottazzo and coworkers used immunofluorescence to detect serum antibodies specific for pancreatic islets. They prepared sections of pancreas to which they added serum from patients with multiple endocrine deficiencies. Following incubation and washing of the sections, the investigators added a fluorescent antibody to human IgG and mapped the location of immunofluorescence.

Thirteen sera (of 171 tested) contained antibodies that bound islet cells. Ten of the donors with positive sera presented with diabetes. The authors ruled out the possibility that the antibodies were against insulin. In their conclusion, Bottazzo and colleagues state that "the finding of these new antibodies certainly makes it easier to believe in an autoimmune form of diabetes mellitus." Subsequent investigators identified other autoantibodies associated with type 1 diabetes including antibodies against insulin in children recently diagnosed with the disease (Palmer et al., 1983) and antibodies to glutamic acid decarboxylase (Baekkeskov et al., 1990).

Several animal models of type 1 diabetes exist including infection of mice with encephalomyocarditis virus (Craighead and McLane, 1968), injection of mice with streptozotocin (Like et al., 1978), and injection of rabbits with xenogeneic insulin (Klöppel et al., 1972). During the 1970s, researchers described two spontaneously occurring animal models of type 1 diabetes. In 1977, Azima Nakhooda and colleagues at the University of Toronto, Canada, identified type 1 diabetes in an outbred colony of Wistar rats. These rats are termed BB (for BioBreeding) and the disease they develop is characterized by hyperglycemia, hypoinsulinemia, and hypoketonemia. These symptoms are similar to those seen in humans presenting with type 1 diabetes. In 1980, Susumu Makino and coworkers at the Shionogi Research Laboratories in Aburahi, Japan, developed a second model of spontaneously occurring diabetes called the nonobese, diabetic (NOD) strain of mice.

These models serve as tools in investigating the genetics, etiology, pathophysiology, and treatment of the disease. Autoreactive T and B lymphocytes as well as macrophages and NK lymphocytes infiltrate the islets in these spontaneously occurring models leading to the development of insulitis and the destruction of the islet cells that precedes the onset of diabetic symptoms.

Thyroiditis

In 1912, Hakaru Hashimoto, a medical student at Kyushu University in Japan, described four females, each presenting with goiter. Lymphocytes and plasma cells infiltrated these thyroid glands, and the parenchyma showed evidence of inflammation and fibrosis. While physicians had recognized goiter for centuries and had identified several different etiologies including infection, cancer, and thyrotoxicosis (hyperthyroidism or Grave disease), the etiology of the goiters associated with this chronic lymphocytic (Hashimoto) thyroiditis was not determined for more than 40 years.

Noel Rose (1927–), working as a postdoctoral fellow in the laboratory of Ernest Witebsky at the University of New York in Buffalo, performed experiments that unraveled the etiology of Hashimoto disease. Witebsky suggested to Rose that he pursue studies on the immunological specificity of the thyroid gland. Rose purified the principle antigen of the thyroid, thyroglobulin, from several different animal species, injected rabbits with the purified protein, and tested the resulting antibodies for organ specificity and cross-reactivity. In his initial studies, Rose found that rabbits produced antibodies against thyroglobulin from all species tested except the rabbit. He postulated that circulating thyroglobulin in the injected animals bound any antibody produced and removed it from the serum. To address this possibility, Rose removed thyroids from individual rabbits, prepared thyroglobulin from these thyroids, and injected it back into the thyroid gland donor.

Since the amount of thyroglobulin that could be obtained from a single thyroid was minimal, Rose incorporated the thyroglobulin into Freund's complete adjuvant (CFA—an oil in water emulsion containing inactivated and dried mycobacteria) to enhance the immunogenicity of the antigen. He immunized three groups of animals with this mixture and completely thyroidectomized, hemithyroidectomized, and sham thyroidectomized. To Rose's surprise all three groups of rabbits produced antibodies specific for rabbit thyroglobulin. In addition, when Rose evaluated the thyroid glands of the hemi- and sham-thyroidectomized animals histologically, he found them to be extensively infiltrated with mononuclear cells (Rose and Witebsky, 1956; Witebsky and Rose, 1956).

Rose and his collaborators, including John Paine, chair of the surgery department at Buffalo, extended these studies to other animal species including dogs. Once again the researchers detected antibodies to thyroglobulin in the dogs when CFA was used as an adjuvant. Mononuclear cells infiltrated thyroids from the injected animals. Observation of this infiltrate led Paine to remark that the organs resembled those seen in thyroids removed from patients with Hashimoto thyroiditis. This comment inspired the next experiment. Rose and his collaborators used a sensitive tanned cell hemagglutination assay to determine if sera from patients with Hashimoto disease bound human thyroglobulin. The investigators tested 12 sera, four of which were strongly positive (Witebsky et al., 1957). As Rose concluded in an essay published in 2006, "(t)his finding now seemed to close the circle. Not only was it possible to immunize animals experimentally with thyroglobulin and induce thyroiditis, but we could also demonstrate the presence of antibodies to thyroglobulin in human patients with chronic thyroiditis."

Idiopathic (Immune-Mediated) Thrombocytopenia

Idiopathic (immune-mediated) thrombocytopenia (ITP), a rare disease characterized by decreased platelet levels, leads to increased bleeding and bruising. Patients presenting with ITP were originally treated by splenectomy to remove the organ responsible for eliminating old platelets from the circulation. The evidence for the role of autoantibodies in this disease derives from an experiment performed by two hematology fellows who used each other as experimental subjects.

William J. Harrington (1924–1992) received his MD from Boston College University Medical School in 1947. In 1950, he was a hematology fellow at Barnes Hospital in St. Louis; one of his patients was diagnosed with ITP. He hypothesized that a serum factor was destroying the platelets. To test this hypothesis, Harrington and another hematology fellow, James W. Hollingsworth, transfused a unit of the patient's blood into Harrington who was ABO compatible with the patient. Within a few hours, Harrington's platelet count plummeted, and he had a seizure. His platelet count recovered after 5 days; during this time he showed many of the signs and symptoms of ITP (Harrington et al., 1951). The experiment was repeated on several other members of the Hematology Division of Barnes Hospital with similar results.

Harrington and his coworkers concluded that an autoantibody specific for a platelet antigen destroyed platelets in ITP. In 1961, Harrington and Grace Arimura confirmed this hypothesis when they described a platelet agglutinin in the serum of a majority of ITP patients. Although this was suggestive of the autoimmune nature of the disease, final proof emerged in 1969 when Simon Karpatikin and Gregory Siskind at the New York University School of Medicine reported the existence of an IgG in a patient's serum that disturbed platelet integrity as measured by activation of platelet factor 3. Subsequently investigators described several different autoantibodies to cell surface antigens on platelets.

The conclusion that antibodies destroyed platelets in patients with ITP led to an investigation of the mechanism of platelet removal. In the mid-1960s, investigators identified receptors for antibodies on the surface of macrophages. These Fc receptors bound immunoglobulin and activated the macrophage to initiate phagocytosis (Berken and Benacerraf, 1966). When antibodies bind platelets and then macrophages, the complex is phagocytized, and the platelets are quickly removed from the circulation. As the process continues the removal of the platelets outstrips the ability of the hematopoietic precursors to produce new platelets to replace them.

Systemic Lupus Erythematosus (SLE)

SLE, a chronic, multisystem, inflammatory disease, affects primarily females between the ages of 15 and 50 years. The disease can take a relapsing–remitting course and is characterized by the presence of antigen–antibody complexes that attach to endothelial cells of small blood vessels particularly in skin, joints, and kidney. These complexes activate the complement system resulting in the induction of an inflammatory response leading to pathology.

Almost 2500 years ago, Hippocrates described a disease resembling SLE characterized by cutaneous ulcers that he called herpes esthiomenos (Smith and Cyr, 1988; Mallavarapu and Grimsley, 2007). Other physicians described a similar disorder; these clinicians introduced the term lupus (wolf) during the tenth century to describe the erosive rash seen on the face that resembled the animal. The term lupus was used loosely during the next several centuries to refer to cutaneous manifestations resulting from several different etiologies.

The initial clinical description of SLE is attributed to Laurent Theodore Biett, a physician in Paris during the early 1800s. His student, Pierre Louis Alphee Cazanave, published this description in 1833 and coined the term lupus erythematosus. Ferdinand von Hebra in 1866 described the facial rash as resembling a butterfly (Mallavarapu and Grimsley, 2007).

These early clinical descriptions concentrated on the cutaneous lesions of the disease. In the mid-1800s, two Viennese physicians, Ferdinand von Hebra and Moritz Kaposi, documented systemic symptoms of the disease, including lymphadenopathy, fever, weight loss, arthritis, and anemia. In 1895, William Osler confirmed these observations in a study of 29 patients with skin disease and systemic involvement. Osler (1849–1919) is considered by some the father of modern medicine. He received his medical training at McGill University in Montreal, Canada, and pursued additional studies in Europe before returning to McGill to join the faculty.

In 1884, he moved to the University of Pennsylvania where he stayed until he was recruited to be one of the four original faculty members of the new Johns Hopkins University Medical School in Baltimore, Maryland. In addition to authoring a classical textbook of medicine (*The Principles and Practice of Medicine*), Osler is recognized as an innovator in medical education for insisting that students be exposed to patients early in their education and for introducing the concept of the medical residency.

Osler noted that SLE involved organ systems other than the skin including renal, cardiovascular, and pulmonary. Subsequent reevaluation of the 29 patients described in Osler's original publications reveals that only two of them had SLE based on current criteria for diagnosis (Scofield and Oates, 2009). In spite of what we recognize today as a diagnostic error, the legacy of Osler continues to exist, and he is credited with reinvigorating the study of SLE. During the ensuing 50 years, clinicians detailed the systemic manifestations of SLE including the observation that patients with SLE do not always present with a facial rash.

The initial indication that an immunologic process might be involved in SLE emerged from the description of the LE cell (Hargraves et al., 1948). LE cells, large phagocytic cells, contain vacuoles stained with hematoxylin, a basic dye that stains negatively charged compounds such as nucleic acids dark blue. Malcolm Hargraves and his colleagues at the Mayo Clinic in Rochester, Minnesota, aspirated bone marrow from patients with SLE and reported the presence of LE cells. These cells are now known to be macrophages or neutrophils that have phagocytized denatured nuclei from dying or dead cells. Further investigation by Hargraves showed that incubation of bone marrow cells from healthy individuals with plasma from SLE patients induced the formation of LE cells.

Investigators hypothesized that the plasma factor was an antibody. They demonstrated that this factor migrated electrophoretically in the 7S gamma globulin fraction. In 1957, three groups of researchers simultaneously identified antibody to DNA in the serum of lupus patients.

Halsted Holman and Henry Kunkel at the Rockefeller Institute for Medical Research in New York demonstrated that the serum factor from SLE patients is

- absorbed by treating the serum with cell nuclei and
- eluted from the nuclei and precipitated by an antibody to gamma globulin.

Holman and Kunkel (1957) performed parallel experiments with nucleoprotein they extracted in 1M NaCl. This nucleoprotein, which contained DNA and histone, absorbed the activity from SLE serum just as cell nuclei had. Treatment of the nucleoprotein with DNase destroyed this activity. Based on their studies the authors conclude that "the L.E. serum factor has an affinity for nuclear nucleoprotein and that desoxyribonucleic acid is involved in the bond. The fact that the L.E. serum factor is a γ-globulin that appears to react with antiserum to normal γ-globulin suggests that the factor may be an antibody."

In 1957, Ruggero Ceppellini and his colleagues working at the University of Turin, in Italy and Maxime Seligmann working at the Saint Louis Hospital in Paris independently made similar observations. Both groups characterized the factor present in the serum of lupus patients that induced the LE cell as antibody to cell nuclei, most likely to DNA. Although subsequent clinical investigations have identified several additional autoantibodies in some lupus patients, these results led to the development of diagnostic tests for SLE.

In 1959, Marianne Bielschowsky and colleagues at the University of Otago Medical School in Dunedin, New Zealand, described several mouse models of autoimmune disease that aided subsequent studies of the mechanisms by which autoantibodies cause pathology (reviewed in Bielschowsky and Goodall, 1970). Initially Bielschowsky and coworkers differentiated these outbred mice by coat color. They developed several different inbred strains with variable expression of autoimmunity.

One hybrid, derived by crossing New Zealand Black (NZB) with New Zealand White (NZW) mice, dies of renal failure by 8–10 months of age (Helyer and Howie, 1963). All of the hybrid mice test positive for LE cells, and their kidney pathology mimics that seen in patients with lupus nephritis. Immunofluorescent staining of sections of kidneys from NZB/W mice with rabbit antibodies to mouse serum demonstrated a pattern of fluorescence similar to that seen in kidneys from patients with SLE (Aarons, 1964). Studies of this animal model confirmed that SLE is an autoimmune disease and that the pathophysiology involves deposition of antigen–antibody complexes in small blood vessels in the glomeruli of kidneys, the synovial membranes of joints, and other organs.

Rheumatoid Arthritis (RA)

Rheumatoid arthritis (RA), a chronic, systemic disease characterized by an autoimmune-induced inflammatory attack on the joints of the body, leads to distinctive disfigurement of the hands and feet. RA has been described in the human population in literature and art for millennia (Entezami et al., 2011). Hippocrates as well as ancient Greek, Roman, and Byzantine physicians described patients who may have been suffering from RA. In addition, a number of artists from the Renaissance depict subjects with hand deformities that are similar to those seen in contemporary patients with the disease. A famous painting by Peter Paul Rubens, *The Three Graces*, contains an example of possible RA in the hand of one

of the Graces. Finally, as reviewed by Entezami and colleagues, paleopathology (the study of disease in human remains) provides clues to the ancient origins of RA.

In 1800, Augustin Jacob Landré-Beauvais (1772–1840) presented a dissertation to the medical faculty at the School of Medicine in Paris for his MD degree. In this dissertation, he described a number of patients who presented with severe joint pain. Although he concluded that the disease was related to gout, he differentiated the signs and symptoms in his patients from those diagnosed with gout. This unique disease was characterized by

- the predominance of the disease in women,
- the involvement of several joints,
- the chronicity of the disease, and
- the effect the disease had on the general health of the patient.

Alford Garrod, an English physician practicing in the mid-1800s, demonstrated that patients with gout have elevated levels of serum uric acid. Patients with other joint diseases, including those with RA, express levels of serum uric acid within established reference ranges for healthy individuals. This differentiated gout and RA as distinct diseases. Archibald Garrod, one of Alford Garrod's sons, coined the term RA to refer to the disease originally described by Landré-Beauvais (Garrod, 1890). Immunologists and clinicians now agree that RA is an inflammatory disease of the synovial membrane lining the joints; however, the initiating event resulting in this inflammatory process remains unknown although several lines of evidence implicate an autoimmune etiology.

In 1940, Emil Waaler (1903–1998) in Sweden detected an agglutination activating factor in the serum of some patients with RA by adding patients' serum to sheep erythrocytes that had first been treated with a low concentration of antibodies specific to the red cells. The factor in the patient's serum agglutinated the erythrocytes. Waaler showed that the factor in RA sera migrated electrophoretically with the globulin fraction of serum, the fraction know to contain antibody.

Published at the beginning of World War II in a Swedish medical journal, this paper was effectively lost to clinical rheumatologists in much of the world. In 1948, Noel Rose and coworkers rediscovered this factor when they performed experiments identical to those carried out by Waaler. The serum factor responsible for the activity was called rheumatoid factor (RF), and the original clinical test developed to detect RF was called the Waaler–Rose test.

RF comprises a group of antibodies with specificity for the Fc region of IgG molecules. While primarily IgM, these antibodies may be IgG or IgA as well. The role of RF in the pathogenesis of RA remains unknown. Moreover, clinicians demonstrated that a positive RF assay is not specific for RA but may be present in patients with other autoimmune diseases and even in unaffected individuals. Despite this, the detection of RF in a patient with joint pain constitutes one of the criteria for diagnosing RA.

Since the original description of RF, investigators have detected a large number of other antibodies to self in patients with RA including ones specific for cartilage proteins, collagen, enzymes, heat shock proteins, and ribonucleoprotein. Many of these antibodies are also present in patients with other autoimmune diseases including SLE, Sjögren syndrome, and autoimmune muscle disease, and are, therefore, not disease specific. Recently researchers have detected antibodies in patients with RA that react to proteins containing the amino acid citrulline, a modification of the amino acid, arginine.

Gerard Schellekens and coworkers at the University of Nijmegen, the Netherlands, initially described antibodies to citrullinated proteins in 1998. This group investigated the fine specificity of antibodies to keratin since the presence of such antibodies appeared to be relatively specific for RA. The antigen recognized by these antibodies is filaggrin, a component of cells of the skin.

The formation of the cellular cytoskeleton requires enzymatic cleavage and dephosphorylation of profilaggrin to filaggrin. This reaction is accompanied by conversion of some of the arginine residues of filaggrin to citrulline. To test if citrulline is important in the epitope recognized by antibodies to keratin, Schellekens and colleagues constructed several synthetic peptides in which citrulline replaced arginine. They designed an assay to detect the presence or absence of antibodies in sera from RA patients and found antibodies to citrulline containing peptides in 76% of sera tested. This finding led to the development of a new clinical laboratory test, the anti citrullinated peptide antibody test (ACPA), that is more sensitive and specific for RA than is the RF test.

Despite the detection of a large number of different antibodies to self in patients with RA, the role of these antibodies in the etiology and pathogenesis of the disease remains elusive. In fact some investigators speculate that antibodies represent an epiphenomenon secondary to a T lymphocyte-mediated response: this has fostered a search for autoreactive T lymphocytes.

In 1976, Arthur Bankhurst and colleagues working at the University of New Mexico, Albuquerque, reported that the predominant cell type infiltrating the synovia of patients with RA is the T lymphocyte. They showed that most of the lymphocytes isolated from the synovia of five RA patients stained with rabbit antibodies to T lymphocytes using immunofluorescence.

In 1977, Harold Paulus and colleagues at the University of California, Los Angeles, established long-term fistulas in the thoracic ducts of 13 patients with severe RA. Drainage of thoracic duct lymphocytes improved several objective criteria of the disease including grip strength, duration of morning stiffness, and number of tender joints in nine of these patients. The fistulas in the other four patients failed to provide adequate lymph drainage. Reinfusion of these lymphocytes exacerbated the disease, and some of the reinfused lymphocytes migrated to inflamed joints. Once the investigators ceased draining lymphocytes from the thoracic duct, acute RA recurred. The authors concluded that "some of the lymphocytes in the thoracic duct lymph are essential for the continued activity of inflammation associated with rheumatoid arthritis."

Previous research demonstrated that thoracic duct lymphocytes are predominately thymus-dependent T lymphocytes. Beginning in the 1980s, investigators characterized functional subpopulations of T lymphocytes based on the expression of cell surface molecules (CD4 and CD8) and on the cytokines produced (Chapter 22); many of the T lymphocytes infiltrating inflamed synovia from RA patients have a CD4$^+$, T_H1 phenotype, a cell implicated in helping CD8$^+$ cytotoxic T lymphocytes.

In 1996, Anders Bucht led a group of researchers that evaluated the expression of immunoregulatory cytokines expressed by lymphocytes isolated from synovial fluid from joints of patients with RA. These investigators demonstrated that synovial fluid lymphocytes expressed mRNA for IFN-γ, TGF-β, IL-10, and IL-12 while they failed to detect mRNA for IL-4. The presence of mRNA for IFN-γ and for IL-12 in the absence of an mRNA for IL-4 suggests that the T lymphocytes in the joint are skewed toward a T_H1 rather than a T_H2 response (Chapter 23).

In 2008, J. Claude Bennett from Biocyst Pharmaceuticals in Birmingham, Alabama, reviewed recent research on the role of T lymphocytes in RA and concluded that not only are the T_H1-inducing cytokines, IL-12 and IL-18, present in synovial fluids but that IL-18 levels correlate with the severity of symptoms and response to therapy. In addition, mice incapable of synthesizing IL-12 or IL-18 show decreased incidence and severity of collagen-induced arthritis, a model used to study human RA (Bennett, 2008).

T_H17 lymphocytes, a recently described subset of CD4$^+$ lymphocytes, have also been implicated in the pathogenesis of RA. T_H17 cells produce several cytokines including IL-17, IL-6, TNF-α, and IL-22 that are involved in the inflammatory response. In 1999, Martine Chabaud and coworkers at Hôpital Edouard Herriot in Lyon, France, detected production of IL-17 by lymphocytes from synovial fluid isolated from patients with RA. These results and others led J. Claude Bennett to conclude in his 2008 review that there is "overwhelming evidence that the T cell, particularly the T_H17 subset plays a role in the pathogenic process of RA."

Despite this assertion, the identity of the initial immunologic insult leading to the inflammatory response in RA remains unknown. A variety of therapies have been developed that provide relief of symptoms but do not cure the disease. Anti-inflammatory pharmaceuticals modify the disease process and are used early in its course. More recently researchers developed biological reagents that target the postulated underlying immune mechanisms. These include monoclonal antibodies and soluble receptors specific for TNF-α, a key proinflammatory cytokine (Chapter 38). Other successful therapeutics depend on interrupting the molecular events involved in initiation of an immune response and include monoclonal antibodies to CD20, a cell surface molecule on antibody-producing B lymphocytes, and a soluble receptor that inhibits the interaction between T lymphocytes and antigen-presenting cells.

CONCLUSION

More than 80 different diseases, some of which physicians identified centuries ago, involve an autoimmune etiology. Ehrlich and Morgenroth in the early part of the twentieth century rejected the concept of pathological autoimmune responses. With a few exceptions, this hypothesis influenced clinical immunology for 50 years despite Donath and Landsteiner describing the presence of antibodies to self-red blood cells in patients with PCH. The finding of RF in patients with RA, of antibodies to nuclear material in SLE, and of antibodies to thyroglobulin in patients with Hashimoto thyroiditis finally disproved the concept of "horror autotoxicus" and affirmed the etiology of autoimmune disorders.

Initially investigators concluded that autoantibodies produced the pathology associated with autoimmune diseases. However, beginning in the 1990s, the role of T lymphocytes as a major actor in some of these disorders has been clarified. A question still not totally resolved is how the immune system overcomes self-tolerance to initiate autoimmune responses.

Burnet, in his clonal selection theory, hypothesized that maturing lymphocytes are sensitive to elimination if they express a cell surface receptor with specificity for self-antigens. Virtually all immunologists accept this hypothesis (Chapter 21). Other mechanisms of eliminating self-reactive lymphocytes include downregulation of responses by T_{REG} lymphocytes and immunoregulatory cytokines (Chapters 20, 21, and 22). Current hypotheses about the mechanisms responsible for breaking self-tolerance invoke genetics (many human autoimmune diseases are associated with the expression of a limited number of human leukocyte-associated antigens), infections (viral and bacterial), and environmental insults including smoking and exposure to chemicals.

Evidence that a disease is autoimmune in nature requires demonstration of several criteria that were developed by Ernest Witebsky in the 1950s. These criteria can be restated based on our current knowledge of the adaptive immune system as follows:

- antibodies or sensitized T lymphocytes with specificity for self-antigens must be isolated from a patient with the disease;
- the antigen against which these antibodies or T lymphocytes are reactive must be identified;
- injection of this antigen into an experimental animal must induce specific antibodies or sensitized T lymphocytes; and
- experimental animals injected with this antigen must demonstrate pathological changes in the corresponding tissues that are basically similar to those in the human disease.

Many of these criteria have been met for several autoimmune diseases identified since the 1960s. However, the relative roles of antibody and T lymphocytes in initiating the pathology of these disorders remain unresolved. In addition, recent evidence that some of these disorders are autoinflammatory in nature (Chapter 30) rather than autoimmune provides ample questions for future investigations.

References

Aarons, I., 1964. Renal immunofluorescence in NXB/NZW mice. Nature 203, 1080–1081.

Baekkeskov, S., Aanstoot, H., Christgal, S., Reetz, A., Solinera, M., Cascalho, M., Folli, F., Richter-Oleson, H., Camilli, P.-D., 1990. Identification of the 64K autoantigen in insulin-dependent diabetes as the GABA-synthesizing enzyme glutamic acid decarboxylase. Nature 347, 151–156.

Bankhurst, A.D., Husby, G., Williams, R.C., 1976. Predominance of T cells in the lymphocytic infiltrates of synovial tissues in rheumatoid arthritis. Arthritis Rheum. 19, 555–562.

Banting, F.G., Best, C.H., Collip, J.B., Campbell, W.R., Fletcher, A.A., 1922. Pancreatic extracts in the treatment of diabetes mellitus: preliminary report. Can. Med. Assoc. J. 12, 141–146.

Bennett, J.C., 2008. The role of T lymphocytes in rheumatoid arthritis and other autoimmune diseases. Arthritis Rheum. 58, S53–S57.

Berken, A., Benacerraf, B., 1966. Properties of antibodies cytophilic for macrophages. J. Exp. Med. 123, 119–144.

Bielschowsky, M., Goodall, C.M., 1970. Origin of inbred NZ mouse strains. Cancer Res. 30, 834–836.

Bielschowsky, M., Helyer, B.J., Howie, J.B., 1959. Spontaneous hemolytic anemia in mice of the NZB/BL strain. Proc. Univ. Otaga Med. Sch. 37, 9.

Bottazzo, G.F., Florin-Christensen, A., Donaich, D., 1974. Isle-cell antibodies in diabetes mellitus with autoimmune polyendocrine deficiencies. Lancet 304, 1279–1283.

Bucht, A., Larsson, P., Weisbrot, L., Thorne, C., Pisa, P., Semdegard, G., et al., 1996. Expression of interferon gamma (IGN-γ) IL-10, IL-12 and transforming growth factor-beta (TGF-β) mRNA in synovial fluid cells from patients in the early and late phases of rheumatoid arthritis (RA). Clin. Exp. Immunol. 103, 357–367.

Ceppellini, R., Polli, E., Celada, F., 1957. A DNA-reacting factor in serum of a patient with lupus erythematosus diffuses. Proc. Soc. Exp. Biol. Med. 96, 572–574.

Chabaud, M., Durand, J.M., Buchs, N., Fossiez, F., Page, G., Frappert, L., Miossec, P., 1999. Human interleukin 17: a T cell-derived pro-inflammatory cytokine produced by the rheumatoid synovium. Arthritis Rheum. 42, 963–970.

Craighead, J.E., McLane, M.F., 1968. Diabetes mellitus: induction in mice by encephalomyocarditis virus. Science 162, 913–914.

Donath, J., Landsteiner, K., 1904. Uber paroxysmile Hamoglobinurie. Muchen. Med. Wochenschr. 51, 1590–1593.

Ehrlich, P., Morgenroth, J., 1901. Uber Hämolysine. Berl. Klin. Wochenschr. 38, 251–257.

Entezami, P., Fox, D.A., Clapham, P.J., Chung, K.C., 2011. Historical perspective on the etiology of rheumatoid arthritis. Hand Clin. 27, 1–10.

Garrison, F.H., 1925. Historical aspects of diabetes and insulin. N. Y. Acad. Med. 1, 127–133.

Garrod, A.E., 1890. Treatise on Rheumatism and Rheumatoid Arthritis. Charles Griffin and Co., London.

Hargraves, M.M., Richmond, H., Morton, R., 1948. Presentations of two bone marrow elements: "tart" cell and "LE" cell. Proc. Staff Meet. Mayo Clin. 23, 25–28.

Harrington, W.J., Arimura, G., 1961. Immune reactions of platelets. In: Johnson, S.A., Monto, R.W., Rebuck, J.W., Horn, R.C. (Eds.), Henry Ford Hospital Symposium: Blood Platelets. Little Brown and Co., Boston, MA, pp. 659–670.

Harrington, W.J., Minnich, V., Hollingsworth, J.W., Moore, C.V., 1951. Demonstration of a thrombocytopenic factor in the blood of patients with thrombocytopenic purpura. J. Lab. Clin. Med. 38, 1–10.

Hashimoto, H., 1912. Zur kentniss der lymphomatosen veränderung des schilddrüsse (struma lymphomatusa). Arch. Klin. Chir. 97, 219–249.

Helyer, B.J., Howie, J.B., 1963. Renal disease associated with positive lupus erythematosus tests in a cross bred strain of mice. Nature 197, 197.

Holman, H.R., Kunkel, H.G., 1957. Affinity between the lupus erythematosus serum factor and cell nuclei and nucleoprotein. Science 126, 162–163.

Karpatikin, S., Siskind, G.W., 1969. In vitro detection of platelet antibody in patients with idiopathic thrombocytopenic purpura and systemic lupus erythematosus. Blood 33, 795–812.

Klöppel, G., Altenahr, E., Freytag, G., 1972. Studies on ultrastructure and immunology of the insulitis in rabbits immunized with insulin. Virchows Arch. 356, 1–15.

Landré-Beauvais, A.J., 1800. Doit-on admettre une nouvelle espèce de goutte sous la denomination de goutte asthénique primitive? Translated and reprinted as: 2001 the first description of rheumatoid arthritis. Unabridged text of the doctoral dissertation presented in 1800. Joint Bone Spine 68, 130–143.

Like, A.A., Appel, M.C., Williams, R.M., Rossini, A.A., 1978. Streptozotocin-induced pancreatic insulitis in mice: morphologic and physiologic studies. Lab. Invest. 38, 470–485.

Makino, S., Kunimoto, K., Muraoka, Y., Mizushima, Y., Katagiri, K., Tochino, Y., 1980. Breeding of a non-obese, diabetic strain of mice. Jikken Dobutsu 29, 1–13.

Mallavarapu, R.K., Grimsley, E.W., 2007. The history of lupus erythematosus. South. Med. J. 100, 896–898.

Nakhooda, A.F., Like, A.A., Chappel, C.I., Murray, F.T., Marliss, E.B., 1977. The spontaneously diabetic Wistar rat: metabolic and morphologic studies. Diabetes 26, 100–112.

Opie, E.L., 1901a. On the relation of chronic interstitial pancreatitis to the islands of Langerhans and to diabetes mellitus. J. Exp. Med. 5, 397–428.

Opie, E.L., 1901b. The relation of diabetes mellitus to lesions of the pancreas. Hyaline degeneration of the islands of Langerhans. J. Exp. Med. 5, 527–540.

Osler, W., 1895. On the visceral complications of erythema exudativum multiforme. Am. J. Med. Sci. 110, 629–646.

Palmer, J.P., Asplin, C.M., Clemons, P., Lyen, K., Tatpati, O., Raghu, P.K., Paquette, T.L., 1983. Insulin antibodies in insulin-dependent diabetes before insulin treatment. Science 222, 1337–1339.

Paulus, H.E., Machleder, H.I., Levine, S., Yu, D.T., MacDonald, N.S., 1977. Lymphocyte involvement in rheumatoid arthritis: studies during thoracic duct drainage. Arthritis Rheum. 20, 1249–1262.

Rose, H.M., Ragan, C., Pearce, E., Lipman, M.O., 1948. Differential agglutination of normal and sensitized erythrocytes by sera of patients with rheumatoid arthritis. Proc. Soc. Exp. Biol. Med. 68, 1–6.

Rose, N.R., 2006. Life amidst the contrivances. Nat. Immunol. 7, 1009–1011.

Rose, N.R., Witebsky, E., 1956. Studies on organ specificity. V. Changes in thyroid glands of rabbits following active immunization with rabbit thyroid extract. J. Immunol. 76, 417–427.

Schellekens, G.A., de Jong, B.A.W., van den Hoogen, F.H.J., van de Putte, L.B.A., 1998. Citrulline is an essential constituent of antigenic determinants recognized by rheumatoid arthritis-specific autoantibodies. J. Clin. Invest. 101, 273–281.

Schwentker, F.F., Rivers, T.M., 1934. The antibody response of rabbits to injections of emulsions and extracts of homologous brain. J. Exp. Med. 60, 559–574.

Scofield, R.H., Oates, J.C., 2009. The place of William Osler in the description of systemic lupus erythematosus. Am. J. Med. Sci. 338, 409–412.

Seligmann, M., 1957. Leuco-préceiitines II. Mise en evidence d'une reaction de precipitation entre des extraits leucocytaires et le serum de maladies atteints de lupus érythémateux disséminé. Vox Sang. 2, 270–282.

Smith, S.D., Cyr, M., 1988. The history of lupus erythematosus; from Hippocrates to Osler. Rheum. Dis. Clin. North Am. 14, 1–14.

von Mehring, J., Minkowski, O., 1890. Diabetes mellitus nach pancreas exstirpation. Arch. Exp. Pathol. Pharmakol. 26, 371–387.

Waaler, E., 1940. On the occurrence of a factor in human serum activating the specific agglutination of sheep blood corpuscles. Acta Path. Microbiol. Scand. 17, 172–188.

Witebsky, E., Rose, N.R., 1956. Studies on organ specificity. IV. Production of rabbit thyroid antibodies in rabbit. J. Immunol. 76, 408–416.

Witebsky, E., Rose, N.R., Terplan, K., Paine, J.R., Egan, R.W., 1957. Chronic thyroiditis and autoimmunization. JAMA 164, 1439–1447.

TIME LINE

1500 BCE	Egyptian and Indian physicians describe diabetes
500 BCE	Hippocrates describes a disease resembling systemic lupus erythematosus (SLE)
1000	The term lupus (wolf) introduced to describe the characteristic facial rash seen in SLE
1800	Augustin J. Landré-Beauvais publishes initial description of patients with rheumatoid arthritis
1833	Pierre L. A. Cazanave publishes initial clinical description of SLE
1890	Archibald Garrod uses the term rheumatoid arthritis to refer to the inflammatory joint disease
1890	Joseph von Mering and Oscar Minkowski induce diabetes in a dog by pancreatectomy
1895	William Osler confirms Kaposi's description of the systemic manifestations of SLE
1901	Eugene Opie describes the relationship between pathology in the islets of Langerhans and type 1 diabetes

1901	Paul Ehrlich and Julius Morgenroth propose the concept of "horror autotoxicus"
1904	Julius Donath and Karl Landsteiner demonstrate the autoimmune nature of paroxysmal cold hemoglobinuria
1912	Hakaru Hashimoto publishes report of inflammatory thyroid disease in four female patients presenting with goiter
1922	Frederick Banting and colleagues reverse diabetes by injecting an extract of pancreatic beta cells
1923	Frederick Banting and John McLeod awarded the Nobel Prize in Physiology or Medicine "for their discovery of insulin"
1940	Emil Waaler describes the presence of an antibody in RA patients that binds other antibodies
1948	Noel Rose and colleagues rediscover Waaler's antibody and call it rheumatoid factor
1948	Malcolm M. Hargraves and colleagues describe LE (lupus erythematosus) cells in bone marrow aspirates of SLE patients

1950	William Harrington and James Hollingsworth prove that idiopathic thrombocytopenia purpura is caused by a serum factor (subsequently identified as antibody to platelets)
1956	Noel Rose and Ernest Witebsky induce autoimmune thyroiditis in rabbits by injecting thyroglobulin
1957	Ernest Witebsky publishes criteria that must be met to prove a disease is autoimmune
1957	Halsted Holman and Henry Kunkel, Ruggero Ceppellini and coworkers, and Maxime Seligmann independently present evidence for the presence of antinuclear antibody in SLE
1974	Gian Franco Bottazzo and colleagues report the presence of antibodies to islet of Langerhans cells in type 1 diabetes
1976	Arthur Bankhurst and colleagues provide evidence that synovia of RA patients are infiltrated by T lymphocytes
1998	Gerard Schellekens and coworkers describe importance of citrulline in the epitopes recognized by autoantibodies in RA patients

35

Lymphoproliferative Diseases

INTRODUCTION

During the 1800s the practice of medicine changed from a clinical presentation and observational discipline to one that incorporated technological advances. The microscope, invented by Anton van Leeuwenhoek in the 1600s, became a mainstay in the study of pathology during the nineteenth century primarily through the efforts of Rudolf Virchow. William Hewson in London described lymphocytes in the spleen and thymus in the 1770s, and Gabriel Andral in France and William Addison in England described white cells in the blood in the 1840s. Beginning in the early nineteenth century several clinicians published cases of patients who presented with aberrations of the cells of the blood stimulating later studies that uncovered malignancies of these cells.

Physicians in the 1800s knew that enlargement of the spleen and lymph nodes often signaled disease although most patients with palpable spleens were diagnosed with nonmalignant disorders including infection, anemia, and malaria. During the 1800s some clinicians associated splenomegaly with the occurrence of cancers in the bloodstream, and the concept of malignantly transformed white blood cells became an additional diagnosis for physicians. The cells of the blood arise from pluripotent stem cells through hematopoiesis.

Hematopoietic stem cells differentiate into either myeloid precursors or lymphoid precursors that, in turn, generate the mature, functional cells of the peripheral blood. Myeloid precursors are the progenitors of erythrocytes, polymorphonuclear leukocytes (neutrophils), eosinophils, basophils, monocytes, and platelets. Lymphoid precursors differentiate into T, B, and NK (natural killer) lymphocytes.

Hematopoiesis involves alternating rounds of proliferation and differentiation both of which involve gene activation. Differentiation requires stimulation by soluble factors (cytokines) that induce gene transcription. These events are under homeostatic regulation providing sufficient but not excessive numbers of mature cells. During the past two centuries, clinicians described several pathologies in which aberrant control of hematopoiesis and differentiation results in overproduction of one or another cell type leading to pathology.

Based on the precursor cell involved, these pathologies are classified as either myeloproliferative or lymphoproliferative. Myeloproliferative syndromes include both malignant and nonmalignant conditions such as chronic myelogenous leukemia, polycythemia vera, essential thrombocytosis, and myelofibrosis. Lymphoproliferative disorders are classified as acute lymphoblastic leukemia, chronic lymphocytic leukemia, lymphoma, and monoclonal gammopathies.

Cancer is a genetic disease and as such can affect any nucleated cell. The genetic events leading to cancer (malignant transformation) occur in lymphocytes at all stages of differentiation from embryonic stem cells to fully mature antibody and cytokine secretors. Clinicians recognized many of these disorders prior to the immunologists' description of the adaptive immune system. Lymphocytes are particularly susceptible to mutations that can lead to the development of cancer since they upregulate various genes both during differentiation in central lymphoid organs (thymus and bone marrow/bursa) and following activation by antigen.

Consequently, clinicians have described patients presenting with a seemingly large number of different hematological cancers. In an attempt to characterize these disorders and to systematize treatment, pathologists and oncologists devised several classification systems based on the histological appearance of the malignant cells. While initially useful, contemporary research on the genetics and molecular biology of these tumors now provides an improved basis for differentiating the tumors, predicting outcome, and designing optimal therapeutic regimens.

Clinicians and pathologists initially divided lymphoproliferative diseases into lymphomas, leukemias, and monoclonal gammopathies (paraproteinemias) defined as follows:

- Lymphomas are malignancies of lymphocytes that form solid tumors in various organs including peripheral lymphoid organs such as spleen and lymph nodes and any organ where lymphocytes are found.
- Leukemias are malignancies of white blood cells including progeny of both the myeloid and lymphoid precursor cells. Lymphocytic leukemia consists of malignantly transformed B, T, or NK lymphocytes circulating in peripheral blood and lymphatic vessels and resident in many of the lymphatic organs.
- Monoclonal gammopathies are malignancies of immunoglobulin-secreting B lymphocytes and plasma cells.

Many of the original descriptions of these malignancies date from the 1800s. Thomas Hodgkin in 1832 published the initial description of patients with lymphoma. Subsequent characterization of other patients with lymphoma led to a classification scheme dividing the disease into two entities termed either Hodgkin lymphoma or non-Hodgkin lymphoma. Leukemia as a clinical entity was recorded several times during the early nineteenth century before Rudolf Virchow introduced the term leukemia in 1856. Multiple myeloma, a neoplasm of antibody-producing plasma cells, was initially described by Samuel Solly in 1844 based on his observations of a patient whose bone marrow contained numerous large cells with a unique staining pattern.

LYMPHOMA

Thomas Hodgkin (1798–1866) received his MD from the University of Edinburgh Medical School in Scotland in 1823. After additional training in Paris, Hodgkin

returned to a medical practice at Guy's Hospital Medical School in London. In 1832 he published an extensive description of the autopsies of patients with enlargement of the spleen and lymph nodes (Aisenberg, 2000). Samuel Wilks (1824–1911), a pathologist at Guy's Hospital in London, referred to these cancers as Hodgkin lymphoma when he reevaluated Hodgkin's original case descriptions and added several additional cases (Wilks, 1865).

In 1878 W.S. Greenfield at the University of Edinburgh, Scotland, described enlarged cells with multiple nuclei in the lymphoid tissue of patients with Hodgkin lymphoma. Twenty years later Dorothy Reed-Mendenhall and Carl Sternberg independently characterized these cells that are now considered pathognomonic of the disease and are called Reed–Sternberg cells (Sternberg, 1898; Reed, 1902). Reed–Sternberg cells are large, abnormal lymphocytes that often contain more than one nucleus (Figure 35.1). Originally Reed–Sternberg cells were thought to be infected with *Mycobacterium tuberculosis*. Current evidence suggests that they are transformed B lymphocytes. Reed-Sternberg cells constitute a rare cell type that confirms the diagnosis; the predominant cells described in histological sections of lymph nodes from patients with Hodgkin lymphoma are lymphocytes and inflammatory cells.

Carl Sternberg (1872–1935) studied at the University of Vienna, Austria, and received his MD in 1896. He worked in the pathology institute at Rudolf Hospital in Vienna where he compared tuberculosis, leukemia, and lymphoma. In 1898 in biopsies derived from patients with Hodgkin disease he described large multinucleated cells now termed Reed–Sternberg.

Dorothy Reed-Mendenhall (1874–1964) received her MD degree from Johns Hopkins Medical School in 1900 as one of the first female graduates, interned with William Osler, and obtained a fellowship in the department of pathology at Johns Hopkins with William Welch. In 1902 Reed studied histological sections from patients

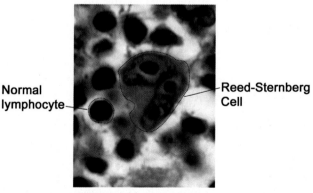

FIGURE 35.1 Photograph of a Reed–Sternberg cell compared to a nonmalignant lymphocyte in a blood smear from a patient with Hodgkin lymphoma (https://visualsonline.cancer.gov/details.cfm?imageid=7172).

diagnosed with Hodgkin disease and described the large multinucleated cell that characterizes this disorder. The presence of these cells in several patients with Hodgkin lymphoma led Reed to conclude that Hodgkin disease is not a form of tuberculosis.

Clinicians described a large number of lymphomas in the 100 years following Wilks' introduction of the term Hodgkin lymphoma. Several classification systems to describe these malignancies evolved. Some of these schemes divided lymphomas into Hodgkin and non-Hodgkin lymphomas. Approximately 90% of all lymphomas are non-Hodgkin lymphomas that lack Reed-Sternberg cells. Both Hodgkin and non-Hodgkin lymphomas encompass a diverse group of diseases.

In 1958 Denis Parsons Burkitt, a British surgeon working at the Makerere College Medical School in Kampala, Uganda, described a unique tumor in the jaws of several African children. He originally identified these tumors as sarcomas; however, further study revealed that these tumors are a form of non-Hodgkin lymphoma, many of which contain the genome of the Epstein–Barr virus. Burkitt lymphoma is a malignant transformation of B lymphocytes.

In 1974 Robert J. Lukes and Robert Collins from the University of Southern California, Los Angeles, classified lymphomas based on their relationship to nonmalignant lymphocytes. Their proposal, based on morphological and functional criteria, related "malignant lymphomas to the B and T lymphocytic systems and alterations in lymphocyte transformation." Based on data available at the time separating B and T lymphocytes into functionally distinct populations (Chapter 13), they proposed a similar division of several of the lymphomas. Figure 35.2 presents Lukes and Collins' scheme.

In 1979 J.A. Habershaw and colleagues, working at St Bartholomew's Hospital in London, phenotyped non-Hodgkin lymphomas from 157 patients and correlated these data with the histological classification of the tumors. They used an array of markers including rosetting with sheep erythrocytes to detect T lymphocytes, rosetting with sheep erythrocytes coated with IgG or IgM to detect cells expressing Fc receptors, and rosetting with sheep erythrocytes coated with C3d to detect cells expressing complement receptors. They also determined the presence of surface and cytoplasmic immunoglobulin, and the expression of a human T lymphocyte antigen, Ia antigen (detecting class II HLA molecules), and an antigen found on acute lymphocytic leukemia (ALL). These researchers compared the expression of these cell surface and intracellular markers with the pathological classifications presented by Rappaport and by Kiel (a modification of the scheme developed by Lukes and Collins) and concluded that non-Hodgkin lymphoma affects both T and B lymphocytes and can be divided into two broad categories:

- tumors of immature lymphocytes with lymphoblastic histology and phenotypes of T and B lymphocytes; and
- tumors of mature B lymphocytes arrested at various stages of differentiation.

Researchers performing parallel studies showed that the malignantly transformed cells in 95% of patients presenting with Hodgkin lymphoma are B lymphocytes.

While early classification systems to differentiate lymphomas relied on the morphology of the transformed lymphocytes, today investigators depend on an array of immunophenotypic and genetic differences between these tumors for characterization. In 2008 the World Health Organization published a classification system

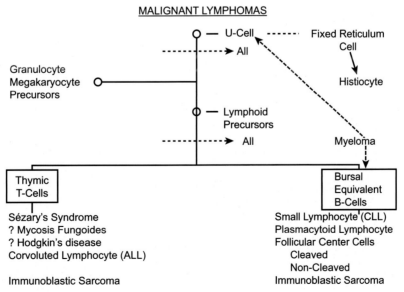

FIGURE 35.2   Scheme relating several lymphomas to the differentiation of T and B lymphocytes. U cell = hematopoietic stem cell. *From Lukes and Collins (1974).*

of neoplasms of the hematopoietic and lymphoid tissues that maintains the designations of Hodgkin and non-Hodgkin lymphoma but includes lymphocyte type (T, B, NK), maturational state, and genetic mutations to determine prognosis and develop therapeutic interventions (Swerdlow et al., 2008; Campo et al., 2011).

LEUKEMIA

In 1811 Peter Cullen (1769–unknown), a surgeon in Scotland, described a case of "splenitis acutus" characterized by milky serum obtained by blood-letting. While Cullen attributed the milky appearance of the blood to rapid absorption of fat, subsequent observations by other physicians suggested that this appearance of the blood was due to the accumulation of large numbers of white blood cells. In retrospect, this represents the initial description of leukemia (Kampen, 2012).

Between 1827 and 1833, three French clinicians, Alfred Armand Louis Marie Velpeau (1795–1867), Jacques Charles Collineau (1783–1860), and A. Duplay, described patients with similar signs and symptoms. These physicians likewise reported milky blood that they attributed to the presence of pus. In 1844 Alfred François Donné reported that "milky" blood contained cells. Microscopic observation of this blood showed that these cells looked similar to the cells found in blood from a healthy patient and hence were neither pus nor fat.

John Hughes Bennett (1812–1875), trained as a physician in Edinburgh, Scotland, compared the microscopic appearance of blood cells from patients presenting with various diseases. In 1845 he published a "Case of hypertrophy of the spleen and liver in which death took place from suppuration of the blood" in the *Edinburgh Medical and Surgical Journal* (referenced in Bennett's obituary, 1875). Bennett described this disease as leucocythemia, observations that are recognized today as the initial description of leukemia as a blood disorder.

Rudolf Virchow (1821–1902) studied medicine at the Friedrich-Wilhelms Institute in Berlin, Germany, and received his MD in 1843. Virchow expanded the cell theory of Theodor Schwann contending that the cell is the basic building block of the body and that every cell derives from a preexisting cell. Virchow firmly established the field of cellular pathology through his investigations of various clinical disorders. Although he spent most of his career at Charité Hospital in Berlin, he also served as Chair of Pathological Anatomy at the University of Wurzberg from 1849 to 1856. In 1857 he returned to Berlin to become Chair of Pathological Anatomy and Physiology at the Friedrich-Wilhelms University as well as the director of the Pathological Institute at Charité Hospital.

In 1845 Virchow published a description of a patient who presented with leg edema, splenomegaly, diarrhea, and nose bleeds. She died 3 months later, and at autopsy Virchow noted a decreased number of red blood cells accompanied by an increase in the number of white blood cells. He also reported that the white blood cells were not granular in nature. In 1856 he termed this disease "leukämie" and differentiated splenic from lymphatic leukemia.

Leukemia represents a broad array of heterogeneous pathologies. According to the American Cancer Society (http://www.buzzle.com/articles/history-of-leukemia.html) by 1913 four major classes of leukemia were differentiated based on morphological differences and maturational stages of the cells:

- chronic lymphocytic leukemia (CLL);
- acute lymphocytic leukemia (ALL);
- chronic myelogenous leukemia (CML); and
- acute myelogenous leukemia (AML).

The availability of cell surface markers, particularly those detected by monoclonal antibodies, permitted identification of the malignant cells in CLL and ALL. In 1982 Robert Schroff and colleagues at the University of California, Los Angeles, used a panel of monoclonal antibodies reactive with lymphocyte subsets from healthy individuals to determine cell surface expression on lymphocytic leukemias. Schroff's group used antibodies specific for HLA-DR (a class II HLA molecule), total T lymphocytes (CD3$^+$), cytotoxic T lymphocytes (CD8$^+$), and helper T lymphocytes (CD4$^+$) and demonstrated that cells from patients with leukemia are heterogeneous but that most could be related to nonmalignant lymphocytes. In general, leukemias classified as acute by morphological and clinical criteria express cell surface molecules similar to immature lymphocytes while chronic lymphocytic leukemias express a more mature phenotype.

In 1983 Robert Dillman and collaborators at the University of California, San Diego, performed similar experiments with the cells from 81 patients with chronic lymphocytic leukemia. They tested these cells for expression of the E-rosette receptor to detect T lymphocytes, surface immunoglobulin to detect B lymphocytes, a human T lymphocyte antigen, and a class II HLA molecule. Results confirmed those of Schroff and his coworkers demonstrating that chronic lymphocytic leukemias express a mature phenotype. Twenty-five years later in 2008, Dillman revisited this publication and reviewed the phenotypes of several chronic lymphocytic leukemias detected by monoclonal antibodies specific for CD markers on the malignant cells. Table 35.1 presents these data.

These phenotypic differences as well as genetic abnormalities that lead to the malignant state provide

TABLE 35.1   Immunophenotypic Cell Surface Markers for Malignant Leukemias

Type of lymphocyte	Surface immunoglobulin	CD5	CD19	CD20	CD10	CD11c	CD22	CD23	CD43	CD103
CLL/SLL	+	+	+	+	–	–	–	+	+	–
MCL	++	+	+	+	±	–	+	–	+	–
HCL	++	–	+	+	–	+	+	–	–	+
LPL	++	–	+	+	–	–	+	–	–	–
SML	++	–	+	+	–	–	+	–	–	–
FCL	++	–	+	+	+	–	+	–	–	–

Abbreviations: CLL, chronic lymphocytic leukemia; SLL, small lymphocytic lymphoma; MCL, mantle cell lymphoma; HCL, hairy cell leukemia; LPL, lymphoplasmacytic lymphoma; SML, splenic marginal zone lymphoma; FCL, follicular cell lymphoma. From Dillman (2008).

the framework for further classification of the lymphocytic leukemias (Swerdlow et al., 2008; Campo et al., 2011). Clinicians rely on this classification scheme to select the most appropriate and efficacious therapy.

MONOCLONAL GAMMOPATHY (PARAPROTEINEMIA)

Several of the lymphomas and leukemias consist of malignantly transformed B lymphocytes at various stages of differentiation. Even though immunoglobulin is routinely detected on the surface of these B lymphocytes or in their cytoplasm, most fail to secrete immunoglobulin either in vivo or in vitro. There are, however, patients who present with an excess of immunoglobulin in their plasma. This immunoglobulin, which can be of any isotype, is usually homogeneous suggesting that it derived from a single clone of transformed lymphocytes.

Based on the immunoglobulin isotype secreted, these malignancies are termed either multiple myeloma or Waldenström macroglobulinemia. Multiple myelomas are those malignancies in which the transformed B lymphocyte synthesizes and secretes immunoglobulin of the IgG, IgA, IgE, or IgD isotype. Since the cells responsible for secreting these isotypes have differentiated to plasma cells, these cancers are also known as plasma cell neoplasms. Variants of multiple myeloma exist in which the malignant B lymphocytes synthesize and secrete only heavy or light chains.

Malignantly transformed B lymphocytes classified as lymphoplasmacytic lymphomas secrete exclusively IgM. Patients diagnosed with IgM-secreting monoclonal gammopathies, also termed Waldenström macroglobulinemia, present with bleeding, peripheral neuropathies, hyperviscous blood, and cardiovascular problems.

Multiple Myeloma

In 1844 Samuel Solly described several patients characterized by fatigue, bone pain, a history of spontaneous fractures, renal failure, and/or anemia. Upon postmortem examination of one of these patients, Solly described the bone marrow as having been replaced with a red substance containing large cells with one or two nuclei and a bright colored nucleolus. Based on the involvement of bones in the presenting signs and symptoms, Solly called the disease "mollities ossium" or softening of the bone.

Other clinicians described additional patients with similar findings during the ensuing 50 years. Another of these patients provided a urine sample in which his physician, William McIntyre, detected a unique protein (McIntyre, 1850). McIntyre sent a sample of urine to Henry Bence Jones, a pathologist at St George's Hospital in London. With the urine sample, McIntyre included a note stating that the urine had a high specific gravity and that the urine became opaque when boiled and cleared when cooled (Kyle and Rajkumar, 2008). Bence Jones confirmed these findings and suggested that the patient had "albumosuria" (Bence Jones, 1848). The identity of this urine protein was not deciphered for over 100 years.

In 1873 J. von Rustizky described a patient with a disease similar to the one reported by Solly and gave the disease the name multiple myeloma (Wright, 1900). Twenty-five years later, James H. Wright working at the Massachusetts General Hospital described an additional patient with a similar presentation and suggested that the malignantly transformed cell in multiple myeloma is, in fact, a plasma cell. The patient described by Wright presented with a tumor of the sternum and ribs and "albumose" of the urine. At autopsy Wright observed that the tumors were composed of large numbers of cells that stained like plasma cells. Wright concluded that "multiple myeloma is … a neoplasm originating … in the plasma cells."

The relationship between the tumor cell and the clinical findings remained a mystery until well into the twentieth century. In 1928 W.A. Perlzweig and colleagues at Johns Hopkins University, Baltimore, Maryland, reported a patient with multiple myeloma who had almost twice the amount of serum protein as do unaffected individuals. Most of the increase in serum proteins was found in the euglobulin fraction, and the authors suggested that this may be related to a reaction to a foreign protein. In 1939 Lewis Longsworth and colleagues at the Rockefeller Institute for Medical Research in New York used serum electrophoresis to detect a unique protein in serum of patients with multiple myeloma. These investigators analyzed serum and plasma from patients diagnosed with a variety of diseases including pneumonia, peritonitis, peritonsillar abscess, rheumatic fever, lymphatic leukemia, nephrosis, aplastic anemia, obstructive jaundice, and multiple myeloma. They compared the electrophoretic patterns of these plasmas with plasma from unaffected donors and observed that plasma from multiple myeloma patients had a narrow, homogeneous protein band in the globulin region that constituted significantly more protein than that seen in the electrophoretic patterns of plasma from unaffected individuals or of individuals with any of the other pathologies.

In 1952 Gail Miller and her colleagues at the Institute for Cancer Research at the Lankenau Hospital in Philadelphia, Pennsylvania, compared the electrophoretic pattern of proteins found in the serum of myeloma patients with that of proteins extracted from myeloma cells of the same patient and demonstrated that the abnormal serum proteins most likely were produced by the malignant cells. In 1955 Henry Kunkel and his group at the Rockefeller Institute for Medical Research in New York further evaluated the serum proteins of myeloma patients and concluded that these serum proteins were similar to gamma globulin from unaffected individuals. Each myeloma protein was immunologically unique suggesting individual specificity (Slater et al., 1955). A large number of similar studies allowed Kunkel to conclude in 1968 that myeloma proteins "may actually represent antibodies for which in most instances the antigen is unknown."

The identity of the unique protein in urine from myeloma patients (known as Bence Jones protein) had yet to be unraveled. In 1956 Leonhard Korngold and Rose Lipari working at the Sloan Kettering Institute for Cancer Research and Cornell University in New York identified Bence Jones protein found in urine from myeloma patients as immunoglobulin light chains. Korngold and Lipari used gel diffusion assays to compare the relationships between Bence Jones proteins, abnormal serum proteins from patients with multiple myeloma, and gamma globulin from unaffected individuals. They demonstrated that an antibody against Bence Jones proteins also reacted against the myeloma protein from the same patient and against gamma globulin in serum from control donors.

Investigators speculated that the source of Bence Jones proteins might be either breakdown products or precursors of the myeloma proteins. Finally, in 1962 Gerald Edelman and Joseph Gally at the Rockefeller Institute in New York compared the amino acid sequences of Bence Jones proteins and light chains from the myeloma protein of the same patient and showed that the two proteins were identical.

By the 1960s the following facts about multiple myeloma were established:

- myeloma proteins are immunoglobulins,
- Bence Jones proteins are isolated light chains, and
- Bence Jones proteins and the light chains of myeloma protein in any given patient are identical.

Waldenström Macroglobulinemia

Jan Waldenström (1906–1996) received his MD from the University of Uppsala, Sweden, in 1937. During his career he described several hematologic conditions including chronic active hepatitis, pulmonary hemosiderosis, and benign hypergammaglobulinemic purpura. In 1944 while working at the University of Uppsala he reported two patients who presented with spontaneous bleeding from the nose and mouth, lymphadenopathy, normochromic anemia, increased erythrocyte sedimentation rate, thrombocytopenia, hypoalbuminemia, low serum fibrinogen, and increased numbers of lymphoid cells in the bone marrow. Waldenström detected a unique serum protein in these patients that he characterized as a macroglobulin with a molecular weight of approximately 1 million daltons. Immunologists now agree that this macroglobulin is monoclonal IgM. Since most of the malignantly transformed B lymphocytes are lymphoblasts rather than plasma cells, the disorder is classified as a lymphoplasmacytic lymphoma (Swerdlow et al., 2008; Campo et al., 2011).

Waldenström also described patients with increased gamma globulin detected by electrophoresis and divided them into two groups: those with a narrow band of gamma globulin he deemed to have a monoclonal gammopathy while patients whose serum contained a broader band he reasoned had a polyclonal gammopathy (reviewed in Waldenström, 1961). He demonstrated that while many of the patients with a monoclonal pattern on electrophoresis had multiple myeloma, some of them showed no signs of malignancy. Further study revealed that up to 3% of individuals over the age of 65 years have a monoclonal increase of gamma globulin in their serum.

The consequence of this monoclonal gammopathy of undetermined significance (MGUS) remains unknown: some of these patients will eventually develop multiple myeloma while a significant percentage will die of other causes with no sign of malignancy.

CONCLUSION

Clinicians describe three distinct groups of lymphoproliferative diseases, lymphomas, leukemias, and monoclonal gammopathies. These disorders are characterized by phenotypically different cell types at varying stages of maturation. Physicians and pathologists first described and clarified these disorders in the nineteenth century based on morphology. Since the 1980s, immunologists employed monoclonal antibodies to detect expression of various cell surface markers on these malignant cells while geneticists and molecular biologists unraveled the underlying etiology of these malignancies. These discoveries lead to unique therapeutic interventions including monoclonal antibodies and dendritic cell vaccines (Chapter 38).

Researchers investigating lymphoid malignancies advanced basic knowledge of the adaptive immune system in several ways including

- deciphering the structure of the immunoglobulin molecule and its component chains,
- deducing the mechanisms responsible for immunoglobulin synthesis and secretion, and
- documenting the developmental history of lymphocytes.

Continued investigation of the lymphocytes involved in these malignancies provides critical information about targets for new therapies as well as understanding the disease process itself. The realization that tumors that appear morphologically similar actually may result from mutations in different genes has ushered in the era of personalized medicine where individual treatments can be designed for patients based on the molecular characteristics of their tumor.

References

Aisenberg, A.C., 2000. Historical review of lymphomas. Br. J. Haematol. 109, 466–476.

Annonymous, John Hughes Bennett Obituary, 1875. Br. Med. J. 2, 473–478.

Bence Jones, H., 1848. On a new substance occurring in the urine of a patient with "mollities ossium". Philos. Trans. 138, 55–62.

Burkitt, P., 1958. A sarcoma involving the jaws in African children. Br. J. Surg. 46, 218–223.

Campo, E., Swerdlow, S.H., Harris, N.H., Pileri, S., Stein, H., Jaffe, E.S., 2011. The 2008 WHO classification of lymphoid neoplasms and beyond: evolving concepts and practical applications. Blood 117, 5019–5032.

Dillman, R.O., 2008. Immunophenotyping of chronic lymphoid leukemias. J. Clin. Oncol. 26, 1193–1194.

Dillman, R.O., Beauregard, J.C., Lea, J.W., Freen, M.R., Sobol, R.E., Royston, I., 1983. Chronic lymphocytic leukemia and other chronic lymphoid proliferations: surface marker phenotypes and clinical correlations. J. Clin. Oncol. 1, 190–197.

Edelman, G.M., Gally, J.A., 1962. The nature of Bence-Jones proteins: chemical similarities to polypeptide chains of myeloma globulins and normal gamma-globulins. J. Exp. Med. 116, 207–227.

Greenfield, W.S., 1878. Specimens illustrative of the pathology of lymphadenoma and leucocythemia. Trans. Pathol. Soc. Lond. 29, 272–304.

Habershaw, J.A., Catley, P.F., Stansfeld, A.G., Brearley, R.L., 1979. Surface phenotyping, histology and the nature of non-Hodgkin lymphoma in 157 patients. Br. J. Cancer 40, 11–34.

Hodgkin, T., 1832. On some morbid appearances of absorbent glands and spleen. Med-Chirurg. Trans. 17, 68–114.

Kampen, K.R., 2012. The discovery and early understanding of leukemia. Leuk. Res. 36, 6–13.

Korngold, L., Lipari, R., 1956. Multiple myeloma proteins III. The antigenic relationship of Bence Jones proteins to normal gamma-globulin and multiple-myeloma serum proteins. Cancer 9, 262–272.

Kunkel, H.G., 1968. The "abnormality" of myeloma proteins. Cancer Res. 28, 1351–1353.

Kyle, R.A., Rajkumar, S.V., 2008. Multiple myeloma. Blood 111, 2962–2972.

Longsworth, L.G., Shedlovsky, T., MacInnes, D.A., 1939. Electrophoretic patterns of normal and pathological human blood serum and plasma. J. Exp. Med. 70, 399–413.

Lukes, R.J., Collins, R.D., 1974. Immunologic characterization of human malignant lymphomas. Cancer 34, 1488–1503.

McIntyre, W., 1850. Case of mollities and fragilitas ossium, accompanied with urine strongly charged with animal matter. Med. Chir. Trans. Lond. 33, 211–232.

Miller, G.L., Brown, C.E., Miller, E.E., Eitelman, E.S., 1952. An electrophoretic study on the origin of the abnormal plasma proteins in multiple myeloma. Cancer Res. 12, 716–719.

Perlzweig, W.A., Delrue, G., Geschicter, C., 1928. Hyperproteinuria associated with multiple myelomas: report of an unusual case. JAMA 90, 755–757.

Reed, D.M., 1902. On the Pathological Changes in Hodgkin's Disease with Especial Reference to its Relation to Tuberculosis, vol. 52. Johns Hopkins Hospital Reports, The Johns Hopkins Press, Baltimore, MD, pp. 45–80.

Schroff, R.W., Foon, K.A., Billing, R.J., Fahey, J.L., 1982. Immunologic classification of lymphocytic leukemias based on monoclonal antibody-defined cell surface antigens. Blood 59, 207–215.

Slater, R.J., Ward, S.M., Kunkel, H.G., 1955. Immunological relationships among the myeloma proteins. J. Exp. Med. 101, 85–108.

Solly, S., 1844. Remarks on the pathology of mollities ossium with cases. Med. Chir. Trans. Lond. 27, 435–461.

Sternberg, C., 1898. Uber eine eigenartige unter den Bilde der Pseudoleukamic verlaufende Tuberculose des lymphatischen Apparates. Ztschr. Helk 19, 21–90.

Swerdlow, S.H., Campo, E., Harris, N.L., Jaffe, E.S., Pileri, S.A., Stein, H., Thiele, J., Vardiman, J.W., 2008. WHO Classification of Tumors of Haematopoietic and Lymphoid Tissues, fourth ed. WHO Press, p. 439.

Virchow, R., 1845. Weisses Blut. In: Virchow, R. (Ed.), Gesammelte Abhandlungen zur Wissenschaftlichen Medizin. Meidinger, Frankfurt, pp. 145–154.

Virchow, R., 1856. Die leukämie. In: Virchow, R. (Ed.), Gesammelte Abhandlungen zur Wissenschaftlichen Medizin. Meidinger, Frankfurt, pp. 190–212.

Waldenström, J., 1944. Incipient myelomatosis or 'essential' hyperglobulinemia with fibrinogenopenia – a new syndrome? Acta Med. Scand. 67, 216–247.

Waldenström, J., 1961. Studies on conditions associated with disturbed gammaglobulin formation (gammopathies). Harvey Lect. 56, 211–231.

Wilks, S., 1865. Cases of Enlargement of the Lymphatic Glands and Spleen (or Hodgkin's Disease) with Remarks, vol. 11. Guy's Hospital Reports, pp. 56–67.

Wright, J.H., 1900. A case of multiple myeloma. J. Boston Soc. Med. Sci. 4, 195–204.

TIME LINE

1832	Thomas Hodgkin provides details of the autopsies of four patients with enlarged spleens and lymph nodes
1844	Samuel Solly describes a multiple myeloma, a disease characterized by large cells replacing normal bone marrow
1847	Rudolf Virchow describes two patients with transformation of peripheral blood white cells and coins the term leukemia
1848	Henry Bence Jones describes a unique protein in the urine of patients with multiple myeloma
1865	Samuel Wilks first uses the term Hodgkin lymphoma
1898–1902	Carl Sternberg and Dorothy Reed-Mendenhall independently describe an enlarged cell in lymphoid tissue of patients with Hodgkin lymphoma
1900	James H. Wright suggests that the transformed cell in multiple myeloma is a plasma cell
1939	Lewis Longsworth and colleagues report the presence of a large amount of serum protein in patients with multiple myeloma
1944	Jan Waldenström describes two patients with macroglobulinemia
1956	Leonhard Korngold and Rose Lipari demonstrate that Bence Jones proteins are related to serum myeloma proteins
1958	Denis Burkitt describes several children in Africa with a tumor in their jaw; this tumor is now termed Burkitt lymphoma
1962	Gerald Edelman and Joseph Gally report that Bence Jones proteins are isolated immunoglobulin light chains
1974	Robert Lukes and Robert Collins propose a classification scheme for lymphomas that relates malignant cells to nonmalignant lymphocytes at various stages of differentiation
1979	J.A. Habeshaw and colleagues phenotype cells from 157 patients with non-Hodgkin lymphomas
1982	Robert Schroff and coworkers use monoclonal antibodies to classify lymphocytic leukemias
1983	Robert Dillman and collaborators immunophenotype cells from chronic lymphocytic leukemias
2008	The World Health Organization updates its classification of lymphoid neoplasms incorporating information about morphology, anatomical location, age of presentation, prognosis, CD expression, and immunogenetics

36

Transplantation Immunology

INTRODUCTION

Tissue and organ transplantation have a long history most of which involves failure (Billingham, 1963). For centuries physicians speculated about the possibility of replacing missing or diseased parts of the body with transplants from healthy donors. For example, Cosmas and Damien reputedly performed the first recorded transplant almost 2000 years ago when they replaced the leg of a soldier who had been injured in battle with that of a Moor. This surgery has been depicted by numerous artists including the Italian Renaissance painter Fra Angelico (Figure 36.1).

Other cultures recount similar stories. The Indian surgeon Sushrutha is reported to have performed rhinoplasty on individuals who had had the tips of their nose cut off as punishment (Saraf and Pariher, 2006). Similarly, during the Renaissance, Italian surgeons developed techniques for transplanting skin, including skin removed from cadavers. Starting in the 1800s, physicians grafted skin to repair wounds due either to burns or to traumatic injury; these efforts have been recorded in the medical literature, and often the skin survived long enough to allow healing to occur. The United States Department of Health and Human Services lists 1869 as the year of the first skin transplant (http://organdonor.gov/legislation/timeline.html).

Despite these anecdotes, physicians faced two challenges prior to widespread use of organ transplantation including

- grafts require a blood supply necessitating methods to anastomose blood vessels and
- transplants between members of an outbred species including humans induce an adaptive immune response that must be controlled.

Alexis Carrel (1873–1944) demonstrated the feasibility of suturing blood vessels in the early 1900s (Carrel and Guthrie, 1906). This advance allowed the subsequent development of methods to transplant vascularized organs such as kidneys and hearts. Carrel received his medical degree from the University of Lyon in 1900. In 1902, he immigrated to the United States and performed most of his experimental studies at the Rockefeller Institute for Medical Research in New York. In 1902, he published a technique for the end-to-end anastomosis of blood vessels. These studies resulted in the awarding of the Nobel Prize in Physiology or Medicine in 1912 "in recognition of his work on vascular suture and the transplantation of blood vessels and organs" (http://www.nobelprize.org/nobel_prizes/medicine/laureates/1912/carrel-bio.html).

The second obstacle facing transplant surgeons has yet to be fully resolved. Physicians early in the twentieth century realized that while autografts (grafts from

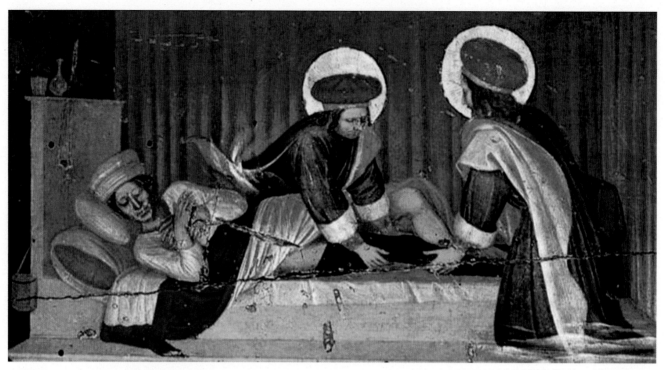

FIGURE 36.1   Cosmas and Damien transplant the leg of a Moor to a soldier injured in battle. "The Healing of Justinian by Saint Cosmas and Saint Damien" is a painting by Fra Angelico.

one part of the body to another) are often successful, allografts (grafts between two members of an outbred population) are invariably rejected. This suggested that foreign grafts stimulated the adaptive immune response; however, it was not until Peter Medawar performed his classic studies in the 1940s that most immunologists accepted the concept that graft rejection is an immunological reaction. This chapter relates the journey toward a solution to this challenge.

CLINICAL EXPERIENCE WITH TRANSPLANTATION

Eduard Konrad Zirm (1863–1944) performed a cornea graft in Moravia, Czechoslovakia, in 1906; this is the initial report of a successful human transplant. Although unrecognized at the time, the eye is an immunologically privileged site, and the cornea is avascular; therefore, antigens that might stimulate an adaptive immune response do not reach the recipient's immune system. As a result the transplant failed to activate an adaptive immune response, and the cornea survived.

Joseph E. Murray and colleagues performed the first successful kidney transplant 50 years later in 1954 (Merrill et al., 1956). Murray (1919–2012), trained as a physician at Harvard Medical School and as a surgeon at

Peter Bent Brigham Hospital in Boston, Massachusetts, became interested in transplantation during his military experience working with soldiers suffering from extensive burns. Some of these patients required transplantation with allogeneic skin, which often led to rejection. He observed that skin grafts between identical twins healed successfully.

The kidney graft between 23-year-old monozygotic twins succeeded because it failed to induce an immune response due to the genetic identity of donor and recipient. The recipient lived with the donated kidney for 8 years before dying of a recurrence of chronic nephritis, his original diagnosis.

In addition to performing the initial successful kidney graft, Murray played a major role in introducing immunosuppressive drugs to transplant recipients and is credited with the initial use of 6-mercaptopurine in a transplant setting. These achievements led to the awarding of the 1990 Nobel Prize in Physiology or Medicine to Murray. He shared this award with E. Donnall Thomas "for their discoveries concerning organ and tissue transplantation in the treatment of human disease."

E. Donnall Thomas (1920–2012) trained at Harvard as a hematologist and met Murray while both were residents at Peter Bent Brigham Hospital. During this time, Thomas participated in the postoperative care of the original renal transplant patient. He subsequently performed seminal studies on bone marrow transplantation in both experimental animals and humans. In 1957 while working in Cooperstown, New York, he performed the initial transplantation of human bone marrow, and in 1959 he successfully treated leukemia by transplanting marrow between monozygotic twins.

In 1967, Christian Barnard in Cape Town, South Africa, performed the first successful cardiac transplant. The graft, from an unrelated individual, functioned well, but the patient died 18 days after surgery. His death was attributed to pneumonia most likely due to the immunosuppressive drugs with which he was treated posttransplant. Barnard (1922–2001), a cardiac surgeon, received his medical training at the University of Cape Town. He studied at the University of Minnesota where he became acquainted with Norman Shumway (1923–2006), the father of cardiac transplantation. Shumway, working at Stanford University in Palo Alto, California, developed the technique for cardiac transplantation in the 1950s and carried out the first successful heart transplant in a dog in 1958. In 1968, he performed the first successful human heart transplant in the United States.

In the 1960s, several other milestones in transplantation included (http://organdonor.gov/legislation/time line.html)

- 1962–1963: lung, liver, and kidney harvested from deceased donors;
- 1966: first successful pancreas transplant;
- 1967: first successful liver transplant and first combined liver/pancreas transplant; and
- 1968: first successful allogeneic bone marrow transplant.

Discoveries in basic immunology led to collaboration between transplant surgeons and clinical immunologists that enhanced success of organ transplantation. These studies demonstrated that

- graft rejection is an adaptive immune response,
- mediated by T lymphocytes, and
- activated by foreign histocompatibility (HLA) antigens.

IMMUNOLOGY OF TRANSPLANT REJECTION

Early studies of transplantation rejection involved grafting tumors between experimental animals. C.O. Jensen in 1902 reported the transfer of a tumor through 19 generations of mice (Chapter 16). Approximately 50% of tumor recipients accepted the tumor. Jensen and others established that the "race" of the recipient mouse determined success or failure of the tumor transplant. These early studies also demonstrated that some transplanted

tumors grew for a time and then regressed while in other mice the tumors appeared not to grow at all. Billingham in 1963 summarized two main points derived from these early studies:

- Mice in which tumor grafts had grown and subsequently regressed were resistant (immune) to a second injection of the same tumor.
- Mice could be rendered resistant to the injection of a foreign tumor if they were first injected with nonmalignant tissue from the same donor prior to tumor grafting.

Up until the early 1940s, virtually all the research on transplantation derived from studies on the transfer of tumors. The advent of World War II stimulated studies on skin transplantation due to an increased number of patients, including members of the armed forces presenting with life-threatening burns. Transplantation of skin to cover the burn areas and protect against infections became an important part of the treatment plan.

In the early 1940s, The Medical Research Council of the United Kingdom asked Peter Medawar to investigate why skin taken from one individual failed to survive when transplanted to an unrelated recipient. Medawar observed that when donor and recipient were related, skin grafts exchanged between them were more likely to survive than when donor and recipient were unrelated. Analysis of the reaction leading to graft failure revealed characteristics similar to other adaptive immune responses including specificity and memory (Medawar, 1944).

In 1943, Gibson and Medawar reported the presence of antibodies in the serum of both humans and rabbits that had rejected foreign grafts. Medawar concluded erroneously that the immunological reaction responsible for graft rejection was due to the action of antibodies. Other investigators made similar observations and reached similar conclusions (reviewed in Hildeman and Medawar, 1958).

Histological evaluation of graft rejection, however, revealed infiltration of the graft with lymphocytes, a picture resembling that seen in delayed skin hypersensitivity reactions. Medawar in 1944 published a description of the fate of skin autografts and allografts in rabbits. Both autografts and allografts went through a period of healing during which time the grafts became vascularized. Subsequently, autografts assumed a healthy appearance. After a few days, allografts became red and edematous, and an inflammatory response developed characterized by invasion with lymphocytes and monocytes. As the inflammatory response continued, the graft became necrotic. All allografts eventually sloughed with a mean survival time of 10.4 ± 1.1 days.

Additionally Medawar observed that

1. a second graft from the original donor went through an accelerated sequence of events resulting in a mean survival time for second set grafts of 6.0 ± 0.6 days, while

2. a graft from an unrelated rabbit was rejected with a mean survival time of approximately 10 days.

Medawar concluded that the foreign skin elicited an immune response and that "(t)he mechanism by which foreign skin is eliminated belongs to the general category of actively acquired immune reactions."

Medawar and his group summarized other findings:

• a latent period exists between the placement of a graft and the development of graft rejection;
• the intensity of the graft rejection is dependent on the dose of foreign tissue transplanted;
• rejection of a graft induces immunologic memory;
• sensitization to a graft is systemic;
• the immune response induced by a graft is specific for the donor; and
• the immune response induced by one tissue (i.e., skin) extends to other tissues from the same donor.

These conclusions form the basis for subsequent studies that led to the identification of the antigens responsible for inducing the transplant rejection. These antigens, expressed on virtually all cells of the body, are coded for by genes in the major histocompatibility complex (MHC) of the species.

ANTIGENIC STIMULUS FOR GRAFT REJECTION

Ernest E. Tyzzer working at Harvard University, Cambridge, Massachusetts, demonstrated that tumors from Japanese waltzing mice grew successfully in other Japanese waltzing mice but failed to grow when transferred to albino mice. F_1 hybrids between Japanese waltzing mice and albino mice accepted the tumor. While some F_2 hybrid mice (produced by breeding two F_1 mice) accepted the tumor, others rejected it suggesting that acceptance or rejection of tumors may be genetically determined although the identification of the specific genes remained unknown (Tyzzer, 1909).

Tyzzer (1875–1965) received his MD from Harvard in 1902. From 1902 to 1905, he pursued parasitological research and the natural course of smallpox infection. In 1905, he became Director of Research for the Harvard Commission where he studied spontaneous tumors in mice, and, with Clarence Little, the genetics of the susceptibility to transplantable tumors.

Little (1888–1971) earned his PhD from Harvard. As an undergraduate he became interested in genetics and developed inbred strains of mice. Little joined Tyzzer's laboratory to study the genetics of cancer susceptibility and resistance.

When Little joined Tyzzer's laboratory, he brought with him the highly inbred strains of mice he had developed and repeated the tumor transfer experiment. Little and Tyzzer obtained similar results except that a small percentage of the F_2 generation (1.6%) was susceptible to tumor growth (Little and Tyzzer, 1916). Based on this result, Tyzzer and Little (1916) calculated that approximately 12 genes are involved in determining susceptibility or resistance to the tumor in mice (Chapter 16).

In 1936, Peter Gorer first identified the antigen responsible for transplant rejection. Gorer (1907–1961), trained as a physician at Guy's Hospital in London and pursued research at the Lister Institute for Preventive Medicine in London where he studied the association between factors responsible for resistance to tumors and blood group antigens. Gorer postulated that cells from different inbred strains of mice express unique antigens, which can be differentiated by antibodies. Initially Gorer discovered that his own (human) serum contained antibodies that discriminated the erythrocytes of three inbred strains of mice (Gorer, 1936a). He then raised rabbit antibodies to the erythrocytes of these strains and identified three antigens, I, II, and III, that were differentially distributed in the strains (Gorer, 1936b). When Gorer transplanted tumors from mice expressing antigen II into mice lacking this antigen, he observed rapid tumor rejection and the appearance of antibodies to antigen II in the serum of the recipient mice (Gorer, 1937).

Gorer continued characterization of antigen II when he collaborated with George D. Snell at the Jackson Laboratory, Bar Harbor, Maine. Snell (1903–1996) earned his PhD from Harvard University in Cambridge, Massachusetts, in 1930. He investigated tumor resistance genes that he called histocompatibility genes. Gorer used the antibodies he had developed against antigen II to test various inbred and hybrid strains of mice and showed that antigen II is coded for by one of the histocompatibility genes described by Snell. Gorer and Snell collaborated to further characterize the gene coding for this antigen; they named this gene and the antigen that it codes H-2 (histocompatibility-2) (Gorer et al., 1948). Subsequent studies showed that antigens coded for by H-2 genes serve as targets for the rejection of foreign tissue grafts. Other investigators defined the genetic region containing the H-2 gene and termed it the MHC.

Based on these studies, George Snell was awarded the Nobel Prize for Physiology or Medicine in 1980. Jean Dausset and Baruch Benacerraf were corecipients of this prize, which was awarded "for their discoveries concerning genetically determined structures on the cell surface that regulate immunological reactions" (Chapters 16 and 20). Gorer died in 1961 and therefore was ineligible for the prize awarded in 1980.

MECHANISM OF GRAFT REJECTION

Peter Medawar demonstrated that rejection of a skin allograft is due to an immunological reaction. Initially he surmised erroneously that graft rejection is due to antibodies detectable in the serum of the graft recipient (Gibson and Medawar, 1943; Medawar, 1944). This conclusion was reasonable at that time because investigators had yet to differentiate the two effector mechanisms of the adaptive immune response, antibody and sensitized T lymphocytes (Chapter 3).

Nicholas Avrion Mitchison (1928–) working at Edinburgh University in Scotland suggested that activated lymphocytes are responsible for tumor graft rejection. Mitchison earned his PhD from New College at Oxford, England, where he worked with Peter Medawar. In 1955, Mitchison demonstrated that lymphocytes derived from the lymph nodes draining a tumor allograft transfer the immune response to the tumor to naïve animals while serum transferred from the tumor-bearing animal failed to elicit rejection. Mitchison further observed that the transferred cells caused rejection rather than indirectly inducing a response in recipient cells. Mitchison concluded that tumors are immunogenic and activate a cell-mediated immune response.

Medawar's group (Brent et al., 1958) reinvestigated the mechanism responsible for rejection of nonmalignant tissue grafts. They injected lymphoid cells from the regional lymph nodes of guinea pigs that had rejected an allograft into the skin of the original graft donor. They hypothesized that lymphocytes activated during graft rejection would react to skin antigens and induce a local response at the injection site. In fact, an inflammatory response resembling a tuberculin reaction occurred within 5–8h at the site of the injection. Serum from these guinea pigs failed to elicit a similar response when injected into the donor's skin.

While these and other studies implicated lymphocytes rather than antibodies in graft rejection, formal proof required investigators to demonstrate graft rejection following transfer of lymphocytes from animals that had rejected a graft to naïve animals. Such studies were performed by several research groups, but the results were equivocal. Finally, Rupert Billingham (1921–2002) and his colleagues working at the Wistar Institute in Philadelphia, Pennsylvania, demonstrated in 1963 that lymphocytes could indeed transfer the potential to reject allogeneic skin grafts.

Billingham and colleagues injected neonatal mice of one inbred strain with cells from a second strain (the alien strain in Figure 36.2), thus inducing immunologic unresponsiveness (tolerance) (Chapter 8). Animals rendered immunologically tolerant by this protocol accept skin grafts from the alien strain indefinitely. Billingham and coworkers transplanted tolerant mice with skin from the alien strain and used those who still had healthy grafts 50 days later as test animals. They injected these tolerant mice intraperitoneally with lymphoid cells derived from nontolerant mice of the same strain that were rejecting or had rejected skin grafts from the alien strain and observed the fate of the tolerated grafts.

Table 36.1 illustrates the results obtained when lymphocytes from either nongrafted mice or from mice grafted with a foreign skin were injected into tolerant mice bearing a successful skin graft. Lymphocytes from nongrafted mice caused rejection of the tolerated graft but only when large numbers were used. Lymphoid cells from grafted animals triggered rejection when infused into the tolerant rats at a much lower concentration. Injection of serum from grafted animals into tolerant animals failed to induce graft rejection.

Billingham and coworkers identified the cell responsible for graft rejection in parallel studies in inbred strains of rats. They transferred thoracic duct cells from rats rejecting a skin graft to tolerant animals bearing successful allogeneic skin grafts. Thoracic duct cells are composed of more than 95% lymphocytes and proved as effective at transferring reactivity to accepted skin grafts on unresponsive animals as were cells from lymph node (Billingham et al., 1963). This observation argues that lymphocytes rather than other cell types present in lymph nodes, such as macrophages and neutrophils, are responsible for graft rejection.

CONTROL OF GRAFT REJECTION

The first successful kidney transplant in humans (Merrill et al., 1956) demonstrated that the procedure was technically feasible; however, this initial success was tempered by the fact that the donor and recipient were monozygotic twins. By contrast allogeneic grafts invariably fail due to the stimulation of a cell-mediated immune response by the host to antigens coded by foreign histocompatibility genes. To overcome these rejections, investigators proposed several approaches for controlling graft rejection. Identification of human histocompatibility (HLA) antigens, coded for by the MHC genes, as the inducers of the graft-destroying immune response drove efforts to detect these antigens and to match donor and recipient as closely as possible. Beginning in 1964, researchers organized a series of International Histocompatibility Workshops during which investigators shared reagents and techniques (http://igdawg.org/ihiw/index.html). It soon became evident

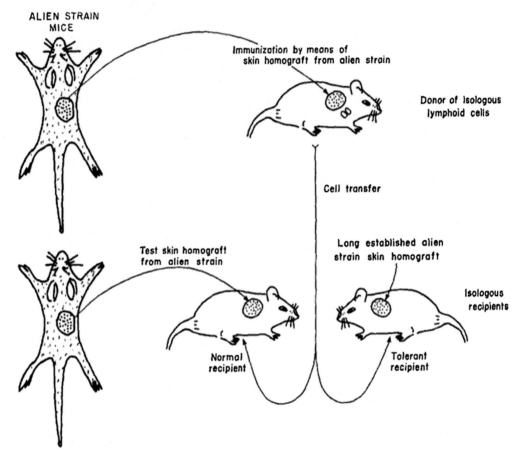

FIGURE 36.2   Experimental design used by Billingham et al. (1963) to demonstrate the ability of lymphocytes to transfer sensitivity to foreign skin grafts. Neonatal mice of one inbred strain (A) were injected with lymphocytes of a second strain (the alien strain) to induce immunologic tolerance. Normal strain A mice received skin grafts from alien strain mice. At various times during the rejection of this graft, lymphocytes from the grafted mice were harvested and injected into normal or tolerant strain A mice bearing skin grafts from the alien strain. The fate of the grafts on the injected mice was followed. *From Billingham et al. (1963).*

that the genes coding for histocompatibility antigens are highly polymorphic and, in an outbred population, the possibility of finding two individuals expressing the same HLA antigens is exceedingly unlikely.

While HLA antigen matching improved the success rate of organ transplants, researchers focused on methods to control the activation of the adaptive immune response. These include whole-body irradiation of the recipient prior to transplantation, induction of immunologic unresponsiveness or tolerance, and the use of immunosuppressive therapies including a variety of nonspecific and specific drugs. During the last half of the 20th century, investigators deployed several drugs to control graft rejection: azathioprine, methotrexate, prednisone, cyclophosphamide, cyclosporine A, tacrolimus, rapamycin, and mycophenolate mofetil.

Azathioprine (Imuran) is a prodrug for 6-mercaptopurine, a purine analog that inhibits DNA synthesis. George Hitchings (1905–1998) and Gertrude Elion (1918–1999) working at the Burroughs-Welcome Company (now Glaxo-Smith-Kline) developed 6-mercaptopurine in the late 1940s as an anticancer drug (Elion, 1989).

George H. Hitchings earned a PhD from Harvard in 1933 and worked in academia for 10 years before joining Burroughs-Welcome as the founding member of the department of biochemistry. There he developed drugs that interfered with the synthesis of DNA. He and his colleagues designed drugs that are used in treating patients with viral and bacterial infections (acyclovir and trimethoprim), gout (allopurinol), leukemia (thioguanine and 6-mercaptopurine), and allogeneic transplants (azathioprine).

Gertrude Elion earned her Master's degree in chemistry at New York University. While she did not earn a doctoral degree, she received several honorary degrees including a PhD from the Polytechnic University of New York and an honorary Doctor of Science degree from Harvard. Elion initially had difficulty getting a position as a chemist until World War II provided more opportunities for women. In 1944, she was hired by Burroughs-Welcome to work with Dr Hitchings.

TABLE 36.1 Transfer of Skin Graft Rejection to Normal or Tolerant Mice Using Lymphocytes. Tolerant A Strain Mice Bearing a Successful Allogeneic Skin Graft Were Injected With Various Numbers of Lymph Node Cells From Syngeneic Mice That Either Were Unmanipulated (Normal) or Were Rejecting a Skin Graft (Sensitized)

Isologous donors			Tolerant A strain mice		
Status	Immunizing stimulus	Number of cells transferred ($\times 10^6$)	Number tested	Survival times of grafts after cell transfer	MST[a]
				days	days
Normal	–	240	3	12 (2)[b], 14	12
		120	3	20, >100 (2)	
		30	6	>100 (6)	
		15	5	18, 19, 56, >100 (2)	
		5	6	>100 (6)	
Sensitized[c]	CBA skin	240	5	9 (4), 10	9
		120	5	8 (3), 10 (2)	8
		60	8	9 (4), 10 (4)	9
		30	6	11 (3), 14, 17, 25	12
		20	5	9 (5)	9
		15	8	10 (2), 11 (2), 17, 18, 22 (2)	12
		10	8	10, 11 (3), 24, 25, 55, >100	12
		5	12	15 (2), 16, 17, 19 (2), 20, 24, 25, 39 (2), 45	21

[a]Median survival time.
[b]Numbers in parentheses indicate number of animals.
[c]Suspensions of regional node cells were prepared from sensitized donors 11 days after they had been grafted with CBA skin.
From Billingham et al. (1963).

Robert Schwartz and colleagues at the New England Hospital in Boston, Massachusetts, described the immunosuppressive properties of azathioprine in 1958. They injected rabbits simultaneously with human serum albumin (HSA) and azathioprine. Treated rabbits failed to make antibody to HSA.

In 1960, Roy Yorke Calne working at the University of Cambridge, England, treated dogs who had received kidney allografts with azathioprine and demonstrated that such treatment prolonged the survival of these transplants.

In 1961, Joseph Murray at Harvard Medical School in Boston, Massachusetts, treated a recipient of a kidney transplant derived from a cadaver with azathioprine. The patient survived for more than a month with a functioning kidney but succumbed due to drug toxicity. A second recipient treated with half the dose survived with a functioning kidney for 3 weeks prior to succumbing to drug toxicity.

Murray and his colleagues published the results of their studies in 1962 comparing the fate of kidney grafts in patients subjected to whole-body irradiation with grafts performed in patients treated with azathioprine. Of 12 patients treated with whole-body irradiation, one survived for 3.5 years after receiving a kidney from his nonidentical twin brother (who may have shared HLA antigens). The transplanted kidney in 5 of the remaining 11 recipients regained renal function early after transplant; however, all of these grafts eventually failed. Of six graft recipients that were treated with azathioprine, five kidneys regained function and the patients survived between 3 and 120 days. Parallel studies on renal transplants in dogs treated with azathioprine confirmed that "(c)hemical suppression of the immune response in both the experimental animal and the human seems promising." The Food and Drug Administration (FDA) approved azathioprine in 1968. Elion and Hitchings were awarded the Nobel Prize in Physiology or Medicine in 1988 for development of the first immunosuppressive drug, azathioprine. They shared the prize with James W. Black "for their discoveries of important principles for drug treatment." Black (1925–2010) discovered two drugs, propranolol, a beta blocker for treatment of heart disease, and cimetidine for the treatment of stomach ulcers.

Yellapragada Subbarao working at Lederle Laboratories, Philadelphia, Pennsylvania, developed a second immunosuppressive drug, methotrexate, an inhibitor of folic acid. Methotrexate, originally developed as a chemotherapeutic agent, proved effective against both leukemias and lymphomas as well as against tumors of the breast, head and neck, lung, and others. Methotrexate is also prescribed for patients with certain autoimmune diseases including rheumatoid arthritis and psoriasis, to induce therapeutic abortions in women with ectopic pregnancies, and for patients undergoing allogeneic bone marrow transplantation to decrease severity of graft-versus-host disease (GvH).

Clinicians transplant allogeneic bone marrow following accidental exposure to high levels of radiation or in patients with leukemia whose bone marrow has been ablated. In these situations the transplanted bone marrow is not subject to rejection by the recipient but rather is likely to induce a GvH response that rejects the recipient. E. Donnall Thomas and his group working at the Mary Imogene Bassett Hospital in Cooperstown, New York, performed the first successful bone marrow transplants in 1957 using two sets of identical twins as donor and recipient; however, more than a decade passed before the procedure became practical using allogeneic donors.

Subsequently, Thomas and his group at the University of Washington pursued animal research simultaneously with their clinical investigations (Storb et al., 1970). They exposed outbred dogs to a lethal dose of total body irradiation and infused them with allogeneic bone marrow and leukocytes. They established three experimental groups:

1. five dogs received no immunosuppressive treatment,
2. nine dogs received methotrexate for 6 days, and
3. ten dogs received methotrexate for up to 102 days after transplant.

All of the dogs in the first group died within 14 days from GvH disease while the dogs in groups 2 and 3 survived longer before GvH disease developed. One of the dogs in group 2 survived for 136 days while three of the dogs in group 3 survived for more than 180 days. These results demonstrated that bone marrow transplantation might be feasible in humans using an intensive treatment plan with methotrexate. Currently methotrexate is used as prophylaxis against GvH disease following allogeneic bone marrow or hematopoietic stem cell transplantation.

In 1963, Thomas Starzl and his group at the University of Colorado in Denver reported the use of high doses of prednisone (a synthetic corticosteroid) in patients postrenal transplantation. Ten patients received daily azathioprine following allogeneic kidney grafting. Once the patients developed a rejection crisis diagnosed by decreased renal function, Starzl and his group added prednisone to the protocol. The inclusion of high-dose prednisone reversed the threat of rejection in eight of the 10 patients reported.

Cyclophosphamide (Cy) is a nitrogen mustard alkylating agent that functions by cross-linking DNA thus inhibiting cell proliferation. Cy, originally designed as an antitumor drug, is effective in patients with autoimmune diseases including systemic lupus erythematosus, rheumatoid arthritis, and multiple sclerosis and in recipients of allogeneic grafts.

The drugs used in the first decades of transplantation had been developed initially as chemotherapeutic agents for cancer patients. Accordingly, they fail to target only lymphocytes and induce significant adverse reactions including anemia, thrombocytopenia, neutropenia, diarrhea and constipation, nausea and vomiting, loss of appetite, edema, fatigue, and others. During the 1970s and 1980s, researchers sought novel drugs that target lymphocytes specifically and achieved several successes.

Jean Francois Borel and coworkers at Sandoz in Basel, Switzerland, discovered the immunosuppressive activity of cyclosporine A (CyA) in 1976. CyA, isolated from extracts of the fungus *Cylindrocarpon lucidum,* was initially screened for activity as an antibiotic. Borel and colleagues studied the immunosuppressive properties of this extract using several measures of immune competence including antibody production and rejection of skin grafts in mice, control of GvH disease in mice and rats, and induction of two experimental autoimmune diseases in rats, experimental allergic encephalomyelitis and Freund's adjuvant-induced arthritis.

Borel and colleagues injected mice and rats with sheep erythrocytes followed 1 day later with an oral dose of CyA. They reported a dose-dependent decrease in serum hemagglutination titers and in the number of antibody-forming lymphocytes detected in mouse spleens using the hemolytic plaque assay. CyA also delayed skin graft rejection in mice and decreased GvH reactions in both mice and rats. Treatment of rats with CyA daily following injection of emulsified spinal cord prevented the development of experimental allergic encephalomyelitis, a model for the study of multiple sclerosis. Likewise rats receiving a daily oral dose of CyA were protected from developing arthritis following injection of complete Freund's adjuvant into a footpad. The researchers compared these results with parallel ones using other immunosuppressive drugs, including cyclophosphamide and azathioprine.

The authors conclude that "cyclosporine A suppresses both humoral and cellular immunity" and argue for additional "investigation in clinical indications like organ transplantation, autoimmune diseases, skin lesions of delayed hypersensitivity and chronic rheumatoid arthritis." During the next few years, several investigators studied CyA in models of graft rejection in a variety of species. Roy Yorke Calne and his group at the University of Cambridge, England, used CyA in human recipients of foreign organ grafts in 1978. Calne and his group reported that five of seven recipients of cadaveric kidneys treated with intramuscular injections of CyA were released from the hospital with functioning allografts. Additional investigators used this drug in recipients of other allografts. Thomas Starzl at the University of Pittsburgh, Pennsylvania, successfully treated recipients of liver transplants starting in 1981. CyA was approved by the FDA in 1983 for patients receiving kidney, liver, and heart transplants. In addition it is used to treat GvH reactions in recipients of bone marrow and hematopoietic stem cell transplants and to treat patients with rheumatoid arthritis, psoriasis, and dry eyes.

When first used in the clinical setting, the mode of action of CyA was unknown. While not cytotoxic to lymphocytes, several investigators demonstrated that the drug preferentially inhibits T lymphocytes while sparing B lymphocytes. Other studies showed that CyA inhibits cytokine secretion by T lymphocytes. In 1984, Martin Krönke and collaborators at the National Cancer Institute, Bethesda, Maryland, reported that in vitro treatment of a human leukemic T lymphocyte line with CyA inhibited the expression of the gene coding for T cell growth factor (IL-2). Investigators now agree that CyA binds to an intracellular protein, cyclophilin. The complex of CyA and cyclophilin inhibits calcineurin, an activator of transcription of IL-2 genes in T lymphocytes.

Toru Kino and collaborators working at the Fujisawa Pharmaceutical Company in Osaka, Japan, in 1987 isolated a second immunosuppressive agent with a similar mode of action. FK-506 (tacrolimus), isolated from the supernatant of cultures of *Streptomyces tsukubaensis* inhibits adaptive immune responses in mice including

- mixed lymphocyte reactions in vitro,
- antibody production in vivo,
- delayed hypersensitivity reactions, and
- localized GvH reactions.

The FDA approved tacrolimus in 1994 for patients receiving liver transplants. This approval has subsequently been extended to cover patients receiving other allogeneic transplants including kidney, heart, pancreas, lung, and bone marrow.

In 1975, Claude Vézina and colleagues working at the Ayerst Research Laboratories in Montreal, Canada, isolated a chemical from cultures of *Streptomyces hygroscopicus* from Easter Island soil samples that inhibited the growth of several fungi. They named the active ingredient rapamycin based on the name, Rapa Nui, given to Easter Island by the native Polynesian inhabitants. Initially investigators developed rapamycin as an antifungal drug; however, studies by Martel and colleagues in 1977 at Ayerst Research Laboratories demonstrated that the drug was immunosuppressive in rats. Administration of rapamycin inhibits the development of experimental allergic encephalomyelitis and adjuvant-induced arthritis and the production of IgE-like antibodies.

Twelve years later in 1989, Roy Yorke Calne and coworkers at Addenbrooke's Hospital in Cambridge, England, extended these observations and demonstrated that intramuscular injection of rapamycin following allogeneic heart transplants extends graft survival. Companion investigations of kidney grafts in pigs and dogs showed a similar prolongation of graft survival. These results led to clinical trials of rapamycin (sirolimus) in recipients of allografts and approval of the drug by the FDA in 1999.

Rapamycin inhibits the response of T lymphocytes to IL-2. As a result, rapamycin and the calcineurin inhibitors such as CyA and tacrolimus inhibit the immune response by different mechanisms, and they are sometimes administered in conjunction. One advantage of rapamycin is relatively low nephrotoxicity and hence it can be prescribed long term in recipients of allogeneic transplants.

In 1943, W.H. Wilkins and G.C.M. Harris working at Oxford University, England, identified a substance in fluids derived from cultures of *Penicillium brevicompactum* that exhibited bacteriostatic properties. Howard Florey and Margaret Jennings at Oxford identified mycophenolic acid as the chemical responsible for this inhibition (1946). During the ensuing 45 years, several investigators reported that mycophenolic acid and a chemically modified derivative termed mycophenolate mofetil (MMF) possessed antifungal, antibacterial, antiviral, and immunosuppressive properties. MMF is a purine antagonist that interferes with the synthesis of guanine in lymphocytes; in the absence of guanine, cells cannot proliferate. Other somatic cells can synthesize guanine using a salvage pathway thus MMF is relatively specific for lymphocytes.

In 1991, Klaus Platz and colleagues at the University of Wisconsin in Madison and Syntex Research in Palo Alto, California, used MMF along with cyclosporine and prednisone in outbred dogs who had received allogeneic kidney transplants. This triple therapy increased the mean survival time of the grafts from approximately 8 days to over 120 days. Clinical trials of MMF combined with cyclosporine and corticosteroids proved successful during the late 1980s and early 1990s and led to FDA approval of the therapy in May, 1995.

CONCLUSION

Successful organ transplantation required solving two challenges. The first problem involved the practical hurdles of transplanting living tissue into a recipient. This included not only maintaining organ viability once removed from the donor but also technical skills of anastomosing blood vessels to provide the transplant with a circulatory system. Once these hurdles were overcome, a second major obstacle remained, control of the adaptive immune response to the foreign tissue.

Investigators characterized antigens responsible for inducing an adaptive immune response against tumors and allogeneic transplants and demonstrated that they preferentially stimulate T lymphocytes, thereby inducing a cell-mediated response. Strategies to inhibit T lymphocytes evolved from nonspecific protocols involving whole-body irradiation to relatively specific treatments exemplified by cyclosporine A and tacrolimus.

Clinical transplantation today faces two problems limiting its wider application—graft rejection and graft availability. The problem of graft survival is amenable to the development of ever more specific immunosuppressant drugs although every drug currently in use puts the patient at increased risk of infection.

The number of potential recipients of lifesaving transplants vastly outnumbers the number of individuals willing to donate. Thus even if the issue of rejection could be solved, the number of transplants available remains limited. One advance in this area includes ongoing work to grow organs in vitro using stem cells derived from the prospective recipient. Organs produced via such a procedure would share histocompatibility antigens with the recipient and resist rejection. Early success in growing blood vessels, ears, and kidneys has been reported, and additional advances are expected.

References

Barnard, C.N., 1967. The operation. A human cardiac transplant: an interim report of a successful operation performed at Groote Schuur Hospital, Cape Town. S. Afr. Med. J. 41, 1271–1274.

Billingham, R.E., 1963. Transplantation: past, present and future. J. Invest. Derm. 41, 165–180.

Billingham, R.E., Silvers, W.K., Wilson, D.B., 1963. Further studies on adoptive transfer of sensitivity to skin homografts. J. Exp. Med. 118, 397–419.

Borel, J.F., Feurer, C., Gubler, H.U., Stählein, H., 1976. Biological effects of cyclosporin A: a new antilymphocytic agent. Agents Actions 6, 468–475.

Brent, L., Brown, J., Medawar, P.B., 1958. Skin transplantation immunity in relation to hypersensitivity. Lancet 272, 561–564.

Calne, R.Y., 1960. The rejection of renal homografts. Inhibition in dogs by 6-mercaptopurine. Lancet 275, 417–418.

Calne, R.Y., Lim, S., Samaan, A., Collier, D.St.J., Pollard, S.G., White, D.J.G., Thiru, S., 1989. Rapamycin for immunosuppression in organ allografting. Lancet ii, 227.

Calne, R.Y., Thiru, S., McMaster, P., Craddock, G.N., White, D.J.G., Evans, D.B., Dunn, D.C., Pentlow, B.D., Rolles, K., 1978. Cyclosporin A in patients receiving renal allografts from cadaver donors. Lancet 312, 1323–1327.

Carrel, A., Guthrie, C.C., 1906. Anastomoses of blood vessels by the patching method and transplantation of the kidney. J. Amer. Med. Assoc. 47, 1648–1651.

Elion, G.B., 1989. The purine path to chemotherapy. Science 244, 41–47.

Gibson, T., Medawar, P.B., 1943. The fate of skin homografts in man. J. Anat. 77, 299–310.

Gorer, P., 1936a. The detection of hereditary genetic difference in the blood of mice by means of human blood group A serum. J. Genet. 32, 17–31.

Gorer, P., 1936b. The detection of antigenic differences in mouse erythrocytes by the employment of immune sera. Brit. J. Exp. Pathol. 17, 42–50.

Gorer, P., 1937. The genetic and antigenic basis of tumor transplantation. J. Pathol. Bacteriol. 44, 691–697.

Gorer, P., Lyman, S., Snell, G.D., 1948. Studies on the genetic and antigenic basis of tumor transplantation. Linkage between a histocompatibility gene and "fused" in mice. Proc. Roy. Soc. Lond. B Biol. Sci. 135, 499–505.

Kino, T., Hatanaka, H., Hashimoto, M., Nishiyama, M., Goto, T., Okuhara, M., Kohsaka, M., Aoshi, H., Imanaka, H., 1987. FK-506, a novel immunosuppressant isolated from a Streptococcus. I. Fermentation, isolation and physic-chemical and biological characteristics. J. Antibiot. 40, 1249–1255.

Krönke, M., Leonard, W.J., Depper, J.M., Arya, S.K., Wong-Staal, F., Gallo, R.C., Waldman, T.A., Greene, W.C., 1984. Cyclosporin A inhibits T-cell growth factor gene expression at the level of mRNA transcription. Proc. Nat. Acad. Sci. U.S.A. 81, 5214–5218.

Little, C.C., Tyzzer, E.E., 1916. Further experimental studies on the inheritance of susceptibility to a transplantable tumor, carcinoma (J.W.A.) of the Japanese waltzing mouse. J. Med. Res. 33, 393–453.

Martel, R.R., Klicius, J., Galet, S., 1977. Inhibition of the immune response by rapamycin, a new antifungal antibiotic. Can. J. Physiol. Pharmacol. 55, 48–51.

Medawar, P.B., 1944. The behavior and fate of skin autografts and skin homografts in rabbits. A report to the War Wounds Committee of the Medical Research Council. J. Anat. 78, 176–199.

Medawar, P.B., 1958. The Croonian Lecture. The homograft reaction. Proc. Roy. Soc. Lond. B 149, 145–166.

Merrill, J.P., Murray, J.E., Harrison, J.H., Guild, W.R., 1956. Successful homotransplantation of the human kidney between identical twins. J. AMA 160, 277–282.

Mitchison, N.A., 1955. Studies on the immunological response to foreign tumor transplants in the mouse. J. Exp. Med. 102, 157–177.

Murray, J.E., Merrill, J.P., Dammin, G.J., Dealy, J.B., Alexander, G.W., Harrison, J.H., 1962. Kidney transplantation in modified recipients. Ann. Surg. 156, 337–355.

Saraf, S., Paihar, R., 2006. Sushruta: the first plastic surgeon in 600 BC. Internet J. Plas. Surg. 4(2). http://ispub.com/IJPS/4/2/8232.

Schwartz, R., Stack, J., Dameshek, W., 1958. Effect of 6-mercaptopurine on antibody production. Proc. Soc. Exp. Biol. Med. 99, 164–167.

Starzl, T.E., Klintmalm, G.B., Porter, K.A., Iwatsuki, S., Schröter, G.P., 1981. Liver transplantation with use of cyclosporine and prednisone. New Eng. J. Med. 305, 266–269.

Starzl, T.E., Marchioro, T.L., Waddell, W.R., 1963. The reversal of rejection in human renal homografts with subsequent development of homograft tolerance. Surg. Gynecol. Obster. 117, 385–395.

Storb, R., Epstein, R.B., Graham, T.C., Thomas, E.D., 1970. Methotrexate regimens for control of graft-versus-host disease in dogs with allogeneic marrow grafts. Transplantation 9, 240–246.

Thomas, E.D., Lochte, H.L., Lu, W.S., Ferrebee, J.W., 1957. Intravenous infusion of bone marrow in patients receiving radiation and chemotherapy. N. Eng. J. Med. 257, 491–496.

Tyzzer, E.E., 1909. A study of inheritance in mice with reference to their susceptibility to transplantable tumors. J. Med. Res. 21, 519–573.

Tyzzer, E.E., Little, C.C., 1916. Studies on the inheritance of susceptibility to a transplantable sarcoma (J.w.B.) of Japanese waltzing mice. J. Cancer Res. 1, 387–389.

Vezina, C., Kudelski, A., Sehgal, S.N., 1975. Rapamycin (AY-22,989), a new anti-fungal antibiotic I. Taxonomy of the producing streptomycete and isolation of the active principle. J. Antibiot. 28, 721–726.

Zirm, E., 1906. Eine erfolgreiche totale keratoplastik. Arch. Ophthalmol. 64, 580–593.

TIME LINE

2600 BCE   The Indian surgeon Sushruta performs skin grafts

1902   C.O. Jensen describes the resistance of mice to the transfer of tumors

1906   Eduard Zirm performs the first successful transplantation of cornea

1909   Ernest Tyzzer demonstrates that resistance to tumor transfers is genetic

1912   Alexis Carrel awarded the Nobel Prize in Physiology or Medicine for his work on suturing blood vessels

1916   Clarence C. Little and Ernest Tyzzer estimate that about 12 genes are responsible for determining resistance or susceptibility to tumor transfers

1936   Peter Gorer reports antigenic difference on cells of different mouse strains

1937   Peter Gorer demonstrates a role for antigen II in rejection of tumors

1944   Peter Medawar provides evidence that foreign skin grafts are rejected by an adaptive immune response

1948   Peter Gorer and George D. Snell show that antigen coded for by the H-2 genes serves as a target for graft rejection

1954   Joseph E. Murray and colleagues perform first successful kidney transplant between identical twins

1957   E. Donnall Thomas and coworkers perform the first transplantation of human bone marrow

1958   Peter Medawar and colleagues demonstrate that graft rejection can be transferred by lymphocytes but not by serum antibodies

1961   Joseph Murray and colleagues use the immunosuppressive drug, azathioprine, for the first time on recipients of kidney transplants

1967   Christian Bernard performs the first successful human cardiac transplant

1975   Claude Vézina and colleagues describe the antifungal agent, rapamycin, from a soil sample from the Easter Islands

1976   Jean Francois Borel and collaborators report the immunosuppressive properties of the fungal metabolite, cyclosporine A

1977   R.R. Martel and colleagues report the immunosuppressive properties of rapamycin

1978   Roy Yorke Calne and coworkers report the use of cyclosporine A in patients receiving cadaveric kidney grafts

1980   George Snell, Jean Dausset, and Baruj Benacceraf awarded the Nobel Prize in Physiology or Medicine "for their discoveries concerning genetically determined structures on the cell surface that regulate immunological reactions"

1988   Gertrude Elion and George Hitchings, developers of the drug azathioprine, awarded the Nobel Prize in Physiology or Medicine "for their discoveries of important principles for drug treatment"

1989   Roy Yorke Calne and coworkers describe the immunosuppressive properties of rapamycin in dogs and pigs receiving allogeneic renal transplants

1990   Joseph E Murray and E. Donnall Thomas awarded the Nobel Prize in Physiology or Medicine for their discoveries in transplantation in treating human diseases

1995   FDA approves mycophenolate mofetil to treat patients postrenal transplantation

Tumor Immunology

INTRODUCTION

The success of vaccines that stimulate the adaptive immune response and decrease the incidence of infectious disease inspired similar attempts to develop innovative therapies to treat cancer. The literature is replete with anecdotes about physicians injecting patients with malignant tissue to induce a protective immune response against the future development of tumors or to selectively attack already existing tumors (Ichim, 2005). Sometimes these efforts met with success, more often with failure.

In 1891, William B. Coley, MD (1862–1936), practicing at what would later become the Memorial Sloan Kettering Institute in New York, reviewed the medical records of patients whose tumors spontaneously regressed and noted that in many instances, tumor regression followed recovery from an elevated fever due to bacterial infection. While unsure how these infections resulted in the regression of the tumors, Coley postulated that the elevated temperature induced by the infections was detrimental to the continued growth of the malignancy. In an attempt to mimic these results, Coley injected a mixture containing killed *Streptococcus pyogenes* and *Serratia marcescens* directly into inoperable tumors (Coley, 1893); these efforts met with varied success including some patients who were "cured." Coley continued to treat cancer patients with this mixture (Coley's toxin), until he retired in 1933.

In 1909, Paul Ehrlich first suggested that tumors might be recognized as foreign by the immune system (Himmelweit, 1957). At that time the relationship between cancer and healthy tissue was unknown, and the concept of tumor-specific antigens had not been developed. Investigators asked whether tumors developed from cells of the tissue or organ affected or if tumor cells arose de novo somewhere else in the body. Despite this, Ehrlich hypothesized that tumors arose spontaneously and that the immune system targeted these aberrant growths for destruction.

Almost 50 years later, F. Macfarlane Burnet (1957a,b) and Lewis Thomas (1959) independently reintroduced the concept that the immune system played a primary role in eliminating cancer. In a relatively pessimistic review, Burnet, director of the Walter and Eliza Hall Institute of Medical Research in Melbourne, Australia, concluded that "(t)here is little ground for optimism about cancer." He does, however, argue that any therapeutic approach must be based on dissimilarities between the tumor cells and the host cells. He suggested that "in many instances there is sufficient antigenic difference to be effective" and that it "is by no means inconceivable that small accumulations of tumour cells may develop and because of their possession of new antigen potentialities provoke an effective immunological reaction, with regression of the tumour and no clinical hint of its existence."

Lewis Thomas (1913–1993), an immunologist/essayist/medical administrator, received his MD from Harvard

A Historical Perspective on Evidence-Based Immunology
http://dx.doi.org/10.1016/B978-0-12-398381-7.00037-X

in 1937. Following a neurology residency, he pursued academic research at Johns Hopkins University, Tulane University, and the University of Minnesota. He served as Dean of the medical schools at Yale and New York University and as president of the Memorial Sloan Kettering Cancer Institute in New York. At a symposium on Cellular and Humoral Aspects of the Hypersensitive States sponsored by the New York Academy of Sciences in 1957, Thomas discussed a presentation by Peter Medawar on the relationship of allograft rejection to delayed hypersensitivity reactions. Thomas questioned why the immune system had developed this allograft rejection mechanism and speculated that "the phenomenon of homograft rejection will turn out to represent a primary mechanism for natural defense against neoplasia" (Thomas, 1959).

Subsequent investigations confirmed that malignantly transformed cells differ from their healthy counterparts by their growth potential, the genes that are transcribed, and the cell-surface molecules expressed. When investigators realized that malignant and nonmalignant cells express different and unique cell-surface antigens, they sought additional evidence to support this immunosurveillance hypothesis. This hypothesis postulates that the adaptive immune system recognizes tumors as foreign and responds to eliminate them. Supporting evidence includes the following:

- Cancer primarily affects the very young and the elderly, stages of life when the immune system is either immature or in decline.
- Tumors arise more often in patients receiving immunosuppressive therapy to prevent graft rejection than in the general population (Penn, 1988). The types of tumors in immunosuppressed patients are different than in the general population with a higher incidence of tumors of lymphocytes.
- Malignancies occur in patients infected with the human immunodeficiency virus (HIV) with a higher incidence than they do in uninfected individuals. These tumors appear late in the infection when acquired immunodeficiency syndrome (AIDS) develops.
- Tumors infiltrated with T lymphocytes are more likely to regress and even disappear than are tumors without lymphocytic infiltration.

This chapter reviews a selection of experiments that further support the immunosurveillance hypothesis including

- tumors express cell-surface molecules (antigens) that differ from those present on the corresponding nonmalignant cell;
- tumor-specific antigens activate both innate host defense mechanisms and the adaptive immune response;

- immune responses directed against tumors inhibit cell growth and/or metastasis as well as destroy the tumor cells; and
- tumors transplanted to an animal previously exposed to tumor antigens fail to grow indicating the animal is protected from tumor development.

Therapeutic measures to decrease the cancer burden on patients include:

- development of vaccines,
- induction of innate immunity,
- passive infusion of cells and molecules of the adaptive immune response, and
- regulation of the adaptive immune response.

TUMOR ANTIGENS

In 1911 Paul Uhlenhuth working at the University of Greifswald in Germany developed precipitin assays that demonstrated species specificity of antigens including those associated with blood. He used rabbit antibodies to egg albumins to differentiate the albumins from several species of birds. He also showed that a rabbit antibody against chicken blood would precipitate chicken serum but would not react with serum from other animals including horse, donkey, sheep, cow, or pigeon. He refined this methodology and used antibodies to differentiate blood from different species (Chapter 2).

Subsequently other researchers showed that different tissues expressed unique antigens detectable by rabbit antibodies. Prior to these investigations, most scientists believed, erroneously, that injection of muscle into a foreign animal induced the same antibody as did injection of the lens of the eye. The realization that different tissues of an animal elicited antibodies of unique specificities suggested to some investigators that tumors also might express unique antigens.

Researchers characterized tumor-specific antigens while developing techniques for the clinical detection of tumors in patients. Garri Abelev and colleagues working at the Department of Immunology and Oncology of the Gamaleya Institute of Epidemiology and Microbiology, Moscow, U.S.S.R., identified the first tumor-associated antigen in 1963. Abelev (1928–2013) earned his doctorate in biological sciences from Moscow State University and subsequently joined the laboratory of Lev Alexandrovich Zilber, a pioneer in the study of viral oncogenesis. Abelev and his colleagues investigated secretory products of rodent liver tumors (hepatomas) and reported that mouse and rat hepatomas synthesize and secrete a glycoprotein (α-globulin) that is normally found only in fetal and embryonic serum. This protein, which can be detected in the serum of tumor-bearing animals and in humans with hepatomas, is called alpha-fetoprotein (AFP) and is the most abundant protein in the fetus. AFP functions like serum albumin during fetal life, decreases following birth, and is associated with several tumors thus leading to the development of one of the first clinical assays for detecting and tracking cancer.

While not tumor-specific, AFP is elevated in patients with liver tumors including hepatocellular carcinoma in adults and hepatoblastoma in children. AFP may be elevated in women carrying a fetus with neural tube defects and in individuals presenting with germ line tumors of the testes and ovaries. Today AFP levels are sometimes measured to monitor patient response to therapy and to detect recurrence of these cancers.

In 1965 Phil Gold and Samuel O. Freedman at McGill University in Montreal, Canada, described a second tumor-associated antigen in patients with colon cancers. Gold and Freedman prepared an extract from both non-malignant and cancerous tissue obtained from patients undergoing colon resection or at autopsy. These investigators injected rabbits with malignant tissue to induce antibodies and absorbed the rabbit serum with healthy colon to remove antibodies to nonmalignant tissue, thus providing a reagent that contained antibodies reacting solely with an antigen expressed by malignant colon tissue.

Gold and Freedman (1965a) injected neonatal rabbits with human colon tissue to induce immunological tolerance. As adults, these rabbits failed to produce antibodies to healthy human colon. Similarly treated rabbits synthesized and secreted antibodies when injected with human colon cancer cells. These antibodies reacted with malignant tissue from colon cancer patients and led the authors to conclude that "pooled tumor extracts contained tumor-specific antigens not present in normal colonic tissue."

In parallel studies Gold and Freedman (1965b) showed that the antibodies induced by injecting rabbits with colon cancer reacted with other tumors of the gastrointestinal tract. In addition, the antigens detected by these antibodies are expressed by tissues of the gastrointestinal tract of the fetus. The authors concluded that the genes coding for these carcinoembryonic antigens (CEA) are expressed during embryonic life, suppressed during differentiation, and reexpressed following malignant transformation of the cells.

AFP and CEA are tumor-associated antigens expressed by some fetal tissue during embryological development. As a result, immunological tolerance to these antigens develops during fetal life, and adaptive immune responses against these antigens are difficult to induce clinically. Thus while useful as markers these antigens are not appropriate candidates for the induction of immune-mediated cancer therapy.

Contemporary research focuses on identification of tumor-associated antigens that are not expressed by nonmalignant tissue or during fetal life. Investigators search for tumor-associated antigens that are useful in immunization (vaccination) protocols. Examples of such antigens comprise products of mutated genes including proto-oncogenes (i.e., *SRC, MYC, RAS*), tumor suppressor genes (i.e., *p53*), or genes that are mutated due to infection with an oncogenic virus (i.e., human papilloma virus (HPV)).

ADAPTIVE IMMUNE RESPONSES TO TUMORS

The description of tumor-specific antigens suggested that protective immune responses against these antigens might be induced. Studies of tumor transplantation in mice and rats demonstrated that tumors are immunogenic (Chapter 16). In 1909 Ernest Tyzzer working at Harvard transferred spontaneously arising tumors between Japanese waltzing mice and albino mice. He reported that a tumor that can be successfully transplanted in Japanese waltzing mice fails to grow when transplanted to albino mice. F_1 hybrids between Japanese waltzing mice and albino mice proved as susceptible as the original tumor host to the transplanted tumor. These studies led to the discovery of genetically regulated transplantation antigens coded for by genes in the major histocompatibility complex (MHC).

Genetically determined histocompatibility antigens expressed by nonmalignant and malignant cells are identical and therefore are not useful targets for an adaptive immune response. Experiments performed during the 1950s demonstrated, however, that a protective adaptive immune response could be induced to tumor antigens. In 1953 E.J. Foley working at the Schering Corporation, Bloomfield, New Jersey, injected inbred mice intramuscularly with cells from a chemically induced, transplantable sarcoma. Once the tumor became palpable, he ligated the blood supply to the tumor; in some mice the tumor disappeared. Foley reinjected mice in which the tumor could no longer be palpated with additional sarcoma cells derived either from the original tumor or from a second, chemically induced tumor. Mice receiving cells from the original sarcoma in this second injection remained free of cancer suggesting that an antitumor response had been induced by the original tumor. This response was tumor-specific as evidenced by the growth of tumors in mice injected with a second sarcoma.

Richmond Prehn and Joan Main working at the National Cancer Institute in Bethesda, Maryland, employed a similar experimental protocol in 1957. These investigators amputated the limb bearing the growing tumor rather than ligating the blood supply to the tumor. The mice from which the growing tumor was removed proved refractory to a second injection of the same sarcoma.

In 1964 Richard Riggins and Yosef Pilch working at the National Cancer Institute in Bethesda, Maryland, showed that a spontaneously arising tumor also induced systemic immunity. Riggins and Pilch injected two groups of inbred mice intramuscularly with either a spontaneously arising adenocarcinoma of the breast or a chemically induced fibrosarcoma. Once the tumors grew to approximately 1 cm in diameter the leg bearing the growing tumor was amputated. Seven days later Riggins and Pilch challenged the mice with an injection of either adenocarcinoma or sarcoma cells and compared the percentage of mice that subsequently developed a palpable tumor. Results presented in Table 37.1 show that both the spontaneously arising adenocarcinoma and the chemically induced fibrosarcoma tumors induced tumor-specific immunity. Riggins and Pilch compared mice immunized with adenocarcinoma to mice immunized with fibrosarcoma and concluded that the adenocarcinoma more efficiently induced a protective adaptive immune response.

IMMUNOTHERAPEUTIC APPROACHES

Additional studies demonstrated that tumor-associated antigens are expressed by many if not all tumors and that these antigens induce adaptive immune responses. These results inspired a search for possible immunotherapies. In 1891 Coley reported the spontaneous regression of sarcomas in some patients who recovered from infection with *S. pyogenes* (erysipelas). Coley attributed these successes to nonimmunological mechanisms including the induction of fever or competition between tumor growth and the growth of bacteria. Based on these observations, Coley in 1893 developed a mixture of killed *S. pyogenes* and *S. marcescens* (Coley's toxin) that he injected into inoperable tumors. Coley's toxin was developed at a time when little was known about the immunogenicity of tumors or the functioning of the immune system. Based on current understanding of the immune system, the most likely explanation for Coley's results is that the bacterial infection nonspecifically induced an inflammatory response that destroyed the tumor. Some contemporary researchers speculate that the lipopolysaccharide released by Gram-negative bacteria stimulates the production of TNF-α, which activates inflammation.

TABLE 37.1 Evidence That Transplanting Spontaneously Arising or Chemically Induced Tumors Into Syngeneic Mice Induced an Anti-Tumor Immune Response. Tumors Were Introduced Into the Hind Limb of Mice and Allowed to Grow Until Palpable. Following Amputation of the Tumor-Bearing Limb, the Mice Were Re-Injected With the Same or Different Tumor and the Growth of the Transplanted Tumor Observed. The Decreased Percentage of Tumors Seen in Mice Previously Immunized With the Same Tumor Was Interpreted as Indication That the Immunized Animals Mounted an Immune Response

| | Challenging tumor[a] | | | |
| | Spontaneous carcinoma | | Fibrosarcoma | |
Experimental groups	Tumor/total mice	Percent	Tumor/total mice	Percent
Experiment 1:				
Immunized with spontaneous carcinoma	33/55	60	50/52	96
Nonimmunized amputated controls	49/55	89	60/63	95
Untreated controls	26/30	87	24/29	83
Experiment 2:				
Immunized with fibrosarcoma	55/59	93	4/52	8
Nonimmunized amputated controls	53/55	95	51/55	93
Untreated controls	25/25	100	29/31	94
Experiment 3:				
Immunized with fibrosarcoma				
1. amputated 20h prior to challenge			54/58	93
2. no amputation prior to or after challenge			58/60	97
Untreated controls			16/18	89

[a]*In each experiment the same tumor cell suspension used to challenge the immunized animals was used in the control groups.*
From Riggins and Pilch (1964).

Support for these observations derived from studies performed in the 1970s and 1980s on the effect of injecting bacillus Calmette–Guérin (BCG) directly into cancers of the bladder. BCG is a vaccine against tuberculosis prepared from an attenuated strain of live *Mycobacterium bovis*. In 1908 Albert Calmette and Camille Guérin, working at the Pasteur Institute in Lille, France, cultured virulent strains of *M. bovis* on different culture media. They discovered one medium on which the tubercle bacillus became less virulent. Following more than 10 years of continued subculturing of this strain, Calmette and Guérin produced a strain that is used as a vaccine in many countries where tuberculosis is endemic although it has never been recommended or approved for use in the United States.

Melvin Silverstein and his colleagues at the University of California, Los Angeles, in 1974 published a report of a single patient with melanoma metastatic to the bladder. Silverstein and coworkers injected BCG directly into the bladder tumor. This treatment led to regression of the tumor as revealed by biopsies that showed granuloma formation (Silverstein et al., 1974). These granulomas contained macrophages, dendritic cells (DCs), neutrophils, and other cells leading to the conclusion that an inflammatory response induced by BCG eliminated the tumor.

This report along with similar observations over the next several years led David Lamm and colleagues at the University of Texas Health Science Center, San Antonio, in 1980 to design a clinical trial to evaluate the efficacy of BCG in treating bladder cancer. Investigators treated patients with surgery alone or with surgery followed with an intravesical injection of BCG. Results showed a lower recurrence rate of the tumor in patients treated with surgery plus BCG injection compared to patients who only had their bladder tumor resected. In 1998 the Food and Drug Administration (FDA) approved intravesical treatment of patients with BCG as a therapy for certain types of bladder cancer.

Two additional advances in cancer immunotherapy occurred in the 1970s:

- Georges J.F. Köhler and César Milstein developed hybridoma technology for the production of monoclonal antibodies of defined specificity, which led to the creation of unique, tumor-specific antibodies that, when passively infused in patients, destroyed their tumors.
- Research groups led by John Erickson at Vanderbilt University in 1975 and by Robert Gallo working at Litton Bionetics Research Laboratory and the National Institutes of Health in Bethesda, Maryland, identified and isolated a T-cell growth factor (IL-2—Chapter 25) that permitted the continuous growth and expansion of T lymphocytes in vitro.

This technology provided other investigators a method to produce large numbers of autologous, tumor-specific T lymphocytes that could be reinfused into the patient to react against their tumors.

Monoclonal Antibodies

Georges J.F. Köhler (1946–1995) and César Milstein (1927–2002) described a technique for the continued culture of clones of antibody-forming cells in 1975. This work, performed while Köhler was a postdoctoral fellow in Milstein's laboratory in Cambridge, has revolutionized several areas of contemporary biology and medicine including the development of targeted antibodies to specific cancers.

Milstein received his early training at the University of Buenos Aires in Argentina. In the late 1950s he moved to Cambridge where he earned his PhD in 1960. During this time he collaborated with Fred Sanger, who was awarded the Nobel Prize in Chemistry in 1958 for "his work on the structure of proteins, especially that of insulin." Milstein spent the bulk of his research career in Cambridge switching his interests from enzymology to immunology. His primary interest was the structure of the antibody molecule and the mechanism responsible for generating antibody diversity.

Köhler earned a PhD in 1974 from the University of Freiburg, Germany, for studies performed in the laboratory of Fritz Melchers at the Basel Institute for Immunology. Köhler's dissertation for his PhD demonstrated that a mouse generated up to 1000 different antibodies to a single epitope on a protein. In an attempt to limit this diversity, Köhler moved to Cambridge where he pursued postdoctoral training with Milstein. The two biologists conceived the idea of fusing antibody-forming lymphocytes from a mouse with mouse myeloma cells to develop long-lived antibody-forming cells that produced a single antibody.

In 1962 Michael Potter and Charlotte Boyce working at the National Cancer Institute in Bethesda, Maryland, injected BALB/c mice intraperitoneally with mineral oil to induce clones of B lymphocytes secreting immunoglobulin of a single specificity. By the early 1970s, a large number of these induced myelomas had been isolated; however, most of these clones synthesized and secreted immunoglobulin whose antibody specificity remained unknown.

Köhler and Milstein hybridized one of these clones with spleen cells from a mouse immunized with sheep erythrocytes. They fused the cells with Sendai virus and incubated the resulting mixture in tissue culture medium containing hypoxanthine, aminopterin, and thymidine (HAT). These cultures contained three populations of cells—unfused lymphocytes from the mouse, unfused myeloma clones, and hybrid cells consisting of mouse lymphocytes fused with myeloma clones. Culturing these cells in HAT tissue culture medium selected for the hybrid cells since

- normal mouse lymphocytes die in culture due to a life span of 5–7 days and
- myeloma clones fail to survive in HAT medium since the aminopterin inhibits folate metabolism that is necessary for DNA synthesis and cell division.

Clones resulting from the fusion of myeloma cells and normal lymphocytes survive due to the provision of enzymes coded for by genes in the normal cell partner that provide a salvage pathway for the production of DNA.

Köhler and Milstein isolated clones of antibody-forming cells (hybridomas) that synthesized and secreted two different immunoglobulins: one derived from the myeloma cell used as the fusion partner and a second that bound and lysed sheep erythrocytes. Subsequent improvements of the technology included developing a myeloma cell line that did not secrete immunoglobulin. They then fused this nonimmunoglobulin-secreting myeloma with B lymphocytes from an immunized mouse to produce hybridomas whose only product was a monoclonal antibody of known specificity.

Köhler and Milstein concluded that "such cultures could be valuable for medical and industrial use." The British government, sponsor of the work, failed to patent the technique. The scientific community, however, soon appreciated the importance of a method to generate cell lines synthesizing and secreting large quantities of monoclonal antibodies. Awards were bestowed for this invention, initially just to Milstein, the senior investigator, but subsequently to Köhler as well (Wade, 1995). These awards culminated in the awarding of the Nobel Prize for Physiology or Medicine in 1984 to Köhler and Milstein for "the discovery of the principle for production of monoclonal antibodies."

Development of hybridomas that produce monoclonal antibodies is an essential tool employed by the pharmaceutical and biotech industries. In 1994, the FDA approved rituximab, the first monoclonal antibody to treat cancer patients. Rituximab, a mouse antibody specific for CD 20, a molecule expressed by both malignant and nonmalignant B lymphocytes, was originally approved to target B-cell non-Hodgkin lymphoma. Subsequently, it is approved to also treat chronic lymphocytic leukemia and the autoimmune diseases, rheumatoid arthritis, granulomatosis with polyangiitis, and microscopic polyangiitis.

Other monoclonal antibodies, developed and approved for use in patients with tumors, include ones targeting breast cancer, metastatic colorectal cancer, melanoma, head and neck cancer, nonsmall cell lung cancer, chronic lymphocytic leukemia, large cell lymphoma, acute myelogenous leukemia, and Hodgkin lymphoma. Table 37.2 lists some of the monoclonal antibodies approved by the FDA to treat patients with cancer.

Each approved monoclonal antibody inhibits tumor growth by one or more of the following mechanisms:

- induction of antibody-dependent cell-mediated cytotoxicity,
- inhibition of tumor vascularization,
- activation of complement,
- induction of apoptosis,
- delivery of radioisotopes or drugs to the tumor, or
- inhibition of signals that downregulate ongoing adaptive immune responses.

While cancer immunotherapy with specific monoclonal antibodies led to survival of many patients, the mechanism by which the immune system actually eliminates tumors naturally is most likely through activation of T lymphocytes, particularly cytotoxic T lymphocytes. Beginning in the mid-1980s investigators focused on the role of T lymphocyte-mediated therapies against malignancies, which led to the development of several new therapeutic interventions.

Lymphokine-Activated Killer Cells

Isolation and characterization of IL-2 (T lymphocyte growth factor) in the mid-1970s resulted in successful long-term growth of thymus-derived lymphocytes in vitro. Simultaneously investigators described several functionally distinct populations of T lymphocytes including CD4$^+$ helpers and CD8$^+$ cytotoxic lymphocytes (Chapter 23). Cytotoxic T lymphocytes provide protection against virally infected cells and reject foreign transplants. Another postulated role for cytotoxic T lymphocytes is the destruction of tumors. The availability of IL-2 provided investigators a tool to study lysis of autologous tumor cells by cytotoxic T lymphocytes. Steven Rosenberg and colleagues at the National Cancer Institute in Bethesda, Maryland, developed several immunotherapeutic methods to inhibit the growth of cancer cells based on isolation of a patient's T lymphocytes that are activated and expanded in vitro followed by infusion back into the patient.

Rosenberg (1940 to present) received his medical degree in 1963 from Johns Hopkins University in Baltimore, Maryland, and earned a PhD in biophysics from Harvard, Cambridge, Massachusetts, in 1969 while completing a surgical residency. In 1974 he was appointed Chief of Surgery at the National Cancer Institute (NCI) of the National Institutes of Health, Bethesda, Maryland. He subsequently became the Head of the Tumor Immunology Section in the Surgery department at NCI.

Early in his career, Rosenberg and colleagues demonstrated that mouse spleen cells grown in tissue culture medium supplemented with IL-2 contain lymphocytes

TABLE 37.2 List of Monoclonal Antibodies Approved by the FDA to Treat Cancer Patients. The Disease Listed in the Indication Column Refers to the Cancer for Which the Antibody Was Initially Approved. Subsequent Clinical Trials Have, in Many Cases, Broadened This List

Name	Target	Indication	Year
Rituximab	CD20	Non-Hodgkin lymphoma	1997
Trastuzumab	HER2	Breast cancer	1998
Ibritumomab	CD20	Non-Hodgkin lymphoma	2002
Cetuximab	EGF receptor	Colorectal cancer	2004
Bevacizumab	VEGF	Colorectal cancer	2004
Panitumumab	EGF receptor	Colorectal cancer	2006
Ofatumumab	CD20	Chronic lymphocytic leukemia	2009
Ipilimumab	CTLA-4	Metastatic melanoma	2011
Brentuximab	CD30	Hodgkin lymphoma	2011
		Anaplastic large cell lymphoma	
Pertuzumab	HER2	Breast cancer	2012
Obinutuzumab	CD20	Chronic lymphocytic leukemia	2013
Ramucirumab	VEGF receptor 2	Gastric cancer	2014
Pembrolizumab	PD1	Melanoma	2014
Blinatumomab	CD19 and CD3	Acute lymphoblastic leukemia	2014
Nivolumab	PD1	Melanoma	2014
		Nonsmall cell lung cancer	
Dinutuximab	GD2	Neuroblastoma	2015

HER2, human epidermal growth factor receptor; EGF, epidermal growth factor; VEGF, vascular endothelial growth factor; CTLA-4, cytotoxic T lymphocyte antigen 4; PD1, programmed cell death protein 1; GD2, a disialoganglioside expressed on neuroblastoma and other neuroectoderm-derived tumors.

cytotoxic to mouse tumors (Yron et al., 1980). They extended this observation to humans when they reported the existence of a population of cytotoxic T lymphocytes that lysed patients' own tumor cells in vitro (Lotze et al., 1981). These investigators isolated lymphocytes from the peripheral blood of cancer patients and cultured them in the presence of IL-2. They tested these lymphocytes for cytotoxicity by incubating them with ^{51}Cr-labeled tumor cells derived from the same patient. Lymphocytes expanded in IL-2 caused significant lysis of tumor cells (Grimm et al., 1982). Rosenberg and his colleagues called the lymphocytes lymphokine-activated killers (LAK) and suggested that similar lymphocytes exist in vivo and that in vitro cultured cells may be useful in the development of tumor immunotherapy.

Rosenberg and his colleagues generated LAK cells in vitro and treated patients with metastatic cancer (Rosenberg et al., 1985). They isolated peripheral blood lymphocytes from patients and cultured them with IL-2 to induce proliferation. Patients received their own lymphocytes by intravenous infusion with or without additional IL-2. Twenty-one of 55 patients treated with LAK cells plus IL-2 showed some regression of their tumor. However, few lymphocytes in the LAK preparations possessed immunologic specificity for the patient's tumor. To overcome this limitation, Rosenberg and his group developed a second approach in which they isolated lymphocytes from the targeted tumor rather than from the peripheral blood. They postulated that tumor-specific lymphocytes preferentially infiltrate the tumor rather than circulate in peripheral blood.

Tumor-Infiltrating Lymphocytes

Investigators observed that tumors highly infiltrated with lymphocytes are more likely to undergo spontaneous regression than are similar tumors lacking lymphocytic infiltration. Studies in mice demonstrated that such tumor-infiltrating lymphocytes (TILs) are 50–100 times more cytotoxic for the tumor than are lymphocytes isolated from the peripheral blood of the same animal (Rosenberg et al., 1986).

Rosenberg and his colleagues transplanted tumors (sarcoma or adenocarcinoma) to inbred mice. Following a growth period, these investigators surgically removed the tumors, enzymatically treated them to isolate a mixture of single lymphocytes and tumor cells, and cultured this mixture with IL-2. Under these conditions, tumor cells died and colonies of TILs remained that were further expanded in tissue culture medium containing IL-2.

Rosenberg's group compared the cytotoxic potential of TILs and LAKs in mice bearing transplanted tumors that had metastasized to their lungs or livers. They treated tumor-bearing mice either with LAKs plus IL-2 or with TILs plus IL-2. Mice infused with TILs plus IL-2 developed fewer lung and liver metastases than did mice infused with LAKs plus IL-2.

Infusion of mice with TILs (as well as with LAKs) induced the regression/disappearance of small metastases; such treatment failed to destroy larger metastatic foci in the liver or lungs. To enhance the activity of TILs, investigators treated some mice that had large metastases simultaneously with TILs and cyclophosphamide, a treatment known to eliminate some lymphoid populations. High-dose cyclophosphamide (100 mg/kg) given in combination with TILs and IL-2 led to disappearance of large metastases in most of the mice.

The researchers speculated that in this model cyclophosphamide functioned by eliminating a host component that interfered with the success of TIL therapy. They theorized that suppressor T lymphocytes downregulated the normal adaptive immune response to tumors and that cyclophosphamide eliminated this inhibition thus permitting the infused TILs to function more efficiently. Subsequent studies (Chapter 24) showed that suppressor T lymphocytes as then envisioned do not exist. However, immunologists now know that expansion of T lymphocytes in vitro with IL-2 preferentially expands a population of T_{REG} cells. In the further development of TILs as an immunotherapy for cancer patients, recipients are routinely treated with lymphoablative therapy prior to TIL infusion. Such pretreatment most likely eliminates the T_{REG} cells and enhances the activity of the injected cytotoxic cells (Gattinoni et al., 2006).

Other Immune System Approaches to Cancer Treatment

Other approaches to immunotherapy currently include the following:

- Vaccination—Oncologists and tumor immunologists seek vaccines to protect populations against cancer. Approximately 20% of cancers worldwide have been traced to infectious microorganisms including Epstein–Barr virus (a proportion of gastric cancers, nasopharyngeal carcinoma, non-Hodgkin and Hodgkin lymphomas), *Helicobacter pylori* (gastric cancers), hepatitis B and C viruses (hepatocellular carcinoma), and (HPV—cervical, oral-pharyngeal, and anal cancers). Two vaccines, the HPV vaccine and the hepatitis B virus (HBV) vaccine, are recommended by the Centers for Disease Control and Prevention.

- In 1975, Harald zur Hausen proposed that infection with HPV is linked to the future development of cervical cancer. By 1984, zur Hausen and his colleagues isolated several strains of HPV from human cervical carcinoma biopsies including strains 16 and 18 now known to be responsible for 70% of all cervical cancers (zur Hausen, 2008). The FDA approved one HPV vaccine in 2006 that has decreased the incidence of HPV infection as well as the number of new cervical cancer cases. This work was recognized by the awarding of the Nobel Prize in Physiology or Medicine in 2008 to zur Hausen "for his discovery of human papilloma viruses causing cervical cancer." The prize was shared with Luc Montagnier and François Barré-Sinoussi "for their discovery of human immunodeficiency virus."

- In 1965 Baruch Blumberg and Harvey Alter identified a previously unrecognized antigen in the serum of an Australian with leukemia. In 1968 Alfred Prince at New York Hospital-Cornell Medical Center showed that this antigen was derived from HBV; this led to the discovery that chronic infection with HBV is the number one risk factor for the development of primary liver cancer. Maurice Hilleman and his group working at Merck and Company in New Jersey isolated this antigen from infected individuals and developed a vaccine against hepatitis B (Buynak et al., 1976; Hilleman et al., 1983). The FDA approved this blood-derived vaccine in 1981, and its use decreased the incidence of liver cancer. In 1986 a recombinant vaccine raised in yeast was approved and the blood-derived vaccine discontinued. The FDA has called the hepatitis B vaccine the first anticancer vaccine.

These antiviral vaccines prevent infections with oncogenic viruses and thus decrease tumor incidence. Both the HPV and the HBV vaccines induce antibody that inhibits the viruses from infecting susceptible cells.

Researchers continue their efforts to develop therapeutic vaccines against already established tumors. These vaccines will require that tumor-associated antigens be presented by antigen presenting cells (APCS) expressing class I and class II histocompatibility molecules to CD8+ T lymphocytes. The most efficient APC is the DC (Chapter 29), which expresses both class I and class II molecules and can present antigenic peptides to both CD4+ and CD8+ T lymphocytes.

In 1996 Frank Hsu and colleagues at Stanford University Medical Center in California reported the treatment of cancer patients with DCs. They isolated DCs from patients with non-Hodgkin lymphoma (a malignancy of B lymphocytes) and incubated them in vitro with immunoglobulin possessing the idiotype of the lymphoma. Idiotype refers to the unique antigenic determinant associated with the immunoglobulin molecule expressed by the specific lymphoma cells. Four patients who were refractory to other treatments received autologous DCs pulsed with immunoglobulin three or four times at 4-week intervals. Two weeks after the intravenous infusion of DCs the patients received a subcutaneous injection of soluble immunoglobulin idiotype as antigen. All patients responded to these injections by the induction of T lymphocytes specific for the idiotype. Three of the four patients showed either total or partial regression of their tumors.

Other investigators developed similar protocols for other types of cancer including melanoma, pancreatic cancer, prostate cancer, renal cell carcinoma, brain cancer, colorectal carcinoma, glioblastoma, lung cancer, and acute myelogenous leukemia (Vachelli et al., 2013). Several of the ongoing clinical trials combine these DC-based vaccines with chemotherapy.

In 2010 the FDA approved a vaccine, sipuleucel-T, designed to activate T-lymphocytes to antigens expressed by prostate tumors. Researchers cultured APCs including DCs from patients with metastatic prostate cancer with the antigen (prostatic acid phosphatase) conjugated to granulocyte-macrophage colony-stimulating factor (GM-CSF). They subsequently infused the APCs into the patient to activate the patient's own T lymphocytes to destroy any cells expressing the antigen (Kantoff et al., 2010).

The future development of vaccines to cancer must overcome two hurdles:

- Many tumors are only weakly immunogenic allowing them to sneak past the adaptive immune response and
- The tumor environment does not provide the necessary factors such as cytokines and growth factors for the induction of an efficient adaptive immune response.

To confront these obstacles, investigators developed techniques for the isolation of genes coding for several components of the adaptive immune response. Researchers transfect these genes into cells subsequently used as immunotherapeutic agents. These studies have proceeded along two pathways:

- Tumor cells transfected with genes coding for molecules including cytokines and cell-surface receptors become potential vaccines and

- Immunocompetent cells (particularly T lymphocytes) transfected with genes coding for receptors that bind known tumor antigens for reinfusion into cancer patients.

Investigators transfect tumor cells with genes coding for one or more of several cytokines (IL-2, IL-4, IL-6, IL-7, IFN-γ, or TNF-α), for costimulatory receptors (CD80/86), or for growth stimulating factors (GM-CSF) (Dranoff et al., 1993). These transfected tumor cells induce a therapeutic response in tumor-bearing animals. While such cells induce both a local and systemic response against melanoma in mice, for example, similar progress in human patients has yet to be achieved.

Modification of T lymphocytes by gene transfer led to some success in the clinic with cancer patients (Grubb et al., 2013). Researchers transfected autologous T lymphocytes with genes coding for receptors specific for antigens present on the patient's tumor as well as for costimulatory molecules, then transfused these cells into the patient. Approximately 30% of the patients treated with these manipulated cells experience complete remissions.

Several investigators developed methods to augment immune responses to tumors by overcoming naturally occurring regulation of the adaptive immune response. They hypothesized that the adaptive immune response is stimulated by antigens on malignantly transformed cells but that the response is short-circuited by immunoregulatory mechanisms. These investigators suggested that if they switch off these regulatory mechanisms (immune checkpoints), the adaptive immune response might eliminate the nascent tumor.

Two mechanisms inhibit the effectiveness of an antitumor immune response:

- Stimulation of T_{REG} cells by IL-2 in the activation of TILs. This inhibition can be ameliorated by treating the recipient with lymphoablative therapy prior to infusing TILs.
- Down-regulation of activated T lymphocytes by the expression of cell-surface molecules that send a negative signal to the nucleus inhibiting further gene transcription. Investigators have described several different regulatory molecules including cytotoxic T lymphocyte antigen-4 (CTLA-4), programmed cell death protein-1 (PD1), and lymphocyte activation gene 3 (LGA3). CTLA-4 (CD 152), a cell-surface receptor upregulated and expressed in activated T lymphocytes, binds CD80/86 on APCs. Interaction of CD 152 with CD 80/86 provides a negative signal to the T lymphocyte and inhibits further activity of the cell.

James Allison and his colleagues at the University of Texas, MD, Anderson Cancer Center, Houston (reviewed in Peggs et al., 2006; Sharma and Allison, 2015), proposed that inhibition of this negative signal might allow an activated antitumor response to continue rather than be terminated. Allison and coworkers developed a monoclonal antibody (ipilimumab) specific for CD152. Preclinical experiments followed by clinical trials confirmed this hypothesis, and ipilimumabe received FDA approval in 2011 for treating patients with metastatic melanoma that cannot be surgically removed. Additional blockers of immune checkpoint inhibitors including monoclonal antibodies to PD-1 are approved or being tested clinically (http://immune-checkpoint.com/what/news-and-more/).

CONCLUSION

In 1909 Paul Ehrlich proposed a protective role of the immune response against cancer. Lewis Thomas and F. Macfarlane Burnet independently reintroduced this concept in the 1950s when they hypothesized the existence of cancer immunosurveillance. As the studies outlined in this chapter indicate, solid experimental evidence confirms the validity of Ehrlich's original proposal. This evidence includes

- innate host defense mechanisms can be stimulated to inhibit the growth of existing tumors;
- tumor-associated antigens, expressed by many tumors, activate the adaptive immune response and serve as targets for antibodies and T lymphocytes;
- exposure of experimental animals to transplantable tumors induces a specific immune response;
- immunotherapies including LAKs and TILs result in regression of some tumors;
- monoclonal antibodies specific for tumor-associated antigens inhibit the further growth of tumors;
- vaccines against HBV and HPV decrease the incidence of tumors associated with these viral infections; and
- treatments that interfere with the downregulation of antitumor responses produce a favorable outcome for some patients.

These studies represent an impressive beginning leading to therapies that should, over the next decades, result in innovative cancer treatments.

References

Abelev, G., Perova, S., Khramkova, N., Postnikova, Z., Irlin, Y., 1963. Production of embryonal (alpha) globulin by transplantable mouse hepatomas. Transplantation 1, 174–180.

Blumberg, B.S., Alter, H.J., 1965. A "new" antigen in leukemia sera. JAMA 191, 541–546.

Burnet, F.M., 1957a. Cancer-a biological approach. I. The process of control and II. The significance of somatic mutation. Br. Med. J. 1, 779–786.

Burnet, F.M., 1957b. Cancer-a biological approach. III. Viruses associated with neoplastic condition and IV. Practical applications. Br. Med. J. 1, 841–847.

Buynak, E.B., Roehn, R.R., Tytell, A.A., Bertrand, A.U., Lawpon, G.P., Hilleman, M.R., 1976. Vaccine against human hepatitis B. JAMA 235, 2832–2834.

Coley, W.B., 1891. Contribution to the knowledge of sarcoma. Ann. Surg. 14, 199–220.

Coley, W.B., 1893. The treatment of malignant tumors by repeated inoculations of erysipelas: with a report of ten original cases. Am. J. Med. Sci. 10, 487–511.

Dranoff, G., Jaffee, E., Lazenby, A., Golumbek, P., Levitsky, H., Brose, K., Jackson, V., Hamada, H., Pardoll, D., Mulligan, R.C., 1993. Vaccination with irradiated tumor cells engineered to secrete murine granulocyte-macrophage colony-stimulating factor stimulates potent, specific, and long-lasting anti-tumor immunity. Proc. Nat. Acad. Sci. U.S.A. 90, 3539–3543.

Foley, E.J., 1953. Antigenic properties of methylcholanthrene-induced tumors in mice of the strain of origin. Cancer Res. 13, 835–837.

Gattinoni, L., Powell, D.J., Rosenberg, S.A., Restifo, N.P., 2006. Adoptive immunotherapy for cancer: building on success. Nat. Rev. Immunol. 6, 383–393.

Gold, P., Freedman, S.O., 1965a. Demonstration of tumor-specific antigens in human colonic carcinoma by immunological tolerance and absorption techniques. J. Exp. Med. 121, 439–462.

Gold, P., Freedman, S.O., 1965b. Specific carcinoembryonic antigens of the human digestive system. J. Exp. Med. 122, 467–481.

Grimm, E.A., Mazumder, A., Zhang, A., Rosenberg, S.A., 1982. Lymphokine-activated killer cell phenomenon. Lysis of natural killer-resistant fresh solid tumor cells by interleukin 2-activated autologous human peripheral blood lymphocytes. J. Exp. Med. 155, 1823–1841.

Grubb, S.A., Kalos, M., Barrett, D., Aplenic, R., Porter, S.L., Rheingold, S.R., Teachey, D.T., Chew, A., Hauck, B., Wright, J.F., Milone, M.C., Levine, B.L., June, C.H., 2013. Chimeric antigen receptor-modified T cells for acute lymphoid leukemia. New Eng. J. Med. 368, 1509–1518.

Hilleman, M.R., McAleer, W.J., Buynak, E.B., McLean, A.A., 1983. Quality and safety of human hepatitis B vaccine. Dev. Biol. Stand. 54, 3–12.

Himmelweit, F. (Ed.), 1957. The Collected Papers of Paul Ehrlich, vol. 2. Pergamon Press, London.

Hsu, F.J., Benike, C., Fagnoni, F., Liles, T.M., Czerwinski, D., Taidi, B., Engleman, E.G., Levy, R., 1996. Vaccination of patients with B-cell lymphoma using autologous antigen-pulsed dendritic cells. Nat. Med. 2, 52–58.

Ichim, C.V., 2005. Revisiting immunosurveillance and immunostimulation: implications for cancer immunotherapy. J. Trans. Med. 3, 18. http://dx.doi.org/10.1186/1479-5876-3-8.

Kantoff, P.W., Higano, C.S., Shore, N.D., Berger, R., Small, E.J., Penson, D.F., Redfern, C.H., Ferrari, A.C., Dreicer, R., Sims, R.B., Xu, Y., Frohlich, M.W., Schellhammer, P.F., 2010. Sipuleucel-T immunotherapy for castration-resistant prostate cancer. N. Eng. J. Med. 363, 411–422.

Lamm, D.L., Thor, D.E., Harris, S.C., Reyna, J.A., Stogdill, V.D., Radwin, H.M., 1980. Bacillus Calmette-Guerin immunotherapy of superficial bladder cancer. J. Urol. 124, 38–42.

Lotze, M.T., Grimm, E.A., Mazumder, A., Strausser, J.L., Rosenberg, S.A., 1981. Lysis of fresh and cultured autologous tumor by human lymphocytes cultured in T-cell growth factor. Cancer Res. 41, 4420–4425.

Peggs, K.S., Quezada, S.A., Korman, H.J., Allison, J.P., 2006. Principles and use of anti-CTLA4 antibody in human cancer immunotherapy. Curr. Opin. Immunol. 18, 206–213.

Penn, I., 1988. Tumors of the immunocompromised patient. Annu. Rev. Med. 39, 63–73.

Potter, M., Boyce, C., 1962. Induction of plasma cell neoplasms in strain BALB/c mice with mineral oil and mineral oil adjuvants. Nature 193, 1086–1087.

Prehn, R.T., Main, J.M., 1957. Immunity to methylcholanthrene-induced sarcomas. J. Nat. Cancer Inst. 18, 769–778.

Prince, A., 1968. An antigen detected in the blood during the incubation period of serum hepatitis. Proc. Nat. Acad. Sci. U.S.A. 60, 814–821.

Riggins, R.S., Pilch, Y.H., 1964. Immunity to spontaneous and methylcholanthrene-induced tumors in inbred mice. Cancer Res. 24, 1994–1996.

Rosenberg, S.A., Lotze, M.T., Muul, M., Leitman, S.L., Chang, A.E., Ettinghausen, S.E., Matory, Y.L., Skibber, J.M., Shlori, E., Vetto, J.T., Seipp, C.A., Simpson, C., Reichert, C.M., 1985. Observations on the systemic administration of autologous lymphokine-activated killer cells and recombinant interleukin-2 to patients with metastatic cancer. New Eng. J. Med. 313, 1485–1492.

Rosenberg, A.A., Spiess, P., Lafreniere, R., 1986. A new approach to the adoptive immunotherapy of cancer with tumor-infiltrating lymphocytes. Science 233, 1318–1321.

Sharma, P., Allison, J.P., 2015. Immune checkpoint targeting in cancer therapy: toward combination strategies with curative potential. Cell 161, 205–214.

Silverstein, M.J., deKernion, J., Morton, D.L., 1974. Malignant melanoma metastatic to the bladder. Regression following intratumor injection of BCG vaccine. JAMA 229, 688.

Thomas, L., 1959. Discussion of a presentation by Medawar, P.B. In: Lawrence, H.S. (Ed.), Cellular and Humoral Aspects of the Hypersensitive States. Harper & Brothers, New York, pp. 529–532.

Tyzzer, E.E., 1909. A study of inheritance in mice with reference to their susceptibility to transplantable tumors. J. Med. Res. 21, 519–573.

Uhlenhuth, P., 1911. On the biological differentiation of proteins by the precipitin reaction with special reference to the forensic examination of blood and meat. J. Roy. Inst. Public Health 19, 641–662.

Vachelli, E., Vitale, I., Eggermont, A., Fridman, W.H., Fucikova, J., Cremer, J., Galon, J., Tartour, E., Zitvogel, L., Kroemer, G., Galluzzi, L., 2013. Trial watch: dendritic cell-based interventions for cancer therapy. Oncoimmunology 2 (10). http://www.ncbi.nlm.nih.gov/pmc/articles/PMC3841205/pdf/onci-2-e25771.pdf.

Wade, N., 1995. Georges Kohler, 48, medicine nobel winner. N.Y. Times, 144, p. 26. Obit. http://www.nytimes.com/1995/03/04/obituaries/georges-kohler-48-medicine-nobel-winner.html.

Yron, I., Wood, T.A., Spiess, R.J., Rosenberg, S.A., 1980. In vitro growth of murine T cells. V. The isolation and growth of lymphoid cells infiltrating syngeneic solid tumors. J. Immunol. 125, 238–245.

zur Hausen, H., 2008. Harald zur Hausen - Biographical. http://www.nobelprize.org/nobel_prizes/medicine/laureates/2008/hausen-bio.html.

zur Hausen, H., Gissmann, L., Steiner, W., Dippold, W., Dreger, I., 1975. Human papilloma viruses and cancer. Bibl. Haematol. 43, 569–571.

TIME LINE

1891	William Coley reports an association between recovery from infection with *Streptococcus pyogenes* and tumor regression
1893	Coley develops a bacterial-based treatment (Coley's toxin) for the treatment of inoperable tumors
1909	Paul Ehrlich postulates that the immune response protects the individual from spontaneously arising tumors
1953; 1957	E.J. Foley, Richmond Prehn, and Joan Main demonstrate the induction of an antitumor immune response in experimental animals
1957; 1959	Lewis Thomas and F. Macfarlane Burnet introduce the concept of immune surveillance of tumors
1963	Garri Abelev reports the presence of alpha fetal protein in the sera of animals with hepatomas—first example of a tumor-associated antigen
1965	Phil Gold and Samuel Freedman describe the association of carcinoembryonic antigen with colon cancer
1974	Melvin Silverstein and colleagues use intralesional injection of BCG to treat melanoma metastatic to the bladder
1975	Georges Köhler and César Milstein describe the methodology for the production of monoclonal antibodies
1975	Harald zur Hausen proposes that HPV infection is linked to future development of cervical cancer
1980	David Lamm and colleagues present results of a phase I trial of BCG injection locally in patients with bladder cancer; this leads eventually to FDA approval of this therapy
1981	FDA licenses a vaccine for hepatitis B virus —first cancer vaccine
1984	Köhler and Milstein awarded the Nobel Prize in Physiology or Medicine
1985	Steven Rosenberg and colleagues introduce the use of lymphokine-activated killers in patients
1986	Rosenberg and colleagues develop antitumor therapy employing tumor-infiltrating lymphocytes
1997	FDA approves the use of rituximab, the initial monoclonal antibody to be approved for use in cancer patients
2006	FDA approves a vaccine against human papilloma virus, a major cause of cervical and other cancers
2010	FDA approves sipuleucel-T for treatment of patients with prostate cancer
2011	FDA approves ipilimumab for treatment of patients with metastatic melanoma

Therapies That Manipulate Host Defense Mechanisms

INTRODUCTION

Clinical immunologists manipulate the adaptive immune system both to enhance immune responses to potential pathogens and to cancers and to suppress potentially harmful immune-mediated pathologies. Even before the discovery of microorganisms, physicians developed vaccines to prevent infectious diseases. In the late 1700s, Edward Jenner in Gloucestershire, England, introduced the smallpox vaccine to western medicine. A century later, William Coley working in New York devised Coley's toxin that he injected into inoperable cancers thus inducing an inflammatory response that sometimes led to tumor regression. During the twentieth century, immunologists elucidated the mechanisms responsible for several immune-mediated hypersensitivities including allergies, asthma, serum sickness, and anaphylaxis and used this knowledge to improve immunosuppressive therapies. For example, in 1911, Leonard Noon and John Freeman at St Mary's Hospital in London, England, experimented with vaccinating patients with increasing doses of ragweed pollen, a precursor to the contemporary practice of desensitization (Jackson, 2003).

In the last decades of the twentieth century, immunologists applied emerging concepts of molecular biology and genetics to the development of new vaccines against several infectious agents such as pertussis, pneumococcus, shingles, and human papilloma virus (HPV). Simultaneously, clinicians devised several procedures, including stem cell transplantation and gene therapy, to reconstitute the immune system for patients with congenital or acquired immunodeficiency disorders.

Current procedures to manipulate the adaptive immune response include

- active immunization,
- passive transfer of immunity,
- immunosuppression, and
- reconstitution of immunodeficiency disorders.

A Historical Perspective on Evidence-Based Immunology
http://dx.doi.org/10.1016/B978-0-12-398381-7.00038-1

As the study of immunology evolves, additional critical information about homeostatic host defense mechanisms and immunopathologies will stimulate innovative interventions aimed at manipulating both innate host defense mechanisms and adaptive immune responses.

ACTIVE IMMUNIZATION

Active Immunization Against Infectious Microorganisms

Exposure to pathogens such as bacteria or virus induces an immune response characterized by antibody production or activation of specifically sensitized T lymphocytes. These products of the adaptive immune system kill or neutralize the pathogen. However, this process, referred to as active immunization, requires several days, and if the microorganism is fast growing, the individual may become ill and even die before the adaptive immune system is triggered to provide protection to the individual.

Vaccines provide a method to induce active immunization prior to natural exposure to a potential pathogen. In the pre-vaccine era, the morbidity and mortality of many childhood infections took a significant toll. For example, in the 1920s between 100,000 and 200,000 children in the United States became ill with diphtheria each year resulting in 13,000–15,000 deaths. Since 2000, only five cases of diphtheria have been reported in the United States (http://www.cdc.gov/vaccines/pubs/pinkbook/dip.html). Similar statistics are available for other vaccine-preventable infections.

The World Health Organization (WHO) in 1980 declared the eradication of naturally occurring smallpox. Vaccines exist for other pathogens including polio, measles, mumps, rubella, diphtheria, tetanus, and pertussis (Table 2.2) and have been successfully deployed around the world. At the end of 2013, the WHO reported that approximately 84% of children worldwide were immunized against these diseases thereby preventing between 2 and 3 million deaths (http://www.who.int/mediacentre/factsheets/fs378/en/).

Investigators employed several approaches to develop successful vaccines. Edward Jenner observed that individuals who had contracted cowpox were protected when exposed to smallpox. In 1879, Louis Pasteur developed a vaccine for chicken cholera from an attenuated or weakened strain of *Pasteurella multocida*. Pasteur in 1885 attenuated the rabies virus to develop a therapeutic vaccine that could be used postexposure. Other strategies include the use of

- toxoid to induce immunity to toxins from *Corynebacterium diphtheriae* and *Clostridium tetani;*
- live, attenuated viruses (measles, mumps, and rubella);

- killed viruses (polio, hepatitis A, influenza);
- killed bacteria (typhoid, cholera, plague);
- polysaccharides (*Pneumococcus, Meningococcus*); and
- recombinant vaccines (hepatitis B, HPV).

Vaccines represent one of the most successful public health initiatives. The WHO sets goals to increase the number of children immunized against vaccine-preventable infections; however, in developing countries, this goal is challenged by limited resources, competing health priorities, and distrust of outsiders. In developed countries, vaccine rates have declined due to complacency and to promulgation of erroneous information about potential adverse side effects including the false reports associating measles vaccine with development of autism.

During the 1970s and 1980s, immunologists and pharmaceutical companies developed few new vaccines. The emergence of new infectious diseases, including the human immunodeficiency virus (HIV) and Ebola, as well as renewed interest in eliminating some infectious diseases such as tuberculosis, malaria, and leishmaniasis that affect individuals primarily in developing countries and for which effective vaccines do not exist, reinvigorated vaccine research and development.

In the twenty-first century, new vaccines are needed to protect an increased population of elderly individuals who have decreased immune capability. Additionally, some existing vaccines cannot readily be used in developing countries due to cost and requirements for expensive and specialized equipment for storage or administration.

To enhance vaccine efficacy, investigators pursue several new approaches. In the past, researchers attenuated or killed the disease-causing pathogen to produce a vaccine; today vaccines are more likely to consist of isolated antigens or even of the genetic material coding for the relevant antigens. This approach produces more effective stimulants of the immune response and at the same time decreases the potential for pathogenic adverse reactions.

Active Immunization Against Tumors

Investigators employ two approaches to active immunization against tumors:

- prevention, in individuals who are cancer free, and
- therapeutic, in individuals presenting with tumors.

The use of vaccines to prevent cancer is not a new idea. Christine Ichim of the University of Toronto, Canada, relates two anecdotes of early attempts to provide protection against cancer. In 1777, the surgeon ministering to the Duke of Kent injected himself with malignant tissue as prophylaxis while in 1808 the physician to Louis XVII of France injected himself with breast cancer in hopes of reversing a sarcoma (Ichim, 2005). Written records fail to show evidence for success of either trial.

Approximately 20% of cancers worldwide are caused by infectious microorganisms including hepatitis B virus (HBV), human papilloma virus (HPV), Epstein–Barr virus, hepatitis C virus, and *Helicobacter pylori*. Scientists developed vaccines specific for HBV and HPV, and adoption of these vaccines greatly decreased subsequent tumor formation.

Chronic infection with hepatitis B is a major risk factor for the development of primary liver cancer. In 1981, the United States Food and Drug Administration (FDA) approved a vaccine against the HBV and the Center for Disease Control and Prevention recommends that all newborns receive the first dose at birth. The vaccine induces antibody synthesis that inhibits infection of liver cells by HBV.

Infection with certain strains of HPV is responsible for most cases of cervical cancer as well as many cases of anal, penile, and oropharyngeal cancer. In 2006, the FDA approved a vaccine against four strains of HPV that is recommended for both males and females older than 11 years of age. Both HBV and HPV vaccines are recommended for individuals who are not yet infected.

Researchers also design vaccines for patients with preexisting tumors. Accordingly, these vaccines are therapeutic rather than preventive. Coley's toxin (a mixture of killed *Streptococcus pyogenes* and *Serratia marcescens*) injected directly into tumors and BCG (Bacillus Calmette-Guerin) injected directly into the bladder of patients with resected bladder cancer both induce an inflammatory response in the environment leading to tumor destruction (Chapter 37). Several problems with continued development of therapeutic vaccines include the following:

- At the time of diagnosis, the number of malignant cells often exceeds 100,000, and the immune system, starting with few specific cells, is at a competitive disadvantage.
- Tumors fail to present antigen to the cells of the adaptive immune system due either to an absence of the expression of class I or class II histocompatibility molecules or to a lack of expression of costimulatory molecules such as CD80/86 that are required for efficient activation of T lymphocytes.
- Many tumors are poorly immunogenic and do not naturally stimulate a robust immune response. In addition, some tumors secrete immunosuppressive factors.

Despite these hurdles, pharmaceutical and biotech companies continue to focus on therapeutic vaccines to tumors. While preventive vaccines (against infectious microorganisms as well as against cancer-causing pathogens) are usually designed to induce antibody responses to inhibit the initial interaction with somatic cells, therapeutic cancer vaccines require induction of a robust cell-mediated response including activation of CD8[+] cytotoxic T lymphocytes and NK lymphocytes. One promising approach is to stimulate antitumor responses by autologous dendritic cells (DCs).

Dendritic Cells (DCs) as a Therapeutic Agent

Ralph Steinman and colleagues working at the Rockefeller University in New York discovered DCs during the 1970s and 1980s. Steinman characterized these cells and demonstrated that they function as highly efficient antigen-presenting cells involved in the activation of T lymphocytes (Chapter 29).

Investigators today focus on designing tumor vaccines as well as vaccines to potential pathogenic microorganisms. The use of DCs in tumor vaccines is covered in Chapter 37.

DCs in Infectious Diseases

Most vaccines are designed to work best if administered to individuals prior to exposure to the infectious pathogen. The epidemic of the human immunodeficiency virus (HIV) provides a challenge to this strategy. Infected individuals carry HIV as a latent virus in their CD4[+] T lymphocytes for a prolonged period of time. As a result, an optimal vaccine candidate would both protect uninfected individuals as well as eliminate the virus in individuals already infected. An approach using DCs to activate such an immune response has produced some encouraging preliminary results.

In 2004, Wei Lu and collaborators at the University of Paris, France, and the University of Pernambuco in Recife, Brazil, reported a successful trial of a DC-based vaccine in HIV-infected patients. They pulsed autologous DCs with inactivated HIV isolated from the infected patient. Following a short time in culture, Lu and coworkers re-infused these DCs into the patient. Eight of the 18 patients treated with this therapy demonstrated 90% or greater suppression of plasma viral loads for at least 1 year. Researchers correlated the decrease in viral loads with an increase in the number of HIV-specific T lymphocytes (both CD4[+] and CD8[+]). Although several other investigators have reported similar results, no DC-based therapy for HIV infection has yet been approved by the United States Food and Drug Administration (FDA) (de Freitas e Silva et al., 2014).

PASSIVE TRANSFER OF IMMUNITY

While investigators developed vaccines to pathogens, other scientists attempted to cure infectious disease with passively transferred antibody. The first success story involved treating *Corynebacterium diphtheriae*-infected patients with antibodies to diphtheria toxin raised in horses (von Behring and Kitasato, 1890; von Behring, 1891, Chapter 3). Until the development of a successful vaccine against diphtheria in the 1920s, serotherapy with passively infused antibody was the treatment of choice for this potentially fatal disease.

Investigators raised antibodies to other infectious microorganisms or their products in horses early in the twentieth century. For example, antibodies specific for the toxin of *Clostridium tetani* protected wounded soldiers during World War I (1914–1918) and sporadically after the war until researchers developed a vaccine against tetanus toxin in the 1920s. Similarly, the FDA approved an antibody generated in horses to the neurotoxin produced by the bacterium *Clostridium botulinum* for the treatment of patients with contaminated wounds and for individuals who have ingested contaminated food.

Antibodies to these toxins continue to be available for treatment of unvaccinated, infected patients. These antibodies are produced in horses and as a result, patients treated are at risk of developing their own antibodies against horse serum proteins that can lead to the formation of immune complexes and the development of serum sickness (Chapter 33).

Antibodies obtained from human volunteers specific for rabies, vaccinia (smallpox), varicella, and tetanus are available to treat patients infected with these associated pathogens. A human antibody against the *C. botulinum* neurotoxin is now approved by the FDA for treating infants under the age of 1 year who have been exposed to the toxin (Arnon et al., 2006).

Preventing Erythroblastosis Fetalis

Passive infusion of antibodies has proven efficacious in several noninfectious clinical situations including treatment of autoimmune diseases (i.e., antibodies to inflammatory cytokines in patients with rheumatoid arthritis and Crohn disease) and hypersensitivity reactions (i.e., antibodies to IgE in patients with persistent asthma). Antibody infusion is also used to prevent erythroblastosis fetalis in Rh incompatible pregnancies and represents one of the greatest success stories of clinical immunology.

Erythroblastosis fetalis occurs when mother and fetus possess incompatible red blood cell antigens. This condition results most often when mother and father are incompatible at the Rh (D) antigens expressed on erythrocytes. If the father's red cells express the Rh (D) antigen, he is said to be Rh positive and will transmit the gene for this antigen to the embryo. When the mother lacks the Rh (D) antigen, she is considered Rh negative (Chapter 33).

During pregnancy, some fetal blood crosses the placenta; if fetal red cells express Rh (D) antigen they stimulate the mother's immune system to produce antibody to the Rh (D) antigen. This antibody, initially of the IgM class, switches to IgG upon a second exposure to the antigen. Unlike IgM, IgG is actively transported across the placenta, enters the fetal circulation, binds to fetal red blood cells, and marks them for destruction. Phillip Levine and Rufus Stetson working at Newark Beth Israel Hospital in New Jersey originally described this disease process in 1939.

Usually the mother is not exposed to fetal red blood cells until near, or at the time, of delivery of her first incompatible pregnancy, and hence she fails to produce IgG antibodies to the Rh (D) antigen sufficiently early to put that fetus at risk. However, second and subsequent incompatible fetuses are at risk and may suffer from a series of syndromes ranging from hemolytic anemia to kernicterus to death. In 1943, Phillip Levine noted that Rh-isoimmunization occurred more frequently when the mother and father shared ABO blood types than when they were ABO-incompatible. From this observation, he hypothesized that ABO incompatibility provides some protection against development of antibodies to the Rh (D) antigen.

Other investigators reached similar conclusions including Israel Davidsohn and colleagues working in Chicago, Illinois. In 1956 they injected Rh-negative male volunteers with Rh-positive blood and demonstrated that a higher concentration of antibody to the Rh (D) antigen resulted if the donors and volunteers were ABO-compatible. An explanation for this phenomenon is that naturally occurring isohemagglutinins (antibodies to the A or B red blood cell antigens) in the volunteer's circulation bind and eliminate the Rh-positive red cells before they induce a response.

Ronald Finn and coworkers in Liverpool, England, postulated that injecting antibody to the Rh (D) antigen would similarly eliminate Rh-positive red cells and protect against antibody production. To test this postulate, they injected Rh-negative male volunteers with ^{51}Cr-labeled, ABO-compatible Rh-positive blood. One-half hour later, they injected the volunteers with antibodies specific for the Rh (D) antigen (Finn et al., 1961). They obtained blood samples from the volunteers 2, 5, and 14 days later to determine the percentage of radiolabeled cells remaining.

By 2 days after red blood cell injection, the percentage of radioactive cells in volunteers treated with antibody to the Rh (D) antigen was significantly decreased compared to controls who had not received antibodies. Based on these findings, the authors concluded "our results suggest that it may be possible to prevent most cases of Rh sensitization, and thus in time eliminate Rh haemolytic disease."

Vincent Freda and colleagues working at Columbia University in New York in 1964 tested if treatment of Rh-negative individuals with antibody to the Rh (D) antigen prior to injection of Rh-positive red cells inhibited antibody production. These investigators conducted experiments at Sing Sing prison in Ossining, New York, where they injected nine Rh-negative male volunteers with Rh-positive blood once a month for 5 months. Four of these volunteers received 5 ml of antibody to Rh (D) intramuscularly 1 day prior to injection with Rh-positive blood; the other five volunteers received no antibodies and served as controls. Six months after the last injection, Freda and coworkers detected no antibodies to the Rh (D) antigen in the experimental group while four of the five controls produced a significant antibody response to the Rh (D) antigen.

In a follow-up study, Freda and colleagues injected additional volunteers with Rh-positive blood followed 72 h later with an injection of antibody to the Rh (D) antigen. These volunteers also failed to synthesize and secrete antibodies to the Rh (D) antigen.

These results led to clinical trials in 43 countries including the United States, Canada, England, Argentina, Scotland, and Australia in which Rh-negative women who had just delivered their first Rh-positive infant received Rho(D), a human antibody specific for the Rh (D) antigen (Pollack et al., 1968). In 1967, Freda and colleagues presented results of clinical trials at five study centers (New York—two sites, Long Beach, California, Baltimore, Maryland and Freiberg, Germany). The investigators enrolled 666 postpartum women all of whom were Rh negative who had delivered an Rh-positive, ABO-compatible baby. Of these, 329 received an injection of human antibody to Rh (D) antigen within 72 h of delivery, and 337 served as controls. None of the injected women developed antibodies to the Rh (D) antigen while 46 of the controls produced antibodies. During the course of the trial, 58 of the women became pregnant a second time; 31 of the injected group and 27 controls. None of the babies born of the injected mothers developed erythroblastosis fetalis while 11 babies born of mothers in the control group were affected. The FDA licensed the use of antibody to Rh (D) in 1968.

IMMUNOSUPPRESSION

Throughout the twentieth century, investigators described a number of immune-mediated pathologies including anaphylaxis, asthma, autoimmune disease, and toxic shock syndrome (Chapter 33) that immunologists today attribute to aberrant adaptive immune responses. In addition, activation of the adaptive immune responses interferes with successful therapeutic manipulations such as allogeneic organ transplantation and reconstitution with stem cells. Therapies to control these unwanted or hyperreactive immune responses focus on downregulating or suppressing the adaptive immune system.

Initial methods to manipulate immune responses involved relatively nonspecific reagents. For example, during the early history of organ transplantation, recipients of allogeneic grafts received cytotoxic reagents including azathioprine, methotrexate, prednisone, or cyclophosphamide designed to inhibit rapidly proliferating cells including lymphocytes that might be activated to reject the foreign graft. While effective, these treatments place the patient at increased risk of developing severe infections, anemia, gastrointestinal disturbances, or cancer. Subsequent advances led to the development of immunosuppressive drugs that target individual components of the immune system. For example, cyclosporine and tacrolimus inhibit the synthesis of IL-2, a T-lymphocyte growth factor, while sirolimus blocks IL-2 receptor-dependent signal transduction. Adoption of these therapeutic agents resulted in fewer adverse reactions in transplant recipients and longer survival times although a percentage of patients still present with life-threatening infections (Chapter 36).

Immune-mediated diseases including hypersensitivities (i.e., allergy, asthma, immune complex diseases—Chapter 33) and autoimmunity (i.e., type 1 diabetes, systemic lupus erythematosus, multiple sclerosis—Chapter 34) result from overreactive adaptive immune responses and are amenable to immunosuppressive therapies. Immunologists continue to devise several unique means of downregulating the response including monoclonal antibodies and biologics that inhibit inflammatory cytokines.

Monoclonal Antibodies

Georges J.F. Köhler (1946–1995) and César Milstein (1927–2002) published their landmark paper describing a technique for the continued culture of clones of antibody-forming cells in 1975. This work, performed while Köhler was a postdoctoral fellow in Milstein's laboratory in Cambridge, England, has revolutionized several areas of contemporary biology and medicine including the development of targeted therapies. The background of this discovery is presented in Chapter 37. Table 38.1 lists some FDA-approved monoclonal antibodies for indications other than cancer.

Muromonab, the first monoclonal antibody to be approved by the FDA, is a mouse antibody directed against CD3, a molecule expressed by human T lymphocytes. Approved in 1986, muromonab is indicated for recipients of solid organ grafts who become resistant to the immunosuppressive effects of steroids.

A potential problem with treating humans with a mouse monoclonal antibody is the risk that the patient will synthesize antibodies to the mouse immunoglobulin. This can lead to decreased efficacy of the monoclonal antibody as well as to the possible development of serum sickness.

TABLE 38.1   List of FDA-Approved Monoclonal Antibodies for Non-oncological Indications

Name	Target	Indication	Year
Muromonab	CD3	Kidney graft rejection	1986
Abciximab	GPIIb/IIIa	Blood clots in angioplasty	1994
Basiliximab	IL-2 receptor	Kidney transplantation	1998
Palivizumab	RSV	Prevent RSV infection	1998
Adalimumab	TNF	Rheumatoid arthritis	2002
Omalizumab	IgE	Asthma	2003
Natalizumab	Alpha-4 integrin	Multiple sclerosis	2004
Ranibizumab	VEGF	Macular degeneration	2006
Eculizumab	C5	Paroxysmal nocturnal hemoglobinuria	2007
Certolizumab	TNF	Crohn's disease	2008
Ustekinumab	IL-12/23	Psoriasis	2009
Golimumab	TNF	Rheumatoid and psoriatic arthritis Ankylosing spondylitis	2009
Canakinumab	IL-1β	Muckle–Wells syndrome	2009
Tocilizumab	IL-6 receptor	Rheumatoid arthritis	2010
Denosumab	RANK ligand	Bone loss	2010
Raxibacumab	*Bacillus anthracis*	Anthrax infection	2012
Siltuximab	IL-6	Castleman disease	2014
Vedolizumab	α4β7 integrin	Ulcerative colitis; Crohn's disease	2014
Secukinumab	IL-17a	Psoriasis	2015

TNF, tumor necrosis factor.

To protect against the production of potentially pathogenic antibodies, investigators manipulated monoclonal antibodies so that portions of the molecule are derived from human immunoglobulin amino acid sequences. Examples include basiliximab, a chimeric human–murine monoclonal antibody, in which the constant region of the heavy chain of the mouse antibody is replaced with a human constant region, and daclizumab, a humanized monoclonal antibody, in which the entire molecule except the hypervariable regions is human. Both chimeric and humanized monoclonal antibodies are less immunogenic in patients than are mouse monoclonal antibodies.

During the 1990s, investigators generated several humanized and chimeric monoclonal antibodies specific for tumor necrosis factor (TNF). For example, in 1993, David Knight and colleagues working at Centocor in Malvern, Pennsylvania, developed a mouse–human chimeric monoclonal antibody specific for TNF-α. This antibody, infliximab, is a mouse monoclonal antibody in which the mouse immunoglobulin constant regions are replaced with human constant regions.

In 1994, Michael Elliott and collaborators from England, Germany, Austria, and the Netherlands conducted clinical trials of infliximab in patients presenting with rheumatoid arthritis. Patients treated once with infliximab had decreased subjective and objective markers of rheumatoid arthritis when compared to patients treated with placebo. The authors concluded "the results provide the first good evidence that specific cytokine blockade can be effective in human inflammatory disease and define a new direction for the treatment of rheumatoid arthritis."

Treatment of inflammatory conditions with humanized or chimeric monoclonal antibodies requires lifelong injection of the antibody. While humanized and chimeric monoclonal antibodies are less immunogenic than mouse antibodies, the potential still exists for the patient to experience adverse reactions including accelerated clearance and formation of immune complexes leading to type III hypersensitivity reactions including serum sickness. During the 1990s, researchers devised two methods to derive totally human monoclonal antibodies: antibody phage display and transgenic mice.

Antibody phage display involves genetic engineering of bacteriophage to express the variable regions of H and L chains of human immunoglobulins. Selection of phages that bind antigen is followed by infection of *Escherichia coli* with the phages to generate human monoclonal antibodies of the appropriate specificity (Barbas et al., 1991; Breitling et al., 1991; McCafferty et al., 1990). In 1994, Laurent Jespers and coworkers in Cambridge, England, synthesized a fully human monoclonal antibody specific for TNF-α using phage display. This antibody bound TNF-α with the same affinity as did a mouse monoclonal antibody to TNF-α.

Collaboration between the Cambridge group and BASF Bioresearch Corporation in Worcester, Massachusetts, led to the development of a fully human monoclonal antibody to TNF-α called D2E7. By 1999, Joachim Kempeni of Knoll AG-BASF Pharma in Ludwigshafen, Germany, summarized the results of early clinical trials using this monoclonal antibody. These studies included safety testing as well as efficacy following a single or multiple injections of the antibody. Between 40% and 70% of patients receiving the highest doses of the antibody responded with decreased joint swelling and other indications of rheumatoid arthritis compared to 19% of patients receiving placebo. Kempeni concluded "these early data suggest that the fully human anti-TNF-α mAb D2E7 is safe and effective as monotherapy." Subsequent development of this antibody (adalimumab) led to FDA approval in 2002 for several indications including rheumatoid arthritis, psoriatic arthritis, ankylosing spondylitis, Crohn disease, chronic psoriasis, and juvenile idiopathic arthritis.

In 1994, Larry L. Green and colleagues working at Cell Genesys, Inc. in Foster City, California, inserted human heavy and kappa light chain genetic loci contained on yeast artificial chromosomes into the mouse germ line. These mice produce human antibodies, and when Green and coworkers immunized them, the mice synthesized and secreted antibodies specific for the injected antigen. Lymphocytes synthesizing these antibodies could be hybridized using classical techniques. Other investigators produced similar transgenic mice that are currently employed by pharmaceutical and biotech companies to generate human monoclonal antibodies.

In 2008 the WHO convened a meeting of the International Nonproprietary Names Working Group to develop policies for naming monoclonal antibodies. Among other recommendations this group agreed that names for all monoclonal antibodies would end in "-mab." Preceding this suffix, a 1 to 3 letter substem B indicates the biological origin of the molecule. Relevant substem B designations are as follows: "o" = mouse, "u" = human, "xi" = chimeric, and "zu" = humanized (http://www.who.int/medi cines/services/inn/generalpoliciesmonoclonalantibodie sjan10.pdf).

Anti-Inflammatory Biologics

Beginning in the 1980s, immunologists in academic settings and at pharmaceutical and biotech companies focused on biological agents that decreased the severity of inflammation associated with several autoimmune diseases including rheumatoid arthritis, Crohn disease, and psoriasis. Their efforts succeeded, and the FDA approved several biologics that interrupt the inflammatory response targeting several mediators.

Lloyd Old and colleagues at Memorial Sloan Kettering Cancer Institute in New York identified TNF in 1975 (Carswell et al., 1975—Chapter 25). In addition to inducing necrosis in tumors, TNF is a potent proinflammatory cytokine. The cell surface receptor to which TNF binds was identified and cloned by two groups of scientists in 1990 (Loetscher et al., 1990; Schall et al., 1990).

In 1990, Bruce Beutler and coworkers at the Southwestern Medical School, University of Texas, Dallas, constructed a cDNA of the extracellular domain of this receptor attached to a DNA sequence coding for the Fc portion and hinge region of a mouse immunoglobulin (Peppel et al., 1990). These researchers inserted DNA into Chinese hamster ovary cells that secreted a chimeric protein with TNF inhibitory properties. In preliminary studies, Beutler and colleagues compared the level of inhibition created by this chimeric protein with the amount of inhibition produced by three monoclonal antibodies specific for TNF; the chimeric protein was between 100 and 10,000 times as effective as the antibodies in the assay system used.

In 1993, Kendall Mohler and colleagues at Immunex in Seattle, Washington, demonstrated that injecting mice with soluble TNF receptors chimerized to the Fc region of mouse IgG protected the mice from an otherwise lethal dose of lipopolysaccharide. Dimeric forms of the receptor proved more efficient than monomeric forms. These studies led to the development of an FDA-approved drug, etanercept, which acts as a competitive inhibitor of TNF-α in several inflammatory diseases including rheumatoid arthritis, psoriasis, ankylosing spondylitis, psoriatic arthritis, and juvenile idiopathic arthritis.

Investigators developed additional biological inhibitors of inflammatory responses for patients with rheumatoid arthritis. These include agents blocking the inflammatory cytokine, IL-1, and monoclonal antibodies to the IL-6 receptor (tocilizumab).

In 1984, Zenghua Liao and coworkers working at Albert Einstein College of Medicine in the Bronx, New York, and Giuseppe Scala and collaborators at the National Cancer Institute, Bethesda, Maryland, independently described a naturally occurring inhibitor of interleukin 1. Liao's group identified this inhibitor in urine using an in vitro assay of IL-1-induced proliferation of thymus cells. These investigators characterized this inhibitor as a low molecular weight protein (20–40 kDa) that is specific for IL-1 and is not cytotoxic to thymus cells.

Scala and coworkers isolated a similar inhibitor from the culture medium of a human B-lymphocyte line that had been transformed by Epstein–Barr virus. They detected the inhibitor and determined its effect on the in vitro stimulation of human thymus cells by IL-1. Scala's group demonstrated that the inhibitor they isolated while specific for IL-1 has a molecular weight of approximately 95 kDa, considerably larger than that reported by Liao and coworkers.

Further characterization revealed that several human cells including lymphocytes and epithelial cells secrete these naturally occurring inhibitors called IL-1 receptor antagonists (IL-1ra). IL-1ra binds to the IL-1 receptor and interferes with signaling by IL-1. Since IL-1 is a potent inflammatory cytokine involved in several disease processes including rheumatoid arthritis, biotech companies identified this as a therapeutic target to control chronic inflammatory diseases.

A recombinant form of IL-1ra produced by *E. coli* is virtually identical to the natural molecule. The FDA approved IL-1ra (anakinra) in 2001 for use alone or with methotrexate in the treatment of rheumatoid arthritis. Other examples of IL-1-blocking agents to treat autoimmune and autoinflammatory diseases include a soluble decoy IL-1 receptor (rilonacept) and a monoclonal antibody specific for IL-1β (cankinumab) (Dinarello et al., 2012).

RECONSTITUTION OF IMMUNODEFICIENCIES

A number of primary (congenital) immunodeficiencies (PID) result from mutations in genes coding for proteins involved in the adaptive immune response (Chapter 32). As a result, patients with these diseases present with an increased incidence of infections. Methods of reconstituting the immune system in patients with PID can be categorized into three approaches:

- replacement therapy,
- hematopoietic stem cell transplantation, and
- gene therapy.

Replacement Therapy

In 1952, Ogden C. Bruton described a case of agammaglobulinemia in an 8-year-old boy. This X-linked disease, characterized by a decrease in mature B lymphocytes and a corresponding serum immunoglobulin level below the established reference range, is caused by a mutation in the gene coding for a tyrosine kinase responsible for the maturation of pre-B lymphocytes into more mature forms. While Bruton was unaware of the underlying genetic defect in this disease, he provided protection against most infections by infusing the patient periodically with pooled human gamma globulin. This treatment proved

the therapy of choice for this individual and for others diagnosed with this disease until the advent of bone marrow transplantation.

In 1968, an 8-month-old male with a form of severe combined immunodeficiency (SCID) (Swiss-type agammaglobulinemia) presented with thymic dysplasia, lymphopenia, and underdeveloped peripheral lymphoid organs. Richard Hong and colleagues working with Robert Good's group at the University of Minnesota and Humphrey Kay's group in London, England, injected this child with maternal blood plus fetal thymus and liver cells. Initially this treatment corrected many of the immunological defects—the white blood cell and lymphocyte counts rose, small lymphocytes appeared, a previously accepted skin graft was rejected, plasma cells were detected in the bone marrow, a yeast infection cleared, and peripheral blood lymphocytes responded in vitro to typhoid antigen. Unfortunately, a graft-versus-host (GvH) reaction occurred, and the patient died 15 days after infusion of fetal cells. The investigators concluded that reconstitution of patients with immunodeficiency might be possible although they recommended treatment with stem cells in future attempts.

Infants born with thymic aplasia (DiGeorge syndrome) fail to develop an adaptive immune response against viral infections and other intracellular pathogens. They also lack antibodies due to the failure of helper (CD4+) T lymphocytes to mature (Chapter 32). Shortly after the initial description of this defect, Humphrey Kay and colleagues in London reconstituted the adaptive immune response of DiGeorge patients with fetal thymus transplants (August et al., 1968; Cleveland et al., 1968). While this resulted in some immunologic reconstitution, subsequent efforts were aimed at either hematopoietic stem cell transplantation or gene therapy.

Hematopoietic Stem Cell Transplantation

In the early 1950s, researchers rescued experimental animals exposed to lethal doses of irradiation with bone marrow transplantation. Clinicians adopted this procedure, treating patients with a variety of diseases including immunodeficiencies. In 1957, E. Donnall Thomas and colleagues performed the first successful human bone marrow transplantation (Chapter 36). In 1970, Mortimer Bortin of Marquette School of Medicine, Milwaukee, Wisconsin, reviewed the results of 203 human bone marrow transplants performed between 1939 and 1968. Many of these transplants proved unsuccessful due either to technical reasons or to an incomplete understanding of tissue typing, immunosuppression, and appropriate postoperative care of the recipient. As knowledge about the immune system accumulated, the success rate of stem cell and bone marrow transplantation improved.

A major advance in bone marrow transplantation occurred when Irving Weissman and his group at Stanford University and SyStemix, Inc., Palo Alto, California (Baum et al., 1992; Spangrude et al., 1988), identified a marker (CD34) expressed by hematopoietic stem cells but not by other cells. Clinicians isolate human hematopoietic stem cells from various sources including bone marrow, peripheral blood, and umbilical cord blood based on expression of CD34. The isolated cells are used therapeutically for patients with a variety of pathologies including lymphoma, leukemia, and inherited blood disorders and to rescue patients following chemotherapy or radiotherapy.

The standard treatment for infants with SCID is now bone marrow transplantation. At least 13 different mutations have been identified in patients diagnosed with SCID. The defects caused by these mutations can often be overcome by providing hematopoietic stem cells from allogeneic or related donors. Rebecca Buckley at Duke University in Durham, North Carolina, reviewed her experience in 2011 with this procedure in 166 SCID patients treated during a 28-year period. She concluded "transplantation of rigorously T cell-depleted HLA-identical or HLA-haploidentical bone marrow is highly effective in reconstituting T cell immunity in all of the known genetic types of SCID."

Gene Therapy

Now that gene mutations responsible for most congenital immunodeficiencies are documented, researchers have a third approach to treating patients with PID—namely, to transplant autologous stem cells transduced with a nonmutated copy of the gene. In theory, at least, these transplanted cells should neither induce an adverse immune response nor be activated against host antigens.

In 1990, R. Michael Blaese and W. French Anderson with colleagues at the National Institutes of Health, Bethesda, Maryland, developed a clinical trial involving the transplantation of genetically modified autologous stem cells in patients with one form of SCID. These investigators treated two girls, one 4 year old and one 9 year old diagnosed with SCID caused by mutations in the adenosine deaminase (ADA) enzyme. These two children received autologous stem cells in which an ADA gene from an unaffected individual had been inserted. Four years later, Blaese and colleagues reported that both patients survived with few complications (Blaese et al., 1995). An additional 30 similar transplants during the following 20 years resulted in the development of functional T lymphocytes in the majority of patients to the point where they no longer needed enzyme supplementation.

Other patients with SCID have a mutation in the gene coding for the common γ-chain of the receptor for several different interleukins. Investigators in France and England designed clinical trials to provide these individuals with autologous stem cells transduced with a nonmutated copy of this gene. Unfortunately five of the first 20 patients transplanted with these manipulated stem cells developed T-lymphocyte leukemia, most likely because the gene incorporated randomly into the DNA of the cell within a proto-oncogene (Fischer et al., 2011).

Patients with two other primary immunodeficiencies have been treated successfully with gene therapy. In 1997, Harry Malech and colleagues working at the National Institutes of Health in Bethesda, Maryland, transfused five patients with chronic granulomatous disease with autologous peripheral blood stem cells transduced with a retrovirus containing the $p47^{phox}$ gene, a gene shown to be mutated in these patients. This procedure resulted in the transient appearance of granulocytes that produced NADPH oxidase thus providing protection against *Staphylococci* and other catalase-positive bacteria. Studies to increase engraftment of the transduced stem cells continue.

Wiskott–Aldrich syndrome, a PID characterized by eczema, thrombocytopenia, recurrent infections, and an increased risk of developing cancer and/or autoimmune diseases, results from mutations in a gene coding for a protein involved in regulating cellular cytoskeleton (Wiskott–Aldrich syndrome protein, WASP). In 2013, a group led by Alessandro Aiuti working at various institutions in Milan, Italy, reported treating three patients with autologous stem cells that contained the unmutated gene for WASP. These patients showed stable integration of the gene into their myeloid cells with expression of the protein in platelets and lymphocytes. When followed for up to 2.5 years, the patients became clinically stable showing immunological and hematological improvement.

T REGULATORY (T_{REG}) LYMPHOCYTES AS THERAPEUTIC AGENTS

T_{REG} lymphocytes are required to maintain homeostasis in the adaptive immune response. The discovery of this subpopulation of $CD4^+$ T lymphocytes is presented in Chapter 23. These cells inhibit the development of autoimmune disease and maintain self-tolerance. Based on this observation, numerous investigators suggested the use of T_{REG} lymphocytes in clinical situations characterized by unwanted immune responses including autoimmune disease (Chapter 34), allergies (Chapter 33), allogeneic organ grafts (Chapter 36), and autoinflammatory diseases (Chapter 31). In addition, inhibition of T_{REG} lymphocyte activity is an attractive target in clinical situations where an enhanced adaptive immune response may be desirable including the response to tumors (Chapter 37) and pathogenic microorganisms.

Protocols to enhance T_{REG} lymphocyte activity require isolation of these cells from a mixed population of peripheral blood lymphocytes. Once relatively pure T_{REG} lymphocytes are isolated they can be stimulated in vitro to increase their numbers prior to reinfusion. A number of different protocols have been developed including stimulation with monoclonal antibodies to cell surface molecules (CD3, CD28), cytokines (IL-2), or antigen-presenting cells displaying the desired antigen. Other techniques may be developed to isolate and activate these lymphocytes as clinical trials proceed.

Examples of the use of T_{REG} lymphocytes to downregulate pathogenic immune responses include

- induction of transplant tolerance,
- control of atopic disease (allergy),
- treatment of autoimmune disease,
- inhibition of autoinflammatory disease,
- antitumor immunity,
- graft-versus-host disease in allogeneic stem cell transplantation, and
- infectious disease.

Inhibition of T_{REG} Lymphocytes

Sometimes downregulation by T_{REG} lymphocytes is counterproductive in treating pathologies. One such case is when an ongoing immune response to a tumor is curtailed prior to elimination of all the malignant cells. An approach that has met with success in these situations is to interfere with cell surface molecules expressed on the surface of activated T lymphocytes that send a negative signal to the nucleus thus turning the cell off. Several different such regulatory molecules exist; the one most extensively studied is cytotoxic T-lymphocyte antigen-4 (CTLA-4—CD152). CD152, a cell surface molecule whose expression is upregulated in activated T lymphocytes, binds the costimulatory molecule on antigen-presenting cells, CD80/86. Interaction of CD152 with CD80/86 sends a negative signal to the T lymphocyte and inhibits further activity of the cell.

James Allison and his colleagues working at the University of Texas M.D. Anderson Cancer Center (reviewed in Peggs et al., 2006) developed a monoclonal antibody (ipilimumab) specific for CD152. The FDA approved ipilimumab in 2011 for use in patients with metastatic melanoma that cannot be surgically removed. A similar monoclonal antibody (pembrolizumab) specific for PD-1 has subsequently been approved by the FDA for patients with melanoma or with advanced non-small cell lung cancer.

CONCLUSION

Manipulation of host defense mechanisms originally focused on induction of adaptive immune responses to provide protection against potentially pathogenic microorganisms. Starting with Jenner's introduction of the smallpox vaccine to the Western world in the late 1700s, this approach has evolved leading to the availability of vaccines for more than 30 infectious diseases. Currently vaccination has eradicated smallpox as a threat, and the elimination of polio is anticipated.

The discovery of antibodies and their role in providing protection to some infectious diseases in the late 1880s led to the development of serotherapy. Although this therapeutic maneuver does not alter the homeostasis of the adaptive immune system, it was an important adjunct to clinical treatments during the first two decades of the twentieth century.

Starting in the 1960s, investigators developed a large number of immunotherapies aimed at maintaining homeostasis of the adaptive immune system in both normal and pathological circumstances. The goal of some of these treatments is to correct aberrant immune responses to environmental antigens leading to asthma and allergies as well as to eliminate the pathologies associated with autoimmune diseases.

Major breakthroughs in development of these therapies include an enhanced understanding of the molecular and genetic mechanisms responsible for both normal and abnormal immune responses. In addition, technological advances, such as the production of monoclonal antibodies, methods to regulate the synthesis and/or function of various cytokines, and replacement of mutated genes in immunocompetent cells propelled this field. These advances produced FDA-approved therapies for several clinical pathologies including cancer, allogeneic transplantation, inflammatory autoimmune diseases, and congenital and acquired immunodeficiencies.

Progress in these areas represents an ongoing testimony to coordinating basic science research with clinical application. The use of this bench to bedside approach promises enhanced methods for controlling diseases in a wide variety of clinical disciplines.

References

Anderson, W.F., Blaese, R.M., Culver, K., 1990. The ADA human gene therapy clinical protocol: points to consider response with clinical protocol. Hum. Gene Ther. 1, 331–362.

Arnon, S.S., Schechter, R., Maslanka, S.E., Jewell, N.P., Hatheway, C.L., 2006. Human botulism immune globulin for the treatment of infant botulism. N. Engl. J. Med. 354, 462–471.

August, C.S., Rosen, F.S., Filler, R.M., Janeway, C.A., Markowski, B., Kay, H.E.M., 1968. Implantation of a fetal thymus restoring immunological competence in a patient with thymic aplasia (DiGeorge's syndrome). Lancet 292, 1210–1211.

Barbas, C.F., Kang, A.S., Lerner, R.A., Benkovic, S.J., 1991. Assembly of combinatorial antibody libraries on phage surfaces: the gene III site. Proc. Natl. Acad. Sci. U.S.A 88, 7978–7982.

Baum, C.M., Weissman, I.L., Tsukamoto, A.S., Buckle, A.M., Peault, B., 1992. Isolation of a candidate human hematopoietic stem-cell population. Proc. Natl. Acad. Sci. U.S.A 89, 2804–2808.

Blaese, R.M., Culver, K.W., Miller, A.D., Carter, C.S., Fleishi, T., Clerici, M., Shearer, G., Chang, L., Chiang, Y., Tolstoshev, P., Greenblatt, J.J., Rosenberg, S.A., Klein, H., Berger, M., Mullen, C.A., Ramsey, W.J., Muul, L., Morgan, R.A., Anderson, W.F., 1995. T lymphocyte-directed gene therapy for ADA-SCID: initial trial results after 4 years. Science 270, 475–480.

Breitling, F., Dübel, S., Seehaus, T., Klewinghaus, I., Little, M., 1991. A surface expression vector for antibody screening. Gene 104, 147–153.

Bruton, O.C., 1952. Agammaglobulinemia. Pediatrics 9, 722–728.

Buckley, R.H., 2011. Transplantation of hematopoietic stem cells in human severe combined immunodeficiency: longterm outcomes. Immunol. Res. 49, 25–43.

Carswell, E.A., Old, L.J., Kassel, R.L., Green, S., Fiore, N., Williamson, B., 1975. An endotoxin-induced serum factor that causes necrosis of tumors. Proc. Natl. Acad. Sci. U.S.A 72, 3666–3670.

Cleveland, W.W., Fogel, B.J., Brown, W.T., Kay, H.E.M., 1968. Fetal thymic transplant in a case of DiGeorge's syndrome. Lancet 292, 1211–1214.

Davidsohn, I., Masaitis, L., Stern, K., 1956. Experimental studies on Rh immunization. Am. J. Clin. Pathol. 26, 833–843.

de Freitas e Silva, R., de Castro, M.C.A.B., Pereira, V.R., 2014. Dendritic cell-based approaches in the fight against diseases. Front. Immunol. 5. http://journal.frontiersin.org/Journal/10.3389/fimmu.2014.00078/full.

Dinarello, C.A., Simon, A., van der Meer, J.W.M., 2012. Treating inflammation by blocking IL-1 in a broad spectrum of diseases. Nat. Rev. Drug Discov. 11, 652–653.

Elliott, M.J., Maini, R.N., Feldmann, M., Kalden, J.R., Antoni, C., Smolen, J.S., Leeb, B., Breedveld, F.C., Macfarlane, J.D., Bijl, H., Woody, J.N., 1994. Randomised double-blind comparison of chimeric monoclonal antibody to tumour necrosis factor versus placebo in rheumatoid arthritis. Lancet 344, 1105–1110.

Finn, R., Clarke, C.A., Donohoe, W.T.A., McConnell, R.B., Sheppard, P.M., Lehane, D., Kulke, W., 1961. Experimental studies on the prevention of Rh haemolytic disease. Brit. Med. J. 1, 1486–1490.

Fischer, A., Hacein-Bey-Abina, S., Cavazzana-Calvo, M., 2011. Gene therapy for primary adaptive immune deficiencies. J. Allergy Clin. Immunol. 127, 1356–1359.

Freda, V.J., Gorman, J.G., Pollack, W., 1964. Successful prevention of experimental Rh sensitization in man with an anti-Rh gamma2-globulin antibody preparation: a preliminary report. Transfusion 4, 26–32.

Freda, V.J., Gorman, J.G., Pollack, W., Robertson, J.G., Jennings, E.R., Sullivan, J.F., 1967. Prevention of Rh isoimmunization. Progress report of the clinical trial in mothers. JAMA 199, 383–389.

Green, L.L., Hardy, M.C., Maynard-Currie, C.E., Tsuda, H., Louie, D.M., Mendez, M.J., Abderrahim, H., Noguchi, M., Smith, D.H., Zeng, Y., David, N.E., Sasai, H., Garza, D., Brenner, D.G., Hales, J.F., McGuinness, J.P., Capon, D.J., Klapholz, S., Jakobovits, A., 1994. Antigen-specific human monoclonal antibodies from mice engineered with human Ig heavy and light chain YACs. Nat. Genet. 7, 13–21.

Hong, R., Cooper, M.D., Allan, M.J.G., Kay, H.E.M., Meuwissen, H., Good, R.A., 1968. Immunological restitution in lymphopenic immunological deficiency syndrome. Lancet 292, 503–506.

Ichim, C.V., 2005. Revisiting immunosurveillance and immunostimulation: implications for cancer immunotherapy. J. Trans. Med. 3, 18. http://dx.doi.org/10.1186/1479-5876-3-8.

Jackson, M., 2003. John Freeman and the origins of clinical allergy in Britain, 1903–1950. Stud. Hist. Philos. Sci. Part C 34, 473–490.

Jespers, L.S., Roberts, A., Mahler, S.M., Winter, G., Hoogenboom, H., 1994. Guiding the selection of human antibodies from phage display repertoires to a single epitope of an antigen. Nat. Biotech. 12, 899–903.

Kempeni, J., 1999. Preliminary results of early clinical trials with the fully human anti-TNFα monoclonal antibody D2E7. Ann. Rheum. Dis. 58 (Suppl. I), 170–172.

Knight, D.M., Trinh, H., Le, J., Siegel, S., Shealy, D., McDonough, M., Scallon, B., Moore, M.A., Vilcek, J., Daddona, P., Ghrayab, J., 1993. Construction and initial characterization of a mouse-human chimeric anti-TNF antibody. Mol. Immunol. 30, 1443–1453.

Levine, P., 1943. Serological factors as possible causes of spontaneous abortion. J. Hered. 34, 71–80.

Levine, P., Stetson, P.E., 1939. An unusual case of intra-group agglutination. J. Amer. Med. Assoc. 113, 126–127.

Liao, Z., Grimshaw, R.S., Rosenstreich, D.L., 1984. Identification of a specific interleukin 1 inhibitor in the urine of febrile patients. J. Exp. Med. 159, 126–136.

Loetscher, H., Pan, Y.-C.E., Lahm, H.-W., Gentz, R., Brockhaus, M., Tabuchi, H., Lesslauer, W., 1990. Molecular cloning and expression of the human 55kd tumor necrosis factor receptor. Cell 61, 351–359.

Lu, W., Arraes, L.C., Ferreira, W.T., Andrieu, J.-M., 2004. Therapeutic dendritic-cell vaccine for chronic HIV-1 infection. Nat. Med 10, 1359–1368.

Malech, H.L., Maples, P.B., Whiting-Theobald, N., Linton, G.F., Sekhsaria, S., Vowells, S.J., Li, F., Miller, J.A., DeCarlo, E., Holland, S.M., Leitman, S.F., Carter, C.S., Butz, R.E., Read, E.J., Fleisher, T.A., Schneiderman, R.D., Van Epps, D.E., Spratt, S.K., Maack, C.A., Rokovich, J.A., Cohen, L.K., Gallin, J.I., 1997. Prolonged production of NADPH oxidase-corrected granulocytes after gene therapy of chronic granulomatous disease. Proc. Natl. Acad. Sci. U.S.A 94, 12133–12138.

McCafferty, J., Griffiths, A., Winter, G., Chiswell, D., 1990. Phage antibodies: filamentous phage displaying antibody variable domains. Nat. 348, 552–554.

Mohler, K.M., Torrance, D.S., Smith, C.A., Goodwin, R.G., Stremler, K.E., Fung, V.P., Madani, H., Widmer, M.B., 1993. Soluble tumor necrosis factor (TNF) receptors are effective therapeutic agents in lethal endotoxemia and function simultaneously as both TNF carriers and TNF antagonists. J. Immunol. 151, 1548–1561.

Peggs, K.S., Quezada, S.A., Korman, H.J., Allison, J.P., 2006. Principles and use of anti-CTLA4 antibody in human cancer immunotherapy. Curr. Opin. Immunol. 18, 206–213.

Peppel, K., Crawford, D., Beutler, B., 1990. A tumor necrosis factor (TNF) receptor-IgG heavy chain chimeric protein as a bivalent antagonist of TNF activity. J. Exp. Med. 174, 1483–1489.

Pollack, W., Gorman, J.G., Freda, V.J., Ascari, W.Q., Allen, A.E., Baker, W.J., 1968. Results of clinical trials of RhoGAM in women. Transfusion 8, 151–153.

Scala, G., Kuang, Y.D., Hall, R.E., Muchmore, A.V., Oppenheim, J.J., 1984. Accessory cell function of human B cells. I. Production of both interleukin 1-like activity and an interleukin 1 inhibitory factor by an EBV-transformed human B cell line. J. Exp. Med. 159, 1637–1652.

Schall, T.J., Lewis, M., Koller, K.J., Lee, A., Rice, G.C., Wong, G.H.W., Gatanaga, T., Granger, G.A., Lentz, R., Raab, H., Kohr, W.J., Goeddel, D.V., 1990. Molecular cloning and expression of a receptor for human tumor necrosis factor. Cell 61, 361–370.

Spangrude, G.J., Heimfeld, S., Weissman, I.L., 1988. Purification and characterization of mouse hematopoietic stem cells. Science 241, 58–62.

Thomas, E.D., Lochte, H.L., Lu, W.S., Ferrebee, J.W., 1957. Intravenous infusion of bone marrow in patients receiving radiation and chemotherapy. N. Eng. J. Med. 257, 491–496.

von Behring, E.A., 1891. Untersuchungen über das Zustandekommen der Diphtherie-immunität bei Thieren. Dtsch. Med. Wochenschr. 50, 1145–1148.

von Behring, E.A., Kitasato, S., 1890. Über das Zustandekommen der Diphtheria-immunität und der Tetanus-immunität bei Thieren. Dtsch. Med. Wochenschr. 49, 1113–1114.

TIME LINE

1796   Edward Jenner introduces smallpox vaccine to Western medicine

1890   Emil von Behring and Shibasaburo Kitasato develop serotherapy for treatment of patients infected with diphtheria

1943   Phillip Levine reports that antibody production to the Rh antigen occurs more readily if mother and father share ABO blood types

1943   W.H. Wilkins and G.C.M. Harris identify a bacteriostatic substance in culture fluids from *Penicillium brevicompactum*

1946   Howard Florey and Margaret Jennings identify mycophenolic acid as an antibiotic and immunosuppressant

1952   Ogden C. Bruton infuses pooled immunoglobulin into a patient with agammaglobulinemia

1957   E. Donnall Thomas and colleagues perform the first human bone marrow transplantation

1961   Ronald Finn and coworkers demonstrate that antibody to the Rh antigen inhibits production of additional antibody to Rh

1964   Vincent Freda and colleagues inhibit production of antibody to Rh antigen by injecting antibody up to 72 h after antigen

1968   FDA licenses RhoGAM for use following Rh-incompatible pregnancies

1968   Richard Hong and colleagues reconstitute a patient with Swiss-type agammaglobulinemia with fetal thymus

1968   Humphrey Kay and coworkers transplant fetal thymus in patients with DiGeorge syndrome

1975   Lloyd Old and colleagues identify TNF as a potent inflammatory cytokine

1975   Georges Köhler and César Milstein describe a technique for producing hybridomas that secrete monoclonal antibodies

1980   The World Health Organization declares smallpox eradicated from the world

1981   FDA approves a vaccine for hepatitis B virus—the first cancer vaccine

1984   Zenghua Liao and coworkers and Giuseppe Scala and colleagues describe IL-1 receptor antagonist, a naturally occurring inhibitor of IL-1 (anakinra)

1986   FDA approves the use of a monoclonal antibody specific for CD3 for recipients of solid organ transplants

1990   R. Michael Blaese, W. French Anderson, and coworkers perform the first gene therapy on a patient with severe combined immunodeficiency

1991   Bruce Beutler and coworkers design a soluble TNF receptor that inhibits inflammation (etanercept)

1992   Irving Weissman and colleagues identify CD34 as a marker for human hematopoietic stem cells

1993   David Knight and colleagues develop a mouse–human chimeric monoclonal antibody against TNF-α (infliximab)

1994   Laurent Jespers and coworkers use phage display to select a fully human monoclonal antibody to TNF-α (adalimumab)

1995   FDA approves mycophenolate mofetil for use in renal transplant patients

1996   Frank Hsu and collaborators use dendritic cells (DCs) to treat patients with non-Hodgkin lymphoma

1997   A group led by Harry Malech uses genetically modified autologous stem cells to treat patients with chronic granulomatous disease

2002   FDA approves adalimumab, a human monoclonal antibody specific for TNF-α for treatment of patients with rheumatoid arthritis

2004   Wei Lu and colleagues develop a DC-based vaccine for chronic HIV infection

2006   FDA approves a vaccine against the human papilloma virus

2010   FDA approves sipuleucel-T, a T-lymphocyte vaccine for patients with metastatic prostate cancer

2011   FDA approves ipilimumab, a monoclonal antibody specific for CTLA-4 for use in patients with late-stage melanoma

2013   A group led by Alessandro Aiuti uses genetically modified autologous stem cells to treat patients with Wiskott–Aldrich syndrome

Techniques to Detect and Quantify Host Defenses

INTRODUCTION

Patients presenting with fever, difficulty breathing, joint pain, skin rashes, and sweet-tasting urine have puzzled clinicians for centuries. While these and other signs and symptoms point to a variety of possible underlying etiologies, each of these presentations may herald an immunological disorder. Over the past 150 years, physicians and scientists developed diagnostic techniques that identified the immunological mechanisms responsible for these pathologies with an eventual goal of providing therapeutic interventions.

Exposure of mammals to foreign antigen triggers cell proliferation and gene transcription leading to protein synthesis. Some of these proteins are secreted while others are expressed on cell surfaces. Secreted proteins include antibodies produced by B lymphocytes and cytokines and chemokines synthesized by a variety of cells including B and T lymphocytes. Proteins expressed on cells include receptors for cytokines and chemokines as well as molecules responsible for activating and regulating the immune response. As activated cells mature, unique functional populations emerge. Techniques to detect and quantitate proliferation, gene transcription, and protein synthesis defined immunology as a separate discipline.

Immunologists first developed in vivo techniques to visualize responses to antigens including skin tests. Subsequent studies led researchers to devise tests to detect correlates of these reactions. Some of these methods employ experimental animals while others use in vitro methodology. Over the past 100 years the techniques used to investigate the immune system have evolved from semiquantitative measures to highly analytic processes employing the most up-to-date genetic and molecular biology assays. Many of these techniques are used clinically to diagnose patients presenting with a variety of symptoms including fever,

A Historical Perspective on Evidence-Based Immunology
http://dx.doi.org/10.1016/B978-0-12-398381-7.00039-3

difficulty breathing, joint pain, skin rashes, and sweet-tasting urine. This chapter reviews the history of technique development including

- quantitation of the cells involved in both innate host defenses and adaptive immune responses,
- functional studies of lymphocytes in vitro,
- development of skin tests as an in vivo model of systemic responses,
- detection and quantitation of antibody, and
- quantitative assays using immunologic principles.

THE CELLS OF HOST DEFENSE MECHANISMS

Host defenses depend on the activation of cells found in various anatomical compartments including connective tissue, peripheral lymphoid organs, and blood. Anton van Leeuwenhoek, born Thonis Phillipszoon (1632–1723), worked as a linen draper in Amsterdam where he encountered an early microscope originally described in the 1590s by Hans and Zacharias Jansen (http://www.history-of-the-microscope.org/). In the 1660s he improved this microscope and used it to discover many objects too small to be observed by the naked eye. One of his most celebrated discoveries was of small "animalcules" (bacteria). For this he has been credited as the father of microbiology. In 1675 van Leeuwenhoek discovered red blood cells in humans and several other species. He observed that red blood cells formed sediments upon sitting and lysed when exposed to water (http://www.vanleeuwenhoek.com/#hisdiscoveries).

In 1845 Rudolph Virchow (1821–1902) in Berlin, Germany, and John Hughes Bennett (1812–1875) in Edinburgh, Scotland, independently described the peripheral blood cells of patients with leukemia; this represented the initial characterization of white blood cells including lymphocytes. Likewise in the 1840s

Gabriel Andral in France and William Addison in England reported the presence of white cells in peripheral blood. In the 1870s Paul Ehrlich, during his training at the University of Strasbourg, employed staining techniques to differentiate neutrophils, basophils, and eosinophils (reviewed in Pearson, 2002; Hajdu, 2003).

Virchow popularized the cell theory of disease and differentiated pathologies through correlation with changes in the number of cells in the peripheral blood. Specifically he noted that leukemia patients had an excess of white cells. Quantification of these cells required development of a new instrument.

Louis-Charles Malassez (1842–1909) studied medicine in Paris, eventually assuming the position of head of anatomy at the College of France in 1875. In the 1870s he developed a blood counting chamber that has evolved into the hemacytometer (Verso, 1971). The basic design of this apparatus is a thick microscope slide with an indentation containing a grid of perpendicular lines (Figure 39.1). A coverslip placed over this indentation results in an area of known volume. A dilute cell preparation introduced into this area results in a distribution of these cells across the grid. The number of cells in a portion of the grid is counted. From this count, the concentration of cells in the original sample can be calculated. While quantification of cells of the peripheral blood is now achieved using electronic technology, evaluation of cells in cerebrospinal fluid, analysis of semen, and quantification of bacteria in body fluids such as urine continues to rely on the hemacytometer.

Automation of cell counting depended on the development of the Coulter counter in the late 1940s. Wallace H. Coulter (1913–1998), educated as an electrical engineer at Westminster College and the Georgia Institute of Technology, was contracted by the United States Department of Defense to determine the number of particles in paint used for battleships. During these studies he discovered the Coulter principle. This principle, which Coulter patented in 1953, is based on the deflection of

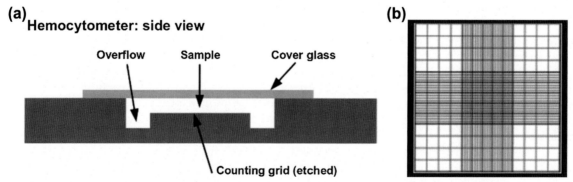

FIGURE 39.1   (a) Side view of a hemocytometer demonstrating the formation of the counting chamber between the counting grid and coverslip. Cells suspended in liquid medium are introduced into the chamber to determine cell number. (http://www.microbehunter.com/the-hemocytometer-counting-chamber/). (b) The counting grid of a hemocytometer that is etched on the chamber. By counting cells in various squares the technician can calculate the concentration of cells in the original sample. (http://www.microbehunter.com/the-hemocytometer-counting-chamber/).

an electrical current by microscopic particles suspended in a liquid traversing a small opening. In 1954 Coulter incorporated this principle into an instrument to detect and count cells of the blood as well as for quality control of various other liquids including paint, chocolate, and beer (Simson, 2013). The Coulter counter is used in hematology laboratories to quantify cells of the peripheral blood.

Subsequent improvements led to instruments able to sort cells using several physical properties. In 1965 Mack J. Fulwyler (1936–2001) working at the Los Alamos Scientific Laboratory in New Mexico developed an electronic particle separator, "a device capable of separating biological cells (in a conducting medium) according to volume." This device incorporated a Coulter counter to measure cell volume. Cells isolated in droplets of tissue culture medium were differentially charged based on volume. Fulwyler recognized the relevance of this electronic particle separator to biology. He separated a mixture of mouse and human red blood cells and fractionated mouse lymphoma cells to obtain those with different cell volumes (size).

In 1972 a group led by Leonard Herzenberg working at Stanford University in Palo Alto, California developed a flow cytometer that detected and separated cells based on their size and granularity (Bonner et al., 1972).

Suspensions of single cells from peripheral blood or lymphoid organs are forced, in a liquid stream, past an electronic detection device permitting physical and chemical characterization. The cells trigger an electric signal, and the stream is broken into droplets optimally containing a single cell. The droplets pass between two charged plates and are deflected according to their associated electric signal. In this way the droplets can be separated and collected. Flow cytometers are widely used in clinical and experimental laboratories to count cells and sort them into discrete populations. While contemporary instruments are increasingly more sophisticated than the original device, the basic principles of cell sorting remain the same.

The Herzenberg laboratory led by Leonard and Leonore Herzenberg refined the methodology and developed the fluorescence-activated cell sorter (FACS). Cells are stained with fluorescent dyes bound to reagents that detect cell surface molecules including CD markers and antigen receptors and analyzed by FACS. Cells are forced in a liquid stream past lasers of various wavelengths that detect fluorescence and separate them into droplets containing individual cells. The FACS was commercialized by several companies including Becton–Dickinson. Due to the large amount of data generated using this technology, computers and programs to analyze the results are critical additions to the instrument. Numerous investigators combine FACS analysis using monoclonal antibodies (developed by Köhler and

Milstein—Chapter 37) with functional assays to describe both healthy host defense mechanisms and aberrations that occur when the immune system becomes pathologic.

FUNCTIONAL STUDIES OF LYMPHOCYTES

Foreign antigen activates lymphocytes triggering cell division, gene transcription, and synthesis and secretion of proteins. Investigators devised techniques to study these phenomena in vitro. This section describes the development of three methods:

- lymphocyte proliferation,
- antibody production by individual lymphocytes, and
- lymphocyte-mediated cytotoxicity.

Lymphocyte Proliferation

James Murphy working at the Rockefeller Institute in New York described antigen-induced lymphocyte proliferation in the 1920s. James Gowans at Oxford University in England confirmed this observation when he studied the disappearing lymphocyte phenomenon (Chapter 4). Initially, immunologists measured proliferation by determining increases in the weight of lymphoid organs or by observing histological sections of lymphoid tissue and counting the number of mitotic figures. By the late 1950s, investigators developed more quantitative methods to detect lymphocyte proliferation using radiolabeled precursors of DNA.

In 1958 Walter L. Hughes and colleagues at the Brookhaven National Laboratory in New York injected mice with tritiated thymidine (^{3}H-TdR) and removed various organs 7–48h later. Autoradiography revealed DNA labeling in cells lining the gastrointestinal tract and in the spleen. Since the base thymidine is incorporated into DNA but not into RNA, investigators concluded that labeled cells were proliferating.

Peter C. Nowell working at the University of Pennsylvania in Philadelphia initially described the mitogenic effects of phytohemagglutinin (PHA) on human lymphocytes in 1960. He investigated possible factors responsible for inducing mitosis in unstimulated cultures of peripheral blood leukocytes from leukemic and control individuals. Factors that failed to alter the baseline mitotic activity included temperature, pH, oxygen or carbon dioxide tension, plasma or cell concentration, or agitation. At that time, Nowell (and other investigators) used the plant lectin, PHA, to agglutinate erythrocytes thus enhancing recovery of leukocytes from heparinized blood. When Nowell isolated leukocytes from erythrocytes using other techniques, no mitosis was observed. Addition of PHA to leukocyte cultures obtained without the use of PHA induced mitosis primarily of monocytes and large lymphocytes. Following three days in vitro, Nowell counted the number of mitotic figures. Comparison with parallel cultures devoid of PHA confirmed that this lectin is mitogenic for human lymphocytes. Subsequent investigators modified this assay by adding ^{3}H-TdR to the culture to simplify detection of proliferating cells. In addition, researchers described other plant lectins with mitogenic properties for human lymphocytes including concanavalin A and pokeweed mitogen.

Within a few years of Nowell's observation, two groups of investigators demonstrated that lymphocytes from antigen-sensitized humans proliferated in vitro to the sensitizing antigen. In 1963 Robert Schrek working at Loyola University, Chicago, Illinois, and G. Pearmain and colleagues in New Zealand demonstrated that peripheral blood leukocytes from patients with a positive tuberculin skin test proliferate in culture to purified protein derivative.

One year later in 1964 Barbara Bain and colleagues at McGill University in Montreal, Canada, mixed peripheral blood leukocytes in vitro from two unrelated individuals and observed some of these cells transform into large basophilic blasts that synthesize DNA and undergo mitosis. Simultaneously, in 1964, Fritz Bach and Kurt Hirschhorn working at New York University showed that lymphocytes from two animals cultured together transform to blast cells and proliferate. Both groups of investigators speculated that this reaction may be related to genetic differences responsible for graft rejection. Today, this assay, termed the mixed lymphocyte reaction, remains a standard test to detect differences in expression of histocompatibility antigens between transplant donors and recipients.

Antibody Production by Individual Lymphocytes

The hemolytic plaque assay (Jerne and Nordin, 1963) detects antibody formation by single lymphocytes. This assay quantifies the number of lymphocytes secreting antibodies to a particular antigen and permits visualization of the antibody-forming cell's morphology. The basic methodology for this technique is covered in Chapter 13.

In 1983 two groups, Jonathon Sedgwick and Patrick Holt working at the Princess Margaret Hospital and the University of Western Australia in Perth, and Cecil Czerkinsky and colleagues at the University of Gothenburg, Sweden, described a second method, the enzyme-linked immunospot (ELISPOT), to detect specific antibody-forming lymphocytes. Both groups harvested spleen cells from immunized mice and incubated them on polystyrene plates that were coated with antigen. Antibody secreted during this incubation bound to the antigen. Once the investigators removed the spleen cells, the antibody was subsequently detected by adding an enzyme-conjugated second antibody specific for IgG. Addition of a substrate that changed color when enzymatically cleaved demonstrates the location of the antigen antibody reaction.

Lymphocyte-Mediated Cytotoxicity

Cytotoxicity by CD8$^+$ T lymphocytes and by natural killer (NK) lymphocytes is most often measured using a ^{51}Cr release assay. This assay derived from methods devised to detect antibody-mediated cytotoxicity against mouse lymphocytes.

In 1964, Arnold Sanderson working at the Microbiological Research Establishment in Wiltshire, England, injected BALB/c mice with lymphocytes from C3H animals. This induced an antibody specific for histocompatibility antigens expressed on C3H cells. He incubated this antibody along with guinea pig complement with C3H lymphocytes labeled with ^{51}Cr and demonstrated release of the radiolabel that he interpreted as indicative of cell lysis.

In 1968 K. Theodor Brunner and colleagues working at the Swiss Institute for Experimental Cancer Research and the University of Lausanne, Switzerland, developed a quantitative assay to measure the cytotoxic activity of sensitized lymphoid cells. These investigators injected DBA/2 mastocytoma cells into C57Bl mice and harvested spleens from the injected mice 9–12 days later. They incubated isolated spleen cells with mastocytoma cells labeled with ^{51}Cr. Incubation of splenic lymphocytes with mastocytoma cells at a ratio of 100 to 1 resulted in the release of up to 90% of the label within 6–9 h. By contrast Brunner and coworkers report while spontaneous release of ^{51}Cr from the mastocytoma cells reached 25% in 24 h, "no lytic effect of normal allogeneic lymphoid cells was noted in any of the experiments" and they conclude that "spleen cells of mice sensitized by a tumor allograft destroy donor target cells in vitro, as indicated by specific ^{51}Cr release."

SKIN TESTS

Foreign antigens injected intradermally or subcutaneously into patients with certain pathologies induce skin reactions that can be used diagnostically. Some responses are observed shortly after the injection of antigen reaching maximum intensity in a few hours in which case they are called immediate hypersensitivity reactions. Other responses require one or more days to develop and are termed delayed hypersensitivity reactions. Immunologists now agree that the immediate skin reactions result from the presence of antibody to the injected antigen while delayed reactions signal the activity of sensitized T lymphocytes.

Immediate Skin Reactions

Immediate skin reactions most commonly diagnose patients presenting with suspected allergies, particularly allergic rhinitis, allergic asthma, food and drug allergies, or stinging insect hypersensitivity. Allergists apply dilute preparations of suspected allergens to the skin and observe the site 15–30 min later. Appearance of a wheal and flare at the site suggests the presence of IgE antibodies to the allergen and is considered positive (Chapter 33).

Other examples of immediate skin tests include assays to determine if an individual had produced antibodies specific for an infectious bacteria or its toxin (the Dick test and the Schick test) and assays to investigate mechanisms of disease (the Arthus reaction and the Prausnitz–Kütsner reaction).

Bela Schick, working at the University of Vienna, Austria, developed the Schick test in 1913 to determine if an individual possessed adequate antibodies to diphtheria toxin to be protected against the disease. He injected patients intradermally with a dilute preparation of diphtheria toxin and observed the injection site. If the injection site became red and swollen, the individual did not have antibodies to the toxin. Alternatively if the person possessed sufficient antibodies, the injection failed to trigger a reaction. Clinicians employed this test to screen populations of individuals until the development of a diphtheria vaccine in the 1920s.

In 1924 George F. Dick and Gladys H. Dick working at the John McCormick Institute for Infectious Diseases in Chicago developed the Dick test to detect susceptibility to scarlet fever. They injected a filtrate of a culture of *Streptococcus* into the skin of three groups of patients:

- those who had a history of scarlet fever,
- those who were convalescing, or
- uninfected controls.

Individuals with no previous history developed erythema at the injection site in 4–6 h reaching a maximum diameter at 18–36 h. Individuals with a history of scarlet fever including those convalescing from the disease failed to show a skin reaction.

To study the mechanism of this reaction, the investigators mixed serum from patients who were recovering from scarlet fever with the *Streptococcus* filtrate and injected this mixture into several uninfected controls. This mixture failed to induce a skin reaction leading the investigators to conclude that the lack of a skin reaction in infected and convalescing individuals is due to a serum factor specific for the *Streptococcus*; immunologists today agree that the serum factor is specific antibody.

The Arthus reaction is an experimental model to investigate the mechanism responsible for immune complex-mediated pathology such as serum sickness or systemic lupus erythematosus. In 1903 Nicholas Maurice Arthus,

working at the Pasteur Institute in Lille, France, repeatedly injected rabbits subcutaneously with horse serum. Following four injections, Arthus noted edema at the injection site. Additional injections resulted in gangrene at the injection site. By contrast, multiple injections of horse serum intravenously led to an anaphylactic reaction. Immunologists now agree that the skin reaction results from the formation of antigen–antibody complexes that induce an inflammatory response (Chapter 33).

In 1921 Otto Prausnitz (1876–1963) and Heinz Küstner (1897–1963) working at the Hygiene Institute of the University of Breslau in Germany reported the transfer of skin hypersensitivity from an allergic to a healthy individual. They collected serum from Küstner, who was allergic to fish, and injected it subcutaneously into Prausnitz. Twenty-four hours later they applied a fish extract locally to Prausnitz' skin and observed an immediate skin reaction characterized by the appearance of a wheal and flare. This Prausnitz–Küstner (P–K) reaction proved useful to demonstrate the pathophysiology of immediate hypersensitivity to various antigens in humans. In fact Kimishige Ishizaka and his coworkers working at the University of Colorado Medical School in Denver employed the P–K reaction in the mid-1960s to identify the antibody isotype responsible for allergy to ragweed pollen (Chapter 33) (Ishizaka et al., 1967).

Delayed Skin Reactions

Delayed skin reactions appear 24–72 h following intradermal injection of antigen. A positive response indicates a T lymphocyte reaction. The classic example is the tuberculin reaction, which has several eponyms including the Mendel–Mantoux test or the Mantoux test. Robert Koch working in Berlin, Germany, isolated *Mycobacterium tuberculosis* and demonstrated it as the causative agent of tuberculosis in the 1880s. By 1890 he isolated a substance, tuberculin, that he touted as a cure for the disease. Rudolph Virchow presented his own findings in 1891 indicating that tuberculin was not a cure for the disease and in fact exacerbated tuberculosis in patients with advanced disease (Sharrer, 2007).

Tuberculin has subsequently assumed an important place in the evaluation of patients infected with *M. tuberculosis*. Koch noted that injection of tuberculin into the skin of individuals who had previously had tuberculosis produced erythema and induration in about 48 h. He did not pursue this finding further; however, several other investigators did. Clemens von Pirquet in Vienna, Austria, reported in 1907 that the application of a drop of tuberculin into a scratch on the skin produced a reaction in those patients who had previously been infected with tuberculosis and distinguished them from those who had not been exposed (Dworetzky and Cohen, 2002; Sharrer, 2007).

In 1908 Felix Mendel in Germany reported similar results when he injected tuberculin into the skin. This technique was improved by Charles Mantoux working in Cannes, France, in 1908. Mantoux injected patients with tuberculin intradermally and observed the resulting erythema and induration 48–72h later. Results obtained from subcutaneous or intradermal injections were more consistent and reproducible than instilling the tuberculin into a scratch, and the Mendel–Mantoux test became the gold standard for identification of individuals who had been exposed to tuberculosis.

MEASUREMENT OF ANTIBODIES

In the nineteenth century, researchers injected animals with antigen, harvested their blood, and detected antibodies by bacterial neutralization, red blood cell agglutination, protein precipitation, or complement activation. Investigators indicated the relative strength of a given antibody by assigning an arbitrary scale often indicated by plus (+) or minus (−) signs thereby providing an estimate of antibody quantity to compare different experimental protocols.

Development of semiquantitative assays to compare the concentration of antibody in individual experimental animals led to the concept of antibody titer. Titer, defined as "the strength of a solution or concentration of a substance as determined by titration" (http://www.merriam-webster.com/dictionary/titer), was first used in the mid-1880s to refer to the concentration of silver or gold in a coin.

Scientists determine an antibody titer by serially diluting serum or some other body fluid thought to contain antibody in physiological saline. These dilutions provide a series of samples containing diminishing concentrations of antibody. Investigators then add a predetermined amount of antigen to each antibody dilution, incubate the mixture using conditions known to produce an antigen–antibody reaction (agglutination, precipitation, lysis, etc.), and record the tubes at various time intervals. The tube with the highest dilution of serum in which an antigen–antibody reaction is visible is considered the end point, and the reciprocal of the dilution is reported as the titer of the antibody in the original serum (i.e., if antibody activity is detected in a tube containing serum diluted 1:16 but is not detected in serum diluted 1:32, the titer is recorded as 16).

In 1915 Simon Flexner and Harold Amoss working at the Rockefeller Institute of Medical Research in New York published one of the first recorded uses of serial dilution of antibody in a study of horse antibodies specific for bacilli responsible for dysentery. Flexner and Amoss injected horses three times with *Shigella dysenteriae* or its toxin to prepare antibodies for serotherapy

of patients infected with the bacteria. They evaluated these antibodies in two different protocols and correlated the results:

- horse antibodies were mixed with bacteria or toxin and injected into guinea pigs to determine protection against infection and
- serial dilutions of horse antibodies were mixed with bacteria and agglutination titers recorded.

Flexner and Amoss demonstrated that horse sera containing antibodies with higher agglutination titers provided enhanced protection against infection.

A serum titer is a semiquantitative measure of the antibody present in the original serum sample. Several factors affect the titer including the affinity of the antibody for antigen, the concentration of antigen included in each of the tubes, and the method used to visualize the results. Despite this, antibody titers are reported in many clinical situations including the results of assays to detect autoantibodies in patients with autoimmune disease and antibodies in individuals with viral infections.

Agglutination of Red Blood Cells (Hemagglutination)

Adolf Creite, a medical student in Göttingen, Germany, in 1869, injected rabbits intravenously with serum from several animals (sheep, cat, chicken, duck, or goat). The injected rabbits developed hematuria (blood in the urine), malaise, and, occasionally, died (Hughes-Jones and Gardner, 2002). Creite observed this phenomenon prior to the initial description of antibody by von Fodor, Nuttall, and von Buchner in the late 1880s. Although Creite failed to comprehend the underlying mechanism for this observation, he speculated that the serum contained some substance that caused the red blood cells to lyse. Subsequently, Creite performed an in vitro experiment in which he added serum from the various animals to a drop of rabbit blood and noted that under the microscope "the cells suddenly flow together in peculiar way forming different shaped, drop-like clusters with irregular branches."

In 1875 Leonard Landois, the director of the Physiological Institute at the University of Greifswald, Germany, reported similar results. Landois transfused animals with blood from different species. He observed that many such transfusions resulted in the lysis of red cells. To determine the source of the lysed erythrocytes he mixed blood from one animal species (i.e., cat) with serum from a second species (dog). In most cases the added red cells lysed; however, when high concentrations of erythrocytes were added, clumping occurred rather than lysis. Landois postulated that a substance existed in the serum that made the membranes of the red cells soft and sticky.

In the 1880s several investigators identified an inducible serum substance immunologists now call antibody (Chapter 2). In 1901 Karl Landsteiner reported the existence of naturally occurring antibodies in the serum of some humans that caused agglutination of erythrocytes from other individuals. Landsteiner received his MD in 1891 from the University of Vienna and pursued a research career at several institutions in Vienna, Holland, and the Rockefeller Institute in New York.

While at the Pathological Anatomy Institute in Vienna, Austria, Landsteiner developed techniques to detect serological differences between individuals. In 1901, Landsteiner mixed serum from one group of humans with red blood cells from a second group of individuals and observed the reaction. As he noted in his Nobel address (1930), "With many samples there was no perceptible alteration, in other words the result was exactly the same as if the blood cells had been mixed with their own serum, but frequently a phenomenon known as agglutination—in which the serum causes the cells of the alien individual to group into clusters—occurred." These observations led to the discovery of the ABO blood groups and the successful development of compatible blood transfusion.

Bacterial Agglutination

In 1889 Albert Charrin and Georges-Henri Roger in France injected rabbits with heated and filtered cultures of *Pseudomonas aeruginosa*. These injections protected the rabbits from subsequent infection with *Pseudomonas*. Blood from these rabbits clumped or aggregated bacteria and rendered them immotile (http://www.microbelibrary.org/library/laboratory-test/3659-bacterial-agglutination).

In 1896 Herbert Edward Durham (1866–1945), working at Guy's Hospital, London, differentiated bacterial species using specific antibodies in an in vitro assay. Durham injected animals with either *Vibrio cholerae*, *Bacillus coli communis* (*Escherichia coli*), or *Bacillus pyocyaneus* (*P. aeruginosa*). Serum removed from these animals and mixed with the bacteria caused specific clumping of the bacteria, loss of motility, and inhibition of growth.

Georges-Fernand-Isidor Widal (1862–1929) used bacterial agglutination to develop a diagnostic test for typhoid fever. Widal studied at the University of Paris and received his MD in 1886. In 1896 working at the Faculty of Medicine in Paris, France, he showed that addition of *Salmonella typhi* to serum from a patient with typhoid fever resulted in agglutination of the bacillus. The Widal test differentiates patients with typhoid fever from those with other diseases including typhus, tuberculosis, and pneumonia and is still used in parts of the world where typhoid fever is endemic.

Precipitation

Precipitation occurs when two soluble substances (i.e., antigen and antibody) interact to form an insoluble complex. Many chemical reactions result in the formation of a precipitate. In immunology, interaction of a soluble antigen with its antibody often produces a precipitate that can be visualized and measured. Precipitation of antigen–antibody complexes depends on the bivalency of antibody molecules and the multivalency of antigens. Binding of several antigen molecules to two or more antibodies leads to the formation of a matrix that settles out of solution.

Michael Heidelberger (1888–1991) earned a PhD in organic chemistry from Columbia University in 1911. He subsequently held positions at the Rockefeller Institute and at Columbia University in New York. In 1929 Heidelberger and Forrest Kendall working at Presbyterian Hospital and the College of Physicians and Surgeons (Columbia University) in New York performed a quantitative study of the precipitin reaction between an antigen (pneumococcal polysaccharide type III) and its specific antibody. By varying the amount of antigen and antibody in different test tubes Heidelberger and Kendall demonstrated that the reaction between antigen and antibody can be explained by postulating three zones—antigen excess, equivalence, and antibody excess (Figure 39.2). These results allowed Heidelberger and Kendall to conclude that antibodies are bivalent. Additionally, they provided a framework to understand immune complex diseases including serum sickness and poststreptococcal glomerulonephritis.

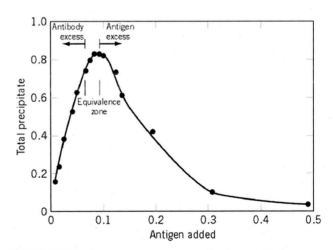

FIGURE 39.2 Precipitin curve constructed by determining the amount of precipitate produced by adding increasing amounts of antigen to a constant concentration of antibody. Three areas are identified—antibody excess, equivalence zone, and antigen excess. *From* http://what-when-how.com/molecular-biology/precipitin-reaction-molecular-biology/.

Precipitin Reactions to Detect Antigen–Antibody Interactions

Starting in the 1940s several investigators modified the precipitation phenomenon to detect antigen–antibody reactions.

- In 1946 Jacques Oudin working at the Pasteur Institute in Paris, France, layered antibody on top of a solution of soluble antigen so there was no mixing of the two. After incubation a white precipitate formed at the interface of the two layers if the top solution contained antibody specific for the antigen.
- Orjan Ouchterlony working at the State Bacteriological Laboratory in Stockholm, Sweden, in 1948 modified this procedure to observe the reaction in a semisolid gel. He prepared a thin layer of agar solution in a petri dish. By including two small cups on the petri dish when he poured the gel, two wells were present once the gel solidified. He filled one of the wells with diphtheria toxin and the second with antibody to diphtheria toxin. Following 48 h of incubation, Ouchterlony observed a white line between the two wells that he interpreted as marking the precipitation of antigen (toxin) with antibody. In 1949 Ouchterlony published additional details of this procedure and demonstrated that if he started with different concentrations of the antigen and antibody in the wells, the precipitin lines formed at different distances from the wells.
- In 1965 G. Mancini from the University of Ferrara, Italy, working with Joseph Heremans from the Catholic University of Louvain in Brussels, Belgium, described a technique to quantify immunoglobulin or other antigens by immunodiffusion. This technique, called radial immunodiffusion, relied on the migration of an antigen from a well through agar into which antibody had been incorporated. The migrating antigen established a concentration gradient. When the antigen and antibody are in optimal proportions (the equivalence zone), precipitation occurs, and a white ring appears around the antigen well. The diameter of this precipitin ring is proportional to the concentration of the antigen originally placed in the well.

Precipitation Combined with Electrophoresis

Electrophoresis provides a semiquantitative measure of the concentration of proteins in a mixture such as serum. Arne Tiselius in Sweden described electrophoresis in 1930 and used it to separate serum proteins in 1937. He demonstrated four serum components that could be separated at pH 8.6—albumin, alpha globulin, beta globulin, and gamma globulin (Chapter 11). The gamma globulin fraction contains immunoglobulins (antibodies) and fails to migrate in the electrical field. All other serum proteins migrate to the anode. Tiselius was awarded the Nobel Prize in Physiology or Medicine in 1948 "for his research on electrophoresis and adsorption analysis, especially for his discoveries concerning the complex nature of serum proteins."

Scientists use electrophoresis to detect myeloma proteins, paraproteins, and polyclonal immunoglobulins in serum as well as Bence Jones proteins in urine and oligoclonal bands in the cerebrospinal fluid of patients with multiple sclerosis.

In 1953 Pierre Graber and Curtis A. Williams working at the Pasteur Institute in Paris, France, described immunoelectrophoresis, a method that combines electrophoresis with gel diffusion. Graber and Williams separated human serum proteins by electrophoresis in an agar gel and then cut a trough in the gel parallel to the migration of the serum proteins. Antibody to serum proteins placed into this trough migrates out and forms precipitin bands where serum proteins interact with specific antibodies. Figure 39.3 depicts an immunoelectrophoresis pattern obtained when human serum is electrophoresed and reacted with antibodies to whole serum or to antibodies specific for various immunoglobulin isotypes or light chains.

Several variations on immunoelectrophoresis have been developed including

- counterelectrophoresis devised in 1959 by Alain Bussard working at the Pasteur Institute in Paris, France;
- crossed electrophoresis developed by Carl-Bertil Laurell working at Malmö General Hospital and the University of Lund, Sweden, in 1965; and
- rocket electrophoresis developed by Carl-Bertil Laurell in 1966.

These specialized techniques detect and quantify

- microbial and nonmicrobial antigens in complex mixtures,
- antibodies to these antigens, and
- serum proteins in individuals presenting with various clinical disorders.

QUANTITATIVE TECHNIQUES USING IMMUNOLOGIC PRINCIPLES

Investigators use immunologic reagents and techniques to detect and quantify other biological molecules including hormones, vitamins, and enzymes.

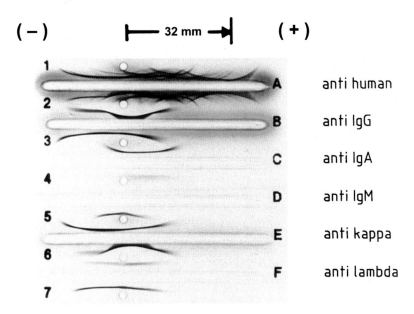

FIGURE 39.3 Photograph of immunoelectrophoresis performed in agar gel. Human serum is first separated by electrophoresis following which troughs are cut in the agar, and antibodies to whole serum, isolated isotypes, or light chains are added. *From* http://dxline.info/diseases /immunoelectrophoresis-serum.

These procedures are based on interactions between the molecules and antibodies and provide highly specific and sensitive assays. Three of these techniques that have advanced both immunology and other disciplines are

- radioimmunoassay,
- enzyme-linked immunosorbent assay (ELISA), and
- nephelometry.

Radioimmunoassay

In 1960 Rosalyn Yalow and Solomon Berson working at the Bronx Veteran's Administration Hospital in New York developed radioimmunoassay, a technique that allows detection and quantitation of minute quantities of substances in human blood and other aqueous samples. Yallow (1921–2011) earned her PhD in physics in 1945 from the University of Illinois, Champaign–Urbana. She taught at Hunter College from 1945 to 1950 and joined the Bronx Veteran's Affairs (VA) Hospital in 1947 to establish the radioisotope service. Solomon Berson (1918–1972) received his MD from New York University in 1945 and joined the radioisotope service at the VA in 1950.

In the 1950s, Yallow and Berson used radioisotopes to determine blood volume, clinically diagnose thyroid disease, and study the kinetics of iodine metabolism in patients injected with animal insulin (http://www.nobel prize.org/nobel_prizes/medicine/laureates/1977/yalow-bio.html). The results of this last study demonstrated that patients injected with animal insulin developed antibodies. This observation led to the development of an assay to measure the concentration of insulin in human blood. The assay involves competition for antibody binding between a known quantity of a radiolabeled substance (i.e., insulin) and an unknown quantity of the same substance in human blood. By establishing concentration curves with known quantities of the unlabeled reagent, Yallow and Berson determined the concentration of insulin. This technique was widely used to detect and measure hormones, vitamins, and enzymes.

The Nobel Committee recognized the development of radioimmunoassay when they awarded the Nobel Prize for Physiology or Medicine to Rosalyn Yalow in 1977 "for the development of radioimmunoassays of peptide hormones." She shared the prize with Roger Guillemin and Andrew Schally "for their discoveries concerning the peptide hormone production of the brain." Solomon Berson died in 1972 and hence was not eligible for the prize awarded in 1977.

Enzyme-Linked Immunosorbent Assay

Radioimmunoassays provided a major advance in identifying and quantifying antigens and antibodies in complex mixtures. However, the use of radioisotopes involved risks that impeded wider application of the technique. In 1971 two groups independently developed an assay to measure antibodies or antigens using an enzyme as the indicator rather than a radioisotope. Bauke van Weemen and Anton Schuurs working in the Netherlands developed a competitive assay to measure the hormone, human chorionic gonadotropin (HCG), in human serum or urine. Eva Engvall and Peter Perlman, working in Sweden, developed a similar assay to measure human IgG.

ELISAs are competitive assays that measure either antigen or antibody concentrations. In one variety antibody specific for the antigen (i.e., HCG) is bound to a plastic surface. A mixture of purified HCG conjugated with an enzyme (i.e., horseradish peroxidase-HRP) and blood or urine containing an unknown amount of HCG is added to the well. The HCG in the two samples competes to bind the antibody; unbound HCG is washed from the reaction. A substrate that changes color when enzymatically cleaved by HRP (i.e., 3,3',5,5'-tetramethylbenzidine) is added to the mixture, and the color change is measured using a spectrophotometer. If the blood or urine contains HCG, it will compete with the enzyme-linked HCG for binding to the antibody, and the amount of color change will be decreased proportionally.

Nephelometry

Nephelometry, a method to detect the concentration of serum proteins including immunoglobulin, is based on the concept that particles in solution will scatter light passing through the solution rather than absorbing the light. Nephelometers record the degree of scatter, and scientists correlate this with the quantity of protein in the solution. The principle of this technique was developed in the early 1900s (Kober and Graves, 1915); however, application to immunology and the clinical laboratory only occurred in the 1970s.

In 1971 L.M. Killingsworth and John Savory working at the University of Florida in Gainesville described a method for the detection and quantitation of immunoglobulin isotypes in human serum. They diluted human serum with saline and mixed these dilutions with antibody specific for IgG, IgA, or IgM. The turbidity of these mixtures was measured in a nephelometer, an instrument that measures the scatter of light from a laser passing through the solution. Known quantities of the immunoglobulin being measured are mixed with the antibody to develop a standard curve from which the concentration of the protein in the unknown sample can be deduced.

Nephelometry is the method of choice in the clinical laboratory to measure the concentration of immunoglobulin isotypes (IgG, IgA, IgM, and IgE) as well as other serum proteins including hemoglobin, C-reactive protein, albumin, haptoglobin, and others. Polyclonal increases in immunoglobulin concentrations are associated with infections, autoimmune diseases, and chronic inflammation, while monoclonal increases suggest multiple myeloma or Waldenström macroglobulinemia. Decreased concentrations may signal immunosuppression, kidney failure, or protein losing enteropathies.

CONCLUSION

Detection and quantitation of the immune response requires several different assay systems that have increased in sophistication during the history of the discipline. Researchers and clinicians have developed a large number of assays to evaluate the immune response both clinically and in experimental settings. These proceeded along several independent paths of investigation:

- In the eighteenth and nineteenth centuries, investigators identified the cells of the peripheral blood that are involved in protecting vertebrates against infections. Shortly thereafter methods to characterize and quantify these cells became available and evolved from microscopic evaluation to automated methods of counting and sorting these cells.
- Several investigators described antibody in the late 1800s that they detected based on unique functions including neutralization, agglutination, and precipitation. Subsequent investigators devised methods to quantify immunoglobulin and antibody in serum and in individual lymphocytes.
- Technical advances in other biological fields (i.e., electrophoresis and electron microscopy; radioisotopes and enzymes to detect and trace cells, antigens, and antibodies; gene manipulation) are incorporated into contemporary techniques that increase knowledge of the adaptive immune response. Development of new technology will allow immunologists to address the questions that remain unresolved (Chapter 40).

References

Arthus, N.M., 1903. Injections répétées de serum du cheval chez le lapin. C. R. Séances Soc. Biol. Filiales 55, 817–820.

Bach, F., Hirschhorn, K., 1964. Lymphocyte interaction: a potential histocompatibility test in vitro. Science 143, 813–814.

Bain, B., Vas, M.R., Lowenstein, L., 1964. The development of large, immature mononuclear cells in mixed leukocyte cultures. Blood 23, 108–116.

Bonner, W.A., Hulet, H.R., Sweet, R.G., Herzenberg, L.A., 1972. Fluorescence activated cell sorting. Rev. Sci. Instrum. 43, 404–409.

Brunner, K.T., Mauel, J., Cerottini, J.C., Chapius, B., 1968. Quantitative assay of the lytic action of immune lymphoid cells on ^{51}Cr-labeled allogeneic target cells in vitro; inhibition by isoantibody and by drugs. Immunology 14, 181–196.

Bussard, A., 1959. D'une technique combinant simultanement l'electrophorese et la precipitation immunologique dans un gel. Biochim. Biophys. Acta 34, 258–260.

Charrin, A., Roger, G.H., 1889. Note sur le développement des microbes pathogenes dans le serum des animaux vacciné. C. R. Soc. Biol. 19, 667–669.

Czerkinsky, C.C., Nilsson, L.A., Nygren, H., Ouchterlony, O., Tarkowski, A., 1983. A solid-phase enzyme-linked immunospot (ELISPOT) assay for enumeration of specific antibody-secreting cells. J. Immunol. Methods 65, 109–121.

Dick, G.F., Dick, G.H., 1924. A skin test for susceptibility to scarlet fever. J. Am. Med. Assoc. 82, 265–266.

Durham, H.E., 1896. On a special action of the serum of highly immunized animals and its use for diagnostic and other purposes. Proc. R. Soc. London 59, 224–226.

Dworetzky, M., Cohen, S.G., 2002. The allergy archives. Clemens von Pirquet, MD (1874–1929). J. Allergy Clin. Immunol. 109, 722–726.

Engvall, E., Perlman, P., 1971. Enzyme-linked immunosorbent assay (ELISA). Quantitative assay of immunoglobulin G. Immunochemistry 8, 871–874.

Flexner, S., Amoss, H.L., 1915. The rapid production of antidysenteric serum. J. Exp. Med. 21, 515–524.

Fulwyler, M.J., 1965. Electronic separation of biological cells by volume. Science 150, 910–911.

Graber, P., Williams, C.A., 1953. Methode permettant l'etude conjugée des propriétes électrophorétiques d'un mélange de proteins. Application du serum sanguine. Biochem. Biophys. Acta 10, 193–194.

Hajdu, S.I., 2003. A note from history: the discovery of blood cells. Ann. Clin. Lab. Sci. 33, 237–238.

Heidelberger, M., Kendall, F., 1929. A quantitative study of the precipitin reaction between type III pneumococcus polysaccharide and purified homologous antibody. J. Exp. Med. 50, 809–823.

Hughes, W.L., Bond, V.P., Brecher, G., Cronkite, E.P., Painter, R.B., Quastler, H., Sherman, F.G., 1958. Cellular proliferation in the mouse as revealed by autoradiography with tritiated thymidine. Proc. Natl. Acad. Sci. U.S.A. 44, 476–483.

Hughes-Jones, N.C., Gardner, B., 2002. Historical review – Red cell agglutination: the first description by Creite (1869) and further observations made by Landois (1875) and Landsteiner (1901). Br. J. Haematol. 119, 889–893.

Ishizaka, K., Ishizaka, T., Menzel, A.E.O., 1967. Physicochemical properties of reaginic antibody. VI. Effect of heat on γE-, γG- and γA-antibodies in the sera of ragweed sensitive patients. J. Immunol. 99, 610–618.

Jerne, N.K., Nordin, A.A., 1963. Plaque formation in agar by single antibody-producing cells. Science 140, 405.

Killingsworth, L.M., Savory, J., 1971. Automated immunochemical procedures for measurements of immunoglobulins IgG, IgA, and IgM in human serum. Clin. Chem. 17, 936–940.

Kober, P.A., Graves, S.S., 1915. Nephelometry (photometric analysis). I. History of method and development of instruments. J. Ind. Eng. Chem. 7, 843–847.

Landsteiner, K., 1901. Über Agglutinationserscheinungen normal menschlichen Blutes. Wein. Klin. Wochenschr. 14, 1132–1134.

Landsteiner, K., 1930. Nobel Lecture: On Individual Differences in Human Blood. Nobelprize.org. Nobel media AB 2014. Web. 1 May 2015. http://www.nobelprize.org/nobel_prizes/medicine/laureates/1930/landsteiner-lecture.html.

Laurell, C.-B., 1965. Antigen-antibody crossed immunoelectrophoresis. Anal. Biochem. 10, 358–361.

Laurell, C.-B., 1966. Quantitative estimation of proteins by electrophoresis in agarose gel containing antibodies. Anal. Biochem. 15, 45–52.

Mancini, G., Carbonara, A.O., Heremans, J.F., 1965. Immunochemical quantitation of antigens by single radial immunodiffusion. Immunochem 2, 235–254.

Mantoux, C., 1908. Intraderm-réaction de la tuberculine. C. R. Acad. Sci. 147, 355–357.

Mendel, F., 1908. Die von Priquet'sche Hautreaktion und die intravenöse Tuberkulinbehandlung. Med. Klinik München 4, 402–404.

Nowell, P.C., 1960. PHA: an initiator of mitosis in cultures of normal human lymphocytes. Cancer Res. 20, 462–466.

Ouchterlony, Ö., 1948. In vitro method for testing the toxin-producing capacity of diphtheria bacteria. Acta Pathol. Microbiol. Scand. 25, 186–191.

Ouchterlony, Ö., 1949. Antigen-antibody reactions in gels. Acta Pathol. Microbiol. Scand. 26, 507–515.

Oudin, J., 1946. Méthode d'analyse immunochemique par précipitation spécifique en milieu gélifié. C. R. Acad. Sci. 222, 115.

Pearmain, G., Lycette, R.R., Fitzgerald, P.H., 1963. Tuberculin induced mitoses in peripheral blood leukocytes. Lancet 281, 637–638.

Pearson, H.A., 2002. History of pediatric hematology oncology. Pediatr. Res. 52, 979–992.

Sanderson, A.R., 1964. Cytotoxic reactions of mouse iso-antisera: preliminary considerations. Br. J. Exp. Pathol. 45, 398–408.

Schick, B., 1913. Die Diphthreictoxin-Hautreaktion del Menschen als Vorprobe des prophylaktischen Diphtherie-heilseruminjection. Munch. Med. Wochenschr. 60, 2608–2610.

Schrek, R., 1963. Cell transformation and mitoses produced by tuberculin PPD in human blood cells. Am. Rev. Resp. Dis. 87, 734–738.

Sedgwick, J.D., Holt, P.G., 1983. A solid-phase immunoenzymatic technique for the enumeration of specific antibody-secreting cells. J. Immunol. Methods 57, 301–309.

Sharrer, T., 2007. Tuberculin, 1890. The Scientist 21. http://www.the-scientist.com/?articles.view/articleNo/25025/title/Tuberculin–1890/.

Simson, E., 2013. Wallace Coulter's life and his impact on the world. Int. J. Lab. Hematol. 35, 230–236.

Tiselius, A., 1937. Electrophoresis of serum globulin. I. Biochem. J. 31, 313–317.

van Weemen, B., Schuurs, A., 1971. Immunoassay using antigen-enzyme conjugates. FEBS Lett. 15, 232–236.

von Pirquet, C., 1907. Tuberkulindiagnose durch cutane Impfung. Berlin Klin. Wochenschr. 44, 644–645.

Verso, M.L., 1971. Some nineteenth century pioneers of haematology. Med. Hist. 15, 55–67.

Widal, F., 1896. On the serodiagnosis of typhoid fever. Lancet 148, 1371–1372.

Yallow, R.S., Berson, S., 1960. Immunoassay of endogenous plasma insulin in man. J. Clin. Invest. 39, 1157–1175.

TIME LINE

1674	Anton van Leeuwenhoek invents the microscope and observes red corpuscles in blood
1840s	Gabriel Andral in France and William Addison in England report the presence of white cells in peripheral blood
1845	Rudolph Virchow and John Hughes Bennett independently describe peripheral blood cells in a patient with leukemia
1869	Adolf Creite describes agglutination of red blood cells by serum from a foreign species
1870s	Louis-Charles Malassez invents a cell counting chamber that evolves into the hemocytometer
1875	Leonard Landois demonstrates red blood cell agglutination
1877	Paul Ehrlich describes the staining properties of the granulocytes and differentiates neutrophils, basophils, and eosinophils
1890	Robert Koch demonstrates that subcutaneous injection of tuberculin identifies patients who have been infected with *Mycobacterium tuberculosis*
1896	Georges-Fernand-Isidor Widal develops an assay to determine if a patient has been infected with *Salmonella typhi*

1901   Karl Landsteiner discovers naturally occurring isohemagglutinins in human serum that react with erythrocytes from other individuals

1901   Jules Bordet develops the complement fixation assay

1903   Nicholas Maurice Arthus describes a skin reaction induced by repeated injections of soluble protein

1907   Clemens von Pirquet develops a scratch test to detect individuals previously infected with *M. tuberculosis*

1908   Charles Mantoux reports that intradermal injection of tuberculin provides a superior assay for detection of tuberculosis infection

1913   Bela Schick devises the Schick test to evaluate level of protection to diphtheria toxin

1924   George and Gladys Dick develop a test to detect susceptibility to scarlet fever

1929   Michael Heidelberger and Forrest Kendall study quantitative aspects of antigen–antibody precipitation reactions

1930   Karl Landsteiner awarded the Nobel Prize in Physiology or Medicine "for his discovery of human blood groups"

1937   Arne Tiselius separates serum proteins by electrophoresis

1946   Jacque Oudin devises a method to visualize antigen–antibody precipitin reactions in a test tube

1948   Örjan Ouchterlony develops a double immunodiffusion method for detecting antigen–antibody reactions based on precipitation

1948   Arne Tiselius awarded the Nobel Prize in Physiology or Medicine "for his research on electrophoresis and adsorption analysis, especially for his discoveries concerning the complex nature of serum proteins"

1953   Wallace Coulter awarded patent on the Coulter principle, the basis for automated counting of cells

1953   P. Graber and C.A. Williams describe immunoelectrophoresis

1958   Walter Hughes and colleagues use tritiated thymidine to visualize cell proliferation

1960   Rosalyn Yalow and Solomon Berson describe radioimmunoassay

1960   Peter Nowell demonstrates that PHA stimulates normal human lymphocytes

1963   Nels Jerne and Albert Nordin describe the hemolytic plaque assay

1964   Barbara Bain and colleagues as well as Fritz Bach and Kurt Hirschhorn demonstrate that culturing leukocytes from unrelated individuals induces DNA synthesis and mitosis

1965   Mack Fulwyler develops an electronic particle separator and uses it to separate a mixture of blood cells

1965   G. Mancini and colleagues develop radial immunodiffusion to quantify antigens

1968   K. Theodor Brunner and colleagues develop a quantitative assay to detect lymphocyte-mediated cytotoxicity

1971   Bauke van Weiman and Anton Schuur as well as Eva Engvall and Peter Perlman independently describe enzyme-linked immunosorbent assay

1972   Leonard Herzenberg and colleagues develop the fluorescence-activated cell sorter (FACS)

1977   Rosalyn Yalow awarded the Nobel Prize in Physiology or Medicine for development of radioimmunoassay

1983   C.C. Czerkinsky and collaborators and Jonathon Sedgwick and Patrick Holt independently describe the ELISPOT assay for quantifying specific antibody-producing cells

CHAPTER

40

The Future of Immunology

INTRODUCTION

Nothing is so dangerous to the progress of the human mind than to assume that our views of science are ultimate, that there are no mysteries in nature, that our triumphs are complete and that there are no new worlds to conquer. *Humphry Davy (1778–1829), Cornish chemist who discovered and characterized several chemical elements including barium, calcium, potassium, sodium, magnesium, strontium, and boron.* http://www.chemheritage.org/discover/online-resources/chemistry-in-history/themes/electrochemistry/davy.aspx

Immunology is a major discipline in the biomedical sciences. Several subdisciplines have emerged including immunochemistry, cellular immunology, immunogenetics, and molecular immunology. Starting with the introduction of vaccination by Edward Jenner in the late eighteenth century, advances in understanding the immune system and its function in disease process have provided the physician with many new tools. A useful question, particularly for beginning students, is what knowledge remains to be discovered.

In 1957, F. MacFarlane Burnet working at the Walter and Eliza Hall Institute of Medical Research in Melbourne,

Australia, proposed the clonal selection theory to explain the mechanism by which antigens induce a specific antibody response. This theory postulates the existence of a large number of antibody-forming cells, each of which is genetically preprogrammed to produce a unique antibody specificity. These antibody-forming cells (lymphocytes) are selected and activated by invading pathogens and other antigens. Immunologists consider the clonal selection theory (Chapter 6), which replaced instruction hypotheses of antibody formation, as the most significant advance in immunology in the twentieth century.

In 1967 Burnet, working at the University of Melbourne in Australia, opened a major symposium at the Cold Spring Harbor Laboratory on Long Island, New York, with a presentation titled "The Impact on Ideas of Immunology." After he described the experiments that led to the acceptance of the clonal selection theory, Burnet predicted that we would shortly uncover the genetics responsible for determining antibody specificity and that this, in turn, would provide an understanding of interactions between a number of biological molecules including enzymes and their substrates and viruses and the receptors on cells they infect.

A Historical Perspective on Evidence-Based Immunology
http://dx.doi.org/10.1016/B978-0-12-398381-7.00040-X

365

On a more pessimistic note, Burnet warned against pursuing some studies in biology in general and immunology in particular since he was convinced that the results of these experiments could lead to consequences threatening society. He stated that scientists "are on the verge of knowing the nucleotide sequences which determine virulence and antigenicity of polio virus… and other small viruses such as yellow fever and foot and mouth disease. These are doomsday weapons in the making." He also suggested that while "detailed analysis of some phage DNA and RNA is well under way…we shall probably always have to be content with general ideas" since "to synthesize a mammalian genome is a task for 1000 million years of evolution, not for a biochemistry laboratory."

Burnet similarly warned against studies that unraveled the regulation of biological interactions as well as investigating the immunological response to cancer. Of the latter, he stated "our present state of population growth is bad enough but if, in addition, we were all to become centenarians it would throw our whole social and economic life into disorder."

At the conclusion of this symposium, Niels Jerne (1967) from the Paul Ehrlich Institute in Frankfurt, Germany, presented a summary titled "Waiting for the End" in which he predicted that the solution of "the antibody problem," that is, an understanding of the mechanisms responsible for the specificity of individual antibody molecules, would soon be solved, and that "we older amateurs had perhaps better sit back, waiting for the End."

Many immunologists interpreted these presentations by a Nobel laureate (Burnet) and a future laureate (Jerne) to suggest that all the major immunological concepts had been discovered and that the only challenge remaining was to wrap up loose ends. However, this symposium occurred prior to characterization of:

- B and T lymphocytes;
- cell interactions in the adaptive immune response;
- mechanisms by which cells of the host defenses recognize foreign material;
- T cell receptor (TCR) structure;
- the concept of major histocompatibility complex (MHC) restriction;
- lymphocyte maturation including the roles of the thymus and bursa of Fabricius;
- positive and negative selection of T lymphocytes in the establishment of immunologic tolerance;
- functional populations of T lymphocytes (CD4+ and CD8+);
- differential expression of MHC-coded molecules;
- functional subpopulations of CD4+ T lymphocytes;
- cytokines and chemokines and their receptors;
- monoclonal antibodies; and
- cluster of differentiation (CD) markers.

In contrast in 1976, Robert Good of the University of Minnesota presented his presidential address to the American Association of Immunologists. Good described several of the important advances made in immunology, particularly related to clinical medicine, during the previous 200 years starting with Jenner and the development of smallpox vaccination. At that time, he offered several predictions concerning the future of immunological research:

- Vaccines against bacterial diseases will replace our reliance on antibiotic treatment.
- Congenital defects of the host defense mechanisms will be treated by "cellular engineering" (i.e., bone marrow transplantation).
- Many of the diseases of aging will be corrected through "macromolecular engineering" to repair the cells of the immune system.
- Diseases involving the molecules active in the immune response and inflammation will be controlled by inhibiting or augmenting the activity of these molecules.
- Methods of immunization will be developed that will inhibit allergic reactions.
- Tissue typing and matching will be perfected allowing successful transplantation as well as the development of new methods to treat autoimmune diseases and virus infections.
- Drugs capable of regulating the host defense mechanisms will be developed and provided orally.
- Methods will be developed allowing local immunization with vaccines thus providing active immunity in the anatomical location of the infection.
- Immunotherapy and immunoprophylaxis against tumors will be developed and will replace our reliance on chemotherapy and radiation therapy.
- Immunotherapy and immunoprophylaxis against many of the infectious diseases (leprosy, malaria, trypanosomiasis, schistosomiasis, and fungal diseases) will be developed.

While many of these predictions have been realized in the years since this presentation, several remain.

In the summer of 1976, a second Cold Spring Harbor Symposium focused on immunology summarized advances during the preceding 10 years. Niels Jerne from the Basel Institute for Immunology in Switzerland presented the opening address, "The Common Sense of Immunology," in which he described the state of the discipline nearly 20 years after publication of the clonal selection theory (Jerne, 1977). He stated "cooperative and suppressive clonal interactions have now become the dominant themes" in immunology. These included not only previously demonstrated cell-to-cell interactions but postulated interactions of cells with soluble factors (idiotypes and anti-idiotypes) as well. In predicting what will transpire in the interval between the 1976 symposium and a subsequent symposium, which he projected to occur in 1985, Jerne envisaged additional studies on embryology, differentiation, membrane structure, network analysis, and other areas that will provide a basis for medical advances.

Gerald Edelman from the Rockefeller University in New York summarized the 1976 symposium by predicting that the immune system would serve as a model for other areas of biology (Edelman, 1977). He stated "the immune system is one of the most startling and beautiful molecular recognition machines" and suggested that neuroscience, developmental biology, and enzymology might gain insights by studying the immune system. Shortly after this symposium, Edelman took his own advice and shifted his research focus to neurobiology.

A third Cold Spring Harbor Symposium focused on "Immunological Recognition" was held not in 1985 but rather in 1989. Charles Janeway from Yale University in New Haven, Connecticut, provided the opening address titled "Approaching the Asymptote? Evolution and Revolution in Immunology." The symposium took place shortly after the structure of the histocompatibility molecules coded for by the class I genes in the MHC had been revealed. In his presentation, Janeway predicted three areas that will be covered in future symposia including "the enzymology of gene rearrangement in somatic cells; pattern recognition by lymphocytes and antigen-presenting cells; and the sociology of lymphocytes."

Jonathan C. Howard of Cambridge University, England, summarized the 1989 meeting and invoked Jerne's "Waiting for the End" presentation from the symposium 22 years previously. Howard suggested that we immunologists are "destined to ask at this stage of the proceedings where we stand in relation to the end, and by the same token, to come to terms with the idea that immunology has an end, a stage when outstanding problems are trivial or no longer distinctive to the field." He predicted that a symposium held in 2000 would focus on whole animal immunology, immunologic memory, the "deployment of lymphocyte populations in space and time in vivo," and immunoregulation. His hope was that this fundamental knowledge could be applied to human immunopathology, particularly autoimmune diseases.

Two more immunology-related symposia held at the Cold Spring Harbor Laboratory covered "Signaling and Gene Expression in the Immune System" in 1999 and "Immunity and Tolerance" in 2013. William E. Paul and colleagues from the National Institutes of Health in Bethesda, Maryland, provided the final presentation to the 2013 symposium in which they developed a synthesis of the mechanisms responsible for regulating the immune system, keeping it from reacting to self and initiating autoimmune disease. This synthesis included a description of advances in immunology (regulatory T lymphocytes,

pattern recognition by dendritic and other cells) that had been described during the previous 15 years.

Tracing this history of symposia during the previous half century permits immunologists to gain perspective on the future. Although much has been learned about host defense mechanisms including the molecular and genetic control of the responses, several major gaps in our knowledge remain. In the speculations that follow, basic science and clinical immunology are separated; however, advances in one area will impinge on progress in the other.

BASIC SCIENCE

Investigators over the previous 150 years determined many of the mechanisms by which the innate host defenses and the adaptive immune responses eliminate potentially pathogenic microorganisms. Despite this history, several aspects of the immune system remain unexplained:

- function of IgD antibodies,
- discrimination of commensal and potentially pathogenic bacteria,
- Natural Killer (NK) and Natural Killer T (NKT) lymphocytes in host defenses,
- functional subsets of lymphocytes,
- gamma–delta T lymphocytes,
- immunological memory, and
- regulation of the innate and adaptive host defenses.

Function of IgD Antibodies

In 1965 David Rowe and John Fahey, working at the National Cancer Institute, Bethesda, Maryland, described a patient with multiple myeloma who possessed a distinctive myeloma protein (Chapter 11). While this immunoglobulin contained light chains similar to those found in IgG, IgA, and IgM, the electrophoretic mobility of the Fc region of the molecule was unlike that of other immunoglobulin isotypes. An antibody specific for this myeloma protein reacted with an immunoglobulin present in control human serum. As a result, Rowe and Fahey concluded that this represented a unique immunoglobulin isotype that they named IgD.

The function of IgD in the adaptive immune response is yet to be ascertained. IgD is present in very low concentrations in serum and is not synthesized in appreciable amounts following immunization although some immunologists report an increase in patients with chronic infections. IgD fails to activate the complement system. Unstimulated B lymphocytes express IgD on their surface along with IgM, and some immunologists speculate that this isotype is responsible for regulating B lymphocyte differentiation.

Discrimination of Commensal and Potentially Pathogenic Bacteria

In 1989, Charles Janeway working at Yale University, New Haven, Connecticut, predicted that macrophages and other phagocytic cells of the innate host defense mechanism express pattern recognition receptors that allow these cells to recognize pathogen-associated molecular patterns. Bruce Beutler at Southwestern Medical School in Dallas, Texas, and Jules Hoffman in Strasbourg, France, confirmed the existence of such receptors in the 1990s. Despite this, immunologists still cannot explain how the immune systems, both innate and adaptive, differentiate between microorganisms that are beneficial or benign from those that are potentially pathogenic and might cause disease. The importance of this distinction is demonstrated by recent observations that certain disorders such as inflammatory bowel disease may result from abnormal immune or inflammatory responses to bacteria present in the gastrointestinal microbiota.

NK and NKT Lymphocytes

NK lymphocytes provide a mechanism by which the innate host defense system lyses virally infected or malignant cells (Chapter 28). NK lymphocytes, a component of the innate host defense mechanisms, are the counterpart of $CD8^+$ cytotoxic T lymphocytes of the adaptive immune system. While the two cell types share cytotoxic mechanisms, the recognition structures expressed by $CD8^+$ T lymphocytes and NK lymphocytes are unique. In the late 1980s, several groups of investigators described a third population of lymphocytes that shares characteristics of both NK and $CD8^+$ T lymphocytes. These NKT lymphocytes recognize a glycolipid presented by a unique class I MHC-coded molecule, CD1d. Since NKT lymphocytes express cell surface markers of both T lymphocytes and NK lymphocytes, investigators hypothesize that they bridge the gap between innate host defenses and adaptive immune responses. However, their role in providing protection against potential pathogens and/or malignantly transformed somatic cells has yet to be unraveled.

Functional Subsets of Lymphocytes

Currently immunologists divide lymphocytes into several populations that can be discriminated based on function and on the expression of CD markers. B lymphocytes synthesize and secrete antibodies while T lymphocytes are cytotoxic and function as regulators of other lymphocytes. T lymphocytes are further divided into $CD4^+$ and $CD8^+$ lymphocytes based on the mechanism by which they interact with antigen. Finally, $CD4^+$ lymphocytes comprise at least five functionally unique subpopulations based on the cytokines involved in their differentiation and the cytokines they secrete once activated (Chapter 23). Additional populations of $CD4^+$ and $CD8^+$ T lymphocytes may yet be discovered.

That cytokines are responsible for the differentiation of subpopulations of $CD4^+$ T lymphocytes provides a target to preferentially increase or decrease these subpopulations in patients. Future investigation on mechanisms to manipulate these populations and to determine their functions will provide clinicians new tools to treat patients with various disorders.

Gamma–Delta T Lymphocytes

Most T lymphocytes express a cell surface receptor (TCR) comprised of two chains—an alpha chain and a beta chain. A minor population (0.5–5%) of lymphocytes that are dependent on the thymus for differentiation express a TCR comprised of two chains (gamma and delta) coded for by genes different from those coding for the alpha and beta chains (Pardoll et al., 1987). These TCRs fail to reflect the diversity of the alpha–beta TCRs, and hence the lymphocytes are less specific. Gamma–delta T lymphocytes are present in relatively high concentrations in the gastrointestinal tract and may be responsible for initial recognition of invading microorganisms. Other functions attributed to these lymphocytes include regulation of the adaptive immune response and bridging the innate and adaptive host defense mechanisms. Activation of gamma–delta T lymphocytes remains to be explained but appears to be independent of antigen presentation by molecules coded for by genes in the MHC.

Immunological Memory

Immunologic memory provides the rationale for the development of vaccines against microbes such as smallpox, polio, diphtheria, and measles that have historically caused epidemics responsible for altering social and economic history. Vaccine development has succeeded for many infectious diseases including eradication of smallpox. Vaccines against several other infectious diseases including tuberculosis, malaria, dysentery, acquired immunodeficiency syndrome, and Ebola are targets for ongoing studies. Future advances in comprehending immunological memory require answers to several questions including

- the identity of the genetic and molecular components required for the maintenance of immunologic memory,
- the differences of memory responses of various populations of lymphocytes involved in the adaptive immune response, and
- methods for enhancing or suppressing the memory response in a variety of clinical situations.

Regulation of the Innate and Adaptive Defense Mechanisms

Immunology since the 1970s has evolved from "a lymphocyte is a lymphocyte" to great excitement about collaboration between B and T lymphocytes to suppressor T lymphocytes and idiotype–anti-idiotype networks and finally to T regulatory lymphocytes. Regulation of ongoing immune responses appears to involve molecules expressed by antigen-presenting cells and T lymphocytes as well as by soluble mediators of intercellular communication. Much remains to be explained about the molecular and genetic stimuli leading to these regulatory interactions.

CLINICAL APPLICATIONS

Manipulation of the immune system to treat clinical disorders is still in its infancy, and hence many opportunities exist to make major contributions. Target diseases include both those caused by abnormal or aberrant immune responses, such as allergies, autoimmune diseases, and auto-inflammatory disorders, as well as those for which immunological intervention might prove useful including destruction of tumors, prevention of allograft rejection, and reconstitution of the host defenses in both congenital and acquired immunodeficiencies.

Basic scientists and clinicians need to collaborate to develop more sophisticated therapies to regulate immune responses. For example, attempts to control the immune-mediated rejection of allogeneic tissue and organ grafts are somewhat more targeted today than they were at the start of the transplant era (Chapter 36), but they still present challenges to the patient and the physician leaving the graft recipient in danger of contracting infections caused by microbes that normally are nonpathogenic.

Various strategies aimed at either augmenting or inhibiting the immune response are available to clinicians. While clinical protocols address both these strategies, future efforts to enhance the specificity of such therapies will yield a more targeted approach. In the following, examples of each strategy are outlined with predictions for future directions.

Augmentation of Immune Responses

Vaccines to infectious diseases continue to be a main priority in the fight against pathogenic microorganisms. Starting with smallpox and continuing to recent successes with vaccines against the human papilloma virus and Ebola, vaccine development is a fruitful endeavor. New diseases will continue to emerge, and old vaccines will need to be updated. During the next decades, vaccines specific for several infectious diseases including malaria, tuberculosis, and human immunodeficiency virus will become available. Advances in understanding T lymphocyte activation will result in vaccines that can be used therapeutically.

Vaccines for other diseases are also in development. As the population ages, the number of individuals presenting with Alzheimer-related dementia is increasing. Efforts to develop a vaccine to induce antibodies to the proteins associated with this disease are underway, and some success has been reported. Other vaccines to be used in treating chronic diseases such as cancer and atherosclerosis provide opportunities for investigators interested in these pathologies.

Inhibition of tumors through the manipulation of the adaptive immune response is an expanding field of investigation. Basic science research has identified several checkpoints by which an ongoing immune response is negatively regulated. Interference with these checkpoints enhances immune responses against malignancies thus permitting the body to rid itself of the malignantly transformed cells (Chapter 37). A first step in this area has been provided by James Allison and colleagues working at the University of Texas, MD Anderson Cancer Center, Houston (Sharma and Allison, 2015). These investigators demonstrated that inhibition of this negative signal allows an activated antitumor response to continue rather than be terminated.

A third application of immune system augmentation is reconstitution of immunocompetence in patients presenting with congenital immunodeficiencies. Initially physicians treated these patients with transplants of the organ or cells responsible for the immune defect. Recently some patients received genes to replace ones that are mutated. While some successes have been reported (Chapter 38) much still needs to be learned about gene therapy so that it becomes a practical procedure.

Inhibition of Immune Responses

More than 20 million Americans suffer from autoimmune diseases. Contemporary therapies involve treating the symptoms (i.e., insulin replacement in patients with type 1 diabetes) or immunosuppression. While some of the immunosuppressive drugs are targeted to specific mediators (i.e., use of monoclonal antibodies for inflammatory cytokines in rheumatoid arthritis), no reversal of disease has been reported. Several questions remain:

- What is the identity of the antigen(s) responsible for eliciting an autoimmune response?
- How do these antigens activate T and/or B lymphocytes?
- How do self-reactive lymphocytes escape tolerance induction? and
- Are there methods for induction of immunologic tolerance?

Another clinical situation amenable to induction of self-tolerance is in the control of transplantation rejection. Starting in the 1950s, the number of recipients of foreign allografts has increased yearly. Treatment of potential rejection used drugs that indiscriminately destroyed lymphocytes and other rapidly proliferating cells leaving the recipient with impaired immune defenses against pathogens. Recent advances produced several drugs with greater specificity (Chapter 38); however, adverse side effects still make organ transplantation risky. An alternate strategy for treating potential graft recipients would be the induction of tolerance to antigens of the donor, thereby allowing successful transplantation with minimal immunosuppression.

Immune-mediated hypersensitivities, particularly allergies, asthma, and other manifestations of IgE-mediated reactions, affect a relatively large proportion of the population. Therapy focuses on avoidance of the offending antigen or relatively nonspecific treatment of symptoms. Occasionally, the antigen (allergen) cannot be conclusively identified. Alternatively, in some individuals a drug (e.g., penicillin) required for therapy becomes immunogenic and induces an IgE response. A second exposure to penicillin might lead to a potentially life-threatening hypersensitivity reaction (anaphylaxis). Additional information about the mechanism responsible for immunoglobulin isotype switching could provide an additional approach for therapeutic interventions.

CONCLUSION

Some historians identify Edward Jenner (1749–1823) as the father of immunology for his development of the smallpox vaccine in 1796. Others give this honor to Louis Pasteur (1822–1895) for his studies validating the germ theory of disease and development of vaccines against rabies and anthrax. In reality, anecdotal evidence for the existence of a host defense system predates both of these scientists.

Beginning in the late 1800s investigators unraveled the physiological mechanisms responsible for protecting vertebrates from potentially pathogenic microorganisms. As a result, immunology began as a subdiscipline of microbiology. The development of the clonal selection theory by F. Macfarlane Burnet in 1957 followed by an explosion of investigations of the cells and molecules involved in the immune system starting in the 1960s fostered the development of immunology as its own discipline in both biology and medicine.

Beginning in the 1950s, several prominent immunologists suggested that all major breakthroughs have been made in the discipline and predicted that future generations of scientists would merely complete a picture that was 95% finished. Some of these prognostications were presented at a series of symposia held at the Cold Spring Harbor Laboratory at approximately 10-year intervals (1967, 1976, 1989, 1999, 2013). These predictions seem premature and, to paraphrase Mark Twain, the reports of the death of immunology are greatly exaggerated.

A number of important problems remain to be addressed by future generations of immunologists, and the likelihood of new advances appears highly probable. Both basic science questions and clinical applications remain to be addressed—some of these are highlighted in this chapter. A student entering this field in the twenty-first century needs to realize that

- new technology drives the types of questions that can be asked, and their application to the immune system provides opportunities for interdisciplinary research;
- new diseases are continually emerging—many of these are infectious and provide problems of prevention and treatment that immunologists are uniquely qualified to address;
- diseases that have been known for centuries (i.e., atherosclerosis, dementia) may well include immunologic mechanisms as a part of their etiology and as a target for therapy; and
- new therapies, some based on immunologic principles, will be developed, and their effect on host defense mechanisms will emerge.

These factors argue that the future of immunologic research remains bright.

References

Burnet, F.M., 1967. The impact on ideas of immunology. Cold Spring Harbor Symp. Quant. Biol. 32, 1–8.

Edelman, G.M., 1977. Summary: understanding selective molecular recognition. Cold Spring Harbor Symp. Quant. Biol. 41, 891–902.

Good, R.A., 1976. Runestones in immunology: inscriptions to journeys of discovery and analysis. J. Immunol. 117, 1413–1428.

Howard, J.C., 1989. Summary: the new pragmatics of immunology. Cold Spring Harbor Symp. Quant. Biol. 54, 947–957.

Janeway, C.A., 1989. Approaching the asymptote? Evolution and revolution in immunology. Cold Spring Harbor Symp. Quant. Biol. 54, 1–13.

Jerne, N.K., 1967. Summary: waiting for the end. Cold Spring Harbor Symp. Quant. Biol. 32, 591–603.

Jerne, N.K., 1977. The common sense of immunology. Cold Spring Harbor Symp. Quant. Biol. 44, 1–4.

Pardoll, D.M., Fowlkes, B.J., Bluestone, J.A., Kruisbeek, A., Maloy, W.L., Coligan, J.E., Schwartz, R.H., 1987. Differential expression of two distinct T-cell receptors during thymocyte development. Nature 326, 79–81.

Rowe, D.D., Fahey, J.L., 1965a. A new class of human immunoglobulin. I. A unique myeloma protein. J. Exp. Med. 121, 171–184.

Rowe, D.S., Fahey, J.L., 1965b. A new class of human immunoglobulin. II. Normal serum IgD. J. Exp. Med. 121, 185–199.

Sharma, P., Allison, J.P., 2015. Immune checkpoint targeting in cancer therapy: toward combination strategies with curative potential. Cell 161, 205–214.

TIME LINE

1967   Cold Spring Harbor Symposium on Quantitative Biology #32 Antibodies

1976   Cold Spring Harbor Symposium on Quantitative Biology #41 Origins of Lymphocyte Diversity

1976   Robert Good presents his presidential address in the annual meeting of the American Association of Immunologists

1989   Cold Spring Harbor symposium on Quantitative Biology #54 Immunological Recognition

1999   Cold Spring Harbor symposium on Quantitative Biology #64 Signaling and Gene Expression in the Immune System

2013   Cold Spring Harbor Symposium on Quantitative Biology #78 Immunity and Tolerance

Index

Note: 'Page numbers followed by "f" indicate figures and "t" indicate tables.'

Printed in the United States
By Bookmasters